A Consumer's Dictionary of Cosmetic Ingredients

ALSO BY RUTH WINTER

A Consumer's Dictionary of Food Additives, 5th Edition

Vitamin E

The Anti-Aging Hormones

Super Soy

A Consumer's Dictionary to Medicines in Food

A Consumer's Dictionary of Medicines: Prescription, Over-the-Counter, and Herbal

A Consumer's Dictionary of Household, Yard, and Office Chemicals

Poisons in Your Food

Ageless Aging

Cancer-Causing Agents

Beware of the Food You Eat

A Consumer's Dictionary of Cosmetic Ingredients

FIFTH EDITION

Ruth Winter, M.S.

Three Rivers Press
New York

To my husband, Arthur Winter, M.D., my daughter, Robin Winter-Sperry, M.D., my sons, Craig and Grant, and my grandchildren, Samantha, Hunter, and Katelynd.

This book provides general information about cosmetic ingredients. If you have particular questions or concerns about any ingredient and your personal health or if you believe you are reacting to a particular cosmetic, you should consult your physician.

Published by Three Rivers Press, a division of Crown Publishers, Inc., 201 East 50th Street, New York, New York 10022. Member of the Crown Publishing Group.

Random House, Inc. New York, Toronto, London, Sydney, Auckland
www.randomhouse.com

THREE RIVERS PRESS is a registered trademark of Random House, Inc.

Printed in the United States of America

Library of Congress Cataloging-in-Publication Data

Winter, Ruth, 1930–
    A consumer's dictionary of cosmetic ingredients / Ruth Winter.
    — 5th ed.
    p.   cm.
Includes bibliographical references.
1. Cosmetics—Dictionaries.   I. Title.
TP983.A55 W57   1999
668'.55'03—dc21
                                                         98-44781
                                                         CIP

ISBN 0-609-80367-0 (pbk.)

10 9 8 7 6 5 4 3 2

Fifth Edition

CONTENTS

INTRODUCTION

Why You Need This Book

You need this book more than ever before!

Cosmetics have always been a low priority at the U.S. Food and Drug Administration, but now its regulatory powers have been weakened to the point where they are almost nonexistent. The Cosmetics Office, which deals with a $36.4 billion dollar cosmetics and toiletries industry, has had its funding cut 50 percent in 1999 and its staff reduced from 27 to 15 people, including secretaries and clerks. The result:

- The Cosmetics Voluntary Registration Program has been suspended in its entirety. This means that those companies who were honorable enough to inform the FDA about the ingredients they were using no longer have anyone to whom to report. (About 35 to 40 percent participated in the program.)

- Consumer and Industry assistance previously provided by the Cosmetics Office has been "significantly reduced or eliminated." The FDA is no longer able to respond to technical inquiries concerning ingredient usage, product formulation, or safety substantiation.

- Laboratory studies have been significantly reduced or suspended.

All this has occurred while claims about the wonders of cosmetics have escalated, and more importantly, while a new category of cosmetics has developed—the *cosmeceutical*.

COSMECEUTICALS—BETWEEN A PHARMACEUTICAL AND A COSMETIC

While the Food, Drug, and Cosmetic Act does not recognize the term "cosmeceutical," the cosmetic industry has begun to use this word to refer to cosmetic products that have druglike benefits. And in some cases, the designation is right!

Potential for cosmeceutical ingredients in the United States alone is $100 million and includes such products as skin peelers, wrinkle creams, emollients, hair growth stimulants, skin lighteners and darkeners, and botanicals.[1] The 75 million baby boomers are the major market for cosmeceuticals. No matter what your age, however, before you spend a penny for a cosmetic "treatment product," you should know about your skin, the largest organ of your body. You will then be better able to judge what cosmetic companies are offering you. Your skin is made up primarily of three parts:

1. The outermost layer of your skin, your *epidermis,* is also called the *horny layer.* Flattened and insensitive, it is continually flaking off. The other layers of your epidermis are alive and receive nourishment from below. The lower layers of your epidermis continually produce new cells that rise to the surface and gradually turn into the horny layer.

2. Your *dermis*—which in Greek means skin—is composed mostly of collagen, a protein substance found in connective tissue, and elastin, which has the ability to stretch and then snap back. Like your epidermis, your dermis is layered. The upper or *papillary layer* is made up of small mounds rich in blood vessels and nerve endings. Your lower level is a thick mesh of connective fiber attached at its base to your subcutaneous (beneath the skin) tissue.

3. Your *subcutaneous layer* consists of connective tissue and fat that protects your inner body structure.

If you are young and your hormones and your oil glands are very active, your skin is supple but may pop out with pimples.

As your skin ages collagen and elastin, the tissues that keep it supple, weaken. Your skin becomes thinner and loses fat, so it looks less plump and smooth. While these changes are taking place, gravity participates by causing your skin to sag. Cosmeticians don't call a wrinkle a wrinkle, however. It's a "dermatologic corrugation"! But no matter what it is called, a wrinkle signifies a pot of gold. So do liver spots, dry skin, and gray hair. People have tried all sorts of concoctions for centuries, even millennia to reverse the signs of aging. Today's arsenal of chemicals, though, is unique. Some products may actually work. The trick is to know which may be based on scientific evidence and which are just fantasy. This book can help you decide.

If the cosmetics really do as promised and change the structure of the skin making it more youthful, then they are drugs. If they don't do what they promise, they are fraudulent. Can they be both a cosmetic and a drug?

---

[1] Thomas Dooley, Ph.D., Director of Molecular Pharmacology, Southern Research Institute, "Sulfotransferases As Molecular Targets for Cosmeceutical Agent Discovery," paper presented at International Business Communications: Drug Discovery and Development Approaches to Cosmeceuticals, Short Hills, N.J., February 12–13, 1998.

The definition of cosmetics, according the Food, Drug, and Cosmetic Act, is:

(1) Articles intended to be rubbed, poured, sprinkled or sprayed on, introduced into, or otherwise applied to the human body or any part thereof for cleansing, beautifying, promoting attractiveness, or altering the appearance and (2) Articles intended for use as a component of any such articles, except that such terms shall not include soap.

To the U.S. government, *a cosmetic improves appearance,* whereas *a drug diagnoses, relieves, or cures a disease.*

Drugs are also subjected to an intensive review and approval process by the FDA while cosmetics are not. If a product has drug properties, it is supposed to be approved as a medicine, a process that costs more than $250 million and usually takes years. The FDA, on the other hand, does not require premarket approval for cosmetics. With the exception of color ingredients that have to be authorized for use, the FDA doesn't, in fact, *approve* the use of any cosmetic ingredient. And anyone can go into the cosmetic business without a license or notification to any regulatory agency.

The over-the-counter drug category, which requires no prescription, contains some products most of us consider cosmetics: fluoride toothpastes; hormone creams; sunscreen preparations; antiperspirants, and dandruff shampoos. Their manufacturers have to follow a monograph—a set of instructions for the product set by FDA expert panels.

As for cosmetics, the agency's regulations were determined more than forty years ago. Cosmetics, therefore, have traditionally received little attention because back then it was wrongly assumed that such products do not really affect our health and safety. The skin was believed to be a nearly perfect barrier that prevented chemicals applied to it from penetrating the body. This belief went unchallenged until the 1960s, when the much-heralded—but unmarketed—miracle drug DMSO proved its ability to carry substances with it through the skin and into the body's tissues and bloodstream. Until it was shown that rabbits' eyes were adversely affected by DMSO, the drug was being promoted as a through-the-skin carrier of all sorts of medication. Today, ironically, an increasingly popular way to deliver drugs is "transdermally." Medications to prevent seasickness or treat angina (chest pains) and hormonal deficiencies are placed in an adhesive disk for delivery through the skin. Would-be ex-smokers today can even get their nicotine "fix" through their skin by wearing a patch rather than through inhaling cigarette smoke. It has now been accepted, furthermore, that all chemicals penetrate the skin to some extent, and many do so in significant amounts.

Good tests for skin penetration are available, yet they are rarely used for cosmetics. Tests to determine the systemic effects or metabolic degradation of a cosmetic ingredient are rarely performed either. Most consumers and the cosmetic companies are concerned with allergic reactions and skin irritations, but what of systemic absorption, toxicity, and chronic effects?

What degree of absorption is there when a cosmetic is left on the face (as a makeup base might be for twelve hours) or spread over the entire body (as suntan lotions may be)? What is the exposure to ingredients that may be used over a number of years?

Pharmaceutical and cosmetic companies are working right now on carriers and solvents for cosmetic products that will either help ingredients penetrate more deeply through the skin or prevent them from entering at all.

The modern age of the cosmeceutical received a boost from the approval of Johnson & Johnson's Retin-A as a topical anti-acne drug in 1973. A serendipitous observation was made that the product not only got rid of pimples, it reduced the appearance of wrinkles. Johnson & Johnson subsequently sought approval for a related Vitamin A product, Renova®. After much controversy, it was recommended for approval by an FDA advisory panel for the treatment of fine wrinkling, mottled hyperpigmentation (liver spots), and roughness associated with photo damage (sun damage) in April 1992.

Medical reports that a Vitamin A derivative could reverse some sun damage and fade wrinkles fueled a whirlwind of interest in the cosmetic field. Some companies rushed to market with Vitamin A products. One of them, Cosmetic Laboratory Sales, took a full-page ad in the tabloid *The Star,* September 28, 1993, promoting "free retinol Vitamin A creme when you purchase Alpha/H, Alpha Hydroxy Creme, Medical Science's New Age Reversal Formula." The ad went on to say that "Direct from leading medical journals, plus fashion magazines like *Vogue* and *Cosmopolitan,* comes the 'bombshell announcement' of a wondrous discovery that can help you grow away lines and signs of age . . . grow in a brand new, smooth-as-silk complexion and make you look 10 to 15—why even a whole generation younger."

By 1997 highly respected companies were in the mix. Neutrogena, for example, introduced its Healthy Skin Antiwrinkle Cream with Retinol®. It contains a combination of moisturizers and vitamin B_5, which is claimed *"increases moisture levels and skin firmness"* and *"evens out skin tone."* It's a big seller.

Many cosmetic companies have been more cautious about their claims for Vitamin A products and instead placed their emphasis on alpha-hydroxy acids *(see)* as a great antiaging ingredient. Since alpha hydroxies are somewhat irritating and may cause increased sensitivity to the sun, the trend, at this writing, is toward beta-hydroxy acids. These contain salicylic acid, long used in acne medicines. Both the alphas and the beta acids are exfoliants that cause the shedding of superficial skin cells. In the youth market, such products are sold to get rid of oily, blackhead-dotted top layers of skin. As one cosmetic manufacturer told me, however, you can grind up apricot pits and rub them on your face and get the same effect.

In the mid-1990s, the number of commercial products containing the acids exploded, going from around five in 1990 to two hundred by 1994.[2]

---

[2]Nathan Childs. "Inflammation Is New Wrinkle in AHA Safety Profile," *Skin & Allergy News,* 29(2):6–7, 1998.

Are these ingredient acids over-the-counter drugs or cosmetics? The cosmetic producers say their exfoliants do not change the structure of the skin, just peel off the dead layers, and therefore the products are cosmetics. Most of the reputable companies says the skin *appears* to be younger, even though they may name their products with names such as "Sudden Change" or "Anti-Wrinkle Treatment" that give the impression of reversing aging.

John Bailey, Ph.D., director of the FDA's Office of Cosmetics and Colors, says the "antiaging" competitive claims war is intensifying, and the FDA is studying the hydroxy acids ingredients being trumpeted.[3] The long-term study of two hydroxy acids most widely used in the cosmetic industry, lactic and glycolic, as far as systemic toxicity and carcinogenicity are concerned, is still in the preliminary stages at the National Institute of Environmental Health Sciences in Research Park, N.C.

Zoe Draelos, M.D., professor of dermatology at Wake Forest University, Winston-Salem, N.C., said at a meeting of cosmetic dermatology in 1998 that "These acids can alter the stratum corneum *(see)* 20 to 30 layers deep, particularly in formulations with a pH of 3 or lower. . . . Even cosmetic products with AHA concentration at or below 10 percent and at a pH of at least 3.5 are penetrating the skin farther than necessary. When patients feel stinging or burning, they think, 'Good, the product is working,' when in fact the pain they feel relates to the fact that the acid has penetrated the dermis and is interacting with the dermal nerve endings. That technically makes AHAs a topical drug."[4]

VITAMINS AGAINST AGING SKIN

The use of vitamins in antiaging creams is burgeoning. Avon's Anew line, for example, offers Formula C Facial Treatment Capsules while Origins' Night-A-Mins Mineral Rich Moisture Lotion contains "invigorating vitamins" including A, B, C, and E.

Vitamins C and E are well proven antioxidants. There is evidence that they fight free radicals, the molecules believed to play a role in the development of aging. Exposures to oxygen and to rays of the sun are among the conditions that can produce free radicals, and Vitamins C and E are being promoted in sunscreens.

The Wrinkling Sun

Sunscreens and sunblockers can arguably be classified as "antiaging" cosmetics. There is overwhelming scientific evidence that the sun can damage the skin, causing premature wrinkling and actinic (solar) keratoses. Actinic keratoses caused by overexposure to ultraviolet rays are manifested as age spots, or "liver spots," which usually appear in middle age and are scaly, often brown-colored lesions that may increase in number as we grow older. The incidence of squamous cell carcinoma in preexisting actinic keratoses is about one in 1,000 annually per individ-

---

[3]John Bailey, Ph.D., personal communication with author, November 8, 1993.
[4]Ibid.

ual. The primary concern of those seeking treatment for actinic keratoses, however, is most often cosmetic rather than medical.

Sunscreens are considered over-the-counter drugs by the FDA. It has become common practice to add sunscreening agents of variable potency to cosmetics to protect against the adverse effects of ultraviolet (UV) radiation exposure. In a study done at Case Western Reserve University, in Cleveland, Ohio, it was shown that cosmetic preparations containing sunscreening agents are protective against the sun's rays and should therefore be encouraged.[5]

It took more than fifteen years, but in 1993 the FDA finally came up with a sunscreen monograph (information required to set OTC regulations). The upper limit of 30 for the Sun Protection Factor (SPF) remained fixed, a decision that undercut efforts by leading marketers to increase ranges into the 40s and beyond with products for children and consumers especially sensitive to solar radiation. The new regulations also curb to some degree the label warnings, discarding the liberal old "prevents cancer of the skin" to versions of "Sun Alert: the sun causes skin damage. Regular use of sunscreens over the years may reduce the chance of skin damage, some types of skin cancer, and other harmful effects due to the sun."

The FDA was believed to be influenced by epidemiologists, who maintain that it is not very healthy for light-complexioned people to expose themselves to long-term ultraviolet radiation (UV), even when protected by sunscreens deemed to be effective. The epidemiologists believe the rising toll of melanoma may well be attributed to the desire to acquire a tan at a time when UV radiation is growing more destructive because of the thinning of the ozone layer.

Dr. Bailey points out that a SPF value of higher than 15 has no meaning because 15 essentially covers the entire period of time that the sun is at its peak in the United States. The higher numbers took into account those people who are nearer to the equator and may be exposed to more intense sunlight.[6]

New products are on the way. Melanin sunscreens that use the substance that naturally colors the skin have been introduced in Spain and Latin America. The developer has applied for its use as a drug in the United States.

So there is a grain of truth in the claims about Vitamin A pharmaceutical creams and exfoliant and sunscreen cosmetics. Dr. Bailey points out that there is a difference between "photoaging" from the sun and chronological aging: "Cosmetics can't do anything about the latter."

The fact is that if cosmetic chemists could put "youth in a bottle," they would deserve the Nobel Prize or at least the Cortez Fountain of Youth Award.

Another big trend that is big not only among youth seekers but young people themselves is toward "natural" cosmetics.

---

[5]C.A. Elmets; A. Vargas; C. Oresajo. "Photoprotective Effects of Sunscreens in Cosmetics on Sunburn and Langerhans Cell Photodamage," *Photodermatology, Photoimmunology and Photomedicine,* June 9, 1992 (3):113–20.
[6]John Bailey, Ph.D., personal communication with author, November 8, 1993.

WHAT'S "NATURAL"?

"Natural" can mean anything to anybody. "There are no standards for what 'natural' means," says Dr. Bailey. "They could wave a tube [of plant extract] over the bottle and declare it natural. Who's to say what they're actually using?"[7]

Revlon, Inc., uses natural plant extracts in its New Age Naturals cosmetics line, says Dan Moriarity, Revlon's director of public relations. "But the base formulas are the same as our conventional products," he says. In addition, because these products contain fragrances, they don't fit Revlon's definition of hypoallergenic, he explains.[8]

"Natural," according to the FDA, implies that ingredients are extracted directly from plants or animal products as opposed to being produced synthetically. There is no basis in fact or scientific legitimacy, the FDA says, to the notion that products containing natural ingredients are good for the skin.

"Natural" doesn't mean pure or clean or perfect either. According to the cosmetic trade journal *Drug and Cosmetic Industry,* "all plants [including those used in cosmetics] can be heavily contaminated with bacteria, and pesticides and chemical fertilizers used to improve crop yields."[9]

Still, as you can determine in this new edition of *A Consumer's Dictionary of Cosmetic Ingredients,* more and more "botanicals" are being added to cosmetics including antiaging products as well as other "treatment" and beautifying ingredients. The European market is particularly focused on finding legendary and newly discovered active botanicals.[10]

The FDA's Dr. Bailey says the agency is concerned about some botanicals being added to cosmetics since little is known about certain plant ingredients.[11]

Besides baby boomers who want to defy aging, what other groups do the cosmetic promoters have in their sights?

CONVINCING US WE STINK AND ARE CONTAGIOUS

Do you smell? Are you covered with germs?

Cosmetic companies for years have been trying to convince us we must mask any natural odors. Women, particularly, were told they needed products to disguise their "feminine odor." Now, the promoters are after both men and women with "body washes." They are in the process of brainwashing us about the need to have special products to clean us, that germs are hiding everywhere. Antibacterials have been added to soaps, deodorants, and toothpastes.

---

[7]Dori Stehlin. "Cosmetic Safety: More Complex Than at First Blush, *FDA Consumer,* May 1995, FDA/CFSAN Consumer.
[8]Ibid.
[9]Ibid.
[10]D. Scholz and G.J. Brooks, "An Ethnobotanical Approach to the Development of Effective Cosmetic Actives," paper presented at Drug Discovery and Development Approaches to Cosmeceuticals, International Business Communications Second Annual International Industry Conference, Short Hills, N.J., February 12–13, 1998.
[11]John Bailey, Ph.D, personal communication with author, July 1, 1998.

Men have been slower to take to body washes than women have but now male bar soap, the largest segment within male personal care, is declining, and male shower gels are climbing.[12]

In the 1980s and early 1990s when women were trying to achieve their place in a "man's world" and men were trying to be more "sensitive," unisex products were big sellers. Most industry experts believe that the great growth in unisex fragrances is over.[13] If we are going to smell, at least we want to smell differently. An interesting investigation by Susan Shiffman, Ph.D., professor of medical psychology at Duke University Medical Center, found that women choose scent to define their territory. She said that in the 1980s, bold, assertive scents with concentrations of up to 40 percent defined a larger territory than the more subtle scents of the 1990s.[14] The softer scents of the 90s send a completely different message. Clingier notes and gentler concentrations (12–15 percent fragrance) perfume the air only inches away from the wearer—pulling others in.

Consort Toiletries updated their packaging in 1997 for men. They made the containers cobalt blue to "communicate a strong masculine image."

The cosmetic marketers have recognized that many men in middle age have to seek a new job or career because of downsizing or burnout. Such men are ripe for products that may make them appear younger and more attractive. Maria Stefanidu, president of Ergo Research Inc., a marketing consulting firm, suggested these men be called "silver peacocks." "Young peacocks," she says, "preen and strut to show off their splendid colors. In the same way, the silver peacocks will show the world and themselves they are still young, attractive, and prepared for a second career or a new business venture. . . . This trend will foster the purchase of grooming aids, hair colors, and new wardrobes."[15]

The cosmetic companies also are trying to entice another group—the ethnics.

Culture and Cosmetics

The African-American consumer spends a disproportionately large amount on cosmetics. African-Americans purchased over $1,260 million in makeup products or 15 percent of the overall market. Black women spent, on average, $107.70 on makeup products during 1997, which was 22 percent more than the national average. No other ethnic group came close to the expenditure per capita. African-American women account for 15 percent of all makeup sales value while representing only 11.4 percent of the overall female population.[16] Of course, the manufacturers are revving up their targeting to this group. When some chains

---

[12]Anthony Bucala, "Overview of the U.S. Cosmetics and Toiletries Market," *Drug and Cosmetic Industry (DCI)*, June 1998, pp. 27–31.
[13]Ibid.
[14]Lesley Jane Seymour. "What Women Want in Fragrance," *DCI*, March 1997, p. 60.
[15]Maria Stefanidu. "The Rise of the 'Silver Peacock': Men's Hair Care Market Ready to Take Off," *DCI*, April 1998, pp. 48–49.
[16]Ibid.

stores put expanded efforts into this market, their sales went up 50–75 percent in this category.[17]

African-Americans are multihued, with at least thirty-five different shades of pigmentation, and there is a considerable variability in hair texture. This accounts for many of their unique skin and hair cosmetic requirements. Dermatologists as well as cosmetic companies are currently investigating the differences in skin sensitivity between whites and blacks and their grooming techniques.

The number one concern of black women, according to the experts, is uneven skin tone, primarily hyperpigmentation, which is dark spots or dark areas on the skin. Other concerns include blemishes, splotchiness, excessive oiliness, dry patches, ashiness, and the quest to find products that are gentle but effective enough to treat these concerns and not trigger any additional damage.[18]

Sensitive skin is a complex problem with genetic, individual, environmental, occupational, and ethnic implications. The development of topical products designed especially for sensitive ethnic skin is now under way.

This edition of *A Consumer's Dictionary of Cosmetic Ingredients* includes some of the unique products traditionally used by Asians, Middle Easterners, and Africans, as well as some of the untoward side effects such as high lead levels from kohl *(see)* and ochronosis *(see)* from the overuse of bleaching creams.

Fragrance companies have also recognized differences in scent preferences among ethnic groups. Orientals like the root extract valerian, which is disliked by most Europeans. The Japanese like camphor, a bark extract, and borneol *(see both)* both of which smell peppery. Camphor is said to keep away the worms that destroy bamboo. It is liked by American introverts, according to research, but disliked by extroverts. Northern Europeans prefer heavier fragrances for use in their cold climes, whereas Mediterraneans like sophisticated floral smells, probably because they love being surrounded by flowers. Most orientals appreciate heavy, spicy, animal perfumes.[19]

THE CHILDREN'S MARKET

While cosmetic companies are increasing marketing to the aging and ethnics, they are also aiming at another group—children. Parents have a vulnerability that the companies tap—getting children to take a bath. When you consider that Bath Time Buddies® by Johnson & Johnson had sales of more than $25 million a year—that's not just small change. L'Oréal Kids packages its 2-in-1 shampoo and conditioners exclusively for kids age three to ten years in bottles in the shape of colorful fish.

By age thirteen, 71.6 percent of female children use blusher, 84.9 percent use lip-gloss, and 94.1 percent use hair conditioner.[20]

---

[17]"Profit Potential of Ethnic HBA," *Outlook,* May 25–27, 1998, p. 4.
[18]Karen Hoppe, Editor. "Black Beauty: A Truly Evolving Market," *DCI,* November 1996, pp. 25–30.
[19]Ruth Winter, *The Smell Book: Scents, Sex, and Society,* New York: J.B. Lippincott, 1976.
[20]"Cosmetics for Children: A Few Ups, Mostly Downs," *DCI,* June 1993, pp. 56–57.

The children's market is estimated at $3 billion to $5 billion and growing 5 to 8 percent a year. One reason: Children now make up one-fifth of the U.S. population, and a growing number of upscale shops and companies are catering to their needs.[21]

Some cosmetic marketers have now decided to put two of the great markets together—blacks and children. They are producing play makeup for black youngsters. Census figures show that 21 percent of the females in the four- to nine-year-old category are black.[22]

BUYER AWARE

"Just because it costs more doesn't mean it's better!"

This has been one of the major themes of all editions of *A Consumer's Dictionary of Cosmetic Ingredients,* but now it is echoing through the colorful, scented halls of the cosmetic, toiletries, and fragrance industry itself. A fierce battle is raging to sell products to a changing population in hard economic times.

When the last edition of this book was published in 1994, there were basically two distinct tiers of cosmetic marketers:

1. *Prestige marketers,* which offered products in fancy containers dabbed on us by trained cosmeticians who provided advice; and

2. *Broad marketers,* from which we could pick out many of the same basic products but with different names in plain self-serve packages in drugstores and supermarkets.

The prestige marketers have been hit hard by the closing of department store chains—their major outlets—and by imitators and "gray marketers."

It costs millions of dollars, for example, to launch a new fragrance from creation to hype, but within a year of a launch, sales are diluted by three or four copycat products that imitate the scent of the original.[23]

The gray marketers, on the other hand, bring overseas goods into the United States. These can be duty-free products of a foreign or U.S. manufacturer or merchandise of a foreign licensee not intended to be sold in this country. Gray marketers take advantage of currency fluctuations. They buy goods at 30 or even 40 percent below wholesale cost and make tremendous profits by holding inventory until the right currency conditions exist to sell to us.[24]

The once-very-particular prestige cosmetic companies, as a result, are now out to sell us their products anywhere they can, from cable TV, direct mail, beauty salons, and, yes, even in the territory of the broad marketers—the supermarket and the drugstore. More and more prestige companies are joining the broad marketers in the use

---

[21]Rhonda Schaffler, CNN, "Personal Care for Kids," March 12, 1997, 11:16 AM EST.
[22]Ibid.
[23]"Cosmetics Through the Looking Glass: Recovery Signs Upbeat, But Diversion and Shifts in Retail Patterns Create Concern," *DCI,* June 1993, pp. 28–39.
[24]"The Fragrance Market," *DCI,* June 1993, p. 42.

of infomercials, which blur the line between a TV program and a commercial. Companies are spending millions of dollars for a thirty-minute cosmetic sales pitch.

Since the last edition of this book two players have entered cosmetic marketing in a big way: specialty stores such as Bath And Body Works, Garden Botanika, and Bed, Bath and Beyond; and the Internet.

Fragrance Counter (http://www.fragrancecounter.com), the leading online retailer of prestige fragrances since 1995, launched Cosmetics Counter (http://www.cosmeticscounter.com), a new commerce web site offering a variety of brand name color cosmetics, beauty treatments, and accessories in the summer of 1998. The Cosmetics Club on the site features a replenishment program that allows you to receive specific products on an ongoing basis.

Elsewhere, from the companies, themselves, you can buy direct on the Internet. For example, you can buy Avon's Anew Alpha Hydroxy face mask at $10.99 or a 1.5 oz jar of Erno Laszlo's AHA Revitalizing Complex at $95. Both employ hydroxy acids.

Eli Katz, senior vice president and general manager of Fragrance Counter and Cosmetics Counter points out that the demand for beauty products online is growing at a rate of about 300 percent for 1998. He points out it gives users the option of selecting products by specific brand or by category. If you want a lipstick, you may click on the Shop-by-brand button and choose the particular brand such as Lancôme or Clinique. You can also type the word "lipstick" in the search bar or click on any of the color, treatments, or accessories buttons to find your lipstick.

You won't have a cosmetician giving you advice and telling you how beautiful your look online but you will save time, a precious commodity in this busy world.

MIRROR MIRROR—WHOSE FAIR?

We have become more savvy consumers. We are reading labels and recognizing that often the only difference between an expensive cosmetic and an inexpensive one is the cost of the package and the hype. There is a 500–1,000 percent spread between cost and sales price in cosmetics. This margin is needed, according to manufacturers, to meet heavy promotional expenses. The industry is the largest advertiser on TV and in magazines. Cosmetic promotions can make Barnum look like an introvert.

Don't feel sorry for the cosmetic, toiletries, and perfume industry, though. As long as they can sell "hope in a bottle," they will prosper. When the third edition of this book was published, in 1989, their sales were $18 billion a year. In the fourth edition published in 1994, sales were $28.6 billion. At this writing, sales are estimated to be $36.4 billion. Makeup is the largest individual market in the cosmetic and toiletries industry, with sales reaching $8.6 billion in 1997, which was 23.7 percent of the entire business. Behind makeup was the fragrance market at $6.7 billion in sales, and third was skin care with nearly $5 billion. Shaving products were $2 billion. The makeup category had the largest number of new product releases in 1997, 55 percent. Skin care accounted for 25 percent, and hair care slid in at 10 percent.[25]

---

[25]Bucala, op. cit.

One major reason cosmetic sales keep climbing, no matter what, is that the cosmetic, toiletries, and fragrance industry is better at tapping into sociological and economic trends than almost any other group, including politicians. The cosmetic marketers have recognized the white, eighteen-to-thirty-five-year-old age group is no longer the most fruitful sales target. The population is getting older. In a little more than five years, women aged thirty-five to fifty-four years will outnumber those eighteen to thirty-four by 10 million. The population, furthermore, is increasingly multihued.

They are masterful at understanding our vulnerabilities and gullibilities. Like the alchemists and medicine men of old, cosmetic companies promise beauty and youth in a bottle. "Rub this into your face, and your wrinkles will disappear," they say, or "Put this on your skin, and you will be irresistible."

If we believe a cream can take away wrinkles or a mascara can make us alluring, what's the harm? So we pay $50 for five cents' worth of ingredients. Maybe the psychological lift is priceless.

On the other hand, cosmetics may cost us more than we really want to pay. If a cosmetic ingredient may cause an allergic reaction or contribute to the cancer burden, that's quite another matter. If we take a drug with side effects, the risk may be worth it because we may need the drug to regain or maintain our health. But although they may be rewarding psychologically, are cosmetics worth any risk?

QUESTIONS ABOUT SAFETY

Cosmetics have received and still receive the lowest priority at the FDA. The agency spends less than 1 percent of its budget on cosmetic safety surveillance.

In September 1980, the National Toxicology Program (NTP) contracted with the National Research Council (NRC) and the National Academy of Sciences for a study[26] with two principal charges:

1. To determine toxicity-testing needs for substances to which humans are exposed so that the federal agencies responsible for the protection of public health will have the information needed to assess the toxicity of such substances.

2. To develop and validate uniformly applicable and wide-ranging criteria by which to set priorities for research on substances with potentially adverse public-health impact.

The study found that there is no toxicity information available for 56 percent of the cosmetic ingredients, 28 percent have less than minimal information, and for only 2 percent is complete health hazard assessment possible.

American and European experts point out the importance of exposure levels in use:

---

[26]Toxicity Testing Strategies to Determine Needs and Priorities, National Research Council (U.S.), National Academy Press, Washington, D.C., 1984.

The assessment of the safety of any cosmetic product clearly relates to the manner of use. This factor is important since it determines the amount of substance that may be ingested, inhaled, or absorbed through the skin or mucous membranes. Consideration of the quantity of ingredients applied in the different products is also important as the following examples illustrate.

- Soap is applied in dilute form and although the area of application may be extensive, the product is rapidly washed off.

- Products used on the lips and mouth will be ingested to some extent.

- Cosmetics used around the eyes and genital regions may come into contact with the conjunctiva or mucosa respectively, resulting in reaction due to the thin epithelial lining of these areas.

- Suntanning products, body lotions or body creams may be applied over a large surface of the body, and the ingredients, often at appreciable concentrations, may remain in contact with the skin over several hours. Suntanning products, due to their extensive skin contact, combined with direct exposure to UV radiation for prolonged periods, require a distinct type of safety evaluation.

Thus, before any safety evaluation and risk assessment of a finished product are made, the degree and route of consumer exposure must be known. This needs to be carried out on a case-by-case basis.

The major companies are safety conscious. Whether driven by altruism, liability, or the bottom line, most companies see the need for safety testing.

The fact is that we must rely largely on the cosmetic companies themselves to protect us and to thoroughly test their products before putting them on the market. The Cosmetic, Toiletries and Fragrance Association (CTFA), in fact, has established its own safety assessment system, the Cosmetic Ingredient Review (CIR). Since 1976, a panel of seven scientists has been conducting an independent review to assess the safety data concerning ingredients. The Cosmetic Ingredient Review panel recommendations are publicly announced without any private review or comment, according to the CTFA. Thus far, members have questioned the safety of several ingredients—such as 6-methyl coumarin and musk ambrette—and these substances have been voluntarily removed by CTFA member companies. As of May 1998, the CIR had released final reports covering 720 ingredients widely used in the industry. Of those, 390 were found safe as used; 228 were safe with qualifications as to product type, area of use, or concentration; 95 had insufficient data for the panel to reach a conclusion; and 7 were found to be unsafe.

The CTFA claims that its members produce 90 percent of the cosmetics produced. We should be grateful that there are scientists testing ingredients for us. However, the cosmetic companies are politically astute. Such self-testing and efforts at self-regulation fend off potential outside regulation by government agencies. And the cosmetics manufacturers contribute heavily to political campaigns, including the presidential.

It is in their own interest, of course, to avoid using an ingredient that might be found at some later date to be potentially harmful. Adverse publicity can instantly kill a product in which millions of dollars have been invested.

ANIMAL TESTS

Many companies have begun to label their products with statements indicating that no animals have been used in testing. *Cruelty free* implies that products have not been tested on animals. Most ingredients have been at some point tested on animals so you may want to look for "no new animal testing," to get a more accurate designation.

The most controversial and widely used animal test is the Draize Eye Irritancy Test, which involves putting drops of the substance in question into the eyes of albino rabbits. Investigators then note if any redness, swelling, cloudiness of the iris, or corneal opacity occurs. In addition, the ability of the eye to repair any damage is noted.

The European Communities (EC) Guidelines state that an "animal study shall not be performed if another scientifically satisfactory method of obtaining the result sought, not entailing the use of an animal, is reasonably and practically available."[27] The EC says, however, "It is a common view among the general public that in order to define the safety of finished cosmetics products it should be sufficient to test them directly on human volunteers. This type of evaluation is sufficient to reveal any acute toxic effects of that product; it is absolutely insufficient for identifying those effects, such as systemic toxicity, carcinogenicity, and teratogenicity for which the only test methods that are currently scientifically acceptable are those developed in animals."

How do many companies claim their products are "cruelty free"?

A cosmetic manufacturer told me that some companies are now paying humans to test cosmetics rather than using four-legged animals. A private labeler who supplies products to many "name" companies, told me his company tests on animals, and the large companies who buy his products then say that they, themselves, do not do animal tests. If, on the other hand, a company uses older cosmetic ingredients that have long ago been tested on animals, they can then say their "new" cosmetic versions have not been tested on animals.

"As far as we know," says Neil Wilcox, D.V.M., director of the FDA's Office of Animal Care and Use, "what these companies do is use, for the most part, old reliable ingredients that have been proven safe [based on past animal data and a history of safe use] and then test the final product on people."[28]

The FDA's Division of Toxicological Review and Evaluation is evaluating two alternatives for the Draize eye test. One is Eytex, manufactured by Ropak Corporation, Irvine, California, a chemical assay that produces opacity similar to

---

[27]N. Loprieno, "Guidelines for Safety Evaluation of Cosmetic Ingredients," *Food Chemistry Toxicology,* 30 (9): 809–15, 1992.
[28]Dori Stehlin, "Cosmetic Safety: More Complex Than at First Blush," *FDA Consumer,* May 1995, Publication No. (FDA) 93-5012.

that of an animal cornea upon exposure to irritants. The other is vertebrate cell cultures from humans and mice.

Draize may be impossible to replace with a single alternative test, says Sidney Green, Ph.D., a toxicologist with the FDA's Center for Food Safety and Applied Nutrition.[29] He explains that because the Draize test measures three different areas of the eye, replacing Draize will probably take a combination of alternative tests, "but we've not seen that combination yet."

Dr. Wilcox notes that for the FDA to approve other methods, those methods will have to produce test results that can be reproduced in other labs. In addition, databases will have to correlate historical animal test results with newer lab results.

"Database development and cooperation [between industry and FDA] is pivotal to the validation process," says the FDA veterinarian.

The cosmetics industry has taken one step toward database development—the Cosmetic Ingredient Review. The basic purpose of the review is to gather information from the scientific literature and from company files on the safety of cosmetic ingredients and make that information publicly available.

If a safety problem with a cosmetic product arises after it's been marketed, the FDA can take action to obtain the manufacturer's safety data on the product. Because there is not yet enough information on alternatives to animal testing to validate their use in ensuring human safety, the FDA, at this point, would only accept animal safety data.

Incidentally, cosmetic manufacturers took the word "animal" out of their ingredient labels but not out of the ingredients. Hydrolyzed animal protein, for example, is now called hydrolyzed collagen *(see)*.

THE STATE OF STATE COSMETIC REGULATIONS

Due largely to consumer pressure, some states have been formulating regulations concerning cosmetics. California and New York are interested in air quality and cosmetic aerosols. Massachusetts opted to ban the sale of cosmetics tested on animals. Oregon insisted on the use of recycled plastic resins in cosmetic bottles. A consumer group, As You Sow, filed a lawsuit in California to require a warning under the state's Proposition 65 concerning nail polish, primarily because of the solvent toluene *(see)*. The Cosmetic, Toiletries and Fragrance Association said it considered the suit frivolous.[30] California consumer advocates were trying to force reformulation of many hair fixatives and adoption of nonaerosol packaging forms for most antiperspirants.

There have been serious injuries reported due to the use of hairsprays containing flammable alcohol combined with an even more flammable hydrocarbon propellant. This produces a potentially lethal product when the user is smoking or when there may be a heating unit or hot curler in a small room. There are now warnings on many hairspray cans that caution the user to avoid flames and smok-

---

[29]Ibid.
[30]"Washington Letter," *DCI,* June 1993, p. 12.

ing while using the product and not to spray themselves in the face or eyes with the aerosol. Dr. Bailey says that the warnings are not consistent, and some of them are not distinguishable from the other matter on the labels. He said that Canada requires the warning on aerosols to be on the front of the can, and the FDA is considering new, more uniform, and distinct warnings on the labels.

ADVERSE REACTIONS FROM COSMETICS

Labels that claim a product is "dermatologist-tested," "sensitivity-tested," "allergy-tested," or "nonirritating" carry no guarantee that you won't have a reaction, and what you have in a bottle is not necessarily what you have on the skin in a few minutes. Alcohol and/or water may evaporate, and you may be left with a very different compound than what is listed on the bottle.

The FDA's Cosmetics Office estimates that it may receive only a small percentage of cosmetic complaints reported by consumers. Complaints, the FDA says, are more often filed with poison control centers, state and local agencies, or with the product manufacturer and/or distributor who are not required to submit their complaint files to the FDA.

This author looked at the 1996 list of problems concerning cosmetics sent to the FDA. Most cited hair care products, particularly hair straighteners and hair colorings. Nail treatments, mouthwashes, depilatories, bubble baths, toothpastes, and mascaras followed.

Although the FDA believes that the industry received about fifty reports for every one made to the FDA, the problems reported to companies are along the same lines—allergies and skin irritations.

As the author of this book, I have received more anecdotal reports from readers about adverse effects from cosmetics than the FDA. My sister and her friend both had severe skin reactions from a new moisturizing lotion. Both had to pay for medical attention by dermatologists, yet I could get neither one to report the reaction to the FDA. They said they would, but as yet they haven't. Neither have their dermatologists reported the incident. If consumers, like my sister and her friend, do develop a skin, hair, or eye reaction, they may just stop using the product and not report it. Frequently, neither the consumer nor the consumer's doctor even associates a physical problem, particularly a systemic one, with the use of a cosmetic.

If you have an adverse reaction, please call the Cosmetics and Colors Automated Information Line 1-(800)-270-8869 for information on how to report adverse reactions to cosmetics, as well as problems such as filth, decomposition, or spoilage.

So we have poor reporting of adverse reactions and a dearth of scientific investigations into the adverse effects of cosmetic ingredients.

Dr. Bailey says: "The agency can't do much about isolated allergic reactions or irritation problems. It's up to the individual to avoid the product that caused the reaction and any other products that contain the offending ingredient."

But that doesn't mean the FDA feels reporting the problem isn't important. "We look for clusters," Dr. Bailey says. "If we see we're getting a number of complaints for the same product, then that is cause for concern."

Unlike reports of allergic or irritation reactions, even one report of an acute injury, usually caused by a contaminated product, results in quick action by the agency. "We'll inspect the establishment, talk to the consumer, talk to the doctor, collect samples, and analyze them to determine the extent of contamination," says Dr. Bailey.

But remember the FDA does not take action unless a consumer or physician reports a problem, and Dr. Bailey says if you do have a problem, report it.

The most difficult issue in the identification of ingredients and contaminants in cosmetics concerns cancer-causing agents. A number of cosmetic ingredients now in use have been shown to be carcinogenic in animals or to cause genetic breaks in cells. Testing for mutagenicity—breaks in the genetic material of bacteria—can screen many chemicals inexpensively and rapidly. Almost all chemicals known to be carcinogenic in humans have been shown to be mutagens in these systems. However, not all mutagens are necessarily carcinogenic. Thus, animal studies, which cost approximately $300,000 to thoroughly test an ingredient, are needed.

All agents that cause cancer in humans cause cancer in rats and mice, with the exception of trivalent arsenic. Whether all chemicals that cause cancer in animals cause cancer in humans is a matter of debate, but many scientists in the cancer field believe they do.

Two contaminants found in cosmetics have been shown to cause cancer. One is *n*-nitrosodiethanolamine (NDELA), which penetrates easily through the skin when in a fatty base. This contaminant appears to be produced by the interaction of two otherwise safe ingredients—for example, the amines (surfactants, emulsifiers, and detergents) and nitrites or nitroso compounds such as in the preservative 2-bromo-2-nitro-propane-1, 3-diol (BNPD). The other carcinogen is 1,4-dioxane, a contaminant of raw materials. It is believed that about one-third of the emulsion-based cosmetics containing polyoxyethylene derivatives have it in amounts ranging from 1 percent to over 25 percent.[31]

In 1998, however, the FDA issued a statement that the agency had become aware of a new National Toxicology Program (NTP) study showing an association between the topical application of diethanolamine (DEA) and certain DEA-related ingredients and cancer in laboratory animals. For the DEA-related ingredient, the NTP study suggests that the carcinogenic response is linked to possible residual levels of DEA. Although DEA itself is used in very few cosmetics, DEA-related ingredients such as oleamide DEA, lauramide DEA, and cocamide DEA *(see all)* are widely used in a variety of cosmetic products. These ingredients function as emulsifiers or foaming agents and are generally used at levels of 1 to 5 percent.[32]

The FDA statement says the agency takes these findings very seriously and is in the process of carefully evaluating the studies and test data to determine the real

---

[31]*FDA's Cosmetics Handbook,* U.S., HHS, Washington, D.C., October 15, 1992, p. 9 and pp. 11–12.
[32]"Diethanolamine in Cosmetic Products," U.S. Food and Drug Administration, Center for Food Safety and Applied Nutrition, Office of Cosmetics Fact Sheet, February 26, 1998.

risk, if any, to consumers. The FDA says that if its evaluation of the NTP data indicates a health hazard exists, it will advise the industry and the public and will consider its legal options under the authority of the Food, Drug and Cosmetic Act. In other words, we will all probably have a few more wrinkles before any "action" is taken.

In 1978, there was a great outcry when it was shown that ingredients in hair dyes caused cancer in animals. The FDA has no power over hair dyes because coal tar colors, which were incriminated, are exempted from the cosmetic act. The FDA was unsuccessful in requiring a warning label on hair-coloring products, and women returned to coloring their hair at the rate of $450 million a year. In the meantime, questions about hair dye ingredients remain (*see* Hair Coloring and Coal Tar).

University of California researchers studying more than 58,000 hairdressers, manicurists, and cosmetologists found that they developed multiple myeloma at four times the rate of the general population. Multiple myeloma is a malignant tumor of the bone marrow. Women aged twenty to sixty-five residing in the Los Angeles area were studied. In 1982, Dr. John Peters and two coauthors said, in the *American Journal of Industrial Medicine,* that among the suspect substances are hair dyes, shampoos, hair conditioners, relaxers, permanent wave solutions, detergents, nail antiseptics, fungi, and bacteria.[33]

Medical researchers have also been trying to find a reason or reasons for the rising incidence of non-Hodgkin's lymphoma (NHL), the cancer that killed Jackie Kennedy Onassis. One area the investigators are studying is the potential connection between hair dyes and NHL. The largest study on this, conducted by the American Cancer Society and reported in 1994, found women who used black hair dye for twenty years or more were more than four times as likely to develop NHL than women who didn't use hair dye. This finding confirms those of other studies. But because only a small fraction of women who dye their hair use black hair dye, this alone cannot contribute significantly to the increase in NHL in recent years, according to the FDA.[34]

Michigan State researchers reported in 1997 that women who have worked as hairdressers are at higher risk of developing a rare form of cancer of the salivary gland. The salivary glands secrete saliva in the mouth which aids digestion. The researchers could not explain why hairdressers are more prone to these cancers but suspect it may be due to inhaled exposure to hairsprays or hair dyes.[35]

A report by National Cancer Institute Researchers published in *American Journal of Public Health*[36] showed an almost doubled risk of multiple myeloma in

---

[33]John Peters, M.D., et al., *American Journal of Industrial Medicine,* September 1982.

[34]Margie Patlak, "Non-Hodgkin's Lymphoma Becomes More Common, More Treatable," *FDA* Consumer, December 1996, pp. 20–22.

[35]Marie Swanson, director of the Cancer Center at Michigan State University, study reported by Michigan State, October 24, 1997.

[36]Linda Morris Brown, M.P.H., et al., "Hair Dye Use in White Men and Risk of Multiple Myeloma," *American Journal of Public Health,* December 1992, p. 200.

men who used hair dyes. In a study reported four years before in the same publication, NCI researchers reported a doubling of the risk for non-Hodgkin's lymphoma and leukemia in men who used hair dye.[37] A study in the same journal, also by NCI researchers, reported women who used hair dyes had a 50 percent higher risk of developing non-Hodgkin's lymphoma than women who never dyed their hair.[38] In the latest report, published in the NCI's own journal, researchers financed by the American Cancer Society, studying more than half a million women from 1982 to 1989, found no increased risk in using hair dye except for those women using permanent black hair dye for more than twenty years. In that case, there were increased risks of developing non-Hodgkin's lymphoma and multiple myeloma.[39]

In 1998, an eight-year retrospective survey of 4,108 persons by a University of San Francisco researcher under a grant from the NIC found hair coloring wasn't linked to any cancers in women. There was a "slightly higher non-Hodgkin's lymphoma in men who used semi-permanent hair dye frequently." The NCI and The American Cancer Society research at this writing continue to study the dark hair dyes and their research results are expected soon.[40]

The controversy about hair dyes and cancer in humans remains. There is growing evidence that hairdressers and cosmetologists are at higher risk for cancers of the breast and urinary tract but whether this is due to dyes, some other substance they use or even cigarette smoke, the final proof is yet to come.[41] Another study in 1997, for example, reported no clear difference in the mutations in the cells of professional hair colorists compared to closely matched controls.[42] In any case, it is wise to be cautious when someone colors your hair in a salon setting. Make sure that person is qualified to do so. The color should be in contact with the skin the shortest time possible.[43]

Another common cosmetic ingredient—talcum powder—has also been cited several times as a possible carcinogen. In 1972, a study by the Office of Product Technology of the FDA showed that of 40 cosmetic talcum powder samples tested, 39 contained 1 percent asbestos or less. Asbestos is a proven human carcinogen. The manufacturers maintain that they have solved the problem of contamination. However, asbestos and talc fibers are similar in composition. Cancer of the ovary was linked to talc use in an article in the journal *Cancer* in 1982. Daniel Cramer, M.D., an obstetrician and gynecologist, found in a study of 215 Boston-area women with

---

[37]Kenneth Cantor, Ph.D., et al., "Hair Dye Use and Risk of Leukemia and Lymphoma," *American Journal of Public Health,* May 1988, p. 60.

[38]Shelia Hoar Zahm, Sc.D., et al., "Use of Hair Coloring Products and Risk of Lymphoma, Multiple Myeloma, and Chronic Leukemia," *American Journal of Public Health,* July 1992, p. 10.

[39]Michael Waldholz, "Use of Hair Dyes Isn't Found to Boost the Risk of Cancer," *Wall Street Journal,* February 1, 1994, p. B7.

[40]E.A. Holly, et al., "Hair-color products and risk for non-Hodgkin's lymphoma: a population-based study in the San Francisco bay area," *American Journal of Public Health,* Dec. 1988 (12): 1767–73.

[41]T. Skov, et al., "Risk for Cancer of the Urinary Bladder Among Hairdressers in the Nordic Countries," *American Journal of Medicine* 2, 1990, pp. 217–23; T.C. Greiner, et al., "Non-Hodgkin's Lymphoma," *Cancer* 75(1 suppl) January 1, 1995, pp. 370–80; L.A. Habel et al., "Occupation and Breast Cancer Risk in Middle-Aged Women," *Journal of Occupational Environmental Medicine* 37(3) March 1995, pp. 349–56.

[42]S. Sardas, et al., "Genotoxicity Studies on Professional Hair Colorists Exposed to Oxidation Hair Dyes," *Mutation Research* 394 (1–3), November 27, 1997, pp. 153–61.

[43]John Bailey, Ph.D., personal communication with author, November 8, 1993.

ovarian cancer that 32 had used talcum powder on their genitals and sanitary napkins when compared with a group of women without cancer. Women who used talc had 328 times the risk of ovarian cancer. In the 1960s, granulomas of the internal organs had been associated with the talc used on surgeons' gloves during operations.

Mouthwash, a simple product that could be either a drug or a cosmetic, was also tied to cancer in 1983. Two reports in the February *Journal of the National Cancer Institute* linked daily use of mouthwash with cancer of the mouth and throat among women usually considered low risk for cancer because they did not smoke or drink alcohol. Ten years later, there was enough evidence that the FDA agreed that formulations having more than 25 percent alcohol do indeed "contribute to user susceptibility to cancer of the mouth." In anticipation of a FDA ruling to lower alcohol content in mouthwash, producers began lowering the alcohol content in 1993.

Dr. Bailey also points out another problem that falls between medical and cosmetic regulations: the permanent tattooing of coloring around the eyes and lips. "None of the colors have been approved for that purpose," Dr. Bailey says. He adds that many people who have the tattooing do not realize how permanent it is. The coloring may be lightened by using a laser, but it can be a hazardous procedure.

BUGGY COSMETICS

Contaminated makeup is the result of either inadequate preservatives or product misuse. But contamination doesn't necessarily translate into serious injury for the user.

"Cosmetics are not expected to be totally free of microorganisms when first used or to remain free during consumer use," according to a 1989 FDA report on contamination of makeup counter samples in department stores. The report was based on a survey that found that over 5 percent of samples collected were seriously contaminated with such things as molds, other fungi, and pathogenic organisms.

Recent studies have shown outbreaks of conjunctivitis (pink eye), which can be precipitated by contaminated eye makeup. One epidemic was caused by mascara shared among a group of women studied. Mascara contaminated with eye *Pseudomonas* has been documented to cause destructive corneal lesions resulting in visual impairment. It is therefore important that you not share mascara or other eye makeup and not allow children to play with makeup that has been used by others. Also, do not use open samples at cosmetic counters. In one survey of makeup counter samples in department stores, the FDA reportedly found that more than 5 percent were contaminated with fungi and other pathogens.[44]

Every time you open a bottle of foundation or case of eye shadow, microorganisms in the air have an opportunity to rush in. But adequately preserved products can kill off enough of the little bugs to keep the product safe.

Occasionally, however, a product will be seriously contaminated. According to FDA data, most cases of contamination are due to manufacturers using poorly designed ineffective preservative systems and not testing the stability of the

[44]Patricia Kloser, M.D., University of Medicine & Dentistry of New Jersey, "Ugly Risks of Beauty Routines," *Medscape Women's Health* 1 (12), 1996.

preservatives during the product's customary shelf life and under normal use conditions.

"Shelf life" or "Expiration date" is the amount of time for which a cosmetic product is good under normal conditions of storage and use, depending on the product's composition, packaging, preservation, and so forth. Expiration dates are, for practical purposes, a rule of thumb, and a product may expire long before that date if it has not been stored and properly handled. On the other hand, products stored under ideal conditions may be acceptable long after the expiration date has been reached. Generally cosmetics are formulated and tested for a shelf life of one to three years under normal storage conditions.

Testing the Testers

There's something else that is definitely taboo when using makeup—sharing!

"Never share, not even with your best friend," says Irene Malbin, CTFA's vice president of public relations. "Sharing cosmetics means sharing germs, and the risk, though small, isn't worth it," says Malbin.

Shared-use cosmetics—the testers commonly found at department store cosmetic counters—are even more likely to become contaminated than the same products in an individual's home, according to the 1989 FDA report.

The FDA followed its 1989 report on makeup testers with a survey of corresponding unopened retail packages. The survey found only negligible contamination, and the agency concluded that the preservatives couldn't handle the challenge of constant use.

"At home, the preservatives have time—usually a whole day—to kill the bacteria that is inevitably introduced after each use," says Bailey. "But in a store, there may be only minutes between each use. The preservatives can't handle it."

If you really want to test a cosmetic before you buy, "you should insist—must insist—on a new, unused applicator," says CTFA's Malbin. She says that some companies use cotton swabs for that purpose.

NAILING NAIL PROBLEMS

Nail problems are about 10 percent of the conditions dermatologists treat. Changes in nails, such as discoloration or thickening, can signal health problems, including liver and kidney disease, heart and lung conditions, anemia and diabetes. Common nail problems include white spots after an injury to the nails, vertical lines under the nails caused by nail injury or certain drugs and diseases and bacterial infections, most often due to injury. Fungal infections cause about half of all nail disorders.[45]

Women who have nail wraps or artificial nails are particularly susceptible to a fungus infection, *onychomycosis*. Before an artificial nail is applied, the surface of the nail is usually abraded with an emery board. This procedure damages the nail surface and creates a possible nidus of fungal infection. Additionally, an emery

---

[45]American Academy of Dermatology Media Backgrounder, 1998.

board used on a fungus-infected nail can introduce the fungal infection to an uninfected nail on the same person or to the next emery board user. Fungal infections can also occur when the woman has her nail tips or wraps in water and collects water in and under the nail.[46] (See Appendix B for precautions for natural and artificial nails.)

SELLING FACTS OR FANTASY

In addition to the FD & C Act, the Fair Packaging and Labeling Act requires an ingredient declaration on every cosmetic product offered for sale to consumers. In addition, these regulations require that ingredients be listed in descending order of quantity. Water, for example, accounts for the bulk of most skin-care products, which is why it usually appears first on these products. If you buy a European product, however, the label may read "aqua," which is what manufacturers in European countries label water. I particularly get a kick out of the European name on the label, *Graveolens sativa* or *Avena sativa*—we call it oatmeal.

Cosmetic companies also do not want the price of their ingredients publicized. If you read labels, you'll see that water and alcohol are two of the most commonly used ingredients. One French perfumer was asked, for example, how much the ingredients in a perfume selling for $230 per ounce in a department store really cost. His answer: "Four to six dollars."

The cosmetic companies have some new gimmicks on their labels to keep you from understanding what is really in the products. Some have the label ingredients listed in a barely contrasting color to the container's so that it is virtually unreadable. Most have the print so small that you need a magnifying glass. A number are now separating the "active" ingredients from the supposedly "inactive." This avoids revealing that the largest ingredients in most cosmetics are water first and then alcohol since the FDA requires the labels to list ingredients in descending order. This way, the minuscule active ingredients are listed in a category above the larger supposedly inactive ingredients.

The argument is sometimes made that while Congress intended to safeguard the health and economic interests of consumers with the Federal Food, Drug, and Cosmetic Act, it also meant to protect a manufacturer's right to market a product free of excessive government regulation. And, in an industry that sells personal image, especially images of beauty and sex appeal, not allowing the puffery claims would certainly hurt the marketing says Dr. Bailey.[47] "Most cosmetics contain ingredients that are promoted with exaggerated claims of beauty, of long-lasting effects to create an image," he says. "Image is what the cosmetic industry sells through its products, and it's up to the consumer to believe it or not."

Advertising of cosmetics, as distinct from labeling, is regulated by the Federal Trade Commission (FTC), not the FDA. The advertising is not supposed to be false or misleading, and the company is supposed to have substantiation for claims

---

[46]Ibid.
[47]Judith Foulke, "Cosmetic Ingredients: Understand the Puffery," *FDA Consumer*, DHHS Publication No. (FDA) 93-5013, reprinted May 1992.

made in ads. Many of the ads, however, are fairy tales for grown-ups—use this product, and you will look younger and be irresistible.

In 1975, the FDA tried to publish regulations defining hypoallergenic to mean a lower potential for causing an allergic reaction but was defeated by two cosmetic companies, Almay and Clinique, which claimed consumers already understood that hypoallergenic products were no panacea against allergic reactions. The courts eventually held for the companies.

Hypoallergenic implies that products making this claim are less likely to cause allergic reaction. There are no prescribed scientific studies required to substantiate this claim, the FDA says. Likewise, the terms "dermatologist-tested," "sensitivity tested," "allergy tested," or "nonirritating" carry no guarantee that they won't cause skin reactions. "Hypoallergenic can mean almost anything to anybody," says Bailey. "Hypo" means "less than," and hypoallergenic means only that the manufacturer feels that the product is less likely than others to cause an allergic reaction. Although some manufacturers do clinical testing, others may simply omit perfumes or other common problem-causing ingredients. But there are no regulatory standards on what constitutes hypoallergenic.

"FDA tried to publish regulations (in 1975) defining hypoallergenic to mean a lower potential for causing an allergic reaction," says Dr. Bailey. "In addition, we were going to require that companies submit information to FDA establishing that in fact their products were hypoallergenic." However, two cosmetic manufacturers, Almay and Clinique, challenged the proposed regulations in court, claiming that consumers already understood that hypoallergenic products were no panacea against allergic reactions. In July 1975, the U.S. District Court for the District of Columbia upheld the FDA's regulations, but the two companies appealed. On December 21, 1977, the U.S. Court of Appeals for the District of Columbia reversed the district court's ruling.

Like hypoallergenic, "natural" and "organic" can mean anything. Many products and drugs are made from plant extracts. As victims of poison ivy know, natural and hypoallergenic are not interchangeable terms.

The FDA is supposed to enforce the rules, not make them. The representatives in Congress and the regulators at the FDA are there to carry out the wishes of the people. If there is not sufficient desire for stronger cosmetic laws, then there won't be stronger laws.

Dr. Bailey says that, with limited funds and personnel, the FDA Office of Cosmetics and Colors must concentrate more on risk than on claims.[48]

LABEL WARNINGS—PAY ATTENTION

Experts in the field of safety often say that consumers do not read, no less pay attention to, warnings on product labels. Misuse of some cosmetic products can cause problems that range in severity from mild rash to skin burns, or from burn-

---

[48]John Bailey, Ph.D., personal communication with author, July 1, 1998.

ing eyes to blindness. Sometimes the label print is too small for those without 20/20 vision. See the list of label warnings in Appendix A.

Choose Your Cosmetics Wisely

Until the time the public demands tighter controls over cosmetics, your greatest protection is your own knowledge. The cosmetic companies are very sensitive to consumer desires, and both the industry and the FDA will respond to reports of untoward effects from a cosmetic. But they can't do so if no one tells them about it.

The purpose of this dictionary is to enable you to look up any cosmetic ingredient under its alphabetical listing to determine if a product is safe or not. You can thereby choose among products on the basis of what is in them and whether or not they do what the advertising claims they do, and at the same time avoid any unnecessary injury to your health. The dictionary includes most of the cosmetic ingredients in common use, a large percentage of which have been kept secret including many of the so-called trade secret ingredients. If a cosmetic company, however, declares an ingredient a trade secret, it does not have to be listed on the label but the list must end with "and other ingredients."

The CTFA won an agreement with the Senate and the Administration which provides the industry with national labeling. The cosmetic companies argued that national uniform labeling is not only good for the cosmetics industry, it is good for the consumer.

For the sake of clarity and ease of use, their many functions are grouped under the following broad categories:

Preservatives

A preservative used in cosmetics is required to offer protection against infection under conditions of use and prevent the decomposition of the product due to microbial multiplication. For example, many kinds of yeast, fungi, and bacteria have been identified in cosmetics. Just the presence of water and various organic components, such as lanolin or cocoa butter, provides an excellent environment for the growth of germs. Furthermore, as consumers we are constantly introducing new germs into open jars, bottles, and boxes. In many instances a product may show no evidence of contamination and yet contain germs that, when in contact with the skin or eyes, may cause infection. A cosmetic preservative should be active at a low concentration, against a wide range of microorganisms, and over a wide acidity/alkalinity range. According to cosmetic chemists, it must also be compatible with other ingredients in the formulation, as well as nontoxic, nonirritating, and nonsensitizing. It should also be colorless, odorless, and stable, as well as economically feasible and easily incorporated into the product.

Parabens and quaternary ammonium compounds *(see both)* are widely used today as preservatives. So are the various alcohols, such as ethyl and isopropyl, and so are the phenols such as *p*-chloro-*m*-cresol. Essential oils, such as citrus and menthol, have been used for hundreds of years as preservatives.

An additional use for preservatives is for fatty products in cosmetic creams and lotions. Such substances are called antioxidants. They prevent the production of off-colors and off-odors. Examples are benzoic acid, BHA, and tocopherols (Vitamin E).

Acids, Alkalies, Buffers, Neutralizers

The degree of acidity or alkalinity (known as the pH) of a product is important in cosmetics because too little or too much of either may irritate the skin. Furthermore, the formulation of a product is dependent upon properly maintaining the intended pH. Citric acid, widely used as the acid, and ammonium carbonate, an alkali, are frequently found in cosmetic formulations. Buffers and neutralizing agents are chemicals added to cosmetic formulas to control acidity or alkalinity in the same way that acids and alkalies might be added directly. Some common chemicals in this class are ammonium bicarbonate, calcium carbonate, and tartaric acid.

Moisture Content Controls

Humectants are necessary to keep many cosmetics from drying out. The contents of an open jar of cream, for instance, may stiffen and crumble without a humectant to keep it soft and pliable. Substances used for this purpose include glycerin and propylene glycol, which keep cleansing lotions and moisturizing creams smooth and spreadable. On the other hand, chemicals may be necessary to keep cosmetics from absorbing moisture from the air and becoming sticky or cakey. Calcium silicate, for instance, is used in powders to prevent moisture absorption.

Coloring Agents

Coloring agents, of course, are extremely important to cosmetics. Without pleasing hues, lipsticks, rouges, and eye makeup would remain on store shelves. Colors of both natural and synthetic origin are extensively employed in cosmetics. However, indiscriminate use of color can cause adverse reactions when used in a cosmetic. For example, coal tar colors are subject to government regulations—although they are exempted from the Cosmetic Act because they were determined to be irreplaceable. Each batch must be certified by the FDA as "harmless and suitable for use."

The World Health Organization, in delineating some 140 different kinds of colorants, found many to be unsafe. Some of the colors originally listed as "harmless" were found to produce injury when fed to animals and were removed from the list. In 1960, the federal government required manufacturers to retest all artificial colors to determine safety.

At present, there are nine colors permanently listed as safe, among them FD & C Blue No. 1 and FD & C Citrus Red No. 2, which have been shown to cause tumors at the site of injection in animals. But the FDA does not consider this significant because the experiment concerned injection by needle and not by ingestion in food or application on the skin. FD & C Red No. 40, one of the most widely used colorings, is also being questioned because it is made from a base known to be carcinogenic and because many scientists feel that it should not have been given permanent listing based solely on the manufacturer's tests.

Almost all cosmetics are colored, but until recently it was frequently impossible for FDA scientists to detect specific colors and quantities employed. Now, with newly developed techniques, FDA scientists are able to analyze finished products and to determine the colors and quantities used.

Among the natural colors widely used in cosmetics are alkanet, annatto, carotene, chlorophyll, cochineal, saffron, and turmeric.

Flavorings

A wide variety of spices, natural extractives, oleoresins, and essential oils are used in cosmetics. In fact, of the 3,000 additives known to be available for use in food, cosmetics, and drugs, 2,000 are flavorings that replace the flavors lost during processing. Of these flavorings, some 500 are natural—that is, they are derived from a wide variety of spices, plant extracts, and essential oils. The balance are synthetics such as amyl acetate, benzaldehyde, and ethyl acetate. Cosmetic products in which flavorings are important include lipsticks, dentifrices, and mouthwashes. Flavorings are employed in amounts ranging from a few parts to 300 parts per million.

Fragrances

In the entire cosmetic industry perhaps the greatest number of creative people are employed in the production of fragrances. It is an ancient art, and the formulas are closely guarded. Even the federal labeling regulations recognize this and require that only the words "perfume" or "fragrance" be added to the label. There may be more than 200 ingredients in a scent. Pleasant aromas are derived from a spectacular number of substances, including plant materials and synthetic chemicals. Perfumers can even improve on nature. Certain natural flower scents, for instance, cannot be extracted, yet the experts, using various chemicals, can reproduce the same aroma we smell from the actual blossom. Because of the complexity of perfume formulas, it is difficult but possible for competitors to break them down and reproduce them.

Since fragrances are intended to vaporize, and they do contain plant and floral derivatives as well as many other chemicals, they frequently cause allergic reactions. A less-frequent side effect of perfume is a skin pigmentation called berloque dermatitis *(see)*. With new awareness that chemicals can be delivered to the body not only through ingestion and absorption through the skin but also by inhalation of scent, federal and industrial scientists are concerned that some of the volatile ingredients in cosmetics may have an adverse systemic effect. In fact, the fixative AETT was voluntarily removed after it was shown to be a nerve toxin in animals. At this writing, there is also concern about another fixative, musk ambrette.

Processing Aids

Many cosmetics fall into this category. One of the largest include surfactants *(see)*, compounds that reduce the friction between two surfaces. A large subdivision of surface-active agents consists of emulsifiers and emulsion stabilizers. Such ingredients help maintain a mixture and ensure consistency. They also influence smoothness, volume, and uniformity. Sodium lauryl sulfate and alumina gel are examples used in moisture creams. Another division of surfactants includes solubilizers and texturizers. Solubilizers mix oil and water. Sodium sulfonate, for instance, is used to disperse oils in shampoos. Texturizers are added to products to give them a desired feel and appearance. An emulsifier may be a texturizer, but a texturizer is not necessarily an emulsifier. For example, acacia is used in hairdressings to thicken them and also to help them hold unruly hair in place. Clarifying and chelating agents are other processing aids that remove extraneous matter from liquids. Tannin, for instance, is used for removing extraneous matter from liquids. Ethylenediamine tetraacetic acid is used to remove calcium, magnesium, and iron soaps from shampoo solutions. Opacifiers, on the other hand, are added to liquids to darken them. The higher alcohols, such as stearyl and cetyl, are frequently used in shampoos for this purpose. Foaming agents, such as dodecylbenzene sulfonic acid, are added to make shampoos foamy.

Texturizers or stabilizers are added to products to give them "body" and maintain a desired texture. For instance, calcium chloride or some other calcium salt is added to canned tomatoes and canned potatoes to keep them from falling apart. Sodium nitrate and sodium nitrite are used in curing meats to develop and stabilize the pink color. Nitrogen, carbon dioxide, and nitrous oxide are employed in pressure-packed containers of certain foods as whipping agents or as propellants. The texture of ice cream and other frozen desserts is dependent on the size of the ice crystals in the product. By addition of agar-agar, gelatin, cellulose gum, or some other gum, the size of the ice crystals is stabilized. Texturizer gums are also used in chocolate milk to increase the viscosity of the product and to prevent the settling of cocoa particles to the bottom of the container. Gelatin, pectin, and starch are used in confectionary products to give a desired texture. Artificially sweetened beverages also need products to give a desired texture; they also need bodying agents because they do not contain the "thickness" normally contributed by sugar. The thickeners employed include such natural gums as sodium alginate and pectins. The foaming properties of brewed beer can also be improved by the addition of texturizers.

For ease of use, this dictionary lists products alphabetically by general use. For example, you can look up eye shadow, mascara, lipstick, eyebrow pencil, and any appearance-improving product to see what is in it. Or you may be interested in grooming products such as dentifrices, mouthwash, nail polish, perfume, eyewash, after-shave lotion, deodorant, depilatory, hair bleach, and so on. Anyone looking for treatment aids would check under cleansing creams, emollients, astringents, hand creams, permanent waves, hair straighteners, skin bleaches, and any other corrective treatment products. In addition, all terms used in this dictionary that might be unfamiliar are also listed alphabetically, such as polymer, reagent, and so on.

How to Use This Book

While unique in content, this dictionary follows the format of most dictionaries. The following are examples of entries with any explanatory notes that may be necessary:

ABIETIC ACID • Sylvic Acid. Chiefly a texturizer in the making of soaps. A widely available natural acid, water-insoluble, prepared from pine rosin, usually yellow and composed of either glassy or crystalline particles. Used also in the manufacture of vinyls, lacquers, and plastics. Little is known about abietic acid toxicity; it is harmless when injected into mice but causes paralysis in frogs and is slightly irritating to human skin and mucous membranes. May cause allergic reactions.

We have learned that abietic acid is also known as sylvic acid, that it is a naturally occurring rosin acid, which as a texturizer maintains a consistency in soaps, and we discovered its noncosmetic uses and its known toxicity. Source material for the comments on toxicity is indicated in the notes at the end of the dictionary.

ALLANTOIN • Used in cold creams, hand lotions, hair lotions, after-shave lotions, and other skin-soothing cosmetics because of its ability to help heal wounds and skin ulcers and to stimulate the growth of healthy tissue. Composed of colorless crystals, soluble in hot water, it is prepared synthetically by the oxidation of uric acid *(see)* or by heating uric acid with dichloroacetic acid. It is nontoxic.

Allantoin, we can see, is a synthetic product derived from uric acid. By looking up uric acid, we learn that it derives from urine and is used as a sunburn preventative.

What to Do if You Have an Adverse Response to a Cosmetic

- Before using any cosmetic, read the label carefully and follow directions exactly. This is especially important when using antiperspirants, depilatories, hair dyes and colorings, home permanents, freckle creams, and skin packs.

- To determine whether you are allergic to a cosmetic, apply a small amount on the inside of your forearm. Leave it on for 24 hours. If you see any adverse effects, such as redness, blisters, or itching, don't use it again.

- If a cosmetic causes any adverse effect—burning, breaking out, stinging, or itching—stop using it. If you are not sure whether it was a cosmetic that gave you your problem or which of several cosmetics affected you adversely, stop the use of all cosmetics. Shampoo your hair with a bland soap to remove all hair preparations. Stop the use of all creams, including cleansing creams, foundation creams, and cold creams. Wash your face with unscented soap. Remove all nail polish.

- If the condition does not clear up or is very uncomfortable, bring the offending or suspected cosmetic to your physician for testing. This includes cosmetic sponges and powder puffs used to apply cosmetics.

- If you recently visited a beauty parlor and had an adverse reaction, return to the shop and obtain the name of the brands used and samples of them.

- If the lips are not involved, the use of lipstick may be continued.

- The cosmetic responsible for your problem may be a relatively new one or it may be one that you have used for years. The fact that all cosmetics have been applied for a long time does not rule out an adverse reaction from any one of them. The development of allergic hypersensitivity may occur at any time. Also, some ingredients in the product may have been changed by the manufacturer.

- Do not let children play with cosmetics. As you will read in this dictionary, some ingredients are toxic, and although others might not hurt an adult, they might harm children.

- Be especially careful in the use of eye cosmetics to avoid possible chemical and mechanical damage to the eyes. Refrain from applying eyeliner to the inner edge of the lid or around the lash line on the lower lid where it can clog tiny oil glands and cause infection. Avoid frosted, pearlized, iridescent, or other glittery types of eye shadow. Ground oyster shells or tinsel used in these products can be harmful if a particle finds its way into the eye, especially if you wear contact lenses. Also consider foregoing "lash-building" and "guaranteed waterproof" products, since many contain nylon and rayon fibers as lash lengtheners. Such fibers can dry, flake off, and fall into the eye.

- Never drive and apply makeup. Not only does it make for dangerous driving, but hitting a bump in the road and scratching your eyeball can cause bacteria to contaminate the cut and could result in serious injury, including blindness.

- Never share makeup. Always use a new disposable applicator when sampling products at a cosmetics counter.

- Never add liquid to a product to bring it back to its original consistency. That includes water and saliva. Adding liquids could introduce bacteria that can easily grow out of control.

- Throw away makeup if the color changes or an odor develops. Preservatives degrade over time and may no longer be able to fight bacteria.

- Do not use eye makeup if you have an eye infection. Throw away all products you were using when you discovered the infection.

- Keep makeup out of sunlight. Light and heat can degrade preservatives.

- Keep makeup containers tightly closed when not in use.

- Never use aerosol beauty products near heat or while smoking because they can ignite. Hairsprays and powder may cause lung damage if inhaled regularly.

- Report any adverse effects from cosmetics to the manufacturer of the product, to the FDA, and to the store where you purchased them. Look up the local Food and Drug Administration office under "United States" in your telephone directory. If you cannot find a local office, write directly to the Food and Drug Administration, Center for Food Safety and Applied Nutrition, Office of Colors and Cosmetics, 200 C Street SW, Washington, DC 20204. You can also call the FDA Cosmetics and Colors Automated Information Line 1-800-270-8869, for information on how to report adverse reactions to cosmetics, as well as problems such as filth, decomposition, or spoilage.

Terminology generally has been kept to a middle road between what is understandable to the technician and to the average interested consumer, while at the same time avoiding oversimplification of data. Once again, if in doubt, look up alphabetically any term listed that seems unfamiliar or whose meaning has been blunted by overuse, such as *isolate, extract, demulcent, emollient,* or even *shampoo.*

The Generally Recognized As Safe List (GRAS) was established in 1958 by Congress. Those substances that were being added to food over a long time, which under conditions of their intended used were generally recognized as safe by qualified scientists, would be exempt from premarket clearance. When a cosmetic ingredient is also a food additive that is listed as GRAS, the designation has been noted by the author even though no premarket clearance is required for cosmetic ingredients.

With *A Consumer's Dictionary of Cosmetic Ingredients,* you will be able to work with current and future labels to determine the purpose and desirability or toxicity of the ingredients listed. For the first time, you will have the knowledge to choose the best cosmetics for you. By checking on a product's ingredients, as listed on the label, you can eliminate many products and choose those that are harmless, even beneficial, and you save money and reward those manufacturers who deserve your purchases. For the first time, with the aid of this book, you will really know what is in the cosmetics you have been using.

A

ABIES • *Alba, Balsamea, Pectinata. Sibirica.* Essential oils derived from a variety of pine trees. They are used as natural flavoring ingredients and to scent bath products. Ingestion of large amounts can cause intestinal hemorrhages.

ABIETIC ACID • **Sylvic Acid.** Chiefly a texturizer in the making of soaps. A widely available natural acid, water-insoluble, prepared from pine rosin, usually yellow and composed of either glassy or crystalline particles. Used also in the manufacture of vinyls, lacquers, and plastics. Little is known about abietic acid toxicity; it is harmless when injected into mice but causes paralysis in frogs and is slightly irritating to human skin and mucous membranes. May cause allergic reactions.

ABIETYL ALCOHOL • See Abietic Acid.

ABITOL • **Dihydroabietyl Alcohol.** Used in cosmetics, plastics, and adhesive. See Abietic Acid.

ABRADE • Scrape or erode a covering, such as skin.

ABSOLUTE • The term refers to a plant-extracted material that has been concentrated but that remains essentially unchanged in its original taste and odor. For example, see Jasmine Absolute. Often called "natural perfume materials" because they are not subjected to heat and water as are distilled products. See Distilled.

ABSORPTION BASES • Compounds used to improve the water-absorbing capacity and stability of creams, lotions, and hairdressings. Lanolin-type absorption bases are mixtures of lanolin alcohols, mineral oil, and petrolatum *(see all)*. Also used as bases are cholesterol and beeswax *(see both)*.

ACACIA • **Gum Arabic. Catechu.** Acacia is the odorless, colorless, tasteless dried exudate from the stem of the acacia tree, grown in Africa, the Near East, India, and the southern United States. Its most distinguishing quality among the natural gums is its ability to dissolve rapidly in water. The use of acacia dates back 4,000 years, when the Egyptians employed it in paints. Its principal use in the confectionery industry is to retard sugar crystallization and as a thickener for candies, jellies, glazes, and chewing gum. As a stabilizer, it prevents chemical breakdown in food mixtures. Gum acacia is a foam stabilizer in the soft drink and brewing industries. Other uses are for mucilage and to give form and shape to tablets. Medically, it is used as a demulcent to soothe irritations, particularly of the mucous membranes. It can cause allergic reactions such as skin rash and asthmatic attacks. Oral toxicity is low, but the FDA issued a notice in 1992 that catechu tincture had not been shown to be safe and effective as claimed in OTC digestive aid products. See also Vegetable Gums and Catechu Black.

ACANTHOPANAX SENTICOSUS • A plant material derived from *Acanthopanax senticosus.* See Ginseng.

ACEFYLLINE METHYLSILANOL MANNURONATE • Used as a skin conditioning ingredient. Prepared from theophylline, an alkaloid *(see)* with caffeine found in tea leaves. Theophylline, however, is usually prepared synthetically. In medicines, it acts as a smooth-muscle relaxant, diuretic, heart stimulant, and vasodilator.

ACER • *Pseudoplantinus. Saccharinum.* Mountain Maple. It acts similarly to tannin *(see).*

ACEROLA • Used as an antioxidant. Derived from the ripe fruit of the West Indian or Barbados cherry, grown in Central America and the West Indies. A rich source of ascorbic acid. Used in Vitamin C. No known toxicity.

ACETAL • A volatile liquid derived from acetaldehyde *(see)* and alcohol and used as a solvent in synthetic perfumes such as jasmine. Also used in fruit flavorings (it has a nutlike aftertaste) and as a hypnotic in medicine. It is a central nervous system depressant, similar in action to paraldehyde but more toxic. Paraldehyde is a hypnotic and sedative whose side effects are respiratory depression, cardiovascular collapse, and possible high blood pressure reactions. No known skin toxicity.

ACETALDEHYDE • **Ethanal.** An intermediate *(see)* and solvent in the manufacture of perfumes. A flammable, colorless liquid with a characteristic odor, occurring naturally in apples, broccoli, cheese, coffee, grapefruit, and other vegetables and fruits. Also used in the manufacture of synthetic rubber and in the silvering of mirrors. It is irritating to the mucous membranes, and ingestion of large doses may cause death by respiratory paralysis. Inhalation, usually limited by intense irritation of the lungs, can also be toxic. Skin toxicity not identified.

ACETAMIDE MEA • **N-Acetyl Acid Amide. N-Acetyl Ethanolamine.** Used as a solvent, plasticizer, and stabilizer *(see all).* Used in hair conditioners and skin creams. Crystals absorb water. Odorless when pure but can have a mousy scent. A mild skin irritant with low toxicity. Has caused liver cancer when given orally to rats in doses of 5,000 milligrams per kilogram of body weight. The CIR Expert Panel *(see)* found that it is safe at concentrations not to exceed 7.5 percent. They found that it may form nitrosamines *(see).*

ACETAMIDOETHOXYBUTYL TRIMONIUM CHLORIDE • See Quaternary Ammonium Compounds.

ACETAMINOPHEN • A coal tar derivative, it is widely used as a pain reliever and fever reducer. It is used as an antioxidant and stabilizer in cosmetics.

ACETAMINOPROPYL TRIMONIUM CHLORIDE • See Quaternary Ammonium Compounds.

ACETAMINOSALOL • Derived from ammonia and salicylic acid *(see both),* it absorbs ultraviolet light.

ACETANILID • **Acetanilide.** A solvent used in nail polishes and in liquid powders to give an opaque matte finish. Usually made from aniline and acetic acid *(see both),* it is of historic interest because it was the first coal tar analgesic and antifever ingredient introduced into medicine. It is a precursor of penicillin and is used as an antiseptic. It is sometimes still used in medicines but is frowned upon by the American Medical Association since there are other related products with less toxicity. It can cause a depletion of oxygen in the blood upon ingestion and eczema when applied to the skin. It caused tumors when given orally to rats in doses of 3,500 milligrams per kilogram of body weight.

ACETARSOL • **Acetarsone.** Used in mouthwashes, toothpaste, and vaginal suppositories. Thick white crystals with a slight acid taste. Soluble in water. The lethal dose in mice is only 4 milligrams per kilogram of body weight. May cause sensitization.

ACETATE • Salt of acetic acid *(see)* used in perfumery and as a flavoring. No known toxicity.

ACETIC ACID • Solvent for gums, resins, and volatile oils. Styptic (stops bleeding) and a rubefacient *(see)*. A clear colorless liquid with a pungent odor, it is used in freckle-bleaching lotions, hand lotions, and hair dyes. It occurs naturally in apples, cheese, cocoa, coffee, grapes, skimmed milk, oranges, peaches, pineapples, strawberries, and a variety of other fruits and plants. Vinegar is about 4 to 6 percent acetic acid, and essence of vinegar is about 14 percent. In its glacial form (without much water) it is highly corrosive, and its vapors are capable of producing lung obstruction. Less than 5 percent acetic acid in solution is mildly irritating to the skin. GRAS for packaging only, not for direct ingredient in product. It caused cancer in rats and mice when given orally or by injection.

ACETIC ANHYDRIDE • **Acetyl Oxide. Acetic Oxide.** Colorless liquid with a strong odor, it is derived from oxidation of acetaldehyde *(see)*. It is used as a dehydrating and acetylating ingredient (*see both* Dehyrated and Acetylated) and in the production of dyes, perfumes, plastics, food starch, and aspirin. It is a strong irritant and may cause burns and eye damage.

ACETOIN • **Acetyl Methyl Carbinol.** A flavoring ingredient and aroma carrier used in perfumery, it occurs naturally in broccoli, grapes, pears, cultured dairy products, cooked beef, and cooked chicken. As a product of fermentation and of cream ripened for churning, it is a colorless, or pale yellow, liquid or a white powder. It has a buttery odor and must be stored in a light-resistant container. No known toxicity.

ACETOLAMIDE • **n-Acetyl Ethanolamine.** Used in hair-waving solutions and in emulsifiers. See Ethanolamines.

ACETONE • A colorless, ethereal liquid derived by oxidation or fermentation and used as a solvent in nail polish removers and nail finishes. It is obtained by fermentation and is frequently used as a solvent for airplane glue, fats, oils, and waxes. It can cause peeling and splitting of the nails, skin rashes on the fingers and elsewhere, and nail brittleness. Inhalation may irritate the lungs, and in large amounts it is narcotic, causing symptoms of drunkenness similar to ethanol *(see)*. In 1992, the FDA proposed a ban on acetone in astringent *(see)* products because it had not been shown to be safe and effective as claimed.

ACETONITRILE • **Methylacyanide.** Colorless liquid with a pleasant odor. Used as a solvent in extraction processes and for separation of fatty acids from vegetable oils. Also used in nail-glue remover. Toxic by skin absorption and inhalation. It is a precursor of cyanide and is extremely hazardous if swallowed, but lab tests may mistake it for alcohol. See also Artificial Nail Remover.

ACETOPHENONE • A synthetic ingredient derived from coal tar, with an odor of bitter almonds, used in strawberry, floral, fruit, cherry, almond, walnut, tobacco, vanilla, and tonka bean flavorings for beverages, ice creams, ices, candy, baked goods, gelatin desserts, and chewing gum. It occurs naturally in strawberries and tea, and may cause allergic reactions.

1-ACETOXY-2-METHYLNAPHTHALENE • A hair coloring. See Naphthalene.

ACETUM • See Vinegar.

ACETYL ACETONE • See Pentane.

ACETYL BENZOYL PEROXIDE • Benzo-benzone. White crystals that decompose slowly. It is an active germicide and disinfectant, and is used for bleaching flour. It is toxic by ingestion, a strong irritant to the skin and mucous membranes.

ACETYL GLUCOSAMINE • Used as a skin conditioning ingredient in cosmetics, glucosamine is found in chitin *(see)*, cell membranes, and protein and sugar complexes in the blood. It has become popular as an antiosteoarthritis medication.

ACETYL GLUTAMIC ACID • Used in skin conditioners. See Glutamic Acid and Acetylated.

ACETYL GLUTAMINE • Used in skin conditioners. See Glutamic Acid and Acetylated.

ACETYL GLYCERYL RICINOLEATE • Used in skin conditioners. See Castor Oil.

ACETYL HEXAMETHYL INDAN • A fragrance ingredient. Derived from coal tar, it may be irritating to the skin and eyes.

ACETYL HEXAMETHYL TETRALIN • Used in perfumes. It is closely related to acetyl ethyl tetramethyl tetralin, which was voluntarily removed from perfumes when it was reported that it caused nerve damage in animals. The "hexyl" component was inserted to make the fragrances less volatile and less allergenic.

ACETYL MANDELIC ACID • A pH *(see)* adjuster, see Carboxylic Acid.

ACETYL METHIONINE • Methenamine. Crystals formed from ethyl acetate. Used to process fat in the manufacture of cosmetics.

ACETYL PROPIONYL • Yellow liquid. Soluble in water. Used as a butterscotch or chocolate-type flavoring. See Propionic Acid.

ACETYL TRIBUTYL CITRATE • See Citric Acid.

ACETYL TRIETHYL CITRATE • A clear, oily, essentially odorless liquid used as a solvent. See Citric Acid.

ACETYL TRIOCTYL CITRATE • Salt of citric acid. See Citric Acid.

ACETYL TRIOCTYL CITRATE PECTIN • Citrus Pectin. A jelly-forming powder obtained from citrus peel and used as a texturizer and thickening ingredient to form gels with sugars and acids. Light in color. It has no known toxicity.

ACETYL TYROSINE • Used in suntan gels, creams, and liquids. Widely distributed amino acid *(see),* termed nonessential because it does not *seem* to be necessary for growth. It is used as a dietary supplement. It is a building block of protein and is used in cosmetics to help creams penetrate the skin. The FDA has asked for further study of this additive that is GRAS. See Acetylated.

ACETYL VALERYL • See Valeric Acid and Acetic Acid.

ACETYLATED • Any organic compound that has been heated with acetic anhydride or acetyl chloride to remove its water. Acetylated lanolins are used in hand creams and lotions, for instance. Acetic anhydride produces irritation and necrosis of tissues in the vapor state and carries a warning against contact with skin and eyes.

ACETYLATED CASTOR OIL • See Acetylated and Castor Oil.

ACETYLATED CETYL HYDROXYPROLINATE • Used in skin conditioners, it is derived from ammonia and amino acids *(see both)*.

ACETYLATED GLYCOL STEARATE • See Acetylated and Glycols.

ACETYLATED HYDROGENATED COTTONSEED GLYCERIDE • See Cottonseed Oil.

ACETYLATED HYDROGENATED LANOLIN • See Lanolin and Hydrogenation.

ACETYLATED HYDROGENATED LARD GLYCERIDE • See Lard.

ACETYLATED HYDROGENATED TALLOW GLYCERIDES • See Tallow and Hydrogenation.

ACETYLATED HYDROGENATED VEGETABLE GLYCERIDE • See Vegetable Oils.

ACETYLATED LANOLIN • An emulsifier and emollient. Repels water better than plain lanolin and does not form emulsions. It is used as a water-resistant film when applied to the skin and reduces water loss through the skin. It is used as an emollient and gives that "velvety feel" to baby products and to skin, hair, and bath preparations such as creams, lotions, powders, and sprays. The CIR Expert Panel *(see)* found it safe. See Lanolin.

ACETYLATED LANOLIN ALCOHOL • The CIR Expert Panel *(see)* found it safe. See Acetylated Lanolin.

ACETYLATED PALM-KERNEL GLYCERIDES • See Acetylated and Palm-Kernel Oil.

ACETYLATED TALLOW • See Acetylated and Tallow.

ACETYLCHOLINE • A chemical neurotransmitter that is released by nerve cells and stimulates either other nerve cells or muscles and organs throughout the body. This neurotransmitter is believed to be involved in memory function. Acetylcholine also dilates the blood vessels and helps to move food through the intestines. In a chloride solution for the eye, it causes contraction of the iris, resulting in contraction of the pupil. Used after eye surgery. No adverse reactions reported for a 1 percent solution.

ACETYLCYSTEINE • Used in skin products as an antioxidant and conditioner. In medicines, it is used to relieve mucous congestion of the nose, sinuses, and airways. Because it alters the action of mucus in the stomach, acetylcysteine has been found to cause digestive problems, especially in people with peptic ulcers.

ACETYLISOEUGENOL • **Isoeugenol acetate.** White crystals with a spicy, clovelike odor, it is used in perfumery, especially for carnation-type odors and for flavoring.

ACETYLMETHIONYL METHYLSILANOL ELASTINATE • An ester of methionine and elastin *(see)*.

ACETYLMETHYLCARBINOL • See Acetoin.

ACETYL-P-AMINOPHENOL • See Phenyl Acetaldehyde.

ACETYLSALICYLIC ACID • See Aspirin.

ACHILLEA MILLEFOLIUM • See Yarrow.

ACID • An acid is a substance capable of turning blue litmus paper red and of forming hydrogen ions when dissolved in water. An acid aqueous solution is one that has a pH *(see)* of less than 7. Citric acid *(see)* is an example of an acid widely used in cosmetics.

ACID AMMONIUM SULFATE • See Quaternary Ammonium Compounds.

ACID BLACK 1 • A diazo dye *(see)*.

ACID BLACK 52 • A monoazo color *(see)*.

ACID BLACK 131 • **Nigrosine.** It is a greenish blue-black. Acid colors are made by adding acids such as adipic *(see)* and tartaric to obtain various shades. Toxicity depends upon ingredients used. See Colors and Acid Dyes.

ACID BLUE 1 • A triphenylmethane color *(see)*.

ACID BLUE 3 • A triphenylmethane color *(see)*.

ACID BLUE 9 • A triphenylmethane color *(see)*.

ACID BLUE 9 ALUMINUM LAKE • See Triphenylmethane Group and Lakes.

ACID BLUE 9 AMMONIUM SALT • A color classed chemically as a triphenylmethane *(see)*. The CTFA adopted name for certified *(see)* batches of this color is FD & C Blue No. 1 *(see)*.

ACID BLUE 62 • Classed chemically as an anthraquinone color *(see)*.

ACID BLUE 74 • An indigoid color.

ACID BLUE 74 ALUMINUM LAKE • See Indigo and Lakes.

ACID BROWN 13 • A coal tar hair coloring. Classed as a nitro coloring.

ACID DYES • The ability of these dyes to color and to remain fast during washing and exposure to light varies greatly. The ones that give the best water and light fastness are the compounds that are combined with metals. They are widely used in inexpensive dyes for plastics, varnishes, and some pigments.

ACID FUCHSIN • See Azo Dyes.

ACID GREEN 1 • A nitro *(see)* color.

ACID GREEN 25 • Classed chemically as an anthraquinone *(see)* color, the name can be applied only to batches of uncertified colors. The CTFA adopted name for certified *(see)* batches of this dye is D & C Green No. 5 *(see)*.

ACID GREEN 50 • A triphenylmethane color. See Triphenylmethane Group and Acid Dyes.

ACID ORANGE 3 • A nitro *(see)* color. A hair dye ingredient, it is mutagenic. Oral cancer-causing studies in rats and mice did yield clear evidence of carcinogenic activity in female (but not in male) rats and in female mice. The results of a skin cancer study in mice exposed to hair dye formulations containing 0.2 percent Acid Orange 3 were negative. The CIR Expert Panel concluded that irritation and sensitization data on Acid Orange 3 are absent. Since the label requirements set by the FDA, however, advise patch-testing instruction, individuals who might have an irritation/sensitization reaction would be able to avoid significant exposure. On the basis of the animal and clinical data, the CIR Expert Panel concluded that Acid Orange 3 "is safe for use in hair dye formulations at concentrations less than 0.2 percent." See also Acid Dyes.

ACID ORANGE 6 • A monoazo color *(see)*. See also Acid Dyes.

ACID ORANGE 7 • A color classed as a monoazo *(see)*. The name can be used only when applied to uncertified batches of this dye. The CTFA adopted name for certified *(see)* batches is D & C Orange No. 4 *(see)*.

ACID ORANGE 24 • A diazo dye *(see)*, the name can be applied only to uncertified batches of this color. The CTFA *(see* Introduction*)* adopted name for certified batches is D & C Brown No. 1 *(see)*.

ACID RED 14 • A monoazo color *(see)*.

ACID RED 18 • A coal tar hair coloring, it is classed as a monoazo color *(see)*.

ACID RED 18 ALUMINUM LAKE • See Acid Red 18 and Lakes.

ACID RED 27 • A monoazo color *(see)*. The name can be used only when applied to batches of color that have not been certified *(see)*. Use of this color certified as FD & C Red No. 2 is prohibited in cosmetic products in the United States. Its use as a cosmetic colorant may also be restricted in other countries.

ACID RED 33 • A monoazo color *(see)*, the name can be applied only to uncertified batches. The CTFA adopted name for certified *(see)* batches is D & C Red No. 33 *(see)*.

ACID RED 35 • A monoazo color *(see)*, it is the disodium salt of napthalenedisulfonic acid. It is very soluble. Determined by NIOSH to be a positive animal carcinogen.

ACID RED 51 • A xanthene color *(see)*, the name can be applied only to uncertified batches of color. The CTFA adopted name for certified *(see)* batches is FD & C Red No. 3 *(see)*. This name can be used only when applied to batches of colors that have not been certified *(see)*. Use of this color certified as FD & C Red No. 3 is prohibited in the United States. Its use as a cosmetic colorant may also be restricted in other countries.

ACID RED 52 • A xanthene color *(see)*.

ACID RED 73 • A diazo dye *(see)*.

ACID RED 87 • A xanthene color *(see)*, it is the sodium salt of Solvent Red 43. The name can be used only when applied to uncertified batches of this dye. The CTFA adopted name for certified *(see)* batches is D & C Red No. 22 *(see)*.

ACID RED 92 • A xanthene color *(see)*, it is the sodium salt of Solvent Red 48. The name can be applied only to uncertified batches of this dye. The CTFA adopted name for certified *(see)* batches of color is FD & C Red No. 28 *(see)*.

ACID RED 95 • A xanthene color *(see)*, it is the sodium salt of Solvent Red 73. The name can be applied only to uncertified batches of this dye. The CTFA adopted name for certified *(see)* batches is D & C Orange No. 11 *(see)*.

ACID RED 184 • A coal tar hair coloring classed as a monoazo color *(see)*.

ACID RED 195 • A coal tar hair coloring classed as a monoazo color *(see)*.

ACID VIOLET 9 • A coal tar dye used in hair coloring, it is classed as a xanthene color *(see)*.

ACID VIOLET 43 • An anthraquinone color *(see)*, the name can be applied only to uncertified batches of this dye. The CTFA adopted name for the certified *(see)* batches of this color is Ext. D & C Violet No. 2 *(see)*.

ACID YELLOW 1 • A nitro color, the name can be applied only to uncertified batches of this dye. The CTFA adopted name for the certified *(see)* batches of this color is Ext. D & C Yellow No. 7 *(see)*.

ACID YELLOW 3 • A mixture of the disodium salts of the mono- and disulfonic acids of indanedione, a class of indirect-acting anticoagulants. The name can be applied only to uncertified batches of this dye. The CTFA adopted name for the certified *(see)* batches of this color is D & C Yellow No. 10 *(see)*.

ACID YELLOW 23 • A pyrazole color *(see)*, the name can be applied only to uncertified batches of this dye. The CTFA adopted name for the certified *(see)* batches of this color is FD & C Yellow No. 5.

ACID YELLOW 23 ALUMINUM LAKE • A coal tar color used in hair dye. See Acid Yellow 23 and Lakes.

ACID YELLOW 73 • Classified as a coal tar dye, the name can be applied only to uncertified batches of this dye. The CTFA adopted name for the certified *(see)* batches of this color is D & C Yellow No. 7 *(see)*.

ACID YELLOW 73 SODIUM SALT • A fluoran color, the name can be applied only to uncertified batches of this dye. The CTFA adopted name for the certified *(see)* batches of this color is D & C Yellow No. 8 *(see)*.

ACID YELLOW 104 ALUMINUM LAKE • An insoluble salt of Sunset Yellow. The name may be used only when applied to batches of uncertified colorants. The CTFA name for certified batches is FD & C Yellow No. 6 *(see)*.

ACIDOPHILUS • **Lactobacillus Acidophilus.** A type of bacteria that ferments milk and is used to treat intestinal disorders. It changes the intestinal flora. Yogurt containing live cultures of these bacteria reportedly decreases by a third the number of vaginal yeast infections in women. Acidophilus is used in emollients in cosmetics; it is also widely used to prevent and to relieve diarrhea, especially when taking antibiotics. See also Yogurt.

ACIDOPHILUS/GRAPE FERMENT • Obtained by the fermentation of grapes by acidophilus *(see)*. Used in antiaging skin creams. See Acidophilus and Grape Extract.

ACINTOL • See Tall Oil.

ACNE • Skin pores become plugged with an oily substance, sebum, and other materials such as pigment, dead cells, and bacteria. If the plug (comedo) remains just beneath the surface, it appears as a very small, round, whitish bump, a "whitehead." If it reaches the skin surface, it looks like a black dot, a "blackhead." In some cases, the plugged pore may burst, thereby releasing its oily contents into the surrounding tissue and causing inflammation. This results in the formation of pimples, pus-filled lesions, or even cysts, cavities containing a sticky fluid. When a makeup product claims that it does not cause comedos, it means it has not been found to plug pores and cause acne.

ACOPHYLLUM NODOSUM • Brown algae. Used in skin conditioners. See Algae.

ACORNS • Akarn. The name means "fruit of the forest trees," and it is the nut of the oak. Acorns are used in teas and in food as a nutrient and to soothe skin. They contain tannins, flavonoids, sugar, starch, albumen, and fats. They were used by American Indians to treat diarrhea and as a food staple.

ACORUS CALAMUS • Sweet Flag. Sweet Sedge. Derived from the herb *Acorus calamus*. The rhizome contains essential oil, mucilage, glycosides, amino acid, and tannins. The oil is obtained by steam distillation of the stem or root and is used as a flavoring ingredient and in perfumery. Calamus root is an ancient Indian and Chinese herbal medicine used to treat acid stomach, irregular heart rhythm, low blood pressure, coughs, and lack of mental focus. Native Americans would chew the root to enable them to run long distances with increased stamina. Externally, it was used to induce a state of tranquility. Banned as a food additive by the FDA.

ACRYL GLUTAMATE • A surfactant. See Glutamate.

ACRYLAMIDE • Colorless, odorless crystals soluble in water and derived from acrylonitrile and sulfuric acid. It is used in the manufacture of dyes and adhesives, and in permanent-press fabrics, nail enamels, and face masks. It is toxic by skin absorption.

ACRYLAMIDE COPOLYMER • A film-former and thickener. See Acrylamide.

ACRYLAMIDE/SODIUM ACRYLATE • A polymer of acrylamide and sodium acrylate monomers. See Acrylamide and Acrylates.

ACRYLAMIDES/DMAPA ACRYLATES/METHOXY PEG METHACRYLATE COPOLYMER • A film-former used in hair fixatives. See Acrylamide and Acrylates.

ACRYLAMIDOPROPYLTRIMONIUM CHLORIDE/ACRYLAMIDE CO-POLYMER • An antistatic ingredient and film used in hair products. See Acrylamide.

ACRYLATES • Salts or esters of acrylic acid used as thickening ingredients and as constituents of nail polishes. Strong irritants. See Acrylic Monomer.

ACRYLATES/ACETOACETOXYETHYL METHACRYLATE COPOLYMER • A film-former and hair fixative. Also used to thicken liquids. See Acrylates.

ACRYLATES/ACRYLAMIDE COPOLYMER • Provides a continuous film for nail enamels or to control film formation in hairsprays. See Acrylates.

ACRYLATES/AMMONIUM METHACRYLATE COPOLYMER • See Acrylates and Ammonium.

ACRYLATES COPOLYMER • Synthetic polymers *(see)* made up of acrylic acid, methacrylic acid or one of their esters *(see)*. Used as a binder, film-former, hair fixative, and suspending ingredient. Widely used in cosmetics in such products as nail polish, blushers, base coats and undercoats, mascara, eye shadows, powders, makeup preparations, deodorants, cleansing products, and hairsprays. See Acrylates.

ACRYLATES/C10-30 ALKYL ACRYLATE CROSSPOLYMER • Synthetic polymers *(see)* used in sunless tanning products. See Alkyl and Acrylates.

ACRYLATES/DIACETONEACRYLAMIDE COPOLYMER • A film-former. See Acrylates Copolymer.

ACRYLATES/OCTYLACRYLAMIDE COPOLYERM • A film-former. See Acrylates Copolymer.

ACRYLATES/STEARETH-50 ACRYLATE COPOLYMER • A thickening ingredient. See Acrylates Copolymer.

ACRYLATES/VA COPOLYMER • A film-former made from acrylates *(see)* and vinyl acetate *(see)*.

ACRYLIC MONOMER • A tough rubbery material first used in fake nails in the cosmetic industry. It was once used to fill teeth. Fake nails usually consist of acrylates, a catalyst such as peroxide, and a plasticizer *(see all)*. To be effective, the compound must be stiff at room temperature. If inhaled, the acrylates can cause allergic reactions in humans. Lethal to rats when inhaled. Can penetrate rubber gloves. May contain hydroquinone benzoyl peroxide and tertiary amines *(see both)*.

ACRYLIC RESINS • Polymers *(see)* of acrylics. Used in waxy oils, base coats, protective coatings, and waterproofing. If inhaled, acrylates *(see)* can cause allergic reactions in humans.

ACRYLINOLEIC ACID • See Cyclocarboxypropyloleic Acid.

ACTINIC DAMAGE • Skin damage caused by the sun.

ACTINIC KERATOSES • AK. Roughness and thickening of the skin caused by overexposure to the sun's ultraviolet rays. Actinic keratoses, also called solar keratoses, age spots, or liver spots, are scaly lesions that are often brown in color. They are caused by exposure to the sun. The lesions usually begin to appear in middle age and may increase in number as individuals grow older. Although sometimes referred to as precancerous lesions, the actual incidence of squamous cell carcinoma in preexisting actinic keratoses is about one in 1,000 annually per individual. The primary concern of patients seeking treatment for actinic keratoses is more often cosmetic than medical.

ACTINIDIA CHINENSIS • Derived from *Acinidia Chinensis,* the Kiwi plant. See Kiwi Extract.

ADANSONIA DIGITATA • Derived from *Adansonia digitata,* cream of tartar tree. The oil is used in skin conditioners. The powder is used as a thickening ingredient.

ADENINE • **Vitamin B4.** Derived from tea or yeast. Used in skin conditioners.

ADENOSINE • White, crystalline powder with mild saline or bitter taste. It is isolated by the hydrolysis of yeast nucleic acid.

ADENOSINE PHOSPHATE • See Adenosine Triphosphate.

ADENOSINE TRIPHOSPHATE • **Adenylic Acid.** An organic compound that is derived from adenosine *(see)*. A fundamental unit of nucleic acid, it serves as a source of energy for biochemical transformation in plants, photosynthesis, and also for many chemical reactions in the body, especially those associated with muscular activity. Used in skin conditioners.

ADEPS BOVIS • Fat from cows. Cannot be used on American labels but is used in European cosmetic labels. United States lists the ingredient as Tallow.

ADEPS SUILLUS • Fat from swine. Cannot be used on American labels but is used on European labels. United States lists the ingredient as Lard.

ADIANTUM CAPILLUS VENERIS • Derived from *Adiantum capillus veneris*. See Maiden Hair Fern Extract.

ADIPIC ACID • **Hexanedoic Acid.** Colorless, needlelike formations, fairly insoluble in water; found in beets. A buffering and neutralizing ingredient impervious to humidity. Used in hair color rinses, nylon manufacture, and plasticizers. Lethal to rats in large oral doses. No known human toxicity.

ADIPIC ACID DIHYDRAZIDE • The CIR Expert Panel *(see)* concludes the available data are insufficient to support the safety of this ingredient as used in cosmetic products. See Adipic Acid.

ADIPIC ACID/EPOXYPROPYL DIETHYLENETRIAMINE COPOLYMER • A "bodying" ingredient and film-former that combines chemically with the amino acid cysteine to give "body" to hair. Shampooing removes it.

ADIPIC ACID/NEOPENTYL GLYCOL/TRIMELLITIC ANHYDRIDE CO-POLYMER • A film-former. See Adipic Acid.

ADONIS VERNALIS • **False Helebore. Bird's Eye.** Found in the lime-rich soil of Eastern and Southern Europe and in Asia, it contains resins and plant hormones. It has been used as a tonic for the heart. It is used in cosmetics in some "antiaging" creams.

ADRENAL GLAND • About the size of a grape, your two adrenal glands lie on top of each of your kidneys. Each adrenal gland has two parts. The first part is the medulla, which produces epinephrine and norepinephrine, two hormones that play a part in controlling your heart rate and blood pressure. Signals from your brain stimulate production of these hormones. The second part is the adrenal cortex, which produces three groups of steroid hormones. The hormones in one group control the levels of various chemicals in your body. For example, they prevent the loss of too much sodium and water into the urine. Aldosterone is the most important hormone in this group. The hormones in the second group have a number of functions. One is to help convert carbohydrates or starches into energy-providing glycogen in your liver. Hydrocortisone is the main hormone in this group. The third group consists of the male hormones androgen and the female hormones estrogen and progesterone.

ADSORBATE • A powdered flavor made by coating liquid flavoring on the surface of a powder such as cornstarch, salt, or maltodextrin *(see)*.

ADSORPTION • The attachment of a substance such as a liquid or gas to the surface of a solid.

AEGOPODIUM PODAGRARIA • Derived from *Aegopodium podagraria*. See Saint John's Wort.

AEROSOL • Small particles of material suspended in gas.

AEROSOL SHAVING CREAMS • See Shaving Creams.

AEROSOLS • Many cosmetic sprays, particularly hair care products and fragrances, are sold in aerosol containers. The first aerosol patent was actually issued in 1899 but was not used until 1940, when insecticides were first packaged in self-dispensing gas-pressurized containers. Freon, the most commonly used group among aerosol gases, is a lung irritant and central nervous system depressant, and in high concentrations can cause coma. More than 100 people, mostly young Americans, have died from sniffing aerosol gases for "kicks." These gases can cause severe irregular heartbeat. In addition to freon, hairsprays contain PVP (polyvinylpyrrolidone—*see*) or shellac. PVP is believed to be cancer causing. In addition, thesaurosis, a condition in which there are foreign bodies in the lungs, has been found in persons subjected to repeated inhalation of hairsprays. The aerosol container can become a lethal weapon, acting as a flame-thrower if near a fire and a shrapnel bomb if heated. It has been known to explode when placed too near a radiator or heater. Also, aerosol gases turn into toxic gases: fluorine, chlorine, hydrogen fluoride, and chloride, or even phosgene, a military poison gas. Aerosol hair dyes and "hot" shave creams were made possible by compartmentalization of the container. However, in the case of the hot shave cream, there was unreliable mixing of the chemicals and skin rashes resulted. In powder products, the inhalation of powder or the silicones can damage the lungs. In 1972, the Society of Cosmetic Chemists reported that powder aerosols evidence a high particle retention in the lungs and profound pulmonary effects. Tests showed large powder particles in 23 separate areas of the lungs. In addition, freon, the propellant, cannot be considered inert—that is, lacking in chemical activity or in an expected biologic or pharmacologic effect. Many products have been placed in hand pump containers because of the concern about aerosols.

AESCULUS HIPPOCASTANUM • See Horse Chestnut.

AFTERBATH LOTIONS • See Cologne.

AFTER-SHAVE LOTIONS • See Shaving Lotions.

AGAR • **Japanese Isinglass.** Used as an emulsifier and emollient in cosmetics and as a substitute for gelatin in foods. Extracted from various seaweeds found in the Pacific and Indian oceans and the Sea of Japan. It is also used as a bulk laxative. It is an occasional allergen.

AGAROSE • Extract of the seaweed *Graceilaria* used in skin conditioners as a humectant and thickener.

AGAVE LECHUGUILLA • **American Aloe.** Native to the warm part of the United States and known by its heavy stiff leaf and tall panicle or spike of candelabralike flowers. The leaves are used for juice, employed in cosmetics as an adhesive, and used in medicines as a diuretic. The fermented juice is popular in Mexico for its distilled spirit (mescal). Some species are cultivated for their fibers, which are used in thread and rope. No known skin toxicity.

AGE SPOTS • See Skin Bleach.

AGRIMONY EXTRACT • An extract of *Agrimonia eupatoria,* an herb found in north temperate regions. It has yellow flowers and bristly fruit. It contains tannins, flavonoids, nicotinic acids, Vitamins B and K, iron, and essential oils. Mentioned in medical literature as early as 63 B.C., it has been used in American folk medicine as an astringent *(see)* and an analgesic, as well as to stop bleeding and to treat inflammations. It is also used in ointments and boluses to shrink hemorrhoids, as a tonic, and to treat abscesses in gout.

AGROPYRON REPENS • Couch Grass Root Extract *(see).*

AHA • Abbreviation for Alpha Hydroxy Acids *(see).*

AHNFELTIA CONCINNA • Derived from *Ahnfeltia concinna.* Used in skin conditioners.

AILANTHUS ALTISSIMA • Derived from *Ailanthus Altissima,* a small family of East Indian and Chinese trees, also called the Tree of Heaven. Used in skin conditioners.

ALANINE • Colorless crystals derived from protein. Believed to be a nonessential amino acid. It is used in microbiological research and as a dietary supplement in the L and DL forms. The FDA has asked for supplementary information. It is now GRAS for addition to food. It caused cancer of the skin in mice and tumors when injected into their abdomens.

ALBUMEN • A group of simple proteins composed of nitrogen, carbon, hydrogen, oxygen, and sulfur that are soluble in water. Albumen is usually derived from egg white and employed as an emulsifier in foods and cosmetics. May cause a reaction to those allergic to eggs.

ALBUMIN • See Albumen.

ALCLOXA • Aluminum Chlorhydroxy Allantoinate. See Allantoin.

ALCOHOL • **Ethyl Alcohol. Ethanol.** Alcohol as a solvent is widely used in the cosmetic field. Many cosmetics consist largely of alcohol: after-shave lotion, bubble bath, cologne, cold cream, deodorant, freckle lotion, face packs, hair lacquer, hair tonic, liquid face powder, mouthwash, nail polish remover, perfume, preshaving lotion, shampoo, shaving cream, skin lotion, spray deodorant, suntan lotion and oil, and toilet water. Alcohol is manufactured by the fermentation of starch, sugar, and other carbohydrates. It is clear, colorless, and flammable, with a somewhat pleasant odor and a burning taste. Medicinally used externally as an antiseptic and internally as a stimulant and hypnotic. "Absolute alcohol" is ethyl alcohol to which a substance has been added to make it unfit for drinking. "Rubbing alcohol" contains not less than 68.5 percent and not more than 71.5 percent by volume of absolute alcohol and a remainder of denaturants, such as perfume oils. Since it is a fat solvent, alcohol can dry the hair and skin when used in excess. Toxic in large doses.

ALCOHOL DENAT • This identifies an approved formula of denaturants in accordance with the European Union's labeling. American manufacturers can use the traditional SD Alcohol *(see)* label or change to this.

ALCOHOL FREE • In the past this has meant that certain cosmetic products do not contain ethyl alcohol (or grain alcohol). Cosmetic products, however, may contain other alcohols, such as cetyl-, stearyl-, and cetearyl alcohol, or lanolin *(see all),* which are known as fatty alcohols.

ALDEHYDE, ALIPHATIC • A class of organic chemical compounds intermediate between acids and alcohols. Aldehyde contains less oxygen than acids and less hydrogen than alcohols. Formaldehyde *(see),* a preservative, is an example of an aldehyde widely used in cosmetics. Benzaldehyde and cinnamic aldehydes are used to scent perfumes. Most are irritating to the skin and gastrointestinal tract.

ALDIOXA • **Aluminum Dihydroxy Allantoinate.** Astringent, antiperspirant prepared with the skin-healing salts of aluminum chlorhydroxy allantoinate *(see).* Used as an astringent, keratolytic, tissue stimulant, and buffer in cosmetics. Nonsensitizing and nonirritating. The CIR Expert Panel *(see)* says that there is not enough information about this additive to judge its safety in cosmetics.

ALDOL • Made from acetaldehyde, which occurs naturally in apples, broccoli, cheese, coffee, grapefruit, and other vegetables and fruits. It is a colorless, thick liquid used in the manufacture of rubber and in perfumes. It has also been used as a sedative and hypnotic in medicine. May cause contact dermatitis.

ALEURITIC ACID • A yellowish solid obtained from shellac *(see).* It is used in perfumes.

ALEURITES MOLUCCANA • **Kukui.** Fatty acids derived from *Aleurites moluccana* are used in skin conditioners. See Kukui Nut Oil.

ALFALFA EXTRACT • **Lucerne.** Extract of *Medicago sativa.* A natural cola, liquor, and maple flavoring ingredient for beverages and cordials. Alfalfa is widely cultivated for forage and is a commercial source of chlorophyll. It is used in cosmetics as a source of proteins and vitamins. No known toxicity.

ALGAE • From seaweed and pond scum. Algae is claimed to prevent wrinkles and to moisturize the skin, but the American Medical Association denies any validity for algae's therapeutic benefits. However, seaweed products are widely used in cosmetics for many purposes. Nontoxic. See Alginates.

ALGIN • The sodium salt of alginic acid *(see).*

ALGINATES • All derivatives of alginic acid are designated "algin" (ammonium, calcium, potassium, and sodium). These gelatinous substances are obtained from certain seaweeds and used as emulsifiers in hand lotions and creams and as thickening ingredients in shampoos, wave sets, and lotions. They are also used as barrier ingredients *(see)* in hand creams and lotions, in the manufacture of celluloid, as an emulsifier in mineral oil, and in mucilage. Sodium alginate from brown seaweed is used as a thickener in dentifrices, but the FDA is testing the sodium form (largest use in ice cream) for short-term mutagenic birth-deforming, reproductive, and subacute effects. Alginates are also used as stabilizers and water retainers in many foods.

ALGINIC ACID • A stabilizer in cosmetics, it is obtained as a highly gelatinous precipitate. The sodium carbonate *(see)* extracts of brown dried seaweeds are treated with acid to achieve a gelatin. Resembles albumen or gelatin *(see both)*. Alginic acid is slowly soluble in water, forming a very thick liquid. No known toxicity.

ALIPHATIC ALDEHYDE • See Aldehyde.

ALIZARIN • **Turkey Red.** Occurs in the root of the madder plant and was known and used in Ancient Egypt, Persia, and India. Today, it is produced synthetically from anthracene, a coal tar. It yields different colors, depending upon the metals mixed with it. Colors used in cosmetics are Turkey red, blue, orange, red, rose, black, violet, lilac, yellow, and dark brown. It is also used to dye wool. Can cause contact dermatitis.

ALKALI • The term originally covered the caustic and mild forms of potash and soda. Now a substance is regarded as an alkali if it gives hydroxyl ions in solution. An alkaline aqueous solution is one with a pH *(see)* greater than 7. Sodium bicarbonate is an example of an alkali that is used to neutralize excess acidity in cosmetics.

ALKALOID • A vegetable substance with an organic nitrogen base capable of combining with acids to form crystalline salts. Alkaloids exert a strong biological response in humans, even in small amounts. Chemical alkaloids end in *-ine,* such as betaine from beets, caffeine from coffee beans, and cocaine from the leaves of the coca plant.

ALKANET ROOT • A red coloring obtained from extraction of the herblike tree root grown in Asia Minor and the Mediterranean. Used as a copper or blue coloring (when combined with metals) for hair oils and other cosmetics. It is also used as a coloring for wines, inks, and sausage casings. May be mixed with synthetic dyes for color tints. Formerly used as an astringent.

ALKANNIN • A red powder and the principal ingredient of alkanet root *(see)*. Used as an astringent in cosmetics and to color cosmetics and food.

ALKANOLAMINES • Compounds used in cold creams and eyeliners as a solvent and to adjust pH *(see)* and composed of alcohols from alkene (a saturated fatty hydrocarbon) and amines (from ammonia). These compounds are viscous, colorless liquids that form soaps from fatty acids *(see)*. Triethanolamine *(see)* is an example.

ALKOHL • A form of kohl *(see)* used in Saudi Arabia.

ALKYL • Meaning "from alcohol," usually derived from alkane. Any one of a series of saturated hydrocarbons such as methane. The introduction of one or more alkyls into a compound makes the product more soluble. The mixture is usually employed with surfactants *(see),* which have a tendency to float when not alkylated.

ALKYL ARYLPOLYETHYLENE GLYCOL ETHER • A dispersant for preshave lotions, but basically a wetting ingredient. It rarely sensitizes or irritates human skin.

ALKYL BENZENE SULFONATE • A detergent used in bubble bath and shampoo. Prolonged feeding to animals showed no evidence of toxicity, but such ingredients are known to be defatting and therefore drying to the skin.

ALKYL SODIUM SULFATES • Used in shampoos because they have cleaning power and wash out of the hair easier than soap. A basic alkyl sulfate shampoo formula: sodium lauryl sulfate, 15 percent; behenic acid 3.5 percent *(see both);* water, 81.5 percent. These sulfates were developed by the Germans when vegetable fats and oils were scarce. A large number have been made. They are prepared from primary alcohols by treatment with chlorosulfuric or sulfuric acid. The alcohols are usually prepared from fatty acids *(see)*. For example, lauric acid makes a soap effective in hard water. If it is reduced to lauryl alcohol and sulfated, it makes sodium lauryl sulfate, a widely used detergent. The alcohol sulfates are low in acute and chronic toxicity, but they may cause skin irritation.

ALKYL SULFATES • These sulfates were developed by the Germans during World War II, when vegetable fats and oils were scarce. A large number have been made. They are prepared from primary alcohols by treatment with sulfuric acid. The alcohols are usually prepared from fatty acids *(see)*. For example, lauric acid makes a soap effective in hard water. If it is reduced to lauryl alcohol and sulfated, it makes sodium lauryl sulfate, a widely used detergent. Alkyl sulfates are used in detergents to thicken and improve foaming. The alcohol sulfates are low in acute and chronic toxicity, but they may cause skin irritation.

ALKYLAMIDO BETAINE COCOAMIDOPROPYL BETAINE • See Coconut Oil and Surfactants.

ALKYLARYLSULFONATE • A detergent. See Bubble Bath.

ALLANTOIN • Used in cold creams, hand lotions, hair lotions, after-shave lotions, and other skin-soothing cosmetics because of its ability to help heal wounds and skin ulcers and to stimulate the growth of healthy tissue. Colorless crystals, soluble in hot water, it is prepared synthetically by the oxidation of uric acid *(see)* or by heating uric acid with dichloroacetic acid. It is nontoxic.

ALLANTOIN ACETYL METHIONINE • See Allantoin.

ALLANTOIN ASCORBATE • Allantoin *(see)* with Ascorbic Acid *(see)* salt.

ALLANTOIN BIOTIN • Allantoin *(see)* with B-complex vitamins.

ALLANTOIN CALCIUM PANTOTHENATE • Allantoin *(see)* with calcium and a B-complex vitamin. A combination of the salt of the B-complex vitamin and the healing ingredient allantoin *(see)*. Used to soothe the skin in emollients. Nontoxic.

ALLANTOIN GALACTURONIC ACID • Allantoin *(see)* and galacturonic acid, which is derived from pectin *(see)*.

ALLANTOIN GLYCYRRHETINIC ACID • See Allantoin and the derivative of licorice root, Glycyrrhetinic Acid.

ALLANTOIN POLYGALACTURONIC ACID • See Allantoin and Galacturonic Acid.

ALLANTOINATE • A salt of Allantoin *(see)*.

ALLERGEN • A substance that provokes an allergic reaction in the susceptible but does not normally affect other people. Plant pollens, fungi spores, and animal danders are some of the common allergens.

ALLERGIC CONTACT DERMATITIS • **ACD.** Skin rash caused by direct contact with a substance to which the skin is sensitive. Symptoms include a red rash, swelling, and intense itching. Blisters may develop and break open, forming a crust. In severe cases, the rash and blisters may spread all over the body. A variety of substances can cause the condition. The most common is poison ivy. Others include industrial chemicals, metals, cosmetics, deodorants, mouthwashes, dyes, certain types of textiles, and medicines, as well as local treatments with ointments and local application of antibiotics. ACD may develop at any age. Its precise prevalence is unknown but is thought to affect a significant percentage of the population. The disease may be acute or chronic. It is less common than skin rashes caused by irritants but more serious because relapses commonly occur and may force a person to change jobs. Symptoms may appear 7 to 10 days after the first exposure to an allergen. More often, the allergic reaction doesn't develop for many years and may require many repeated low-level exposures. Once the sensitivity does develop, however, contact with the triggering allergen will produce symptoms within 24 to 48 hours. An attack builds in severity from 1 to 7 days. Even without treatment, healing often occurs in 1 or 2 weeks, although it may take a month or longer.

The rash does not spread on one's body, nor can it be spread to another person. The extension of the rash is caused by renewed contact with whatever triggered the initial outbreak. Some substances, such as film developers, rubber chemicals, and beryllium, can cause symptoms other than the classic red rash and blisters. In some cases, ACD may look like hives. Detailed questioning about the work and leisure activities and the pattern of the rash often reveals its source. A patch test *(see)* may confirm the diagnosis.

ALLERGIC REACTION • An adverse immune response following repeated contact with otherwise harmless substances such as pollens, molds, foods, cosmetics, and drugs.

ALLERGY • An altered immune response to a specific substance, such as ragweed or pollen, on reexposure to it.

ALLIUM CEPA OR SATIVUM • See Garlic Extract.

ALLYL CAPROATE • See Caprylic Acid.

ALLYL HEPTANOATE • See Heptanoic Acid.

4-ALLYL-2-METHOXYPHENOL • See Eugenol.

ALLYL PELARGONATE • Liquid, fruity odor, used in flavors and perfumes.

ALMOND • *Prunus amygdalus.* The oil is obtained from a small tree grown in France, Spain, and Italy. Almond oil has been reported by researchers to lower cholesterol. It is used as a flavoring ingredient in the United States. It is distilled to remove dihydrocyanic acid (prussic acid), which is very toxic. Almond meal is used to create soothing skin preparations. Almond paste was a favorite early European cleanser. Almonds also contain amygdalin, which serves as the basis of laetrile, a controversial anticancer drug that the FDA will not permit to be sold on the market.

ALMOND MEAL • A powder obtained by pulverizing blanched almonds and used in various cosmetics and perfumes. It is used in skin abrasives. See Bitter Almond Oil for toxicity.

ALMOND MILK • A creamy mixture of blanched almonds, acacia *(see)*, sugar, and water blended to a smooth paste and sieved. Used as a demulcent, especially in organic cosmetics. See Bitter Almond Oil.

ALMOND OIL • Used in brilliantines and spice flavorings. See Bitter Almond Oil.

ALMOND PASTE • A favorite early European cleanser. Made from the dried ripe seeds of the sweet almond. See Bitter Almond Oil for toxicity.

ALMONDAMIDE DEA • Fatty acids from almond *(see)*.

ALMONDAMIDOPROPALKONIUM • Fatty acids derived from almond oil *(see)*. Used as an antistatic ingredient and hair conditioning ingredient.

ALNUS FIRMIFOLIA • Derived from *Alnus firmifolia,* a member of the Alder family found in the Andes and north temperate zones. Has a woody, conelike fruit.

ALOE VERA • *Aloe peryi, Aloe barbadensis.* **First Aid Plant.** A compound expressed from the leaf of the aloe plant, which is a South African lilylike plant. There are more than 300 species. Only a few have been used medicinally. Aloe is employed for its supposed softening benefits in skin creams. It contains 99.5 percent water, aloins, polysaccharides including glucosans, anthraquinones, glycoproteins, sterols, saponins, albumen, essential oil, silica, phosphate of lime, a trace of iron, and organic acids. Used medicinally for more than three thousand years, it is referred to in the Bible. Ancient Egyptian women and today's women use it for softening benefits in skin creams. In the West, aloe gel, which is derived from the thin-walled mucilaginous cells of the plant, is considered an effective healing ingredient for the treatment of burns and injuries. A diluted liquid is taken daily for its enzyme promoting activity. It is used to regulate menstruation and to ease liver problems. It is also used to counteract wrinkles and to regulate female hormones. Used in bitters, vermouth, and spice flavorings for beverages and alcoholic drinks. Cross-reacts with benzoin and Balsam Peru in those who are allergic to these compounds. In 1992, the FDA proposed a ban on aloes in oral menstrual drug products because it has not been shown to be safe and effective for its stated claims. There is no scientific evidence that aloe vera has any benefits in cosmetics according to the American Medical Association.

ALOE VERA GEL • See Aloe Vera.

ALOIN • A mixture of active principles obtained from aloe *(see)*. Yellow crystals with a bitter taste. Cosmetic manufacturers eliminate it from their finished aloe vera gel because of adverse effects on the skin. Banned by the FDA in 1992 as an ingredient in laxatives.

ALPHA BISABOLOL • A synthetic bisabolol *(see)* that is used as an anti-irritant.

ALPHA-GLUCAN OLIGOSACCHARIDE • A carbohydrate used in skin conditioners.

ALPHA-HYDROXY ACIDS • AHA cosmetics are believed to have derived from the "chemical peels" that dermatologists and plastic surgeons have used for years. The peels, typically trichloroacetic acid, phenol, resorcinol, and salicylic acid, help remove undesirable signs of skin aging, such as discoloration, rough-ness, and wrinkling. The chemicals cause the skin to lose its outer layer, or peel off, revealing a fresher-looking layer of skin. Known as chemical exfoliation, the procedure is done in doctors' offices so that doctors can control the process and prevent deep skin burns from the highly acidic solutions. Cosmetic manufacturers began to market similar but milder versions of these chemical peels containing AHAs for salon and at-home use around 1989. They quickly caught on, and by 1992, mass marketing had begun. Typically, AHA products sold to consumers have an AHA concentration of 10 percent or less. The concentration of AHA prod-ucts used by trained cosmetologists may run between 20 and 30 percent, while those used by doctors can range from 50 to 70 percent. The following are the AHAs used in cosmetic products: glycolic acid; lactic acid; malic acid; citric acid; glycolic acid + ammonium glycolate; alpha-hydroxyethanoic acid + ammonium alpha-hydroxyethanoate; alpha-hydroxyoctanoic acid; alpha-hydroxycaprylic acid; hydroxycaprylic acid; mixed fruit acid; triple fruit acid; tri-alpha hydroxy fruit acids; sugarcane extract; alpha hydroxy and botanical complex; L-alpha hydroxy acid; glycomer in cross-linked fatty acids alpha nutrium.

Though sold to consumers mainly in face and body creams and lotions, AHAs also can be found to a lesser degree in other cosmetics, such as shampoos and cuti-cle softeners. Available everywhere, from discount pharmacies to fine department stores, the products typically range in price from a few dollars to as much as $60 a bottle. The FDA has a particular concern about AHAs because, unlike traditional cosmetics, AHAs seem capable of penetrating the skin barrier. In reviewing the limited data on AHAs, the FDA concluded in a 1996 report that certain formula-tions of AHA products can affect the skin in a manner similar to that of chemical peels—that is, increasing cell turnover rate and decreasing the thickness of the outer skin. The effect depends on the product's pH level (a measure of its acid-ity), the AHA concentration, and the AHA vehicle cream, as well as how the prod-uct is used (for example, frequency of use and where on the skin it is applied).

Sun Sensitivity

An additional concern arose as FDA prepared its 1996 report on AHA safety: Some people who had reported adverse reactions cited increased sun sensitivity. In addition, one industry-sponsored study found that participants whose skin was exposed to 4 percent glycolic acid twice daily for 12 weeks developed minimal skin redness with 13 percent less ultraviolet (UV) radiation exposure than normal. Three participants developed minimal redness with 50 percent less UV exposure than normal.

Another study that looked at the effects of glycolic acid on production of sun-burn cells (markers for UV-induced skin damage) found that people who received the AHA product in the presence of UV radiation experienced twice the cell dam-age in areas where the AHA had been applied than those who were treated with the non-AHA product. The FDA's concern is that people who are sensitive to sunlight may be particularly susceptible to UV rays, which can damage the skin and, over a long period, can cause skin cancer.

In 1997, the CIR Expert Panel—the cosmetic industry's self-regulatory body for reviewing and addressing safety of cosmetic ingredients—concluded that the AHA's glycolic acid and lactic acid and their related chemical compounds are safe for use in products intended for consumer use when:

- the AHA concentration is 10 percent or less,
- the final product has a pH of 3.5 or greater (lower numbers indicate greater acidity),
- the final product is formulated in such a way that it protects the skin from increased sun sensitivity or its package directions tell consumers to use sunscreen products.

For AHA products used by trained cosmetologists, the CIR Expert Panel concluded that formulations of glycolic acid and lactic acid at concentrations of 30 percent or less and a pH of 3.0 or greater intended for only "brief" use at one time followed by thorough rinsing and daily use of sun protection are safe.

The panel's conclusions actually serve as guidelines for cosmetic manufacturers, Bailey says. "This means that each manufacturer of an AHA product should conduct appropriate testing on their products to measure whether or not the product increases the sensitivity of the user to UV radiation and, if so, should add sun protection to their product and warn consumers to take extra steps to protect themselves at all times." Meanwhile, the FDA continues to study AHA safety. Later this year, scientists with the National Toxicology Program and the FDA will use hairless mice to study the effect of AHAs on the risk of cancer associated with sunlight and UV radiation. The study will run for about three years. Depending on the outcome of the FDA's investigation, Bailey says, the agency may or may not take action against AHA products. "The absence of action by the FDA to date doesn't mean that there won't be any in the future."

Use with Care

Considering the questionable safety status, the FDA and dermatologists advise consumers who use AHA products to follow these precautions:

- Always protect your skin before going out during the day. Use a sunscreen product with an SPF (Sun Protection Factor) of at least 15. Wear a hat with a brim of at least 4 inches (about 10 centimeters). Cover up with lightweight, loose-fitting, long-sleeved shirts and pants.
- Buy products with adequate label information: for example, a list of ingredients to see which AHA or other chemical acids are in the product; the name and address of the manufacturer or distributor, which can serve as the contact if a problem or question arises; and a statement about the product's

AHA concentration and pH level. The first two pieces of information are mandatory; the third is optional. Consumers can call or write the manufacturer, however, to get information about a product's AHA concentration and pH level.

- Buy only products that comply with the CIR Expert Panel's 1997 recommendations—that is, products with an AHA concentration of 10 percent or less and a pH of 3.5 or greater.

- Do a skin-sensitivity test on a patch of skin if you are a first-time user of any AHA product or are using a different brand or a product with a different concentration or pH than you are used to.

- Follow instructions on the label.

- Do not exceed recommended applications. You won't get "younger" any faster.

Stop using the product immediately if you experience adverse reactions. Signs of adverse reactions include stinging, redness, itching, burning, pain, and bleeding or change in sun sensitivity. Even mild irritation is a sign that the product is causing damage, FDA's Bailey says, despite what the manufacturer may indicate on the product label. "Cosmetics shouldn't sting or cause irritation," he says. See also Salicylic Acid, and Exfoliation.

ALPHA OLEFIN SULFONATE • See Sulfonated Oils.

ALPHA TERPINEOL • See Terpineol.

ALPHA TOCOPHEROL • See Tocopherols and Vitamin E.

ALTHEA ROOT • *Hibiscus Moscheutos.* Marshmallow Root. A natural substance from a plant grown in Europe, Asia, and the United States. The dried root is used in flavorings. The boiled root is used as a demulcent in ointments to soothe mucous membranes. The roots, flowers, and leaves are used externally as a poultice. Nontoxic. The dried root is used in strawberry, cherry, and root beer flavorings for beverages. Nontoxic.

ALTHEA ROSEA POWDER • The dried, crushed flowers of *Althea rosea.* See Marshmallow Root.

ALUM • **Potash Alum. Aluminum Ammonium. Potassium Sulfate.** A colorless, odorless, crystalline, water-soluble solid used in astringent lotions, aftershave lotions, and as a styptic (stops bleeding). Also used to prevent aluminum chloride *(see)* from causing skin irritation in antiperspirants. In concentrated solutions, alum has produced gum damage and fatal intestinal hemorrhages. It has a low toxicity in experimental animals, but ingestion of 30 grams (an ounce) has killed an adult human. It is also known to cause kidney damage. The Food and Drug Administration issued a notice in 1992 that potassium alum and ammonium alum have not been shown to be safe and effective for stated claims in OTC products, including astringent drug products. No specific harmful effects reported in cosmetics.

ALUMINA • A natural or synthetic oxide of aluminum occurring in nature as bauxite and corundum. The aluminum hydroxide *(see)* formed is washed, dried, and used as an extender for cosmetic colors in which opacity is not desired. High concentrations of alumina may be irritating to the respiratory tract, and lung problems have been reported in alumina workers. No known skin toxicity.

ALUMINUM ACETATE • **Burow's Solution.** A mixture including acetic acid and boric acid, with astringent and antiseptic properties, used in astringent lotions, antiperspirants, deodorants, and protective creams. It is also used as a fur dye, in fabric finishes, in waterproofing, and as a disinfectant by embalmers. Ingestion of large doses can cause nausea and vomiting, diarrhea, and bleeding. Prolonged and continuous exposure can produce severe sloughing of the skin. It also causes skin rashes in some persons.

ALUMINUM BEHENATE • The aluminum *(see)* salt of behenic acid *(see)*.

ALUMINUM BENZOATE • See Aluminum Salts and Benzoic Acid.

ALUMINUM BROMOHYDRATE • **Aluminum Bromide.** White, yellowish, deliquescent crystals derived by passing bromine over heated aluminum. The waterless form is highly corrosive to the skin. It is used in bromation, alkylation, and isomerization.

ALUMINUM CAPRYLATE • See Aluminum Salts.

ALUMINUM CHLORHYDROXIDE • See Aluminum Chlorhydrate.

ALUMINUM CHLORHYDROXY ALLANTOINATE • Used in after-shave lotions and other astringents. Also used as a buffer. Nonsensitizing and nonirritating. See Allantoin.

ALUMINUM CHLORIDE • The first antiperspirant salt to be used for commercial antiperspirant products and still the strongest available in effectiveness. It is also antiseptic but can be irritating to sensitive skin, and it does cause allergic reactions in susceptible people. Lethal to mammals upon ingestion of large doses.

ALUMINUM CHLOROHYDRATE • The most frequently used antiperspirant in the United States. Causes occasional infections of the hair follicles. May be irritating to abraded skin and may also cause allergic reactions, but it is considered by cosmetic manufacturers as one of the least irritating of the aluminum salts.

ALUMINUM CHLOROHYDRATE COMPLEX • See Aluminum Chlorohydrate.

ALUMINUM CHLOROHYDREX • A derivative of aluminum chlorohydrate *(see)* combined with propylene glycol, making it soluble in alcohol. It is used in deodorants and in antiperspirants. See Aluminum Salts.

ALUMINUM CITRATE • The salt of aluminum hydroxide and citric acid. See Aluminum Salts.

ALUMINUM DIACETATE • See Aluminum Salts.

ALUMINUM DICETYL PHOSPHATE • An aluminum salt used as an emulsion stabilizer. See Aluminium Salts.

ALUMINUM DICHLOROHYDRATE • An antiperspirant ingredient. See Aluminum Salts.

ALUMINUM DICHLOROHYDREX PEG AND PG • Aluminum dichlorate and propylene glycol in which some of the water molecules have been replaced by the propylene glycol. Used as an astringent. See Aluminum Salts and Propylene Glycol.

ALUMINUM DILINOLEATE • The aluminum salt of dilinoleic acid *(see)*.

ALUMINUM DIMERATE • The aluminum salt of dimer acid. See Aluminum Salts.

ALUMINUM DIMYRISTATE • Used in soaps. See Aluminum Salts and Myristic Acid.

ALUMINUM DISTEARATE • A binder that holds loose powders together when compressed into a solid cake form. On the basis of the available information, the CIR Expert Panel *(see)* concludes that it is safe as a cosmetic ingredient. See Aluminum Stearates.

ALUMINUM FLUORIDE • Less toxic on ingestion than other fluorides, it is used to inhibit fermentation and in toothpaste.

ALUMINUM FORMATE • Used as an antiperspirant to make other aluminum salts less acid and corrosive to fabrics. See Aluminum Salts and Formic Acid.

ALUMINUM GLYCINATE • See Aluminum Salts.

ALUMINUM HYDRATE • **Gloss White.** Usually obtained as a white, bulky, amorphous powder. Practically insoluble in water but soluble in alkaline solution. Used as an adsorbent, emulsifier, and alkali in detergents, antiperspirants, and dentifrices. Used medicinally as a gastric antacid. No known toxicity.

ALUMINUM HYDROGENATED TALLOW GLUTAMATE • The aluminum salt of tallow *(see)* used in face powders.

ALUMINUM HYDROXIDE • Mild astringent and alkali used in antiperspirants, dentifrices, and dusting powders. A white, gelatinous mass used as a drying ingredient, catalyst, adsorbent, and coloring ingredient in many cosmetic processes. A leavening ingredient in the production of baked goods, as well as a gastric antacid in medicine. Practically insoluble in water but not in alkaline solutions. Aluminum hydroxide has a low toxicity but may cause constipation if ingested. No known skin toxicity. See Aluminum Salts and Deodorants.

ALUMINUM ISOSTEARATES/LAURATES/STEARATES • The aluminum salt of a mixture of isostearic acid, lauric acid, and stearic acid *(see all)*. Used as a gelling ingredient. No known toxicity.

ALUMINUM ISOSTEARATES/MYRISTATES • Myristate is the aluminum salt of a mixture of isostearic acid and myristic acid *(see both)*. Used as a gelling ingredient. No known toxicity.

ALUMINUM ISOSTEARATES/PALMITATES • Palmitate is the aluminum salt of palmitic acid *(see)* and isostearic acid *(see)*. Used as a gelling ingredient. No known toxicity.

ALUMINUM LACTATE • The aluminum salts of lactic acid *(see both)*.

ALUMINUM LANOLATE • See Aluminum Salts.

ALUMINUM METHIONATE • See Aluminum Salts.

ALUMINUM MYRISTATES/PALMITATES • Myristate is the aluminum salt of a mixture of palmitic acid and isostearic acid *(see both)*. Used as a gelling ingredient. No known toxicity.

ALUMINUM PALMITATE • White granules, insoluble in water, used as a lubricant and waterproofing material. Employed as an antiperspirant. See Aluminum Salts and Deodorants.

ALUMINUM PCA • The aluminum salt of pyrrolidone carboxylic acid. It is used in skin conditioners. Pyrrolidone is derived from acetylene and formaldehyde. Carboxylic acid is a fatty acid.

ALUMINUM PHENOLSULFONATE • **Aluminum Sulfocarbolate.** Pink powder, soluble in water, used in preshave astringent-type lotions and spray deodorants for its antiseptic and detergent properties. It is also used in dusting powder. See Aluminum Sulfate for toxicity.

ALUMINUM PHOSPHATE • **Aluminum Orthophosphate.** White crystals, insoluble in water. Used in ceramics, dental cements, and cosmetics as a gelling ingredient. Corrosive to tissue.

ALUMINUM POWDER • A color additive composed of finely divided particles of aluminum. Used in face powders and hair colorings. No known toxicity. Permanently listed by the FDA in 1977 for use as a coloring.

ALUMINUM SALTS • **Aluminum Acetate. Aluminum Caprylate. Aluminum Chloride. Aluminum Chlorohydrate. Aluminum Diacetate. Aluminum Distearate. Aluminum Glycinate. Aluminum Hydroxide. Aluminum Lanolate. Aluminum Methionate. Aluminum Phenolsulfonate. Aluminum Silicate. Aluminum Stearate. Aluminum Sulfate. Aluminum Tristearate.** These are both the strong and weak acids of aluminum used in antiperspirants to combat body odors. The smell of sweat is caused by bacterial action on moisture. The salts are believed to prevent perspiration from reaching the skin by impeding the action of sweat and to act as an antibacterial. The strong salts may cause skin irritation and damage fabrics, particularly linens and cottons. Therefore, buffering ingredients are added by cosmetic manufacturers to counteract such adverse effects. The salts are also styptic *(see)*.

ALUMINUM SESQUICHLOROHYDRATE • An aluminum salt used in antiperspirants and cleansing ingredients.

ALUMINUM SESQUICHLOROHYDREX • A complex of aluminum sesquichlorohydrate and polyethylene glycol in which some of the water molecules attached to the metal have been replaced by the polyethylene glycol. In the United States this compound may be used as an active ingredient in over-the-counter drugs and is then called Aluminum Sesquichlorohydrex Polyethylene Glycol Complex.

ALUMINUM SILICATE • A white mass, insoluble in water, obtained naturally from clay or synthesized, used as an anticaking and coloring ingredient in powders. Essentially harmless when given orally and when applied to skin. See Aluminum Salts.

ALUMINUM STARCH OCTENYLSUCCINATE • **Dry Flow®.** See Aluminum Phenolsulfonate.

ALUMINUM STEARATES • Hard, plasticlike materials used in waterproofing fabrics, in thickening lubricating oils, and as a chewing-gum base component and a defoamer component used in processing beet sugar and yeast. Aluminum tristearate is a hard plastic material used as a thickener and coloring in cosmetics. On the basis of the available information, the CIR Expert Panel *(see)* concludes that they are safe as cosmetic ingredients. No known toxicity.

ALUMINUM SULFATE • **Cake Alum.** Colorless crystals, soluble in water, used as an antiseptic, astringent, and detergent in antiperspirants, deodorants, and skin fresheners; also purifies water. It may cause pimples under the arm when in antiperspirants and/or allergic reactions in some people. The Food and Drug Administration issued a notice in 1992 that aluminum sulfate has not been shown to be safe and effective for stated claims in OTC products.

ALUMINUM TRIPALMITATE/TRIISOSTEARATE • See Aluminum Isostearates/Palmitates.

ALUMINUM TRIPALMITATE/TRIMYRISTATE • See Aluminum Myristates/Palmitates.

ALUMINUM TRISTEARATE • An opacifying ingredient and skin "conditioner." Used in mascara, tonics, and other hair grooming products. On the basis of the available information, the CIR Expert Panel *(see)* concludes that it is safe as a cosmetic ingredient. See Aluminum Stearates.

ALUMINUM UNDECYLENOYL COLLAGEN AMINO ACIDS • Used in hair and skin conditioners. See Collagen and Amino Acids.

ALUMINUM ZIRCONIUM TRICHLOROHYDREX GLYC • Aluminum zirconium trichlorohydrate in which glycine is added to replace some of the water molecules that normally cling to metal. It is used in nonaerosol antiperspirants. See Aluminum Salts.

AMALAKI • *Phyllanthus emblica.* An herb used for thousands of years in India to treat coughs and eating disorders and to normalize bowel function. It is also used to treat skin diseases and tumors.

AMARANTH • See FD & C Blue No. 2.

AMARANTHUS CAUDATUS • **Love-lies-Bleeding. Red Cockscomb.** An herb used for digestion, bleeding, diarrhea, menstrual pain, as a douche for vaginal discharge, dysentery, and as a food. It has astringent, nutrient, styptic, and diuretic properties and is high in Vitamins A and C.

AMBER OIL, RECTIFIED • A perfume ingredient distilled from amber, a fossil resin of vegetable origins, and purified. The oil is pale yellow to yellowish brown and volatile, with a penetrating odor and acrid taste. No known toxicity.

AMBERGRIS • Concretion from the intestinal tract of the sperm whale found in tropical seas. About 80 percent cholesterol, it is a gray to black, waxy mass and is used for fixing delicate odors in perfumery. It is also used in a flavoring for food and beverages. No known toxicity.

AMBRETTOLID • Formed in ambrette-seed oil. Used as a flavoring, perfume fixative. No known toxicity.

"AMERCHOL"™ • A series of surface-active lanolin derivatives. Most are soft solids used as emulsifiers and stabilizers for water and oil systems. Emollients in cosmetics.

AMERICAN CENTAURY EXTRACT • Extract of the American centaury plant, *Sabbatia angularis*. A member of the gentian family, it is used by herbalists for jaundice. A bitter compound gives the herb its strong taste and aids digestion and the flow of gastric juices. It is a strong antiseptic for cuts and scratches. Also used as a mouthwash.

AMES TEST • Dr. Bruce Ames, a biochemist at the University of California, developed a simple, inexpensive test using bacteria that reveals whether a chemical is a mutagen. Almost all chemicals that are known carcinogens have also been shown to be mutagenic on the Ames Test. Whether the test can identify carcinogens is still controversial.

AMIDE • Derived from ammonia. Used in cosmetics as thickeners, soil removers, and foam stabilizers. Also used as an anti-irritant to prevent "stinging" of other cosmetic ingredients. Cocoamide DEA is an example.

AMIDO • Denoting a compound that contains ammonia.

AMINE ACID SURFACTANTS • **Acyl Glutamate.** Used as anti-irritants in cosmetics to prevent stinging of some cosmetic ingredients.

AMINE OXIDES • See Amine Acid Surfactants.

AMINES • A class of organic compounds derived from ammonia. They are basic in nature—synthetic derivatives of ammonium chloride, a salt that occurs naturally. Quaternary ammonium compounds *(see)* used in detergents are examples.

AMINO ACIDS • The body's building blocks, from which proteins are constructed. Of the 22 known amino acids, 8 cannot be manufactured in the body in sufficient quantities to sustain growth health. These 8 are called "essential" because they are necessary to maintain good health. A ninth, histidine, is thought to be necessary for growth only in childhood. Widely used in moisturizers and emollients because they are thought to help penetrate the skin.

p-AMINOBENZOIC ACID • See Para-Aminobenzoic Acid.

AMINOBUTYRIC ACID • See Amino Acids and Butyric Acid.

6-AMINOCAPROIC ACID • See Amino Acids and Caproic Acid.

2-AMINO-6-CHLORO-4-NITROPHENOL • A coal tar hair coloring. The CIR Expert Panel *(see)* concludes this ingredient is poorly absorbed through the skin suggesting that any systemic effects were unlikely. The Panel says based on animal tests and clinical data that this ingredient is safe for use at concentrations up to 2 percent.

6-AMINO-m-CRESOL • A coal tar hair coloring. See Phenol.

AMINODIMETHICONE • Used as a skin protectant and in hairsprays. See Dimethicone.

5-AMINO-2,6-DIMETHOXY-3-HYDROXY-PYRIDINE • A coal tar hair coloring. See Phenol.

AMINOETHYLACRYLATE PHOSPHATE/ACRYLATES COPOLYMER • See Acrylates.

2-AMINO-4-HYDROXYETHYLAMINOANISOLE • A coal tar hair coloring. See coal tar.

2-AMINO-3-HYDROXYPYRIDINE • A coal tar hair coloring. See Coal Tar.

4-AMINO-2-HYDROXYTOLUENE • Used in the manufacture of hair dyes. The CIR Expert Panel *(see)* concludes this is a safe ingredient in cosmetics. The Panel says that based on the weight of epidemiological studies with this ingredient, there is no indication of it causing cancer. See Toluene.

2-AMINOMETHYL-p-AMINOPHENOL HCL • A coal tar hair coloring. See Coal Tar and Phenol.

AMINOMETHYL PROPANEDIOL • Crystals made from nitrogen compounds that are soluble in alcohol and mixable with water. Used as an emulsifying ingredient for cosmetic creams and lotions and in mineral oils. No known toxicity.

AMINOMETHYL PROPANOL • An alcohol made from nitrogen compounds; mixes with water. Soluble in alcohol and used as an emulsifying ingredient for cosmetic creams and lotions, and in hairsprays. Used in medicines that reduce body water. Prolonged skin exposure may cause irritation due to alkalinity, but in most commercial products the alkalinity is neutralized. It is used in cosmetics up to 10 percent. The available test data do not exceed 1 percent. Therefore, the CIR Expert Panel *(see)* says that concentrations not exceeding 1 percent are safe for use in cosmetics.

4-AMINO-2-NITROPHENOL • See Aminophenol.

AMINOPHENOL • m-Aminophenol. o-Aminophenol. p-Aminophenol. 2-Amino-5-Nitrophenol. 4-Amino-2-Nitrophenol. 2-Amino-6-Chloro-4-Nitrophenol. p-Aminophenol HCL. Aromatic, colorless crystals derived from phenol *(see)*, used as intermediates *(see)* in orange-red and medium brown hair dyes. Discovered in London in 1854, aminophenols are also used in the manufacture of sulfur and azo dyes *(see)*. Can cause a lack of oxygen in the blood but is less toxic than aniline *(see)* in animals. Solutions on the skin have produced restlessness and convulsions in humans as well as skin irritations. May also cause skin rashes and sensitization, and inhalation may cause asthma. These ingredients have been found to be mutagenic in laboratory tests. They are metabolized in a way similar to acetaminophen (Tylenol) which has been found to have a potential effect on the liver. The CIR Expert Panel *(see)* concluded that although the clinical data for the aminophenols are limited and skin tests in guinea pigs produced some sensitivity, the aminophenols are "safe as cosmetic ingredients in the present practices of use and concentrations."

m-AMINOPHENOL • A hair colorant. See Aminophenol.

p-AMINOPHENOL • A hair colorant. See Aminophenol.

p-AMINOPHENOL HCL • A hair colorant. See Aminophenol.

AMINOPROPYL DIMETHICONE • A hair conditioning ingredient. See Dimethicone.

AMINOPROPYL LAURYLGLUTAMINE • An antistatic ingredient used in hair conditioners. Also used as a cleansing ingredient.

AMMONIA • Liquid obtained by blowing steam through incandescent coke. It is used in refrigerants, in the manufacture of permanent wave lotions and hair bleaches, in the manufacture of detergents, and in cleaning preparations. It may cause hair breakage when used in permanent waves and hair bleaches. It is also used in the manufacture of explosives and synthetic fabrics, herbicides, fertilizers, and pesticides, and is one of the top five inorganic chemicals produced in the United States. It has been shown to produce cancer of the skin in human doses of 1,000 milligrams per kilogram of body weight. It is extremely toxic when inhaled in concentrated vapors, and is irritating to the eyes and mucous membranes. See Ammonium Hydroxide.

AMMONIA WATER • Ammonia gas dissolved in water. Used as an alkali *(see)* in metallic hair dyes, hair straighteners, and protective skin creams. Colorless with a very pungent odor, it is irritating to the eyes and mucous membranes. In strong solution, it can cause burns and blistering.

AMMONIATED MERCURY • **Mercuric Chloride Ammoniated.** A white, odorless powder with a metallic taste used in ointment form to combat skin infections and to treat eye disorders. All forms of mercury are poisonous. Topical application may lead to skin rash and other allergic manifestations. Prolonged use may cause skin pigmentation and, when applied too vigorously, it can be absorbed and result in systemic poisoning. Absorption or ingestion may lead to kidney damage. Ingestion also causes stomach pains and vomiting. No longer permitted in cosmetics except in small amounts as a preservative.

AMMONIUM ACETATE • The ammonium salt of acetic acid *(see)*.

AMMONIUM ACRYLATES COPOLYMER • See Acrylates.

AMMONIUM ALGINATE • See Alginates.

AMMONIUM ALUM • See Alum.

AMMONIUM BENZOATE • White crystals or powder used as a preservative. See Benzoic Acid.

AMMONIUM BICARBONATE • Used as a buffer in thioglycolate cold permanent-waving lotions. Occurs in the urine of alligators. Usually prepared by passing carbon dioxide gas through concentrated ammonia water. Shiny, hard, colorless or white crystals; faint odor of ammonia. Used in baking powder formulas for cooling baths. Used medicinally as an expectorant and to break up intestinal gas. Also used in compost heaps to accelerate decomposition. See Ammonium Carbonate for toxicity.

AMMONIUM BISULFITE • Colorless, water-absorbing powder that is used as a catalyst in hair-waving formulations.

AMMONIUM C12-15 ALKYL SULFATE • See Quaternary Ammonium Compounds.

AMMONIUM C12-15 PARETH SULFATE • **Pareth-25-3 Sulfate.** The ammonium salt of a sulfated polyethylene glycol ether of a mixture of C12-15 fatty alcohols *(see)*. See also Ammonium Sulfate.

AMMONIUM CARBONATE • A white, solid alkali derived partly from ammonium bicarbonate *(see)* and used as a neutralizer and buffer in permanent wave solutions and creams. It decomposes when exposed to air. Also used in baking powders, for defatting woolens, in fire extinguishers, and as an expectorant. Ammonium carbonate can cause skin rashes on the scalp, forehead, or hands.

AMMONIUM CASEINATE • A hair-conditioning ingredient and skin conditioner. See Casein.

AMMONIUM CHLORIDE • Ammonium salt that occurs naturally. Colorless, odorless crystals or white powder, saline in taste, and incompatible with alkalies. Used as an acidifier in permanent wave solutions, in eye lotions, and as a cooling and stimulating skin wash. Industrially employed in freezing mixtures, batteries, dyes, safety explosives, and in medicine as a urinary acidifier and diuretic. Keeps snow from melting on ski slopes. If ingested, can cause nausea, vomiting, and acidosis. As with any ammonia compound, concentrated solutions can be irritating to the skin.

AMMONIUM CITRATE • See Citric Acid.

AMMONIUM COCOMONOGLYCERIDES • See Coconut Oil and Sulfated Oil.

AMMONIUM COCO-SULFATE • Used as an emulsifying ingredient and a cleanser. See Coconut Oil.

AMMONIUM CUMENE SULFONATE • **Benzenesulfonic Acid. Methylated Ammonium Salt.** Derived from coal tar or petroleum, it is used as a solvent. See Coal Tar.

AMMONIUM DICHROMATE • Orange needles used in dyeing red colors and in synthetic perfumes. Irritating to the eyes and skin, and a suspected carcinogen.

AMMONIUM DIMETHICONE COPOLYOL SULFATE • Used as a surfactant and cleansing ingredient. See Dimethicone and Silicone.

AMMONIUM DODECYLBENZENESULFONATE • **Ammonium Lauryl Benzene Sulfonate.** See Quaternary Ammonium Compounds and Surfactants.

AMMONIUM FLUORIDE • Corrosive to tissue. Used in oral care products and as an antiseptic. Also used in mothproofing.

AMMONIUM FLUOROSILICATE • Strong irritant. Used in oral care products. Also used in glass etching, electroplating, and as a disinfectant in the brewing industry.

AMMONIUM GLYCOLATE • A pH *(see)* adjuster widely used in cosmetics such as cold creams, cleansing ingredients, liquids and pads, moisturizing preparations, body and hand preparations (excluding shaving products) and skin care preparations. See Glycolic Acid.

AMMONIUM GLYCYRRHIZATE • The ammonium salt of glycyrrhizic acid *(see)*. See also Quaternary Ammonium Compounds.

AMMONIUM HYDROLYZED ANIMAL PROTEIN • Name changed to ammonium hydrolyzed collagen *(see)*.

AMMONIUM HYDROLYZED COLLAGEN • **Ammonium Hydrolyzed Protein.** The ammonium salt of hydrolyzed animal protein. See Hydrolyzed Collagen and Surfactants.

AMMONIUM HYDROXIDE • **Ammonia Water.** A weak alkali formed when ammonia dissolves in water and exists only in solution. A clear, colorless liquid with an extremely pungent odor. Used as an alkali *(see)* in metallic hair dyes and hair straighteners and in protective skin creams. Also used in detergents and for removing stains. It is irritating to the eyes and mucous membranes. It may cause hair breakage.

AMMONIUM IODIDE • An ammonium salt prepared from ammonia and iodine. White, odorless crystals with a sharp saline taste. The crystals become yellow and brown on exposure to air and light. Used in cosmetics as an antiseptic and preservative and in medicine as an expectorant. See Iodine for toxicity.

AMMONIUM ISOSTEARATE • The ammonium salts of isostearic acid *(see)*. Also see Surfactants.

AMMONIUM LACTATE • Used as a buffering ingredient, skin conditioner, and humectant. See Lactic Acid.

AMMONIUM LAURETH-8 CARBOXYLATE • See Lauric Acid and Polyethylene Glycol. See also Surfactants.

AMMONIUM LAURETH SULFATE • **Ammonium Lauryl Ether Sulfate.** A compound that breaks up and holds oils and soil so they can be easily removed from skin or hair. See Lauryl Alcohol.

AMMONIUM LAUROYL SARCOSINATE • A hair-conditioning ingredient, surfactant, and cleansing ingredient. See Sarcosines.

AMMONIUM LAURYL SULFATE • The ammonium salt of lauryl sulfate derived from the natural coconut alcohols, it is a mild anionic surfactant *(see)* cleanser that is widely used at mild acidic pH values. On the basis of available information, the CIR Expert Panel *(see)* concludes that it is safe as presently used in cosmetic formulations designed for brief use followed by thorough rinsing from the surface of the skin. In products for prolonged contact with skin, concentrations should not exceed 1 percent. See Lauryl Alcohol.

AMMONIUM MONOOLEAMIDO • See Ammonia.

AMMONIUM MYRETH SULFATE • See Sodium Lauryl Sulfate.

AMMONIUM MYRISTYL SULFATE • The ammonium salt of myristyl sulfate. See Myristic Acid.

AMMONIUM NITRATE • **Saltpeter.** Colorless crystals derived from nitric acid. Used in herbicides and insecticides, as an oxidizer in solid rocket propellants, as a nutrient for antibiotics and yeast, and as a catalyst.

AMMONIUM NONOXYNOL-4-SULFATE • Cleansing material that breaks up and holds oils and soil so that they may be removed easily from the skin or hair surface. See Ammonium Sulfate.

AMMONIUM OLEATE • The ammonium salt of oleic acid *(see),* used as an emulsifying ingredient.

AMMONIUM PALM KERNEL SULFATE • A surfactant and cleansing ingredient. See Palm-Kernel Oil.

AMMONIUM PERSULFATE • **Ammonium Salt.** Colorless crystals soluble in water, used as an oxidizer and bleach in dyes and skin lighteners. Also as a disinfectant, deodorant, and preservative. It may be irritating to the skin and mucous membranes. In cosmetics, may make hair brittle. Lethal to rats in large oral doses.

AMMONIUM PHENOLSULFONATE • The ammonium salt of phenol sulfonic acid. See Quaternary Ammonium Compounds.

AMMONIUM PHOSPHATE • **Ammonium Salt.** An odorless, white or colorless crystalline powder with a cooling taste used in mouthwashes. It is also used in fireproofing textiles, paper, and wood. No known toxicity.

AMMONIUM POLYACRYLATE • An emulsion stabilizer. See Acrylates.

AMMONIUM PROPIONATE • A preservative. See Propionic Acid.

AMMONIUM SALICYLATE • See Salicylates.

AMMONIUM STEARATE • **Stearic Acid. Ammonium Salt.** A yellowish white powder used as a texturizer in vanishing creams. No known toxicity. On the basis of the available information, the CIR Expert Panel *(see)* concludes that it is safe as a cosmetic ingredient.

AMMONIUM STYRENE/ACRYLATE COPOLYMER • The ammonium salt of a polymer of styrene and a monomer of acrylic acid and methacrylic acid used as an opacifier. See Acrylates.

AMMONIUM SULFATE • **Ammonium Salt.** A neutralizer in permanent wave lotions, it is odorless and colorless, either crystals or powder. Industrially used in freezing mixtures, fireproofing fabrics, and tanning. Used medicinally to prolong analgesia. No known toxicity when used cosmetically. Rats were killed when fed large doses.

AMMONIUM SULFIDE • A salt derived from sulfur and ammonium, it is used as a neutralizer in permanent wave lotions, as a depilatory, to apply patina to bronze, and in spice flavorings. It has been reported to have caused a death when ingested in a permanent wave solution. Irritating to the skin when used in depilatories.

AMMONIUM SULFITE • Ammonium salt made with sulfuric acid. White, crystalline, soluble in water, almost insoluble in alcohol and acetone. Antiseptic. A preservative in cold permanent waves. See Ammonia for toxicity.

AMMONIUM TALLATE • The ammonium salt of tall oil fatty acids. See Quaternary Ammonium Compounds.

AMMONIUM TARTRATE • See Tartaric Acid.

AMMONIUM THIOCYANATE • Colorless, water-absorbing crystals derived from ammonium cyanide. Used in analytical chemistry, fertilizers, photography, curing resins, and adhesives. See Cyanide.

AMMONIUM THIOGLYCOLATE • The ammonium salt of thioglycolic acid, a liquid with a strong unpleasant odor that is readily oxidized by air. A hair straightener, antioxidant, and depilatory, it can cause severe burns and blistering of the skin. Large doses injected into the stomachs of mice killed them. The CIR Expert Panel *(see)* concludes this ingredient can be used by individuals at concentrations of up to 14.4 percent if it is used infrequently. It is a cumulative irritant and weak sensitizer.

AMMONIUM THIOLACTATE • The ammonium salt of lactic acid *(see)*.

AMMONIUM VA/ACRYLATES COPOLYMER • See Acrylates and Copolymer.

AMMONIUM VINYL ACETATE/ACRYLATES TERPOLYMER • See Acrylates.

AMMONIUM XYLENESULFONATE • **Ammonium salt of xylene.** A lacquer solvent used in nail polishes. Flammable, insoluble in water. It may be narcotic in high doses. Chronic toxicity or skin effects are not known.

AMNIOTIC FLUID • The fluid surrounding the cow embryo *in utero.* It is promoted for benefits similar to those of human placenta (*see* Placental Extract) and has limited use in moisturizers, hair lotions, scalp treatments, and shampoos.

AMODIMETHICONE • The silicone polymer with amino acids. See Amino Acids and Silicones.

AMOMUM AROMATICUM • Derived from *Amomum aromaticum,* an aromatic herb grown in the tropics. It is a member of the Zingiber family. See Ginger Oil.

AMP • The abbreviation for aminomethyl propanol *(see).*

AMP-ACRYLATES COPOLYMER • A film-former. See Acrylates.

AMP ISOSTEAROYL HYDROLYZED COLLAGEN • Collagen *(see)* from animals used in "antiaging" products and other emollients.

AMPD • The abbreviation for aminomethyl propanediol *(see).*

AMPD ACRYLATES/DIACETONEACRYLAMIDE COPOLYMER • **Acrylic Acid, Methacrylic Acid,** and their simple esters. See Acrylates.

AMPD ISOSTEARIC HYDROLYZED PROTEIN • The salt of isostearic hydrolyzed animal protein. See Hydrolyzed Protein.

AMPD-ROSIN HYDROLYZED COLLAGEN • The salt of hydrolyzed collagen *(see).* Used in hair and skin conditioners and as a surfactant and cleansing ingredient.

AMPHO- • Means double or both.

AMPHOTERIC • A material that can display both acid and basic properties. Used primarily in surfactants *(see),* it contains betaines and imidazoles (*see both*).

AMPHOTERIC-2 • A cleansing compound that breaks up and holds oils and soil so that they may be removed easily from skin or hair surface. See Amphoteric.

AMYGDALIN • A glycoside (organic compound) found in bitter almonds, peaches, and apricots. It has been a controversial substance because claims have been made that it can fight cancer in a compound called laetrile. Such claims have been unaccepted by conventional United States scientists but the compound is widely available in Mexico.

AMYL ACETATE • **Banana Oil. Pear Oil.** Obtained from amyl alcohol, with a strong fruity odor. Used in nail finishes and nail polish remover as a solvent, and as an artificial fruit essence in perfume. Also used in food and beverage flavoring and for perfuming shoe polish. Amyl acetate is a skin irritant and causes central nervous system depression when ingested. Exposure of 950 ppm for one hour has caused headache, fatigue, chest pain, and irritation of the mucous membranes. It has been found to stimulate acetylcholine release in the nerve endings and act as a competitive inhibitor of acetylcholine in isolated nerves. Acetylcholine is a nerve messenger and plays a big part in memory functioning. It is used up to 10 percent in fingernail formulations. The CIR Expert Panel *(see)* concludes this is a safe ingredient in cosmetics.

AMYL ALCOHOL • A solvent used in nail lacquers. It occurs naturally in cocoa and oranges and smells like camphor. Highly toxic and narcotic, ingestion of as little as 30 milligrams has killed humans. Inhalation causes violent coughing.

AMYL BENZOATE • A fragrance ingredient. See Benzoic Acid.

AMYL BUTYRATE • Used in some perfume formulas for its apricotlike odor. It occurs naturally in cocoa and is colorless. Also used for synthetic flavorings. No known toxicity.

AMYL CINNAMIC ALCOHOL • A solvent used in nail polish removers, waterproofing, and enamelware. See Cinnamic Acid.

AMYL CINNAMIC ALDEHYDE • Liquid with a strong floral odor suggesting jasmine. Used in perfumes and flavorings. See Cinnamic Acid.

AMYL DIMETHYL PABA • Used in sunscreens to absorb ultraviolet light from sun's rays to help prevent or lessen sunburn while allowing the skin to tan. See Para-Aminobenzoic Acid and Sunscreen Preparations.

AMYL ESTERS • Used in fragrances. See Amyl Alcohol and Ester.

AMYL GALLATE • An antioxidant obtained from nutgalls and from molds. No known toxicity.

AMYL PHENOL • Used in hair-grooming preparations. See Phenol.

AMYL PROPIONATE • Colorless liquid with applelike odor used in perfumes, flavors, and lacquers. No known toxicity.

AMYL SALICYLATE • Derived from salicylic acid. A pleasant-smelling liquid used in sunscreen lotions and perfumes. Insoluble in water. See Salicylates.

AMYL TRICRESOL • A phenol mercury compound used in mouthwashes. See Phenol.

AMYLASE • Used as a texturizer in cosmetics, it is an enzyme prepared from hog pancreas used in flour to break down starch into smaller molecules. Used medicinally to combat inflammation. No known toxicity.

AMYLOPECTIN • **Amioca.** Derived from starch, it is the almost insoluble outer portion of the starch granule. The gel constituent of starch. Used as a texturizer in cosmetics. Obtained from corn. Gives a red color when mixed with iodine and does not gel when mixed with water. No known toxicity.

AMYRIS ACETATE • See Amyris Oil.

AMYRIS OIL • *Amyris balsamifera.* The sweet oil distilled from the wood of a torchwood and used in perfumery.

ANACARDIUM OCCIDENTALIS • **Cashew Nut.** Derived from *Anacardium occidentalis,* a small family of tropical American trees that have kidney-shaped fruit.

ANACYCLUS PYRETHRUM • Derived from *Anacyclus pyrethrum,* a Mediterranean herb with white or yellow flowers. See Pyrethrins.

ANANAS SATIVUS • **Pineapple.** The common juice from the tropical plant. Contains a protein-digesting and milk-clotting enzyme, bromelin. An antiinflammatory enzyme, it is used in cosmetic treatment creams. It is also used as a texturizer. No known toxicity.

AND OTHER INGREDIENTS • Term used to represent those ingredients that have received trade secret status by the U.S. Food and Drug Administration (FDA).

ANETHOLE • A flavoring ingredient used in mouthwashes and toothpastes and as a scent for perfumes. Obtained from anise *(see)* oil and other sources. Colorless or faintly yellow liquid with a sweet taste and a characteristic aniselike odor. Chief constituent of anise. Anethole is affected by light and caused irritation of the gums and throat when used in a denture cream. When applied to the skin, anethole may produce hives, scaling, and blisters.

ANETHUM GRAVEOLENS • See Dill.

ANGELICA • Used in inexpensive fragrances, toothpastes, and mouthwashes. Grown in Europe and Asia, the aromatic seeds, leaves, stems, and roots have been used in medicine for flatus (gas), to increase sweating, and reduce body water. Also used as a flavoring in food. When perfume is applied, skin may break out with a rash and swell when exposed to sunlight. The bark is used medicinally as a purgative and emetic.

ANGOSTURA BARK • Flavoring ingredient from the bark of trees grown in Venezuela and Brazil. Unpleasant, musty odor and bitter aromatic taste. The light yellow liquid extract is used in bitters, liquor, root beer, and spice flavorings for beverages and liquors (1,700 ppm). Used in cosmetics. Formerly used to lessen fever. No known toxicity. GRAS.

ANHYDRIDE • A residue resulting from water being removed from a compound. An oxide—combination of oxygen and an element—that can combine with water to form an acid, or that is derived from an acid by the abstraction of water. Acetic acid *(see)* is an example.

ANHYDROUS • Describes a substance that contains no water.

ANIBA ROSAEODORA • **Rosewood.** See Bois de Rose Oil.

ANIGOZANTHOS FLAVIDUS • See Kangaroo Paw Flower.

ANILINE • A colorless to brown liquid that darkens with age. Slightly soluble in water, it is one of the most commonly used of the organic bases, the parent substance for many dyes and drugs. It is derived from nitrobenzene or chlorobenzene and is among the top five organic chemicals produced each year in the United States. It is used as a rubber accelerator to speed vulcanization, as an antioxidant to retard aging, and as an intermediate *(see);* it is also used in dyes, photographic chemicals, the manufacture of urethane foams, pharmaceuticals, explosives, petroleum refining, resins, adhesive products, paint removers, herbicides, and fungicides. Also used in crayons and shoe polishes. It is toxic when ingested, inhaled, or absorbed through the skin. It causes allergic reactions. It is a potential human cancer-causing ingredient. It caused cancer in mice when injected under the skin or administered orally. It can also cause contact dermatitis. In a 1991 report of a study of 1,749 workers at the Goodyear Tire & Rubber Company plant in Niagara Falls, N.Y., it was revealed that workers exposed directly to aniline had 6.5 times the rate of bladder cancer of the average state resident.

ANILINE DYES • **Coal Tar Dyes.** Aniline is a colorless to brown liquid that darkens with age. A synonym for coal tar *(see)* dyes, it refers to a large class of synthetic dyes made from intermediates *(see)* based upon or made from aniline. It is among the top five organic chemicals produced in the United States. Used in the manufacture of hair dyes, medicinals, resins, and perfumes. It is used in carbons, fur dyeing, rubber, photographic inks, colored pencils, and crayons. Most are somewhat toxic and irritating to the eyes, skin, and mucous membranes but are generally much less toxic than aniline itself. These dyes caused tumors in animals whose skins were painted with them. Can cause contact dermatitis.

ANIMAL COLLAGEN AMINO ACIDS • The word "animal" has been deleted from any name with it, when possible, by the cosmetic manufacturers. See Collagen Amino Acids.

ANIMAL ELASTIN AMINO ACIDS • Now called elastin amino acids. See Elastin and Amino Acids.

ANIMAL KERATIN AMINO ACIDS • Now called keratin amino acids *(see)*.

ANIMAL PROTEIN DERIVATIVE • Used in skin conditioners to attract water, thereby helping to maintain the skin's moisture balance. See Hydrolyzed Collagen.

ANIMAL SKIN LIPIDS • A mixture of fats derived from animal skin.

ANIMAL TISSUE EXTRACT • The mixed extract of the skin, testes, and ovaries of the pig, and the thymus, placenta, and udder of the cow. Also called Epiderm Oil R, it is used in moisturizers and other creams.

ANIONIC SURFACTANTS • A class of synthetic compounds used as emulsifiers in about 75 percent of all hand creams and lotions. An anion is a negatively charged ion that is "surface active." These detergents usually consist of an alkali salt as soap, or ammonium salt of a strong acid. Can be irritating to the skin, depending on alkalinity. See Emulsifiers and Ammonia Water. Used in shampoos. Whether or not it is irritating to the eyes depends on the compound. Sodium Laureth Sulfate, for example, is very irritating, whereas Triethanolamine (TEA) Coco Hydrolyzed Animal Protein is the least irritating.

ANISE • **Anise Seed.** Dried, ripe fruit of Asia, Europe, and the United States. Used in licorice, anise, pepperoni sausage, spice, and vanilla flavorings for beverages, ice cream, ices, candy, baked goods, condiments, and meats. The oil is used for butter, caramel, licorice, anise, rum, sausage, nut, root beer, sarsaparilla, spice, vanilla, wintergreen, and birch beer flavorings for the same foods as above, excepting condiments but including chewing gum and liquors. Sometimes used to break up intestinal gas. Used in masculine-type perfumes, cleaners, and shampoos. Can cause contact dermatitis.

p-ANISIC ACID • A flavoring ingredient. Prepared from methoxybenzene. See benzene.

ANISIDINE. o-ANISIDINE. p-ANISIDINE • Derived from anisole *(see)*. Colorless needles. Used in the manufacture of azo dyes *(see)*. Can be absorbed through the skin. It is an irritant and sensitizer.

ANISOLE • A synthetic ingredient with a pleasant odor used in licorice, root beer, sarsaparilla, wintergreen, and birch beer flavorings for beverages, ice cream, ices, candy, and baked goods. Also used in perfumery.

ANISYL ACETATE • Colorless liquid with a lilac odor used in perfumery. See Anise.

ANISYL FORMATE • Used in perfumery and flavoring. See Formic Acid.

ANNATTO • A vegetable dye from a tropical tree. Yellow to pink, it is used in dairy products, baked goods, margarine, and breakfast cereals. No known toxicity. Permanently listed as a coloring in 1977.

ANNONA MURICATA EXTRACT • **Custard Apple.** Used in skin conditioning products.

ANONA CHERIMOLIA • **Annona Cherimolia.** Derived from *Anona cherimolia*. Cultivated in Mexico and in tropical America. It is native to Peru. Contains alkaloids. Used by herbalists for pain in the back.

ANTHOCYANINS • One of the most important and widely distributed groups of water-soluble natural colors, anthocyanins are responsible for the attractive red, purple, and blue colors of many flowers, fruits, and vegetables. Over 200 individual anthocyanins have been identified, of which 20 have been shown to be naturally present in black grapes, the major source of anthocyanin pigment for food coloration.

ANTHRANILIC ACID • **o-Aminobenzoic Acid.** Yellowish crystals with a sweet taste used in dyes and perfumes. See Benzoic Acid.

ANTHRAQUINONE • A coal tar color produced industrially from phthalic anhydride and benzene *(see both)*. Light yellow slender prisms, which are insoluble in water. May cause skin irritation and allergic reactions. It is also used as an organic inhibitor to prevent growth of cells and a repellent to protect seeds from being eaten by birds. Caused tumors when given orally to rats in doses of 72 milligrams per kilogram of body weight. It can also cause contact dermatitis.

ANTHRISCUS CEREFOLIUM • **Chervil.** A Eurasian herb of the family *umbelliferae* with short beaked fruit. Celery belongs to this family. It is used as a flavoring ingredient and in perfumery.

ANTHYLLIS VULNERARIA • **Kidney Vetch.** A legume with yellowish red flowers.

ANTIFOAMING INGREDIENT • Defoamer. A substance used to reduce foaming due to proteins, gases, or nitrogenous materials that interfere with the manufacture of the product. See Silicones, for example.

ANTIGEN • Any substance that provokes an immune response when introduced into the body.

ANTIMONY COMPOUNDS • **Antimony Potassium Tartrate. Tartar Emetic.** Used in hair dyes. Obtained from ore mined in China, Mexico, and Bolivia, this silver-white brittle metal can cause contact dermatitis, eye and nose irritation, and ulceration by contact, fumes, or dust. It is used medicinally as an emetic and in the manufacture of bullets and metal bearings and to combat worms.

ANTIOXIDANTS • Preservatives that prevent fats from spoiling. Tocopherols and BHA are examples *(see both)*.

ANTIPERSPIRANT • Any substance having a mild astringent action that tends to reduce the size of skin pores and thus restrain the passage of moisture on local body areas. The most commonly used antiperspirant compound is aluminum chlorohydrate. Use of zirconium compounds in antiperspirant sprays has been discontinued because of their suspected carcinogens, though they are permissible in creams. Antiperspirants exert a neutralizing action that give them deodorant properties. The FDA classified them as drugs rather than as cosmetics.

ANTISTATIC INGREDIENTS • Plastic polymers accumulate static electricity, which causes dust and other matter to cling. Cosmetic manufacturers add substances such as polyethylene glycols and quaternary ammonium compounds in an effort to counteract static cling.

AOICTBYN CANNABINUM • **Indian Hemp.** A member of the nettle family, legend has it that it stops bleeding.

AORTA EXTRACT • Extract of the aorta, the major artery in the body of animals. Used in "antiaging" creams.

AOSAINE® • A newer ingredient that consists of elastic fibers of algae *(see)* origin. It is claimed to inhibit elastase and substitutes for elastin *(see both)*. It allegedly traps elastases that have been released during exposure to ultraviolet radiation. Application to the skin is supposed to provide a "smoothness."

APIUM GRAVEOLENS • See Celery.

APPLE • Used in organic cosmetics. See Malic Acid.

APPLE BLOSSOM • Used in perfumes and colognes, it is the essence of the flowers from a species of apple tree. No known toxicity.

APRICOT • Fruit and oil. The tart orange-colored fruit. The oil expressed from *Prunus armeniaca* is used in brilliantine, and the crushed fruit is used as a facial mask to soften the skin. For a do-it-yourself facial mask, soak a cup of dried apricots in water until softened, then mix with a small bunch of grapes and 3 tablespoons of skimmed milk powder. Mix the concoction in a blender, and pat on the neck and face; allow to remain for 15 minutes, followed by a rinse of cool water. No known toxicity.

APRICOT AMIDOPROPYL BETAINE • Fatty acids derived from apricot *(see)*.

APRICOTAMIDOPROPYL ETHYLDIMONIUM ETHOSULFATE • A quaternary ammonium compound *(see)* made from apricots and ethosulfate.

APRICOT EXTRACT • See Apricot.

APRICOT KERNEL OIL PEG-6 ESTERS • A complex mixture formed from esterification *(see)* of Apricot Kernel Oil. See Apricot and PEG.

AQUA • The European name for what Americans list on the label as "water."

ARABIC GUM • See Acacia.

ARACHIDIC ACID • A fatty acid, also called eicosanoic acid, that is widely distributed in peanut-oil fats and related compounds. It is used in lubricants, greases, waxes, and plastics. No known toxicity.

ARACHIDONIC ACID • A liquid, unsaturated, fatty acid that occurs in the liver, brain, glands, and fat of animals and humans. The acid is generally isolated from animal liver. A surfactant and emulsifying ingredient, it is used essentially for nutrition and to soothe eczema and rashes in skin creams and lotions. In one study, thus far, it altered the skin's immune response. The CIR Expert Panel *(see)* says it cannot conclude whether this ingredient is safe for use in cosmetic products until such time that the appropriate safety data have been obtained and evaluated.

ARACHIDYL BEHENATE • A waxy alcohol made from arachidyl alcohol and behenic acid.

ARACHIDYL PROPIONATE • The ester of arachidyl alcohol and N-propionic acid used as a wax and as an emollient. The CIR Expert Panel *(see)* concludes this is a safe ingredient in the present practices of use and concentration. See Arachidic Acid.

ARACHIS HYPOGAEA • See Peanut Oil.

ARALIA NUDICAULIS • **Wild Sarsaparilla.** See Sarsaparilla Extract.

ARBITRARY FIXATIVE • An odorous substance that lends a particular note to the perfume throughout all stages of evaporation but does not really influence the evaporation of the perfume materials in the compound. Oakmoss is an example. See Fixative and Oakmoss.

ARBUTIN • Diuretic and anti-infective derived from the dried leaves of the heath family, genus *Vaccinium,* including blueberries, cranberries, and bearberries, and most pear plants. This may explain why cranberry juice is reputed to ward off and treat urinary tract infections. In cosmetics it is used as an antioxidant and skin conditioner.

ARBUTUS EXTRACT • From the leaves of the evergreen shrub *Arbutus,* found in southern Europe and western North America. It has a white or pink flower.

ARCTIUM, MAJOR and MINOR • **Beggar's Buttons. Burdock Root.** The roots, seeds, and leaves of this common roadside plant contain essential oil. The oil contains nearly 45 percent inulin (sugar) and many minerals. Herbalists use it for skin diseases. In modern experiments, burdock root extract has been shown to have antitumor effects.

ARGANIA SPINOSA • **Spinosa Oil.** See Olive Oil.

ARGEMONE MEXICANA OIL • An oil expressed from the leaves of a Mexican poppy. It is used as a skin and hair conditioning ingredient.

ARGININE • An essential amino acid *(see),* strongly alkaline. The FDA has asked for further information on the nutrient, which plays an important role in the production of urea *(see)* excretion. It has been used for the treatment of liver disease.

ARISTOLOCHIA CLEMATIS • A woody herb with pungent, aromatic roots. Used in fragrances.

ARMENIAN BOLE • A soft, claylike red earth. The pigment is found chiefly in Armenia and Tuscany and is used as a coloring material in face powder. No known toxicity.

ARMERIA MARITIMA EXTRACT • Derived from an herb that grows along the seacoast in temperate climates.

ARNICA • **Wolf's Bane.** Skin fresheners may contain this herb found in the Northern Hemisphere. The dried flower head has long been used as an astringent and to treat skin disorders, especially in tinctures. It has been used externally to treat bruises and sprains. Ingestion leads to severe intestinal upset, nervous disturbances, irregular heartbeat, and collapse. Ingestion of one ounce has caused severe illness but not death. Active irritant on the skin. Not recommended for use in toilet preparations and should never be used on broken skin.

AROMA • This is the term Europeans use instead of listing individual components of a flavor. The United States labels say "flavor."

AROMATHERAPY • The use of scents to relieve everything from stress to a broken heart. Usually promoted by cosmetic manufacturers for bath products and body lotions, it has a long history, and there are some scientific studies now in progress about the use of scent to alter mood.

AROMATIC • In the context of cosmetics, a chemical that has an aroma.

AROMATIC BITTERS • Usually made from the maceration of bitter herbs and used to intensify the aroma of perfume. The herbs selected for aromatic bitters must have a persistent fragrant aroma. Ginger and cinnamon are examples.

ARROWROOT • An ingredient in dusting powders and hair dyes made from the root starch of plants. Arrowroot was used by the American Indians to heal wounds from poisoned arrows. It is used as a culture medium and as a medicine. In cosmetics, it is used to help moisturizers penetrate the skin. No known toxicity.

ARSENIC COMPOUNDS • Arsenic is an element that occurs throughout the universe and is highly toxic in most forms. Its compounds are used in hair tonics and hair dyes and have been employed to treat spirochetal infections, blood disorders, and skin diseases. Ingestion causes nausea, vomiting, and death. Chronic poisoning can result in pigmentation of skin and kidney and liver damage. In hair tonics and dyes, it may cause contact dermatitis. The limit of arsenic in colors is 0.0002 percent. Arsenic can also cause the skin to be sensitive to light and break out in a rash or to swell.

ARTEMIA • Named for the Greek goddess of the forests and hills, this is a genus of crustaceans found in salt lakes and brines of saltworks.

ARTEMISIA ABROTANUM • See Artemisia Capillaris.

ARTEMISIA ABSINTHIUM • See Artemisia Capillaris.

ARTEMISIA CAPILLARIS • **Mugwort.** A shrub native to the Eastern United States. Hippocrates recommended this herb to aid in the delivery of the placenta after childbirth. One of the most commonly used herbal preparations to induce menstruation, the extract has been shown to stimulate uterine muscle. Chinese dry mugwort and then burn it in a therapeutic technique, moxibustion, to treat a variety of ills. Contains volatile oils, tannin *(see)* and the sugar, inulin.

ARTICHOKE EXTRACT • A tall herb, *Cynara scolymus,* that resembles a thistle. It is edible. It is used in cosmetics to "relax" the muscles as it is rubbed on the skin.

ARTIFICIAL • In the context of cosmetics, a substance not duplicated in nature. A scent, for instance, may have all natural ingredients, but it must be called artificial if it has no counterpart in nature.

ARTIFICIAL NAIL REMOVER • Contains acetonitrile, also known as methyl cyanide. May cause skin irritation. Cyanide poisoning from ingestion of such products has been reported.

ARTIFICIAL NAILS • Plastics designed to be pasted or self-adhered to one's natural nails to give the appearance of long, lovely, undamaged fingernails. After application, the artificial nails are cut or filed to desired length and shape. Artificial nails were developed from materials used by dentists to fill teeth. The basic ingredients include a vinyl compound (methyl methacrylate is one of the most commonly used vinyls), a catalyst, and a plasticizer. Allergy and irritation to the skin may develop from ingredients in the fake nails or in the adhesive. Artificial nails can be used to beautify as well as camouflage discolored, thickened, or malformed fingernails. Unfortunately, this group of cosmetics is responsible for both allergic contact dermatitis and nail damage. Speaking at the American Academy of Dermatology's Academy 1997 Meeting in New York, Zoe Diana Draelos, M.D., Clinical Associate Professor, Department of Dermatology, Bowman Gray School of Medicine, Wake Forest University, spoke about the dermatologic problems associated with the latest nail cosmetics. The most popular type of artificial nail is the preformed plastic nail. These come in press-on, preglued forms and in forms requiring glue application. The acrylic glue used is typically methacrylate-based and a possible cause of allergic contact dermatitis. "Stronger nail adhesives are used to provide better adhesion, but can cause the nail plate to separate from the nail bed. In addition, traumatic removal of artificial nails may result in the nail plate splitting into layers," Dr. Draelos said. Preformed nails are not recommended for patients with weak nails, congenital nail deformity, or nail-plate irregularities, since a smooth nail surface is required for adhesion.

For an even more natural-looking nail, many have been opting for sculptured nails. The word "sculptured" is used since the custom-made artificial nail is sculpted on a template attached to the natural nail plate. The sculpted nail fits perfectly, and if well done, can be hard to differentiate from a natural nail. The actual nail is made from acrylic, and mixed with a number of substances in order to form to the shape of each individual nail. Finished nail sculptures require more care than natural fingernails. Damage to the natural nail plate still occurs even if you are conscientious. After two to four months of wear, the natural nail plate becomes yellowed, dry, and thin. Most nail operators prefer to allow the natural nail to grow out and act as a support for the sculpture. However, typically the nails become thin, bendable, and weak. For this reason, it is not advisable to wear sculptured nails for more than three consecutive months. One month should be allowed between applications. "Weak nails, nails plagued with psoriasis, discolored nails, and damaged nail plates can be cosmetically improved with sculptured nails. The skill of the operator is key. Much success has also been seen with silk or linen cloth wraps, which are combined with nail sculptures to add additional strength to the artificial nail or to aid in covering nail defects. Cloth wraps can be used on nails with mild median canal dystrophy (ridges) to bridge the nail edges. Brittle psoriatic nails can also be strengthened," Dr. Draelos stated. However, there are many problems associated with the application and wearing of nail sculptures. An important issue is the failure of states to uniformly license operator training, application techniques, and facility cleanliness. Poorly trained operators may allow liquid acrylic to enter the nail fold, which could result in nail tissue damage. The failure to sterilize equipment or apply antifungal, antibacterial solutions to the nail plate may result in fungal, viral, or bacterial infections.

Allergic contact dermatitis remains an issue. The chemicals typically used are strong sensitizers. It is very important that the nail operator is careful to avoid skin contact. See your dermatologist for patch testing if you suspect you are sensitive or allergic to these substances. Tearing the natural nail plate from the nail bed is a common problem since the bond between the sculpture and the natural nail plate is stronger than the adhesion between the natural nail and nail bed. This also occurs in individuals sensitive to the acrylic. Many are upset at the broken, thinned, yellowed appearance of their nails following sculpture removal. "This is due to interference with the nail's normal vapor exchange, nail-plate trauma during the removal process, and damage to the underlying nail bed," said Dr. Draelos. See Appendix B.

ARYLALCANOIC • Rubefacient *(see)* used in Europe.

ASAFOETIDA EXTRACT • **Asafetida. Devil's Dung.** A gum or resin obtained from the roots or rhizome of *Ferula asafoetida,* any of several plants grown in Iran, Turkestan, and Afghanistan. The soft lumps, or "tears," have a garlicky odor and are used as a natural flavoring. The gums have also been used medicinally as an expectorant and to break up intestinal gas. No known toxicity.

ASARUM SIEBOLDI • **Snakeweed. European Wild Ginger.** It causes profuse discharge of mucus from the nasal passages. The leaves contain a highly aromatic essential oil.

ASCORBIC ACID • **Vitamin C.** A preservative and antioxidant used in cosmetic creams, particularly bleach and lemon creams. Vitamin C is necessary for normal teeth, bones, and blood vessels. The white or slightly yellow powder darkens upon exposure to air. Reasonably stable when it remains dry in air, but deteriorates rapidly when exposed to air while in solution. Nontoxic.

ASCORBYL PALMITATE • A salt of ascorbic acid *(see),* it is used as a preservative and antioxidant in cosmetic creams and lotions to prevent rancidity. Nontoxic.

ASCORBYL STEARATE • See Ascorbyl Palmitate.

ASIATIC ACID • A carboxylic fatty acid that is used as a skin-conditioning ingredient.

ASIMINA TRIOBA • See PawPaw Extract.

ASPARAGINE • A nonessential amino acid *(see).* It is widely found in plants and animals both free and combined with proteins. It is used as a culture medium and as a medicine. In cosmetics, it is used to help moisturizers penetrate the skin. No known toxicity.

ASPARAGUS ROOT EXTRACT • *Asparagus officinalis.* **Sparrowgrass.** The root is used in Chinese medicine as a tonic. In India, it is used as a hormonal tonic for the female reproductive system. It is prescribed for women to promote fertility, relieve menstrual pains, increase breast milk, and generally nourish and strengthen the female reproductive system. It is also used as a tonic for the lungs in consumptive diseases and for wasting in AIDS. Asparagus contains glycosides, asparagine, sucrose, starch, and mucilage. In 1992, the FDA proposed a ban on asparagus in oral menstrual drug products because it has not been shown to be safe and effective for its stated claims.

ASPARTAME • A compound prepared from aspartic acid *(see)* and phenylalanine, with about 200 times the sweetness of sugar, discovered during routine screening of drugs for the treatment of ulcers. The G.D. Searle Company sought FDA approval in 1973. The FDA approved it in 1974, but objections that aspartame might cause brain damage led to a stay, or legal postponement, of that approval. Another problem arose. An FDA investigation of records of animal studies conducted for Searle drug approvals and for aspartame raised questions. The FDA arranged for an independent audit, which took more than two years and concluded that the aspartame studies and results were authentic. The agency then organized an expert board of inquiry and the members concluded that the evidence did not support the charge that aspartame might kill clusters of brain cells or cause other damage. However, persons with phenylketonuria, or PKU, must avoid protein foods such as meat that contain phenylalanine—one of two components of aspartame. The board did, however, recommend that aspartame not be approved until further long-term animal testing could be conducted to rule out a possibility that aspartame might cause brain tumors. The FDA's Bureau of Foods reviewed the study data already available and concluded that the board's concern was unfounded. Aspartame was approved for use as a tabletop sweetener in certain dry foods on October 22, 1981. It also was approved for breath mints, hard and soft; as a flavor enhancer in chewing gum and hard candy; instant coffee and tea beverages; ready-to-serve nonalcoholic beverages, fruit juice–based beverages and concentrates or syrup; as a flavor enhancer for malt beverages containing less than 3 percent alcohol; and frosting, toppings, fillings, glazes, and icings for precooked baked goods.

ASPARTIC ACID. DL & L FORMS • **Aminosuccinate Acid.** A nonessential amino acid *(see)* occurring in animals and plants, sugarcane, sugar beets, and molasses. It is usually synthesized for commercial purposes. No known toxicity.

ASPERGILLUS • A genus of fungi. It contains many species of molds, spores, which produce the antibiotic aspergillic acid. An Aspergillus flavus-Oryzae Group of mold has been cleared by the U.S. Department of Agriculture's Meat Inspection Division to soften tissues of beef cuts, with: "Solutions containing water, salt, monosodium glutamate, and approved proteolytic enzymes applied or injected into cuts of beef shall not result in a gain of more than 3 percent above the weight of the untreated product." It is also used in bakery products such as bread, rolls, and buns. Toxicity is unknown but because of the use of the fungi-antibiotic and monosodium glutamate, allergic reactions would certainly be possible.

ASPERULA ODORATA • See Woodruff.

ASPIRIN • **Acetylsalicylic Acid.** It is the most commonly taken drug in the United States. It is widely used as an analgesic, antifever, and anti-inflammatory. It produces allergic reactions in an estimated 2 persons per 100. Of the people with severe asthma, about 5 to 10 percent are aspirin sensitive. Allergy to aspirin occurs most frequently in people between the ages of 40 and 60 years who have a long history of sinusitis, nasal polyps, and high levels of eosinophils (a type of white blood cell). Allergy to aspirin can cause symptoms that range from rashes, hives, and swelling to asthmatic attacks that may be life-threatening. The onset of severe symptoms may come within 15 minutes after ingesting aspirin, or it may not occur for hours. The exact mechanism of the aspirin reaction remains uncertain because no antibodies to aspirin have been found. However, those allergic to aspirin may also be sensitive to other salicylates *(see)* such as Tartrazine, used in yellow and orange dyes.

ASTRAGALUS MEMBRANACEUS EXTRACT • Actiphyte of Milk Vetch. Astragal Extract. Sinominceur. Earth Powder. An extract of the roots of *Astragalus membranaceus.* From a bright green prostrate perennial herb that has sulfur yellow flowers.

ASTRAGALUS SINICUS AND EXTRACT • Chinese Milk Vetch Extract. Derived from *Astragalus Sincus.* See Astragalus Membranaceus Extract.

ASTRINGENT • Usually promoted for oily skin. A clear liquid containing mostly alcohol, but with small amounts of other ingredients such as boric acid, alum, menthol, and/or camphor. A typical astringent formula: ethanol, 50 percent; sorbitol, 2.5 percent *(see both);* perfume oil, 0.1 percent; menthol, 0.1 percent; boric acid, 2.0 percent *(see both);* water, 44.9 percent. In addition to making the skin feel refreshed, it usually gives a tightened feeling from the evaporation of the ingredients. According to the American Medical Association, there is no evidence that astringents tighten or shrink the pores. Usually toxic when ingested because of denatured alcohol content.

ATELOCOLLAGEN • A collagen *(see)* that has been treated with enzymes to soften it.

ATOPIC DERMATITIS • A chronic, itching inflammation of the skin also called eczema *(see).*

ATRIPLEX NUMMULARIA • A plant material from the salt bush in Australia and Western United States. Used as a stabilizer.

ATTAPULGITE • See Fuller's Earth.

AVENA SATIVA • See Oat Bran and Oatmeal.

AVENS • *Geum urbanum.* **Clove Root. Colewort. Herb Bennet. Wild Rye.** A perennial herb that derives its name from the Spanish for "antidote." It contains essential oils *(see),* tannins *(see),* resin, and organic acids. It is used as an astringent tonic for stomach problems, diarrhea, and leukorrhea, and as a gargle for sore throats.

AVERRHOA CARAMBOLA • Derivative of an East Indian tree widely cultivated in the tropics. Has somewhat acid fruit and is used in Chinese cookery.

AVOCADAMIDOPROPALKONIUM CHLORIDE • A quaternary ammonium compound *(see)* made from avocados.

AVOCADO • *Persea Gratissima.* The pulpy green fruit of the genus *Persea,* originating in South America and Mexico, it is also called Alligator Pear, and the tree has been nicknamed "the testicle tree," because of the shape of its fruit. The avocado is used in folk medicine as an aphrodisiac. An emollient, it is used in "organic" cosmetics for its high fat and Vitamin A and C components. It is also used in shampoos. No known toxicity. The CIR Expert Panel *(see)* concludes this is a safe ingredient in the present practices of use and concentration.

AVOCADOMIDE DEA • A mixture of the fatty acids *(see)* derived from avocado *(see)*.

AVOIDANCE • Measures taken to avoid contact with allergy-producing substances. Since there are no cures for allergies, as of yet, avoiding allergens is the best way to combat them.

AZELAIC ACID • Prepared by oxidation of ricinoleic acid, it occurs in rancid oleic acid. It is used in antiacne preparations.

AZO DYES • Used in nonpermanent hair rinses and tints. Azo dyes belong to a large category of colorings that are characterized by the way they combine with nitrogen. These are a very large class of dyes made from diazonium compounds and phenol. The dyes usually contain a mild acid, such as citric or tartaric acid. They can cause allergic reactions. People who become sensitized to permanent hair dyes containing para-phenylene diamine *(see* Phenylenediamine) also develop a cross sensitivity to azo dyes. That is, a person who is allergic to permanent *p*-phenylenediamine dyes will also be allergic to azo dyes. There are reports that azo dyes are absorbed through the skin.

AZTEC MARIGOLD • **Tagetes.** Extract and Oil. The meal is the dried, ground flower petals of the Aztec marigold, a strong-scented, tropical American herb, mixed with no more than 0.3 percent ethoxyquin, a herbicide and antioxidant. The extract is taken from tagetes peels. Both the meal and the extract are used to enhance the yellow color of chicken skin and eggs. They are incorporated in chicken feed, supplemented sufficiently with yellow coloring xanthophyll. The coloring has been permanently listed since 1963 but is exempt from certification. The oil is extracted from the Aztec flower and used in fruit flavorings for beverages, ice cream, ices, candy, baked goods, gelatin, desserts, and condiments.

AZULENE • A blue to greenish black hydrocarbon. Used as an antiacid in cosmetics. It has shown anti-inflammatory effects but the CIR Expert Panel *(see)* concludes there is insufficient data to support the safety of this ingredient in cosmetic products.

B

BABASSUAMIDE • A mixture of fatty acids derived from Babassu *(see)*. It is used as a hair conditioner, foam booster, and thickening ingredient.

BABASSU • A nondrying edible oil expressed from the kernels of the babassu palm, *Orbignya oleifera,* grown in Brazil. Used in foods and soaps, but it is expensive.

BABASSUAMIDE DEA • Fatty acids derived from Babassu *(see)*.

BABASSUAMIDOPROPALKONIUM • **Chloride.** The quaternary ammonium *(see)* derived from Babassu *(see)*. Used as an antistatic ingredient in hair conditioners.

BABASSUAMIDOPROPYL BETAINE • A compound containing the fatty acids of Babassu *(see)* and betaine *(see)*.

BABY CREAM • Aimed at protecting baby skin against irritation and soothing it, such formulas usually contain mineral oil, paraffin, lanolin, white beeswax, and ceresin. They may also contain many other ingredients, including petrolatum, mineral wax, glyceryl monostearate, methyl- and propylparabens, extract of lanolin, sterol, hydrogenated fatty oils, and spermaceti *(see all)*. Lanolin, lanolin derivatives, beeswax, and the parabens are common allergens, and if your baby develops a rash, consult your physician.

BABY LOTION • Aimed at protecting, soothing, and cleansing the delicate skin of babies. Usually contains antimicrobials, emulsifiers, humectants to retain moisture, thickeners, and often some perfume. The product may also contain lanolin, mineral oil, cetyl alcohol, preservatives, and antioxidants *(see all)*. Few problems are reported by consumers except for an occasional rash. However, a number of the ingredients used can cause allergic responses, particularly the perfumes and the antimicrobials. If your baby develops a rash, read the label and check the product against ingredients listed in this book. Take the information to a physician, who can make the definitive diagnosis.

BABY OIL • Aimed at protecting and soothing baby skin. Usually contains mineral oil, palmitate, lanolin, vegetable oils, and lanolin derivatives *(see all)*. Mineral oil or vegetable oil right from the pantry will do the same job and lessen the chances of allergic contact dermatitis. If you suspect the product is causing a rash, check the ingredients on the label and see if they may be allergens for your child. Take the information to your physician, who can make a definitive diagnosis.

BABY POWDER • Soothes, dries, and protects baby skin from irritation. Usually contains talc, kaolin, zinc oxide, starch, magnesium carbonate *(see all)*, perfume oil, and—although there have been repeated warnings against it—boric acid *(see)*. Cornstarch from your pantry shelf does not carry the problems of talc *(see)* and will work as well and less expensively.

BABY SOAP • Usually a mild sodium soap of coconut and/or palm oil. Some are made of polyunsaturated vegetable oils. Baby soaps may contain colloidal oatmeal, a mild, soap-free sudsing ingredient, lanolin derivatives, and a germ killer such as chlorobutanol. If your baby is known to be allergic to any of the above, check with the company about the soap's ingredients and then check them in the book.

BACITRACIN • **Bactine First Aid Antibiotic. Baciguent. Campho-Phenique. Triple Antibiotic. Mycitracin. Aquaphor. Antibiotic Ointment. Neosporin. Polysporin.** Introduced in 1948, it is used systemically to treat pneumonia or abscesses caused by staphylococci. It is used topically to treat staphylococcic and streptococcic infections of the skin, outer ear, and eyelids. It is combined with other drugs into ointments that have a wide spectrum of bacteria-killing action. Topical bacitracin rarely causes adverse effects. It is used as a germ killer in cosmetics.

BACTERIAL CATALASE • A catalase is an enzyme in plant and animal tissues. It exerts a chemical reaction that converts hydrogen peroxide into water and oxygen. Derived from bacteria by a pure culture fermentation process, bacterial catalase may be used safely, according to the FDA, in destroying and removing the hydrogen peroxide that has been used in the manufacture of cheese—providing "the organism

Micrococcus lysodeikticus from which the bacterial catalase is to be derived, is demonstrated to be nontoxic and non-pathogenic." The organism is removed from the bacterial catalase prior to the use of the catalase, the catalase to be used in an amount not in excess of the minimum required to produce its intended effect.

BAK • See Benzalkonium Chloride.

BALM • A variation of the word "balsam." Usually means a soothing ointment, especially a fragrant one, or a soothing application. See also Melissa Oil.

BALM MINT • **Balm of Gilead.** The secretion of any of several small evergreen African or Asian trees with leaves that yield a strong aromatic odor when bruised. Known in ancient Palestine as a soothing medication for the skin. Used in cosmetics as an unguent that soothes and heals the skin. It is also used for its fragrance in perfumes. No known toxicity.

BALM MINT OIL • A natural fruit and liquor flavoring ingredient for beverages, ice cream, candy, and baked goods. The balm leaves may also be used for flavorings in beverages and cosmetics. May cause allergic reactions.

BALM OF GILEAD EXTRACT • From the buds of *Commiphora opobalsamum.* A small evergreen grown in Africa and Asia. It has been valued since ancient times as an unguent that heals and soothes. Has a fragrant oil.

BALSAM • The natural exudate from tree or plant.

BALSAM CANADA • *Abies balsamea.* An oleoresin used in creams.

BALSAM COPAIBA • The oleoresin *(see)* from South American trees that yield a thick, brown liquid. It has a strong odor and is used in perfumes and soaps and as a film-former.

BALSAM MECCA • **Balsam of Gilead.** Obtained from a twig. Insoluble in water, soluble in alcohol. Used to scent perfume.

BALSAM OREGON • **Douglas Fir Oil.** Resin from *Pseudotsuga menziesi.*

BALSAM PERU • A dark brown, viscous liquid with a pleasant lingering odor and a warm bitter taste. It is used in face masks, perfumes, cream hair rinses, and astringents. Obtained from Peruvian balsam in Central America near the Pacific Coast. Mildly antiseptic and irritating to the skin; may cause contact dermatitis and a stuffy nose. It is one of the most common sensitizers and may cross-react with benzoin, rosin, benzoic acid, benzyl alcohol, cinnamic acid, essential oils, orange peel, eugenol, cinnamon, clove, balsam Tolu, storax, benzyl benzoate, and wood tars.

BALSAM TOLU • An ingredient used in perfumery and soap. Extracted from a tree grown on elevated plains and mountains in South America. Yellowish brown, or brown, thick fluid with a strong odor and taste. Its vapor has been used as an expectorant. See Balsam Peru for toxicity.

BAMBOO • A woody grass of *Bambusa arundinaria, Dendrocalamus,* and related genera. Usually has a hollow stem. Young shoots are used as food. Employed in "organic" cosmetics. Some extracts of bamboo are muscle relaxants—for example, curare is used by the Indians as an arrow poison.

BAMBUSA ARUNDINACEA • See Bamboo.

BANANA • The common fruit, high in potassium *(see)*, used for dry skin by organic cosmetic enthusiasts. A banana face-mask formula: Mash one ripe banana and mix thoroughly with 1 tablespoon of almond meal *(see)* plus 2 tablespoons of yogurt. Spread mixture on face and neck. Leave on for 5 to 10 minutes. Remove with lukewarm water. Nontoxic.

BAPTISIA TINCTORIA • **Wild Indigo.** The root contains alkaloids, glycosides, and resin *(see all)*. It is used by herbalists to treat infections of the ear, nose, and throat. Taken both internally and as a mouthwash, it reputedly heals mouth ulcers and sore gums and helps to control pyorrhea. Internally, it is used by herbalists to aid in reducing fevers, constipation, and swollen glands. Externally, in an ointment, it is used to treat infected ulcers and soothe sore nipples. Used in a douche, herbalists say it helps relieve vaginal discharge. Toxic in large doses, it can cause severe diarrhea and violent vomiting and may affect the heart.

BARIUM HYDROXIDE • See Barium Sulfate.

BARIUM SULFATE • **Blanc Fixe.** The salt of the alkaline earth metal, it is a fine, white, odorless, tasteless powder used as a white coloring and as a base for depilatories and other cosmetics. Barium hydroxide is also used in a similar manner. The barium products are poisonous when ingested and frequently cause skin reactions when applied.

BARIUM SULFIDE • Used in depilatories as a base, it is a grayish white to pale yellow powder. A skin irritant, it causes rashes and chemical burns. Should never be applied to broken or inflamed skin.

BARLEY EXTRACT • *Hordeum vulgare.* **Pearl Barley. Prelate.** The seed is used by herbalists to treat diarrhea and bowel inflammation. Chinese herbalists use it as an anti-inflammatory diuretic for relieving gall bladder ailments, reducing swelling and tumors, and treating jaundice. It contains proteins, prolamines, albumen, sugars, starch, fats, B vitamins, and alkaloids *(see)*.

BARLEY FLOUR • A cereal grass cultivated since prehistoric times. Used in the manufacture of malt beverages, as a breakfast food, and as a demulcent *(see)* in cosmetics. No known toxicity.

BARM • A yeast formed during the fermentation of alcoholic beverages.

BARRIER INGREDIENT • A protective for hand creams and lotions, which acts as a barrier against irritating chemicals, including water and detergents. The water-repellent types deposit a film that acts as a barrier to water and water-soluble ingredients that irritate the skin; oil-repellent types act as barriers against oil and oil-soluble irritants. Silicones *(see)* are widely used as barrier ingredients. Other skin-protective ingredients in barrier ingredients include petrolatum, paraffin, ozokerite vegetables, beeswax, casein, various celluloses, alginic acid, zein, gum tragacanth, pectin, quince seed, bentonite, zinc oxide, zinc stearate, sodium silicate, talc, stearic acid, and titanium dioxide *(see all)*. Covering one's hands with Vaseline or zinc oxide ointment will protect them well and inexpensively.

BASE COAT • Similar to a nail polish *(see)* in form and formulation but does not contain pigment and has an increased amount of resin *(see)*. Applied on the nail under nail polish to help prevent chipping and to allow smoother application of the nail enamel. See Nail Polish for toxicity.

BASIC BLUE 3 • A coal tar hair coloring. An amine color.

BASIC BLUE 6 • **Medola's Blue.** A phenol color. See Basic Dye.

BASIC BLUE 7 • A triphenylmethane color *(see)*.

BASIC BLUE 9 • **Methylene Blue.** Prepared from dimethylaniline and thiosulfuric acid. Dark green, odorless crystals used as a stain in bacteriology, as an ingredient for several chemicals, as a veterinary antiseptic, and as an antidote to cyanide poisoning.

BASIC BLUE 26 • A triphenylmethane color *(see)*.

BASIC BLUE 41 • **Methylbenzothiazolium Chloride.** See Basic Dyes.

BASIC BLUE 47 • A coal tar hair coloring. An anthraquinone color.

BASIC BLUE 99 • **Arianor Steel Blue R.** May cause allergic reaction. See Basic Dyes.

BASIC BROWN 4 • **Basic Brown R. Bismarck Brown 53.** Prepared from toluene-2-4-diamine (*see* Toluene) with nitrous acid, it is a dark, solid brown, which turns reddish brown or violet in solution. Used in hair dyes. See Aniline Dyes for toxicity.

BASIC BROWN 16 • **Arianor Mahogany R.** An azo dye *(see)*.

BASIC BROWN 17 • **Arianor Sienna Brown R.** An azo dye *(see)*.

BASIC DYE • A group of dyes made from soluble salts, minerals acids, and certain organic acids that form insoluble compounds with acidic fibers. They produce very bright colors but lack good fastness. See Aniline Dyes for toxicity.

BASIC GREEN 1 • A triphenylmethane group *(see)* color.

BASIC GREEN 4 • A coal tar color used in hair coloring.

BASIC ORANGE 1 • A coal tar color used in hair coloring. See Toluene.

BASIC ORANGE 2 • A coal tar hair coloring. See Benzene.

BASIC RED 22 • A triazolium dye. See Azo Dyes.

BASIC RED 46 • A coal tar color used in hair coloring.

BASIC RED 76 • See Azo Dyes.

BASIC RED 118 • A coal tar color used in hair coloring. An amine color.

BASIC VIOLET 1 • **Methyl Violet.** A bright violet artificial coloring ingredient. See Aniline Dyes for toxicity.

BASIC VIOLET 3 • **Crystal Violet. Methyl Violet. Gentian Violet.** A triarylmethane color. Dark green powder or greenish pieces with a metallic luster, it is used as an antiseptic and against worms as well as a coloring.

BASIC VIOLET 4 • A coal tar hair coloring.

BASIC VIOLET 10 • A xanthene *(see)* color. The salt of stearic acid is Solvent Red 49. The name can be used only when applied to batches of uncertified color. The CTFA adopted name for certified *(see)* batches is D & C Red No. 19, also called rhodamine B. A basic red dye, it is very soluble in water and alcohol and forms a bluish red fluorescent solution. Used as a dye for paper, wool, and silk, and as a biological stain as well as in cosmetics.

BASIC VIOLET 14 • Triphenylmethane Color.

BASIC YELLOW 11 • A triazolium dye. See Azo Dyes.

BASIC YELLOW 28 • A coal tar color.

BASIC YELLOW 57 • **Arianor Straw Yellow.** See Basic Dyes.

"BASICOL"™ • A series of essential oils intended for replacement of oils of lavender, geranium, lemon, pine, ylang-ylang, neroli, and orris root (see all).

BASIL EXTRACT • The extract of the leaves and flowers of *Ocimum basilicum*, an herb having spikes of small white flowers and aromatic leaves used as a seasoning. A natural flavoring distilled from the flowering tops of the plant has a slightly yellowish color and a spicy odor. No known toxicity. GRAS.

BASROSMA BETULINA • See Buchu.

BASSIA LATIFOLIA • **Llipe Butter.** Derived from a small family of European herbs that are also grown in North America.

BASSWOOD EXTRACT • **Tilia.** Extract of the flowers *Tilia americana*.

BATH LOTION • For after a bath. Usually a cologne with some emollient oil. May also contain isopropyl myristate and fatty acids. The emollient oil also acts as a carrier for the perfume. May cause allergic reactions depending upon your sensitivity and the ingredients used.

BATH OIL • Softens and protects the skin in a foaming or nonfoaming oil. The concentration of perfume in bath oil is usually quite high and may be a source of allergic reactions. The oil is usually a mineral or vegetable oil and includes a surfactant to cause the oil to spread on the surface of the water. A common ingredient of the foaming-type of oil is TEA-lauryl sulfate, and sometimes foam stabilizers, such as saponin or methyl cellulose, are used to give the bubbles longevity; also the usual chemicals that are added are castor oil, isopropyl myristate, alcohol, lanolin, and certified colors. A number of the ingredients may cause allergic contact dermatitis, so if you develop a rash, check the label.

BATH SALTS • Used to color, perfume, and chemically soften bath water, and to perfume the skin. Usually made from rock salt or sodium thiosulfate, which has been sprayed with alcohol, dye, or perfume. Rock salt is common table salt and has been used for treating inflammation of the skin. Sodium thiosulfate ("hypo") has been used to treat certain skin rashes and has a low toxicity. The effervescent-type bath salts are due to the added sodium bicarbonate and tartaric acid. The non-effervescent type may add trisodium phosphate and sodium chloride. Among other chemicals that may be in bath salts are borax, sodium hexametaphosphate, starch, sodium carbonate, and sodium sesquicarbonate (see all). Phosphate and borax may cause caustic irritation of the skin and mucous membranes; boric acid may cause poisoning when ingested or absorbed through the skin.

BATYL ALCOHOL • Derived from glycerin (see), it is isolated from shark oil, bone, and bone marrow. It is soluble in fat solvents. No known toxicity.

BATYL ISOSTEARATE • An ester (see) of batyl alcohol and isostearic acid. See Glycerin.

BATYL STEARATE • An ester (see) of batyl alcohol (see).

BAY LAUREL • *Laurus nobilis.* A tree of the laurel family, bay is native to southern Europe, where it can grow to a height of fifty feet. In Roman times, the aromatic quality of the leaves led the Romans to scatter it in buildings to ward off the plague. The bay was one of 400 remedies used by Hippocrates, and through the centuries herbalists have used it to treat hysteria, ague, sprains, earache, and many other illnesses. Every part of the tree has healing properties, according to herbalists. It is used in "organic" cosmetics. See also Bay Oil.

BAY OIL • Oil of Myrcia. Astringent and antiseptic oil used in hair lotions and dressings, after-shave lotions, Bay Rum, and perfumes. Distilled from the leaves of the bayberry, it contains 40 to 55 percent eugenol *(see)*. May cause allergic reactions and skin irritations.

BAY RUM • The alcoholic, aromatic oil distilled from the leaves of the bayberry and mixed with rum or made by mixing oil from the leaves with alcohol, water, and other oils. Widely used as an after-shave preparation and skin freshener. Also used in hair tonics. The basic formula for Bay Rum: bay oil, 0.20 percent; pimenta oil, 0.05 percent; ethyl alcohol, 50 percent; Jamaica rum, 10 percent; water, 39.75 percent; and caramel coloring. Can cause allergic reactions. See Eugenol for toxicity.

BAYBERRY • *Myrica cerifera.* **Candleberry. Waxberry. Wax Myrtle.** The bark contains volatile oil, starch, lignin, albumen, gum, tannic and gallic acids, astringent resins, and an acid resembling saponin. It is used by herbalists as a stimulant, astringent, and expectorant, and to induce sweating. It has been used to treat uterine prolapse and excessive menstrual bleeding and in a douche to treat vaginal infections. It has also been used to stop bleeding from the bowel and from the gums. A famous patent medicine containing bayberry, Dr. Thompson's Composition Powder, was used by many physicians to treat colds, coughs, and flu. There are several modern versions used by herbalists.

BAYBERRY WAX • Acrid and astringent resin from the dried root bark of the shrub that grows from Maryland to Florida and from Texas to Arkansas. It is used as an astringent in soaps and hair tonics. Formerly used to treat skin ulcers. May be irritating to the skin and cause an allergic reaction.

BEAN PALMITATE • The crushed beans of *Phaseolus* (beans) with palmitic acid *(see)*.

BEARBERRY EXTRACT • *Arctostaphylos uva-ursi.* **Uva-Ursi.** An astringent used to treat bladder problems, it is believed its action is due to the high concentration of the antiseptic arbutin. Arbutin, in passing through the system, yields hydroquinone *(see)*, a urinary disinfectant. Uva-ursi leaves also contain anesthetic principles that numb pain in the urinary system, and the herb has been shown to have antibiotic activity. Crude extracts of uva-ursi reportedly possess some anticancer property. In 1992, the FDA proposed a ban on uva-ursi extract in oral menstrual drug products because it has not been shown to be safe and effective for its stated claims.

BEAUTY MASKS • See Face Masks and Packs.

BEE BALM EXTRACT • An extract of the leaves of *Monarda didyma.* Contains bergamot *(see)*. An orange flavoring extracted from a pear-shaped fruit whose rind yields a greenish brown oil. It is used in a tea for digestive problems and as a tonic. It can stain skin and may cause sensitivity to sunlight. See also Lemon Balm.

BEE POLLEN • A popular compound among naturalists, it contains 19 amino acids, up to 35 percent protein, 12 vitamins, calcium, phosphorous, magnesium, iron, copper, manganese, sodium, potassium, chlorine, and sulfur. It is claimed that it increases stamina. Those who are allergic to bee stings may also be allergic to bee pollen. It is used in "organic" cosmetics.

BEER • Used to rinse hair on the theory that it gives a feeling of increased body and manageability. The sugar and protein in the beer are probably responsible for the stiffening effect but, according to the American Medical Association, champagne would have the same effect. Beer leaves an odor on the hair that, unlike champagne, may, after a while, become quite unpleasant. Nontoxic.

BEESWAX • From virgin bees and primarily used as an emulsifier. Practically insoluble in water. Yellow beeswax from the honeycomb is yellowish, soft to brittle, and has a honeylike odor. White beeswax is yellowish white and slightly different in taste but otherwise has the same properties as yellow beeswax. Used in many cosmetics, including baby creams, brilliantine hair dressings, cold cream, emollient creams, wax depilatories, eye creams, eye shadow, foundation creams, and makeup, lipstick, mascara, nail whiteners, protective creams, and paste rouge. Can cause contact dermatitis. The CIR Expert Panel *(see)* concludes this is a safe ingredient.

BEET EXTRACT • The powdered stem base of the beet used for its reddish color in powders and rouges. No longer permitted as a colorant in the United States.

BEETROOT RED • Obtained from the roots of beets, this color is not approved in the United States but is used in European cosmetics.

BEHENALKONIUM CHLORIDE • See Quaternary Ammonium Compounds.

BEHENAMIDE • An amide *(see)* used as a thickening ingredient and an opacifier.

BEHENAMIDOPROPYL BETAINE • See Quaternary Ammonium Compounds and Betaine.

BEHENAMIDOPROPYL DIMETHYLAMINE • See Quaternary Ammonium Compounds.

BEHENAMINE OXIDE • See Behenic Acid.

BEHENETH-5, -10, -20, -30 • The polyethylene glycol ethers of Behenyl Alcohol. See Polyethylene Glycol and Behenyl Alcohol.

BEHENIC ACID • **Docosanoic Acid.** Colorless, water-soluble constituent of seed fats, animal fats, and marine animal oils. It is a fatty acid *(see)* used to opacify shampoos. No known toxicity.

BEHENOXY DIMETHICONE • See Behenic Acid and Silicones.

BEHENOYL PG-TRIMONIUM • A quaternary ammonium compound *(see)*.

BEHENTRIMONIUM CHLORIDE • See Quaternary Ammonium Compounds.

BEHENYL ALCOHOL • **Docosanol.** A mixture of fatty alcohols derived from behenic acid, a minor component of vegetable oils and animal fats. It is used in cosmetics as an opacifying ingredient, thickener, and emulsifier. Used also in synthetic fabrics and lubricants to prevent evaporation of water, and as an insecticide and antihistamine. Low toxicity.

BEHENYL BEHENATE • The ester *(see)* of behenic acid *(see)*.

BEHENYL BENZOATE • The ester *(see)* of Behenyl Benzoate. See Benzoic Acid. Used as a skin-conditioning ingredient.

BEHENYL BETAINE • See Behenic Acid and Betaine.

BEHENYL ERUCATE • Used in lipstick. See Behenic Acid and Erucic Acid.

BEHENYL HYDROXYETHYL IMIDAZOLINE • See Imidazoline.

BELAMCANDA CHINENSIS • Blackberry Lily. Freckle Face Leopard Flower. A plant material from China that grows in woods and creeks. It is used in Chinese medicine to treat sore throats and soothe mucous membranes.

BELLIS PERENNIS • Daisy Extract. The fresh or dried flowers of this plant, which is cultivated or grows wild all over North America, are used in an infusion or tincture. The flowers contain saponins, tannin, essential oil, flavones, bitter principle, and mucilage *(see all)*. Daisy is used for coughs and inflammations of the mucous lining. It reputedly also helps arthritis, as well as liver and kidney problems.

BENTONITE • A white clay found in the midwestern United States and in Canada. Used to thicken lotions, to suspend makeup pigments, and to emulsify oils, and used in makeup lotions, liquid makeup, and facial masks to absorb oil on the face and reduce shine. Also used as a coloring. Inert and generally nontoxic, but if injected in rats, it can be fatal.

BENZALDEHYDE • Artificial Almond Oil. A colorless liquid that occurs in the kernels of bitter almonds. Lime is used in its synthetic manufacture. As the artificial essential oil of almonds, it is used in cosmetic creams and lotions, perfumes, soaps, and dyes. May cause allergic reactions. Highly toxic.

BENZALKONIUM CHLORIDE (BAK) • A widely used ammonium detergent (*see* Ammonium) in hair tonics, eye lotions, deodorants, mouthwashes, and aftershave lotions. It is a germicide with an aromatic odor and a very bitter taste. Soluble in water and alcohol but incompatible with most detergents and soaps. Used medicinally as a topical antiseptic and detergent. Allergic conjunctivitis has been reported when used in eye lotions. Lethal to frogs in concentrated oral doses. Highly toxic. In 1992, the FDA proposed a ban on the use of benzalkonium chloride to treat insect bites and stings and in astringent *(see)* drugs because it has not been shown to be safe and effective for stated claims in OTC products. It is a skin and eye irritant at concentrations greater than 0.1 percent. It is used in some cosmetic products at up to 5 percent. The CIR Expert Panel *(see)* concludes this is a safe ingredient if used at concentrations up to 0.1 percent.

BENZENE • A solvent obtained from coal and used in nail polish remover. Also used in varnishes, airplane glue, and lacquers, and as a solvent for waxes, resins, and oils. Highly flammable. Poisonous when ingested and irritating to the mucous membranes. Harmful amounts may be absorbed through the skin. Also can cause sensitivity to light in which the skin may break out in a rash or swell. Inhalation of the fumes may be toxic. The Consumer Product Safety Commission voted unanimously in February 1978 to ban the use of benzene in the manufacture of many household products. The commission took the action in response to a petition filed by the Consumer Health Research Group, an organization affiliated with consumer advocate Ralph Nader. Earlier in the year, OSHA and the EPA both cited benzene as a threat to public health. For more than a century, scientists have known that benzene is a powerful bone-marrow poison, causing such conditions as aplastic anemia. In the past several decades evidence has been mounting that it also causes leukemia. Derived from toluene or gasoline, it is used in the manufacture of detergents, nylon, and artificial leather; as an antiknock ingredient in gasoline; in airplane fuel, varnish, and lacquer; and as a solvent for waxes, resins, and oils. It has a chronic effect on bone marrow, destroying the marrow's ability to produce blood cells. Safety standards for cosmetic manufacturing workers and other workers have been set at 10 parts per million during an eight-hour day, but OSHA wants it reduced to 1 part per million.

1,2,4-BENZENETRIACETATE • See Benzene and Triacetic Acid.

BENZETHONIUM CHLORIDE • An antistatic ingredient, deodorant, and cleansing ingredient. See Quaternary Ammonium Compounds.

BENZOATE • See Sodium Benzoate.

BENZOCAINE • **Ethyl Aminobenzoate.** A white, crystalline powder slightly soluble in water and a local anesthetic. Used in eyebrow-plucking creams and after-shave lotions. As an anesthetic, it is reported low in toxicity. However, there are reports of babies suffering from methemoglobinemia (lack of oxygen in the blood) due to absorption of benzocaine through the skin. But it is believed that the absorption was enhanced by inflamed skin or rectal fissures. Systemic central nervous system excitation has been reported in adults. However, scientists feel that the concentrations in most products have no toxic significance, though there are people who are allergic to benzocaine.

BENZODIHYDROPYRONE • **Dihydrocoumarin.** White to light yellow, oily liquid with a sweet odor. Used in perfumery.

BENZOIC ACID • A preservative that occurs in nature in cherry bark, raspberries, tea, anise, and cassia bark. First described in 1608, when it was found in gum benzoin. Used in chocolate, lemon, orange, cherry, fruit, nut, and tobacco flavorings for beverages, ice cream, ices, candy, baked goods, icings, and chewing gum. Also used in margarine. Also an antifungal ingredient. A mild irritant to the skin, it can cause allergic reactions. In 1992, the FDA proposed a ban on benzoic acid in astringent *(see)* drug products because it has not been shown to be safe and effective for its stated claims.

BENZOIN • See Gum Benzoin.

BENZOPHENONES (1–12) • At least a dozen different benzophenones exist. They are used as fixatives *(see)* for heavy perfumes (geranium, for example) and soaps (the smell of "new-mown hay"). Obtained as a white, flaky solid with a delicate, persistent, roselike odor, and soluble in most fixed oils and in mineral oil. Also used in the manufacture of hairsprays and in sunscreens. They help prevent deterioration of ingredients that might be affected by the ultraviolet rays found in ordinary daylight. May produce hives and contact sensitivity. In sunscreens they may cause immediate hives as well as other photoallergic reactions. Toxic when injected. The CIR Expert Panel *(see)* concludes this is a safe ingredient in the present practices of use and concentration.

BENZOQUINE • See Oxyquinoline and Benzoic Acid.

BENZOXYQUINE • **Benzoxiquine. 8-Hydroxyquinoline Benzoate.** A water-soluble salt of benzoic acid *(see)*. Used as an antiseptic. Also used medicinally in the treatment of dysentery. Toxic when ingested. The CIR Expert Panel *(see)* concludes the safety of this ingredient has not been documented and substantiated and that the Panel states that it cannot "conclude that this ingredient is safe for use in cosmetic products until the appropriate safety data have been obtained and evaluated."

BENZOYL BENZENE • A fixative for heavy perfumes such as geranium, especially when used in soaps. See Benzophenones.

BENZOYL PEROXIDE • A bleaching ingredient for flours, blue cheese, gorgonzola, and milk. A catalyst for hardening certain fiberglass resins. A drying ingredient in cosmetics. Toxic by inhalation. A skin allergen and irritant.

BENZYL ACETATE • A colorless liquid with a pear or flowerlike odor obtained from a number of plants, especially jasmine, for use in perfumery and soap. Can be irritating to the skin, eyes, and respiratory tract. Ingestion causes intestinal upset, including vomiting and diarrhea.

BENZYL ALCOHOL • A solvent in perfumes, a preservative in hair dyes, and a topical antiseptic. It is derived as a pure alcohol and is a constituent of jasmine, hyacinth, and other plants. It has a faint, sweet odor. Irritating and corrosive to the skin and mucous membranes. Ingestion of large doses causes intestinal upsets. In sensitive people, it may cross-react with Balsam Peru *(see)*.

BENZYL BENZOATE • Plasticizer in nail polishes, solvent, and fixative for perfumes. Occurs naturally in Balsam Tolu and Balsam Peru and in various flower oils. Colorless, oily liquid or white crystals with a light floral scent and sharp, burning taste. No known toxicity.

BENZYL CINNAMATE • **Sweet Odor of Balsam.** Colorless prisms, used to give artificial fruit scents to perfumes. See Balsam Peru for toxicity.

BENZYL ETHYL ETHER • Colorless, oily liquid; aromatic odor; insoluble in water; miscible in alcohol. Used in flavoring. Narcotic in high concentrations. May be a skin irritant.

BENZYL FORMATE • A synthetic flavoring ingredient used for its pleasant fruit odor in perfumery. Practically insoluble in water. There is no specific data for toxicity, but it is believed to be narcotic in high concentrations.

BENZYL HYALURONATE • A skin conditioner. See Hyaluronic Acid and Benzyl Alcohol.

BENZYL LAURATE • The salt of lauric acid *(see)*.

BENZYL NICOTINATE • See Benzyl Alcohol and Niacin.

BENZYL PARABEN • A preservative. The CIR Expert Panel *(see)* concludes that the available data are insufficient to support the safety of benzyl paraben as used in cosmetics. See Parabens.

BENZYL PROPIONATE • Similar to benzyl acetate *(see)*, but has a sweeter odor. Used in perfumes and as a flavoring.

BENZYL SALICYLATE • **Salicylic Acid.** A fixative in perfumes and a solvent in sunscreen lotions. It is a thick liquid with a light, pleasant odor, and is mixed with alcohol or ether. May cause skin to break out in a rash and swell when exposed to sunlight. See Salicylates.

BENZYLHEMIOFORMAL • A germicide. See Gum Benzoin.

3-BENZYLIDENE CAMPHOR • **Bicyclo [2,2.1] Heptan-2-one.** See Benzaldehyde and Camphor Oil.

BENZYLTRIMONIUM HYDROLYZED COLLAGEN • The benzyl trimethyl ammonium salt of hydrolyzed animal protein. The word "animal" was taken out of the label listings. See Quaternary Ammonium Compounds and Surfactants.

BERBERINE • Mild antiseptic and decongestant in eye lotions. Derived as yellow crystals from various plants. Relatively inactive physiologically, but ingestion of large quantities may cause fatal poisoning. Used as a dressing for skin ulcers.

BERBERIS • **Holly-leafed Barberry. Oregon Grape Root. Mountain Grape.** The dried roots of shrubs grown in the United States and British Columbia. Used medicinally to soothe skin ulcers and to break up intestinal gas. Used in creams as a mild antiseptic and decongestant. See Berberine for toxicity.

BERGAMOT, RED • **Oswego Tea.** A pear-shaped orange whose rind yields a greenish brown oil much used in perfumery and brilliantine hairdressings. It can cause brown skin stains (berloque) when exposed to sunlight and is considered a prime photosensitizer (sensitivity to light). See Berloque Dermatitis.

BERLOQUE DERMATITIS • Some perfumes, which contain oil of bergamot *(see)* and other photosensitizers, may produce increased pigmentation (brown spots) in the area where the perfume has been applied, especially when it is immediately exposed to sunlight. There is no effective treatment, and the pigmentation generally persists for some time.

BETA-CAROTENE • **Provitamin A. Beta Carotene.** Found in all plants and in many animal tissues. It is the chief yellow coloring matter of carrots, butter, and egg yolk. Extracted as red crystals or crystalline powder. It is used as a coloring in cosmetics. Also used in the manufacture of Vitamin A. Too much carotene in the blood can lead to carotenemia, a pale yellow-red pigmentation of the skin that may be mistaken for jaundice. It is a benign condition, and withdrawal of carotene from the diet cures it. Nontoxic on the skin.

BETAGLUCANS • Polysaccharides *(see)* that yield sugars (glucose) on hydrolysis when exposed to water treatment. Betaglucan is in cellulose and is found in edibles such as oat fiber and barley. Used as a thickener and as a skin conditioner.

BETAINES • Occurs in common beets and in many vegetables as well as animal substances. Used in resins, as emulsifiers, detergents, foam boosters, thickeners, and skin and hair conditioners. Has been employed to treat muscle weakness medically. No known toxicity. Coco Betaine *(see)* is an example.

BETA-NAPHTHOL • Used in hair dyes, skin-peeling preparations, and hair tonics. Prepared from naphthalene, which comes from coal tar. Also used in perfumes. Oral ingestion may cause kidney damage, eye injury, vomiting, diarrhea, convulsions, anemia, and death. Fatal poisoning from external applications has been reported. Local application may produce peeling of the skin, which may be followed by pigmentation, also contact dermatitis. See Naphthas.

BETA-SITOSTEROL • Common sterol *(see)* in plants. Isolated from wheat germ, rye germ, or cottonseed oils. Used medically to treat high cholesterol and prostate tumors. It is used in cosmetics as a skin conditioner.

BETA VULGARIS • See Beet Extract.

BETULA • Obtained from the European white birch and a source of asphalt and tar. Used in hair tonics; it reddens the scalp and creates a warm feeling due to an increased flow of blood to the area. Also used in moisturizing creams and astringents. Betula leaves were formerly used to treat rheumatism. See Salicylates.

BHA • See Butylated Hydroxyanisole.

BHT • See Butylated Hydroxytoluene.

BICARBONATE OF SODA • See Sodium Bicarbonate.

BICHLORIDE OF MERCURY • See Mercury Compounds.

BIFIDA FERMENT LYSATE • A product of the fermentation of *Bifida* used as a skin conditioner. See Bifidus Factor.

BIFIDUS FACTOR • *Lactobacillus bifidus.* A bacteria found in the intestinal tract of breast-fed infants. It is prepared from the gastric mucosa of pigs and is used as a dietetic adjuvant in infant foods. It is also used in cosmetic emollients.

BILBERRY EXTRACT • Grown in the Alps and Scandinavia, this fruit is used by folk medicine practitioners to improve night vision. A number of modern studies have shown that bilberry anthocyanins (the blue-coloring chemicals) given orally improve vision in healthy people and also help treat people with eye diseases. The anthocyanins contained in bilberry act to prevent blood vessel fragility and inhibit blood clot formation. It has been reported that bilberry increases prostaglandin *(see)* release from arterial tissue, which dilates blood vessels. Bilberry also contains arbutin *(see),* a diuretic and anti-infective derived from the dried leaves.

BILE SALTS • The salts of bile acids are powerful cleansing ingredients and aid in the absorption of fats from the intestines.

BINDER • A substance such as gum arabic, gum tragacanth, glycerin, and sorbitol *(see all),* which dispenses, swells, or absorbs water, increases consistency, and holds ingredients together. For example, binders are used to make powders in compacts retain their shape; binders in toothpaste provide for the smooth dispensing of the paste.

BIOCIDE • An ingredient to cleanse the skin and prevent odor by inhibiting the growth of bacteria, fungi, or yeast.

BIOFLAVONOIDS • **Vitamin P Complex.** Citrus-flavored compounds needed to maintain healthy blood vessel walls. Widely distributed among plants, especially citrus fruits and rose hips. Usually taken from orange and lemon rinds and used as a reducing ingredient *(see).* No known toxicity.

BIOSACCHARIDE GUM-1 • A fermentation gum derived from Sorbitol *(see),* used as a skin conditioner.

BIOTIN • **Vitamin H. Vitamin B Factor.** A whitish, crystalline powder used as a texturizer in cosmetic creams. Present in minute amounts in every living cell and in larger amounts in yeast and milk. Vital to growth. It acts as a coenzyme in the formation of certain essential fatlike substances and plays a part in reactions involving carbon dioxide. It is needed by humans for healthy circulation and red blood cells. Nontoxic.

BIRCH FAMILY • *Betulaceae.* Used as an astringent in creams and shampoos, it is an ancient remedy. The medicinal properties of the plant tend to vary, depending upon which part of the tree is used. It has been used as a laxative, as an aid for gout, to treat rheumatism and dropsy, and to dissolve kidney stones. It is supposedly good for bathing skin eruptions. The oil is used in food flavorings. See Betula.

BISABOL • **Opopanax.** A myrrh-type gum resin obtained from African trees. No known toxicity.

BISABOLOL • **Dragosantol.** Derived from Chamomile *(see)* or made synthetically, it is an anti-irritant. The CIR Expert Panel *(see)* concludes this is a safe ingredient in the present practices of use and concentration.

BIS-DIGLYCERYL   CAPRYLATE/CAPRATE/ISOSTEARATE/HYDROXY-STEARATE ADIPATE • A gel made from stearic acid and adipic acid.

4,6-BIS (2-HYDROXYETHOXY)-m-PHENYLENEDIAMINE HCL • A coal tar hair coloring.

2,6-BIS (2-HYDROXYETHOXY)-3-5PYRIDINEDIAMINE HCL • A coal tar dye. An amine.

N,N-BIS-2-HYDROXYETHYL-p-PHENELENEDIAMINE SULFATE • It has produced strong sensitization in both guinea pigs and humans. The CIR Expert Panel *(see)* concludes this is a safe ingredient in the present practices of use and concentration. See Phenylenediamine.

BISHYDROXYETHYL BISCETYL MALONAMIDE • A fatty alcohol used as a skin conditioner. See Malonic Acid.

BIS-HYDROXYETHYL RAPESEEDMONIUM CHLORIDE • A quaternary ammonium compound used as an antistatic ingredient. See Ammonium Quaternary Compounds.

BISMARK BROWN • Prepared from phenylenediamine *(see)* and nitrous acid, it is a basic brown color that is used in dyeing silk, wool, and leather. Can cause contact dermatitis.

BISMUTH CITRATE • Coloring restricted to hair dye only. See Bismuth Compounds.

BISMUTH COMPOUNDS • **Subgallate, Subnitrate, Oxychloride.** Bismuth is a gray-white powder with a bright metallic luster. It occurs in the earth's crust and for many years was used to treat syphilis. Bismuth subgallate, a dark gray, odorless, tasteless form, is used as an antiseptic and in dusting powder. Bismuth subnitrate is odorless and tasteless, and is used in bleaching and freckle creams and hair dyes. Bismuth oxychloride is sometimes called "synthetic pearl" and is used as a skin protective. Most bismuth compounds used in cosmetics have a low toxicity when ingested but may cause allergic reactions when applied to the skin. In 1992, the FDA proposed a ban on bismuth subnitrate in fever blister and cold sore treatment products and poison ivy, poison oak, and poison sumac OTC products because it has not been shown to be safe and effective for its stated claims.

BISMUTH OXYCHLORIDE • Permanently listed as a coloring in 1977. See Bismuth Compounds.

BISPHENYLHEXAMETHICONE • A silicone *(see)* used as an antifoaming agent, skin conditioner, and emollient.

BISPYRITHIONE • A germ killer. See Pyrethrum.

BISTORT EXTRACT • The extract of the roots of *Polygonum bistorta,* an herb found in Europe and North America. The roots are used as an astringent. No known toxicity.

BISULFITES • Bisulfite straighteners or curl relaxers are used instead of the thioglycolates *(see* Thioglycolic Acid). They produce changes in the chemical bonds in the hair. The effectiveness of the bisulfite relaxers is similar to that of hot combing, but it is more permanent. The result is equivalent to the caustic alkali straighteners and superior to the thioglycolate method. Less irritating to the scalp and less damaging to the hair than other methods, but should not be used if the scalp or skin is sensitive, scaly, scratched, sore, or tender. Harmful effects frequently result from not following directions. See also Sodium Bisulfite.

BITHIONOL • Used as a germicide in cold creams, emollients, hair tonics, aftershave lotions, and medicated cosmetics. It is closely related to hexachlorophene, which has been banned by the FDA. Bithionol has been removed from many products sold in the United States because it causes a sensitivity to light; the skin breaks out with a rash and may swell.

BITTER ALMOND OIL • **Almond Oil. Sweet Almond Oil. Expressed Almond Oil.** A colorless to pale yellow, bland, nearly odorless, essential and expressed oil from the ripe seed of the small sweet almond grown in Italy, Spain, and France. It has a strong almond odor and a mild taste. Used in the manufacture of perfumes and as an oil in hair creams, nail whiteners, nail polish remover, eye creams, emollients, soaps, and perfumes. Many users are allergic to cosmetics with almond oil. It causes stuffy nose and skin rashes.

BITTER CHERRY EXTRACT • *Prunus cerasus.* Used for its Vitamin C component and as a flavoring and a scent.

BITTER ORANGE OIL • The pale yellow volatile oil expressed from the fresh peel of a species of citrus and used in perfumes and flavorings. May cause skin irritation and allergic reactions.

BITTER PRINCIPLE • Any of a group of chemicals in plants that are very bitter tasting. They differ chemically but most belong to the iris or pine families. Bitter principles reputedly stimulate the secretion of digestive juices and stimulate the liver. They are being investigated scientifically today as antifungals and antibiotics as well as anticancer ingredients. The bitter principle in mallow plants is being investigated as a male contraceptive. Other bitter principles in herbs are used to combat coughs and as sedatives.

BITTERS • Usually refers to an alcohol prepared from parts of bitter herbs. Used as a mild tonic or stimulant to improve appetite. Also used as a flavoring agent.

BIXA ORELLANA • A solvent extraction of *Bixa orellana L. seeds.* A yellow carotenoid *(see)* solution or powder, it is a color additive in ink used for marking foods, and in oleomargarine, poultry, sausage casings, and shortening. May cause contact dermatitis.

BLACK • Inorganic carbon black and iron oxide used to color face powders. Carbon black from carbon or charcoal. Not subject to certification *(see)*. See Colors.

BLACKBERRY • *Rubus fruiticosus*. The berries, leaves, and root bark are used to treat fevers, colds, sore throats, vaginal discharge, diarrhea, and dysentery. The berries contain isocitric and malic acids, sugars, pectin, monoglycoside of cyanidin, and Vitamins C and A. The leaves and bark are said to lower fever; they are astringent and stop bleeding. The leaves are used in "organic" bath products to soothe and refresh the skin. No known toxicity. See Malic Acid.

BLACK COHOSH • **Cimicifuga. Snakeroot. Bugbane.** Used in astringents, it is a perennial herb with a flower that is supposedly distasteful to insects. Grown from Canada to North Carolina and Kansas. It has a reputation for curing snakebite. It is used in ginger ale flavoring. A tonic and antispasmodic. No known toxicity. See also Cohosh Root.

BLACK CURRANT EXTRACT • The extract of the fruit of *Ribes nigrum,* a European plant that produces hanging yellow flowers and black aromatic fruit.

BLACK LOCUST • Extract of *Robinia Pseudocacia*. **Black Locust Extract. Acacia Glycolystat.** The fragrant flowers can be smelled for hundreds of feet in the spring. The bruised foliage mixed with sugar attracts and kills flies.

BLACK MUSTARD EXTRACT • *Brassica nigra. Sinapis alba.* **Koch. Boiss.** A native of Europe and the Americas, it is cultivated in Holland, Italy, and Germany as a condiment. It is used medicinally to treat arthritis, sciatica, and other pains. It was also used as an emetic to counteract ingested poisons. Mustard seeds are used to stimulate appetite. Mustard plasters were a popular treatment for pains and swelling. It is used in footbaths and to treat cold. Mustard is rapidly absorbed and used as a counterirritant *(see)*. It is irritating to the skin and can cause burns that are slow to heal.

BLACK POPLAR • See Poplar Extract.

BLACK THORN • *Prunus Spinosa*. A European tree or shrub that has hard wood and bears small white flowers and small purplish or blue-black astringent fruits. Used in astringents.

BLACK WALNUT EXTRACT • Extract of the leaves or bark of the black walnut tree, *Juglans nigra,* found in eastern North America. It produces nuts with a thick oil and is used as a black coloring.

BLACKSTRAP POWDER • Obtained from sugarcane in the processes of sugar manufacture. It is a natural flavoring ingredient. No known toxicity.

BLADDER WRACK EXTRACT • **Fucus. Sea Wrack.** A common black rockweed used in cosmetics such as tanning lotions. No known toxicity.

BLANC FIXE • See Barium Sulfate.

BLEACH • See Hair Bleach and Skin Bleach.

BLEMISH COVER • Pimple and undereye covers come in stick or cream form. Based on oil, wax, and alcohol. Usually contain titanium dioxide *(see)* and pigments. Applied before makeup to cover marks, dark circles under the eyes, or other minor blemishes.

BLESSED THISTLE EXTRACT • *Cnicus benedictus.* **Holy Thistle.** The thistle contains tannin *(see),* lactone, mucilage *(see),* and essential oil. It is used by herbalists to treat stomach and liver complaints. It reputedly breaks up blood clots, relieves jaundice and hepatitis, and stops bleeding. It increases appetite and lowers fevers. The FDA issued a notice in 1992 that blessed thistle has not been shown to be safe and effective as claimed in OTC digestive aid products or in oral menstrual drugs.

BLETIA HYACINTHINA EXTRACT • It is the extract of the fragrant flower, a tropical orchid. Used in fragrances.

BLOOD ROOT • *Sanguinaria canadensis.* **Redroot. Red Indian Paint. Tetterwort.** The root contains isoquinoline alkaloids including sanguinaria and berberine. Herbalists use it to treat coughs, sore throats, skin eruptions, skin cancer, athlete's foot, and gum disease. The root is emetic and purgative in large doses. In smaller doses it is a stimulant, diaphoretic, and expectorant. See also Berberis.

BLUE ALGAE • See Haslea Ostrearia. A rich source of Vitamin E, zinc, iron, and copper. It reportedly has a soothing effect on the skin. It is used in "antiaging" products.

BLUE COHOSH • **Squawroot. Blueberry Root. Papooseroot.** A tall herb of eastern North America and Asia, it has three pointed leaves and a small, greenish yellow or purple flower. It produces large blueberrylike fruits. The roots were formerly used as an antiseptic. No known toxicity. See also Cohosh Root.

BLUE FLAG • *Iris versicolor.* **Flag Lily. Fleur-de-lis. Liver Lily. Poison Flag. Wild Iris.** The rhizome contains salicylic *(see)* and isophthalic acids, volatile oil, iridin, a glycoside *(see),* gum, resin, and sterols. Herbalists use it as a cathartic and emetic, and to treat liver complaints, swollen glands, hepatitis, jaundice, skin diseases, and loss of appetite. Promoted in herbal medicines as both relaxing and stimulating.

BLUEBERRY EXTRACT • *Vaccinum myrtillus.* See Bilberry Extract.

BLUE NO. 1 • See FD & C Blue No. 1.

BLUE VIOLET • **Ultramarine Blue. Ultramarine Violet.** Used in ivory face powders. Originally made from lapis lazuli. See Ultramarine Blue.

BLUSHER • Used to put color on cheeks and on other parts of the face. Powder blushers are similar to pressed powder in composition but include lake colors *(see).* Stick blushers are similar in composition to lipsticks *(see).*

BODY-NOTE • The main and characteristic overall odor of a perfume. It has a much longer life than the top-note *(see)* and usually contributes to the dry-out *(see).*

BOIS DE ROSE OIL • A fragrance from the chipped wood of the tropical rosewood tree obtained through steam distillation. The volatile oil is colorless or pale yellow, with a light camphor odor. It is also used as a food flavoring. No known toxicity.

BOMBYX • Extract of the silk worm secretions. See Silk.

BONE MARROW LIPIDS • The soft, spongy center of the bone that acts like a factory to produce white blood cells, the primary ingredients of the body's immune system. The fatty substance contained in bovine bone marrow form is used in cosmetics as a skin conditioner and emollient.

BORAGE EXTRACT • The extract of the herb *Borago officinalis*. Contains potassium and calcium. It has emollient properties and is used in a "tea" for sore eyes.

BORAGO • The extract of the herb *Borago officinalis*. Contains potassium and calcium and has emollient properties and is used in a "tea" for sore eyes. Used in cosmetics as a skin conditioner.

BORATES • Widely used as antiseptic ingredients and preservatives in cosmetics in spite of repeated warnings by medical scientists. Acute poisonings have followed ingestion, injection, enemas, lavage of body cavities, and application of powders and ointments to burned and abraded skin. Borates affect the central nervous system, gastrointestinal tract, kidneys, liver, and skin.

BORAX • **Sodium Borate.** A mild alkali found in the Far West, particularly in Death Valley, California. Used in cold creams, foundation creams, hair color rinses, permanent waves, and shaving creams. It is used as a water softener, as a preservative, and as a texturizer in cream products. Also used to prevent irritation of the skin by the antiperspirant aluminum chloride *(see)*. See Boric Acid for toxicity.

BORIC ACID • An antiseptic with bactericidal and fungicidal properties used in baby powders, bath powders, eye creams, liquid powders, mouthwashes, protective creams, after-shave lotions, soaps, and skin fresheners. It is still widely used despite repeated warnings from the American Medical Association of possible toxicity. Severe poisonings have followed both ingestion and topical application to abraded skin. It is used to treat external ear canal infection by inhibiting bacteria present in the ear canal. It is used for temporary relief of chapped, chafed, or dry skin, diaper rash, abrasions, minor burns, sunburn, insect bites, and other skin irritations. Contraindicated in perforated eardrum or broken skin. In 1992, researchers at the Developmental and Reproductive Toxicology Group, U.S. National Institute of Environmental Health Sciences, reported that developmental toxicity of boric acid in mice occurred below maternally toxic levels in rats and mice and adversely affected the fetuses. The Food and Drug Administration issued a notice in 1992 that boric acid has not been shown to be safe and effective for stated claims in OTC products, including astringent *(see)* drug products and fever blister and cold sore treatments and poison ivy, poison oak, and poison sumac drug products. The CIR Expert Panel says based on available data, it is safe as a cosmetic ingredient at less than or equal to 5 percent; however, cosmetic formulations containing free sodium boric acid at this concentration should not be used on infant skin or injured skin.

BORNELONE • **UV Absorber-4.** A compound that protects a cosmetic product from deterioration by ultraviolet light. See Borneol and Pentane.

BORNEOL • Used in perfumery, it has a peppery odor and a burning taste. Occurs naturally in coriander, ginger oil, oil of lime, rosemary, strawberries, thyme, citronella, and nutmeg. Toxicity is similar to camphor oil *(see)*.

BORNYL ACETATE • A colorless liquid derived from borneol *(see),* it is used in perfumery and flavoring and as a solvent.

BORNYL FORMATE • Used in perfumes, soaps, and as a disinfectant. See Borneol.

BORON • Occurs in the earth's crust in the form of its compounds, never as the element. It is used in dietary supplements up to 1 mg. per day. Salts of boron are widely used as antiseptics even though toxicologists warn about possible adverse reactions. Borates are absorbed by the mucous membranes and can cause such symptoms as gastrointestinal bleeding, skin rash, and central nervous system stimulation. The adult lethal dose is one ounce. A preparation promoted as "anti-aging" contains 2 mg. of boron in a vitamin and mineral supplement—it is claimed that it increases the production of testosterone.

BOSWELLIA CARTERII AND SERRATA • *Olibanum.* **Frankincense Extract.** The extract of *Boswellia carterii* of various species. The volatile, distilled oil from the gum resin of a plant found in Ethiopia, Egypt, and Arabia. It was one of the Gifts of the Magi. It is used in cola, fruit, and spice flavorings for beverages, ice cream, ices, candy, and baked goods.

BOTANICALS • Cosmetic ingredients derived directly from plants and include extracts, juices, waters, distillates, powders, oils, waxes, gels, saps, tars, gums, proteins, starches, and resins. They have generally not undergone chemical processing. The FDA expressed concern about this category because many botanicals were showing up on the market about which little is known as far as effects on human physiology.

BOUGAINVILLEA • A woody plant with ornamental tropical red or purple flowers. Used in "organic" cosmetics. May cause hives.

BOXWOOD • *Cornus florida.* **Dogwood. Green Ozier.** A small tree found in all parts of the United States, the bark possesses astringent, stimulant, and tonic properties. The bark was used in the treatment of malaria, especially when the cinchona bark was unavailable.

BOYSENBERRY • *Rubus Deliclosus.* A very large fruit with a flavor like raspberry. Used as a flavoring.

BRAIN EXTRACT and LIPIDS • The extract of bovine brains. Used in "antiaging" creams.

BRASSICA • See Mustard Oil.

BRAZIL NUT OIL • The oil expressed from the nuts of the Brazil nut tree, *Bertholletia excelsa.* Used in skin conditioners and as an emollient.

BRAZILWOOD • **Redwood. Pernambuco Wood.** Grown in Brazil and used in the manufacture of red lake pigment, which produces warm brown shades in hair colorings. See Colors.

BREATH FRESHENERS • Most breath fresheners contain flavoring, artificial sweeteners, water, and alcohol. They are used in glass or plastic bottles that measure out small amounts or are sprayed from aerosols. However, the propellants in the aerosols may be toxic when used in excess. The spray is really propelled mouthwash.

BREVOORTIA • See Menhaden Oil.

BREWER'S YEAST • Originally used by beer brewers, it is a good source of B vitamins and protein. It can cause allergic reactions.

BRIDEWORT • See *Filipendula rubra*.

BRILLIANT BLACK 1 • A diazo *(see)* color.

BRILLIANTINES • Hairdressings that impart a shine to the hair. Cream brilliantines are usually made of mineral oil (25 percent), beeswax, triethanolamine stearate, and water (65 percent). Liquid brilliantine is composed of mineral oil (75 percent) and isopropyl myristate. Solid brilliantines are made of mineral oil, petrolatum, and paraffin. So-called two-layer dressings contain mineral oil, alcohol, and water. They also may contain antiseptics such as cetyl alcohol, cholesterol, gums such as tragacanth, lanolin, oil of bergamot, and other essential oils, olive oil, synthetic oils, synthetic thickeners, and tars. Toxicity depends upon individual ingredients.

BROMATES • A salt of bromic acid, used in permanent wave neutralizers. Bromates are used as maturing ingredients and conditioners in bread. Severe poisoning has followed ingestion and topical application to abraded skin.

BROMELAIN • Bromelin. A protein-digesting and milk-clotting enzyme found in pineapple. Used for tenderizing meat, chill-proofing beer, and as an anti-inflammatory medication. Solutions consisting of water, salt, monosodium glutamate, and approved proteolytic enzymes applied or injected into cuts of beef shall not result in a gain of more than 3 percent of the weight of the untreated product according to the FDA. A search of the toxicology literature concerning this additive has not yet been performed by the FDA's data bank.

BROMELIA BALANSEA • A tropical American plant. See Pineapple Juice.

BROMIDES, POTASSIUM AND SODIUM • A group of sedative drugs now used only rarely. Potassium bromide has been used medically as a sedative and anticonvulsant. Sodium bromide has been used as a sedative and a sleep inducer. The bromides can cause skin rashes. Large doses of the bromides can cause central nervous system depression, and prolonged intake may cause mental deterioration. The use of sodium or potassium bromide in OTC sleep aids was determined to be ineffective in 1991, and manufacturers had to reformulate or have their products banned.

BROMINE • A dark, reddish brown liquid derived from seawater and natural brines by oxidation of bromine salts. Toxic by ingestion and inhalation. It reacts with many metals to form bromides *(see)*.

BROMO ACID • See D & C Red No. 21.

BROMOCHLOROPHENE • A germicide and deodorant agent. See Chlorophene.

BROMOCRESOL GREEN • This coal tar coloring is not listed for use in the United States but is in Europe.

5-BROMO 5-NITRO-1,3-DIOXANE • Bronidox L®. Preservative. May release formaldehyde *(see)*. Significant skin and eye irritation has been observed in animal studies at concentrations higher than 0.1 percent. There is concern that it can form cancer-causing nitrosamines *(see)*. The CIR Expert Panel *(see)* concludes this is "a safe ingredient at concentrations up to 0.1 percent except under circumstances where its action with amines or amides can result in the formation of nitrosamines."

2-BROMO-2-NITROPANE-1,3-DIOL • A preservative. The CIR Expert Panel *(see)* concludes this is "a safe ingredient at concentrations up to 0.1 percent except under circumstances where its action with amines or amides can result in the formation of nitrosamines." See Bronopol®.

BROMOTHYMOL BLUE • This coal tar color is not approved for use in the United States but is in Europe.

BRONOPOL® • **Bronosol.** Odorless crystals from chloroform widely used as a preservative in cosmetics and toiletries. In European tests the incidence of sensitization to this ingredient was considered to be lower than to parabens *(see)*. Solvent used for nail polishes, fats, oils, and dyes. Also used as an intermediate *(see)* in the manufacture of cosmetics and as a propellant. It inhibits the growth of bacteria, fungi, and yeasts. It is used as a preservative for a wide variety of cosmetics, especially shampoos, creams, lotions, rinses, and eye makeup. It can form nitrosamine or nitrosamide when acting with amines or amides such as triethanolamine or its salts. Of 191 samples tested, 77 contained the powerful cancer-causing ingredient N-Nitrosodiethanolamine (NDELA). The preservative also breaks down at neutral and alkaline pHs to produce formaldehyde and one or two or more bromo compounds. Formaldehyde is a suspected carcinogen. Therefore, if you see it listed as an ingredient with another compound ending in "amine" or "amide," don't purchase it. It is fifth on the list of preservatives that cause contact dermatitis, according to the American College of Dermatology Test Trays.

BRONZE POWDER • Any metal such as a copper alloy or aluminum in fine flakes and used as a pigment to give the appearance of a metallic surface. Used in hair coloring to give a shine and as a "frost," or "pearl," in other cosmetics. No known toxicity. Permanently listed as a cosmetic coloring in 1977.

BROOM OIL • *Cytisus scoparius. Sarothamnus scoparius.* **Scoparius. Scotch Broom. Spartium. Witch's Broom.** A shrub, it has long been used by herbalists as a diuretic and cathartic. It is emetic in large doses.

BROWN MUSTARD EXTRACT • See Mustard Oil.

BRUCINE SULFATE • Salt of the poison taken from the seeds of the strychnos shrub. It has a very bitter taste and is used primarily for denaturing alcohols and oils used in cosmetics, and has been patented. As poisonous as strychnine when ingested. On the skin toxicity is unknown.

BRUSHLESS LATHER • See Brushless Shaving Cream.

BRUSHLESS SHAVING CREAM • Not a soaplike lather shaving cream, but a vanishing or cold cream with additional lubricants added. Because lather creams soften the beard and brushless creams do not, one has to towel the face to effect some softening. Brushless creams usually contain 10 to 20 percent stearic acid *(see)*, 3 to 13 percent mineral oil, 0.5 to 2 percent base, up to 5 percent lanolin, up to 0.5 percent gums and thickeners, 6 to 75 percent water, and 0.2 percent preservative. Nontoxic.

BUBBLE BATH • Foams, perfumes, and softens bath water and generally makes bathing something of a special event. Liquid bubble bath may contain TEA-dodecylbenzene sulfonate, fatty acid alkanolamides, perfume, water, and methyl-paraben. Powdered bubble bath may contain sodium lauryl sulfate, sodium chloride, and perfume. The products may also contain any of the following: alcohol, alkyl benzene sulfonate, various colorings, dioctyl sodium sulfosuccinate, propylene glycol, sodium hexametaphosphate, sodium sulfate, and sodium tripolyphosphate. Ingestion of bubble baths may cause gastrointestinal disturbances, and skin irritations have been reported, especially in children. Reports to the FDA concern skin irritation, urinary and bladder infections, toxic encephalopathy with brain damage, stomach distress, irritation and bleeding of the genital area, inflammation of the genitals, and eye injury. In 1977, the FDA required manufacturers to keep alkylarylsulfonate below 10 percent, preferably between 2 and 5 percent. Children should not take prolonged and/or unsupervised bubble baths. Adults may aggravate dryness or inflammation of the skin by taking bubble baths.

BUBULUM • See Neat's-Foot Oil.

BUCHU • **Hottentot Tea. Zulu Bucu.** The dried leaves of *Barosma betulina* or of *Barosma crenulata,* a citrus shrub grown in South Africa. It is widely used in that country for medicinal purposes. Herbalists use it worldwide to treat diseases of the kidney, urinary tract, and prostate. The leaves contain barosma camphor and essential oil. When given warm, it stimulates sweating. In 1992, the FDA proposed a ban on buchu powdered extract in oral menstrual drug products because it has not been shown to be safe and effective for its stated claims.

BUCKBEAN EXTRACT • *Menyanthes trifoliata.* **Meyanthin. Bog-Bean. Water Shamrock.** A common plant in bogs, it is used by herbalists as a tonic and to reduce fever. It is also used to treat skin diseases due to rheumatism. Depending on the strength and dosage, its action ranges from that of a bitter tonic and cathartic to a purgative and emetic. In folk medicine, buckbean was used to treat edema, scabies, and fever.

BUCKTHORN • **Frangula.** A shrub or tree grown on the Mediterranean coast of Africa, it has thorny branches and often contains a purgative in the bark or sap. Its fruits are used as a source of yellow and green dyes. No known toxicity.

BUCKWHEAT • An herb of the genus *Fagopyrum.* Contains rutin, a pale yellow crystal found in many plants, particularly buckwheat. Used as a dietary supplement for capillary fragility. No known toxicity.

BUFFER • Usually a solution with a relatively constant acidity-alkalinity ratio, which is unaffected by the addition of comparatively large amounts of acid or alkali. A typical buffer solution would be hydrochloric acid and sodium hydroxide *(see).*

BUGLE WEED • **Sweet Bugle.** Extract of the various parts of *Lycopus virginicus,* grown in North America. Contains a volatile oil, resin, and tannin. Used in perfumery.

BUGLOSS EXTRACT • Extract of the various parts, including the roots, stems, leaves, and fruit of *Lycopsis arvensis.* Cultivated for its beautiful flowers. See Alkanet Root.

BUMETRIZOLE • An absorbent. See Phenol.

BURDOCK ROOT EXTRACT • *Arctium lappa.* **Cocklebur. Lapp. Bardane. Beggar's Buttons.** The roots, seeds, and leaves contain the essential oil of this common roadside plant. It contains nearly 45 percent inulin and many minerals. Herbalists use it for skin diseases, blood purification, urinary problems, and as a tonic. Cosmeticians use it to soothe the skin. Chinese burdock is used to eliminate excess nervous energy, and the root is considered to have aphrodisiac properties. It is sold in drugstores as an ointment to treat minor burns, cuts, or other skin traumas. It is used by gypsies in a pouch hung around the neck to ward off arthritis. It is also used to induce sweating in an effort to rid the body of toxins. In modern experiments, burdock root extract has been shown to have antitumor effects and to produce an increased flow of urine. No known toxicity.

BUROW'S SOLUTION • See Aluminum Acetate.

BUTACAINE • A topical anesthetic.

BUTADIENE/ACRYLONITRILE COPOLYMER • See Acrylates.

BUTALBITAL COMPOUNDS • Used in the relief of tension or muscle contraction headache and other aches and pains. The active ingredients are aspirin, codeine or acetaminophen, caffeine, and the barbiturate butalbital. The most frequent adverse reactions are drowsiness and dizziness. Less frequent adverse reactions are light-headedness, nausea, vomiting, and gas. May also cause skin reactions.

n-BUTANE • A flammable, easily liquefiable gas derived from petroleum. Used as a propellant or aerosol in cosmetics. The principal hazard is that of fire and explosion, but it may be narcotic in high doses and cause asphyxiation. On the basis of the available animal and human data, the CIR Expert Panel *(see)* concludes that this ingredient is safe as used in cosmetics.

BUTANEDIOIC ACID • See Succinic Acid.

BUTCHER'S-BROOM • A shrub native to Europe, with stiff prickle-tipped, flattened stems resembling true leaves, used in cosmetics. Formerly used as a broom by butchers. No known toxicity.

BUTETH-3 CARBOXYLIC ACID • See Carboxylic Acid and Propylene Glycol.

BUTOXY CHITOSAN • The derivative of Chitosan *(see)* and acetoacetic acid. Used as a film-former and thickening ingredient. See Chitin.

BUTOXYDIGLYCOL • An ether alcohol. See Diethylene Glycol.

BUTOXYETHANOL • **Butyl Cellosolve®.** A solvent for nitrocellulose *(see),* resins, grease, oil, and albumen. It is used as a solvent in hair and nail products. Severe eye irritation occurs in undiluted forms in rabbits. Moderate and no corneal injury were observed at concentrations of 15 percent and 5 percent in liquids. The CIR Expert Panel *(see)* concludes this is safe as used in "rinse-off" and "leave-on" products at concentrations up to 10 percent. See Polyethylene Glycol for toxicity.

BUTOXYETHYL ACETATE • A solvent. See Ethylene Glycol.

BUTOXYETHYL NICOTINATE • An ester of niacin *(see)* used as a skin conditioner.

BUTOXYPROPANOL • A solvent. See Propanol.

BUTTER • In cosmetology, substances that are solid at room temperature but melt at body temperature are called "butters." Cocoa butter is one of the most frequently used in both foods and cosmetics. Newer butters are made from natural fats by hydrogenation *(see),* which increases the butter's melting point or alters its plasticity. Butters may be used in stick or molded cosmetics such as lipsticks or to give the proper texture to a variety of finished products. Nontoxic.

BUTTERMILK • The fluid remaining after butter has been formed from churned cream. It can also be made from sweet milk by the addition of certain organic cultures. Used as an astringent right from the bottle. Apply liberally and let dry about 10 minutes. Rinse off with cool water. Also used as a freckle bleach. Apply one tablespoon of cooking oil or your favorite moisturizer. Mix 7 tablespoons of buttermilk with one tablespoon of grated fresh horseradish (keep it away from your eyes). Combine the ingredients, and apply to your face. Leave on for 15 minutes and rinse off with cool water. Then reapply your moisturizer or oil.

BUTYL- • Derived from butane *(see).*

BUTYL ACETATE • **Acetic Acid. Butyl Ester.** A colorless liquid with a fruity odor used in perfumery, nail polish, and nail polish remover. Also used in the manufacture of lacquer, artificial leather, plastics, and safety glass. It is an irritant and may cause eye irritation (conjunctivitis). It is a narcotic in high concentrations and toxic to man when inhaled at 200 ppm. On the basis of available data, the CIR Expert Panel concludes that this ingredient is safe as presently used in cosmetics.

BUTYL ACETYL RICINOLEATE • See Ricinoleate.

BUTYL ALCOHOL • A colorless liquid with an unpleasant odor, used as a clarifying ingredient *(see)* in shampoos; also a solvent for waxes, fats, resins, and shellac. It may cause irritation of the mucous membranes, headache, dizziness, and drowsiness when ingested. Inhalation of as little as 25 ppm causes pulmonary problems in man. It can also cause contact dermatitis when applied to the skin. The CIR Expert Panel *(see)* concludes this is a safe ingredient in nail products.

n-BUTYL ALCOHOL • Used as a solvent and denaturant.

t-BUTYL ALCOHOL • Denaturant and solvent. See Butyl Alcohol.

BUTYL AMINOETHYL METHYL ACRYLATE • Used in hairsprays. See Acrylates.

BUTYL BENZOIC ACID/PHTHALIC ANHYDRIDE/TRIMETHYLOETHANE COPOLYMER • A polymer *(see)* formed when the water is removed from the phthalic acid and the acid is combined with trimethyloethane monomers.

BUTYL BENZYL PHTHALATE • The aromatic ester that is used as a sanitizer and plasticizer. There are questions about phthalates *(see),* but the CIR Expert Panel *(see)* concludes this is a safe ingredient.

BUTYL ESTER OF ETHYLENE/MALEIC ANHYDRIDE COPOLYMER • A resin *(see)* made from ethylene and maleic anhydride *(see).* Used in hairsprays and setting lotions, and as a thickener in cosmetics. No known toxicity.

BUTYL ESTER OF PVM/MA COPOLYMER • **Butyl Ester of Poly (Methyl Vinyl Ether, Maleic Acid). Spirit Gum.** Plastic material. Formed from vinyl methyl ether and maleic anhydride. Used in hairsprays and setting lotions, and as a thickener. On the basis of available data, the CIR Expert Panel concludes that this ingredient is safe as presently used in cosmetics.

BUTYL GLYCOLATE • A plasticizer in nail lacquers. See Butyl Acetate.

BUTYL GLYCOSIDE • Obtained by the condensation of butyl alcohol with glucose *(see both).* Used as an emulsifier.

t-BUTYL HYDROQUINONE • An antioxidant. A weak depigmenter at 1.0 and 5.0 percent but not at 0.1 percent. The CIR Expert Panel *(see)* concludes this is a safe ingredient if it does not exceed 0.1 percent. See Hydroquinone.

BUTYL P-HYDROXYBENZOATE • Butyl Paraben. Butyl p-Oxybenzoate. Almost odorless, small colorless crystals or a white powder used as an antimicrobial preservative. No known toxicity.

BUTYL LACTATE • A synthetic butter, butterscotch, caramel, and fruit flavoring ingredient for beverages, ice cream, ices, candy, and baked goods. No known toxicity.

BUTYL MYRISTATE • A fatty alcohol used in nail polishes and nail polish removers, lipsticks, and face and protective creams. It is derived from myristic acid *(see)* and butyl alcohol *(see).* More irritating than ethanol *(see),* but less so than some other alcohols.

BUTYL OLEATE • Light-colored liquid with a mild odor. The ester of butyl alcohol and oleic acid *(see both),* it is a plasticizer, particularly for polyvinyl chloride *(see),* and is used in waterproofing, as a solvent and lubricant, and in polishes. In cosmetics, it is used as a skin conditioner and emollient. No known toxicity.

BUTYL PABA • The ester of butyl alcohol and para-aminobenzoic acid *(see both).*

BUTYL PALMITATE • Used in shampoos to leave a gloss on the hair. See Palmitic Acid.

BUTYL PHTHALYL BUTYL GLYCOLATE • See Butyl Glycolate.

BUTYL STEARATE • A synthetic antifoaming ingredient used in the production of beet sugar. Used as a binder and surfactant in cosmetics. Also a synthetic banana, butter, and liquor flavoring for beverages, ice cream, ices, candy, baked goods, chewing gum, and liqueurs. Used as a skin conditioning ingredient. On the basis of the available animal and human data, the CIR Expert Panel *(see)* concludes that this ingredient is safe as used in cosmetics.

BUTYLATED • The introduction of the butyl group—carbon and hydrogen—form butane into a compound to make it less susceptible to damage from oxygen.

BUTYLATED HYDROXYANISOLE • BHA. A preservative and antioxidant in cosmetics, foods, and beverages. White to slightly yellow, waxy solid with a faint characteristic odor. Can cause allergic reactions.

BUTYLATED HYDROXYTOLUENE • BHT. A preservative and antioxidant in cosmetics, foods, and beverages. A white crystalline solid with a faint characteristic odor. Prohibited as a food additive in England. Chemically similar to BHA, it can cause allergic reactions.

BUTYLATED POLYOXYMETHYLENE • A compound from formaldehyde and urea *(see both)*.

BUTYLATED POLYOXYMETHYLENE UREA • Formerly butylated urea-formaldehyde resin. A product of an amino resin mixed with urea and formaldehyde *(see both)*. The word "formaldehyde" was taken out of the label listing for cosmetics.

BUTYLATED UREA-FORMALDEHYDE RESIN • See Butylated Polyoxymethylene Urea.

BUTYLCARBAMATE • The ester of carbamic acid, which occurs in blood and urine of mammals. Used in sunblocks. See Urea.

BUTYLENE GLYCOL • This humectant is most resistant to high humidity and thus valuable in hairsprays and setting lotions. It retains scents and preserves against spoilage. It has a similar toxicity to ethylene glycol *(see)*, which when ingested may cause transient stimulation of the central nervous system, then depression, vomiting, drowsiness, coma, respiratory failure, and convulsions; renal damage may proceed to kidney failure and death. One of the few humectants not on the GRAS list of the FDA, although efforts to place it there have been made through the years.

BUTYLOCTYL BENZOATE • A plasticizer, skin conditioner, emollient, and solvent. The CIR Expert Panel *(see)* concludes this is a safe ingredient. See Benzoic Acid.

BUTYLOCTYL CANDELILLATE • A skin conditioning ingredient and a cover-up. See Candellia Wax.

BUTYLPARABEN • Widely used in cosmetics as an antifungal preservative, it is the ester of butyl alcohol and p-hydroxybenzoic acid. No known toxicity.

BUTYRALDEHYDE • A synthetic flavoring agent found naturally in coffee and strawberries. Used in butter, caramel, fruit, liquor, brandy, and nut flavorings for beverages, ice cream, ices, candy, baked goods, alcoholic beverages, and icings. Used also in the manufacture of rubber, gas accelerators, synthetic resins, and plasticizers. May be an irritant and a narcotic.

BUTYRIC ACID • **n-Butyric Acid. Butanoic Acid.** A clear, colorless liquid present in butter at 4 to 5 percent. It has a strong, rancid butter odor and is used in butterscotch, caramel, and fruit flavorings. It is used in chewing gums and margarines, as well as in cosmetics. It is found naturally in apples, geraniums, rose oil, grapes, strawberries, and wormseed oil. It has a low toxicity but can be a mild irritant. It caused tumors when applied to the skin of mice in 108-milligram doses per kilogram of body weight and cancer when injected into the abdomen of mice in 18-milligram doses per kilogram of body weight. A NIOSH review has determined it is a positive animal carcinogen. It has a low toxicity but can be a mild irritant. GRAS.

BUTYROLACTONE • **Butanolide.** Liquid lactone used chiefly as a solvent for resins. It is also an intermediate *(see)* in the manufacture of polyvinylpyrrolidone *(see)* and a solvent for nail polish. Human toxicity is unknown.

BUTYROSPERMUM PARKII • See Shea Butter.

BUTYRUM • The European Union name for butter, the United States designation for a label.

BUXUS CHINENSIS • See Jojoba Oil.

BUXUS SEMPERVIRENS • See Boxwood.

C

C18–36 ACID • A synthetic mixture of saturated, waxy fatty acids containing 18 to 36 carbons in the alkyl *(see)* chain. See Fatty Acids.

C29–70 ACID • **C29–70 Carboxylic Acids.** A mixture of synthetic aliphatic acids with 29 to 70 carbon atoms in the alkyl *(see)* chain. See Fatty Acids.

C18–36 ACID GLYCOL ESTER • Ester of ethylene glycol *(see)* and C18–36 acid. See Fatty Acids.

C18–36 ACID TRIGLYCERIDE • The triester of glycerin *(see)* and C18–36 acid. See Fatty Acids.

C9–11 ALCOHOLS • **Alkyls.** A mixture of synthetic fatty alcohols with 9 to 11 carbons in the alkyl *(see)* chain. See Fatty Acids.

C12–15 ALCOHOLS BENZOATE • See C12–15 Alkyl Benzoate.

C12–15 ALCOHOLS LACTATE • See C12–15 Alkyl Lactate.

C12–15 ALCOHOLS OCTANOATE • See C12–15 Alkyl Octanoate.

C12–16 ALCOHOLS • A mixture of synthetic fatty alcohols with 12 to 16 carbons in the alkyl *(see)* chain.

C14–15 ALCOHOLS • **Alkyls.** A mixture of synthetic fatty alcohols with 14 to 15 carbons in the alkyl *(see)* chain. See Fatty Acids.

C9–16 ALKANES/CYCLOALKANES • Hydrocarbons *(see)* that are solvents, surfactants, and cleansing ingredients.

C18–28 ALKYL ACETATE • Esters that are skin conditioners and emollients.

C18–38 ALKYL BEESWAX • Skin conditioner. See Beeswax.

C20–40 ALKYL BEHENATE • A skin conditioner. See Behenic Acid.

C12–15 ALKYL BENZOATE • Ester of benzoic acid *(see)* and C12–15 alcohols. See Fatty Acids.

C12–15 ALKYL LACTATE • The ester of lactic acid and C12–15 alcohols. See Fatty Acids.

C12–15 ALKYL OCTANOATE • The ester of octanoic acid *(see)* and fatty alcohols.

C12–15 ALKYL SALICYLATE • A skin conditioner. See Salicylic Acid.

C16–40 ALKYL STEARATE • Skin conditioners and thickening ingredients for compounds.

C15–18 GLYCOL • The long chain diol that has 13 to 16 carbons in the alkyl *(see)* chain. See Fatty Acids.

C18–20 GLYCOL ISOSTEARATE • The ester of isostearate with 16 to 18 carbons in the alkyl chain. See Fatty Acids.

C18–20 GLYCOL PALMITATE • The ester that has 12 to 14 carbons in the alkyl *(see)* chain. See Fatty Acids.

C14-20 ISOALKYLAMIDOPROPYLETHYLDIMONIUM ETHOSULFATE • A Quaternary Ammonium Compound *(see)*.

C8–9, C9–11, C9–13, C9–14, C10–11, C10–13, C11–12, C11–13, C12–14, C13–14, C13–16, AND C20–40 ISOPARAFFINS • Mixtures of aliphatic hydrocarbons with the number of carbons in the alkyl *(see)* chain given by the numbers. See Fatty Acids.

C7-8 ISOPARAFFIN • A hydrocarbon used as a solvent. See Paraffin.

C11–15 PARETH -3, -5, -7, -9, -12, -20, -30, -40 • Mixture of polyethylene glycols, the higher the number the thicker the mixture. See Polyethylene Glycols.

C11–15 PARETH -7 CARBOXYLIC ACID • The polyethylene mixture of carboxylic acid *(see)*.

C11–15 PARETH-12 STEARATE • The ester of pareth-15–12 and stearic acid *(see)*.

C11–15 PARETH-40 • The polyethylene glycol ether *(see)* of a mixture of synthetic fatty alcohols. See Polyethylene Glycol and Fatty Alcohols.

C12–13 PARETH-3, -7 • Polyethylene glycol ether of a mixture of synthetic fatty alcohols and ethylene glycol *(see all)*.

C12–15 PARETH-2, -3, -4, -5, -7, -9, -12 • The polyethylene glycol ethers of fatty alcohols with ethylene oxide. See polyethylene glycol, ethers, and fatty alcohols.

C12–15 PARETH-2 PHOSPHATE • A mixture of the esters of phosphoric acid *(see)* and polyethylene glycol ethers *(see)*.

C14–15 PARETH -7, -11, -13 • The polyethylene glycol ether of a mixture of synthetic fatty alcohols with ethylene oxide *(see all)*.

C30–46 PISCINE OIL • A marine oil derived from fish. It is used as a thickener. No known toxicity.

C10–18 TRIGLYCERIDES • A mixture of fatty acids and glycerin. Used as a thickener. No known toxicity.

CABBAGE EXTRACT • See Cabbage Rose.

CABBAGE ROSE • A fragrant garden rose *Rosa centifolia* with upright branches and large full white or pink flowers. Used in fragrances.

CACTUS • A family of prickly plants, *Cactaceae,* comprising over 1,500 species almost all of which are native to America. It has no leaves but stores a great deal of water. Cacti bear beautiful, short-lived flowers. They are the source of the drug mescaline and some species are edible. Extracts of cacti are used in "organic" cosmetics.

CADE OIL • See Juniper Tar.

CADMIUM CHLORIDE • A white powder, soluble in water, used in photography and in dye, particularly hair dye. Inhalation of the dust is highly toxic, and ingestion can cause death. Caused tumors when injected under the skin in rats and when given intravenously. It also caused cancer in mice when injected under the skin. NIOSH review determined that it was a positive animal carcinogen.

CAFFEIC ACID • An antioxidant. See Carboxylic Acid.

CAFFEINE • Guaranine. Methyltheobromine. Theine. An odorless white powder with a bitter taste that occurs naturally in the coffee, cola, guarana paste, tea, and kola nuts. Obtained as a by-product of caffeine-free coffee. Its current use in cosmetics has not been identified, but it is used as a flavoring in beverages and other foods. It is a central nervous system, heart, and respiratory system stimulant. Can alter blood sugar release and cross the placental barrier.

CAJEPUT • *Melaleuca leucadendron.* **Cajuput. White Tea Tree. Tea Tree.** The spicy oil contains, among other ingredients, terpenes, limonene, benzaldehyde, valeraldehyde, and dipentene. Native to Australia and Southeast Asia, it is used to treat fungus infections such as athlete's foot, and as a liniment for a wide variety of ailments. Herbalists use it to relieve itchy scalp, arthritic pains, and as an antiseptic for cuts.

CAJUPUT • See Cajeput.

CAKE MAKEUP • See Foundation Makeup.

CAKE MASCARA • Mascara based on fats or soap molded forms. It is applied with a brush dipped in water. A more liquid product is used in a cylinder into which a brush is inserted and pulled out, coated with mascara. A typical cake mascara formula: triethanolamine stearate, 54.0 percent; carnauba wax, 25.0 percent; paraffin, 12.5 percent; lanolin, 4.5 percent; carbon black 3.8 percent; propylparaben, 0.2 percent; other, 1.0 percent (see ingredients above under separate listings.) See Mascara for toxicity.

CAKILE MARITIMA • Sea Rocket. A plant of the genus cakile. A succulent herb found along the sandy shore.

CALAMINE • Zinc oxide with about 5 percent ferric oxide that occurs as a pink powder. Used in protective creams, astringents, lotions, ointments, washes, and powders in the treatment of skin diseases; also to impart a flesh color. Some calamine formulations contain significant amounts of phenol *(see),* and ingestion or repeated applications over large areas of skin may cause phenol poisoning. The FDA proposed a ban in 1992 for the use of calamine to treat insect bites and stings and poison ivy, poison oak, and poison sumac because it has not been shown to be safe and effective for stated claims in OTC products. The FDA said calamine could be used as "a skin protectant" but not as an "external analgesic."

CALAMINTHA OFFICINALIS • See Mint.

CALAMUS ROOT EXTRACT • *Acorus calamus.* **Sweet Flag. Sweet Sedge.** The rhizome contains essential oil, mucilage, glycosides, amino acid, and tannins *(see all).* Calamus root is an ancient Indian and Chinese herbal medicine used to treat acid stomach, irregular heart rhythm, low blood pressure, lack of mental focus, and for coughs. Native Americans would chew the root to enable them to run long distances with increased stamina. Externally, it was used to induce a state of tranquility. It is used in "organic" cosmetics.

CALCIFEROL • Vitamin D.

CALCIUM • The adult body contains about three pounds of calcium, 99 percent of which provides hardness for bones and teeth. Approximately 1 percent of calcium is distributed in body fluids, where it is essential for normal cell activity.

CALCIUM ACETATE • Brown Acetate of Lime. A white amorphous powder that has been used medicinally as a source of calcium. Used cosmetically for solidifying fragrances and as an emulsifier and firming ingredient. Also used in the manufacture of acetic acid and acetone *(see both)* and in dyeing, tanning, and curing skins as well as a corrosion inhibitor in metal containers. Low oral toxicity.

CALCIUM ALGINATE • See Alginates.

CALCIUM ALUMINUM BOROSILICATE • A thickening ingredient. See Silicates.

CALCIUM ASCORBATE • See Ascorbic Acid.

CALCIUM BEHENATE • The calcium salt of Behenic Acid (see) used as a wax.

CALCIUM BENZOATE • See Benzoic Acid.

CALCIUM BROMIDE • See Bromides.

CALCIUM CARBONATE • Chalk. Absorbent that removes shine from talc. A tasteless, odorless powder that occurs naturally in limestone, marble, and coral. Used as a white coloring in cosmetics and food, an alkali to reduce acidity, a neutralizer and firming ingredient, and a carrier for bleaches. Also used in dentifrices as a tooth polisher, in deodorants as a filler, in depilatories as a filler, and in face powder as a buffer. A gastric antacid and antidiarrhea medicine, it may cause constipation. No known toxicity.

CALCIUM CARRAGEENAN • See Carrageenan.

CALCIUM CASEINATE • The calcium salt of casein *(see)*.

CALCIUM CHLORIDE • The chloride salt of calcium. Used in its anhydrous *(see)* form as a drying ingredient for organic liquids and gases. An emulsifier and texturizer in cosmetics and an antiseptic in eye lotions. Also used in fire extinguishers, to preserve wood, and to melt ice and snow. Employed medicinally as a diuretic and a urinary acidifier. Ingestion can cause stomach and heart disturbances. No known toxicity as a cosmetic.

CALCIUM CITRATE • See Citric Acid.

CALCIUM CYCLAMATE • Artificial sweetening ingredient about 30 times as sweet as refined sugar, removed from the food market on September 1, 1969, because it was found to cause bladder cancer in rats. At that time 175 million Americans were swallowing cyclamates in significant doses in many products ranging from chewing gum to soft drinks. There has been a concerted effort to bring cyclamates back to the market, but as of this writing, they have not been approved. The FDA's Cancer Assessment Committee's review of all the evidence reportedly indicates that neither cyclamate nor its major metabolic end product—cyclohexylamine—cause cancer. Still listed for use in cosmetics.

CALCIUM DIHYDROGEN PHOSPHATE • A pH adjuster. See pH.

CALCIUM DISODIUM EDTA • Edetate Calcium Disodium. Calcium Disodium Ethylenediamine Tetraacetic Acid. A preservative and sequestrant, white, odorless powder with a faint salty taste. Used as a food additive to prevent crystal formation and to retard color loss. Nontoxic.

CALCIUM FLUORIDE • See Sodium Fluoride.

CALCIUM GLUCOHEPTONATE • An organic salt that is used in skin conditioners.

CALCIUM GLUCONATE • Odorless, tasteless, white crystalline granules, stale in air. Used as a buffer, firming ingredient, sequestrant. It is soluble in water. May cause gastrointestinal and cardiac disturbances. The final report to the FDA of the Select Committee on GRAS Substances stated in 1980 that it should continue its GRAS status with no limitations other than good manufacturing practices. The FDA issued a notice in 1992 that calcium gluconate has not been shown to be safe and effective as claimed in OTC digestive aid products.

CALCIUM HYDROXIDE • **Limewater. Lye.** Used in cream depilatories; also in mortar, plaster, cement, pesticides, fireproofing, as an egg preservative, and as a depilatory. Employed as a topical astringent and alkali in solutions or lotions. Accidental ingestion can cause burns of the throat and esophagus; also death from shock and asphyxia due to swelling of the glottis and infection. Calcium hydroxide also can cause burns of the skin and eyes.

CALCIUM HYPOCHLORITE • A germicide and sterilizing ingredient, it is the active ingredient of chlorinated lime and is used in the curd washing of cottage cheese, in sugar refining, as an oxidizing and bleaching ingredient, and as an algae killer, bactericide, deodorant, disinfectant, and fungicide. Fruits and vegetables are sterilized by washing in a 50 percent solution. Under various names, dilute hypochlorite is found in homes as laundry bleach and household bleach. Household mildew removers contain 5 percent calcium hypochlorite which is twice as toxic as common household sodium hypochlorite bleach. Industrial strength hypochlorite bleaches contain 15 to 20 percent solutions. Occasionally cases of poisoning occur when people mix household hypochlorite solution with various other household chemicals, which causes the release of poisonous chlorine gas. As with other corrosive ingredients, calcium hypochlorite's toxicity depends upon its concentrations. It is highly corrosive to skin and mucous membranes. Ingestion may cause pain and inflammation of the mouth, pharynx, esophagus, and stomach, with erosion particularly of the mucous membranes of the stomach.

CALCIUM IODATE • See Iodine.

CALCIUM LACTATE • White, almost odorless crystals or powder used as a buffer and as such is a constituent of baking powders; also used in dentifrices. In medical use, given for calcium deficiency; may cause gastrointestinal and cardiac disturbances. In 1992, the FDA proposed a ban on calcium lactate in oral menstrual drug products because it has not been shown to be safe and effective for its stated claims.

CALCIUM LIGNOSULFONATE • See Lignoceric Acid.

CALCIUM MONOFLUOROPHOSPHATE • An inorganic salt used in oral care products. See Phosphorous and Fluoride.

CALCIUM MONTANATE • See Montan Wax.

CALCIUM MYRISTATE • An anticaking ingredient, stabilizer in emulsions and thickening ingredient. See Myristic Acid.

CALCIUM NITRATE • See Nitrate.

CALCIUM OXIDE • Lime. Quicklime. White or gray crystals or powder commercially obtained from limestone. Used as an alkali in cosmetics, as an insecticide and fungicide, and for dehairing hides. A strong caustic that may cause severe irritation of the skin and mucous membranes and can cause both thermal and chemical burns.

CALCIUM PANTETHEINE SULFONATE • An organic salt used in skin conditioners. See Pantothenic Acid.

CALCIUM PANTOTHENATE • Pantothenic Acid Calcium Salt. Vitamin B5. The calcium salt of pantothenic acid, found in liver, rice bran, and molasses, and essential for metabolism of carbohydrates, fats, and other important substances. Sweetish taste with a slightly bitter aftertaste, soluble in water, it is a member of the B-complex family of vitamins. It is also found in large amounts in the jelly of the queen bee, the so-called royal jelly of cosmetic advertising fame. It is used as an emollient and to enrich creams and lotions. No known toxicity.

CALCIUM PARABEN • A preservative. See Parabens.

CALCIUM PEROXIDE • See Peroxide.

CALCIUM PHOSPHATE • White, odorless powder used as an anti-caking ingredient in cosmetics and foods. Employed in toothpaste and tooth powder as an abrasive. Practically insoluble in water. No known toxicity.

CALCIUM PROPIONATE • Propanoic Acid, Calcium Salt. White crystals or crystalline solid with the faint odor of propionic acid. A mold and rope inhibitor in breads and rolls, it is used in processed cheese and artificially sweetened fruit jelly. It is used as a preservative in cosmetics and as an antifungal medication for the skin. The FDA has asked for further study for safety.

CALCIUM PYROPHOSPHATE • A fine, white, odorless, tasteless powder used as a nutrient, an abrasive in dentifrices, a buffer, and as a neutralizing ingredient in foodstuffs. No known toxicity.

CALCIUM SACCHARATE • See Saccharin.

CALCIUM SACCHARIN • See Saccharin.

CALCIUM SALICYLATE • See Salicylates.

CALCIUM SILICATE • Okenite. An anticaking ingredient, white or slightly cream-colored, free-flowing powder used in face powders because it has extremely fine particles and good water absorption. Also used as a coloring ingredient. Used in baking powder, in road construction, and in lime glass. Practically nontoxic orally, but inhalation may cause irritation of the respiratory tract.

CALCIUM SODIUM BOROSILICATE • A thickener. See Calcium and Silicates.

CALCIUM/SODIUM PVM/MA • A mixture of calcium and sodium salts with polyvinyl acetate and maleic acids *(see both)*.

CALCIUM SORBATE • A preservative. See Sorbic Acid.

CALCIUM STEARATE • Prepared from limewater *(see)*, it is an emulsifier used in hair-grooming products. Also used as a coloring ingredient, in waterproofing, and in paints and printing ink. Nontoxic. On the basis of the available information, the CIR Expert Panel *(see)* concludes that it is safe as a cosmetic ingredient.

CALCIUM STEAROYL LACTYLATE • It is the calcium salt of the stearic acid ester of lactyl lactate. A free-flowing powder used as a texturizer. Also used to improve the flow of powder. No known toxicity.

CALCIUM SULFATE • **Plaster of Paris.** A fine, white to slightly yellow, odorless, tasteless powder used in toothpaste and tooth powders as an abrasive and firming ingredient. Also used as a coloring ingredient in cosmetics. Used in creamed cottage cheese as an alkali and employed industrially in cement, wall plaster, and insecticides. Because it absorbs moisture and hardens quickly, its ingestion may result in intestinal obstruction. Mixed with flour, it has been used to kill rodents. No known toxicity on the skin.

CALCIUM SULPHIDE • A yellow powder formed by heating gypsum with charcoal at 1000 F. degrees. Employed in depilatories. Used in acne preparations. Also used as a food preservative and in luminous paints. It can cause allergic reactions.

CALCIUM THIOGLYCOLATE • Used in cream depilatories and permanent wave lotions. Odorless or with a faint odor. Also used to tan leather. Chronic application has led to thyroid problems in experimental animals. Some people develop skin problems on the hands or scalp with hemorrhaging under the skin.

CALCIUM UNDECYLENATE • A fine, white powder used to kill bacteria and fungus. See Undecylenic Acid.

CALCIUM XYLENESULFONATE • The calcium salt of xylene *(see)*. Used as a surfactant and to attract water.

CALENDULA EXTRACT AND OIL • Products from the flowers of pot marigolds grown in gardens everywhere. Formerly used to soothe inflammation of skin and mucous membranes, now used in "natural" creams, oils, and powders for babies. Use of this as a colorant is prohibited in the United States. It is widely used, however, in shampoos, soaps, skin fresheners, suntan gels, hair preparations, permanent waves, baby lotions, and face powders.

CALF BLOOD EXTRACT • Used in "antiaging" products.

CALF SKIN EXTRACT • An oil extracted from bovine skin. Used in "antiaging" products.

CALF SKIN HYDROLYSATE • The hydrolysate *(see)* of calf skin derived by acid, enzyme, or other method of hydrolysis. Used in "antiaging" products.

CALIFORNIA NUTMEG EXTRACT • **Stinking Nutmeg Extract.** Derived from *Torreya californica.* See Nutmeg.

CALLUNA VULAGRUS • **Heather. Ling Extract.** A purple evergreen that grows in northern and alpine regions.

CALOMEL • **Mercurous Chloride.** A white, odorless, tasteless, heavy powder used in bleach and freckle creams. It slowly decays in sunlight into mercuric chloride and metallic mercury. Banned in July 1973, when the FDA ordered all mercury cosmetics (except for mercury preservatives in eye products) off the market. In 1996, the Texas Department of Health and the New Mexico Department of Health reported a mercury-containing beauty cream in stores and flea markets. It contained calomel with about 6 to 10 percent mercury by weight. In response to media announcements, 238 persons in the West and Midwest contacted their health department to report use of the cream called "Crema de Belleza-Manning." The health departments said that although the potential health risks asociated with the product were only recognized in 1996, the cream has been produced since 1971 and the prevalence of its use in this country "cannot be accurately estimated."

CALOPHYLLUM OIL • **Santa Maria Tree.** Extract from a tropical tree having thick, shiny feather-veined leaves, clustered white flowers, aromatic resinous juice, and oily seeds. Used in moisturizing creams. No known toxicity.

CAMELLIA OIL • *Camellia Oleifera. Camellia Sinensis. Camellia Japonica.* **Green Tea.** A tropical Asiatic evergreen shrub or small tree with reddish or white flowers. Used to scent perfumes and in "antiwrinkle" creams. No known toxicity. Green tea has many beneficial effects and has reportedly anti-cholesterol, anti-high blood pressure properties. It also contains tannins *(see).* See Tea Tree Oil.

CAMOMILE • See Chamomile.

CAMPHOR OIL • Used in emollient creams, hair tonics, eye lotions, preshave lotions, after-shave lotions, and skin fresheners as a preservative and to give a cool feeling to the skin. It is used as a spice flavoring for beverages, baked goods, and condiments. It is also used in horn-rimmed glasses, as a drug preservative, in embalming fluid, in the manufacture of explosives, in lacquers, as a moth repellent, and topically in liniments, cold medications, and anesthetics. It is distilled from trees at least 50 years old grown in China, Japan, Taiwan, Brazil, and Sumatra. It can cause contact dermatitis. In 1980, The FDA banned camphorated oil as a liniment for colds and sore muscles because of reports of poisonings through skin absorption and because of accidental ingestion. A New Jersey pharmacist had collected case reports and testified before the Advisory Review Panel on OTC Drugs to the FDA in 1980.

CANADA BALSAM • See Balsam.

CANANGA OIL • A natural flavor extract obtained by distillation from the flowers of the tree. Light to deep yellow liquid with a harsh, floral odor. Used in cola, fruit, spice, and ginger ale flavoring for beverages, ice cream, ices, candy, baked goods. May cause allergic reactions.

CANDELILLA WAX • *Euphorbia Cerifera.* Obtained from candelilla plants for use in lipsticks, solid fragrances, and liquid powders to give them body. Brownish to yellow brown, hard, brittle, easily pulverized, practically insoluble in water, slightly soluble in alcohol. Used in emollients to protect the skin against moisture loss. Also used in the manufacture of rubber, phonograph records, in waterproofing and writing inks, and hardens other waxes. No known toxicity. The CIR Expert Panel *(see)* concludes this is a safe ingredient.

CANDIDA BOMBICOLA/SUCROSE/VEGETABLE ACID ESTER FERMENT • Esters of sunflower seed oil, palm kernel acids, and rapeseed oil *(see all).* Used in creams and oils.

CANDLENUT TREE • See Kukui Nut Oil.

CANEKUBA SATIVA • **Gold of Pleasure.** Derived from *Camelina sativa.* See Tea Tree Oil.

CANOLA OIL • A low erucic-acid rapeseed oil *(see)* is used in salad oils because it contains 50 percent less saturated oils than other popular oils. GRAS.

Used as a skin conditioner and a cover-up. Used in hand and face creams, soft soaps, and mud packs. Can cause acnelike skin eruptions.

CANOLAMIDOPROPYL BETAINE • Used as an antistatic ingredient, hair conditioner, and cleansing ingredient. Also boosts foam and thickens liquids. See Betaines.

CANOLAMIDOPROPYL ETHYLDIMONIUM ETHOSULFATE • A quaternary ammonium compound *(see)* used as an antistatic ingredient in hair products.

CANTHARIDES TINCTURE • **Spanish Fly.** Obtained from blister beetles that thrive in Southern and Central Europe and powdered for use in hair tonics and lotions to stimulate the scalp. A powerful irritant to the skin and causes blistering. If ingested, it can cause severe intestinal upset, kidney damage, and death. Long reputed to have aphrodisiac effects.

CANTHARIDIN • Skin vesicant, rubefacient in hair tonic. Can cause allergic reaction. See Cantharides Tincture.

CANTHAXANTHIN • A color additive, it is a synthetic non-provitamin A carotinoid that is easily absorbed by fat. It is taken for the purpose of skin "tanning" and may be provided by tanning salons or by mail order. It is not approved as a prescription or an over-the-counter drug. A report from the Vanderbilt University's Department of Pharmacy cited the case of a healthy young woman who ingested canthaxanthin given to her by a commercial tanning salon. She developed aplastic anemia and died. The frequency of the adverse effects of this ingredient are unknown, the Vanderbilt researchers said, because there is no current way to monitor distribution. See Beta-Carotene.

CAPERS • A natural flavoring from the spiny shrub. The picked flower bud is used as a condiment for sauces and salads. No known toxicity. GRAS.

CAPPARIS SPINOSA • See Capers.

CAPRACYL BROWN 2R • See D & C Brown No. 1.

CAPRAE LAC • **Goat's milk.**

CAPRAMIDE DEA • See Capric Acid.

CAPRIC ACID • Obtained from a large group of American plants. Solid crystalline mass with a rancid odor used in the manufacture of artificial fruit flavors in lipsticks and to scent perfumes. No known toxicity.

CAPROIC ACID • **Hexanoic Acid.** A synthetic flavoring that occurs naturally in apples, butter acids, cocoa, grapes, oil of lavender, oil of lavandin, raspberries, strawberries, and tea. Used in butter, butterscotch, fruit, rum, and cheese flavorings. Used also in the manufacture of "hexyl" derivatives such as 4-hexylresorcinol *(see)*. No known toxicity.

CAPROYL ETHYL GLUCOSIDE • A cleansing ingredient. See Capric Acid.

CAPROYLAMINE OXIDE • See Caprylic Acid and Capric Acid.

CAPRYL ALCOHOL • See Caprylic Acid and Alcohol.

CAPRYL BETAINE • See Caprylic Acid and Betaine.

CAPRYL/CAPRAMIDOPROPYL BETAINE • An antistatic ingredient for hair products and a foam booster. See Betaines.

CAPRYL HYDROXYETHYL IMIDAZOLINE • See Imidazoline.

CAPRYLETH-4 CARBOXYLIC ACID • A cleansing ingredient. See Carboxylic Acid and Polyoxyethylene Compounds.

CAPRYLIC ACID • An oil liquid made by the oxidation of octanol *(see)* for use in perfumery. Occurs naturally as a fatty acid in sweat, fusel oil, in the milk of cows and goats, and in palm and coconut oil. No known toxicity.

CAPRYLIC ALCOHOL • See 1-Octanol.

CAPRYLIC/CAPRIC GLYCERIDES • Emollient. The CIR Expert Panel *(see)* concludes this is a safe ingredient. See Capric Acid and glycerin.

CAPRYLIC/CAPRIC/LAURIC TRIGLYCERIDE • A mixture of triester of glycerin with caprylic, capric, and lauric acids *(see all)*. An oily mixture derived from coconut oil, it is used extensively in cosmetics as a vehicle for pigment dispersions in bath oils, hairsprays, and lipsticks. Also used as an emollient to prevent water loss from the skin. Low toxicity.

CAPRYLIC/CAPRIC/STEARIC TRIGLYCERIDE • A mixture of the triester of glycerin with caprylic, capric, and stearic acids *(see all)*.

CAPRYLOYL COLLAGEN AMINO ACIDS • Caprylic acid *(see)* with amino acids from collagen *(see)*.

CAPRYLOYL HYDROLYZED COLLAGEN • The condensation product of capric acid and hydrolyzed collagen *(see)*. The word "animal" has been removed from this ingredient. Used as a hair conditioner, skin conditioner, and as a cleansing ingredient.

CAPRYLOYL HYDROLYZED KERATIN • The condensation product of caprylic acid and hydrolyzed keratin. Formerly called hydrolyzed animal keratin. Hair conditioning and cleansing ingredient.

CAPRYLYL/CAPRYL GLUCOSIDE • A carbohydrate that acts as a cleansing ingredient in shampoos and cold cream, and in pads. See Capric Acid.

CAPRYLYL GLYCOL • An alcohol that is used in hair conditioners and emollients. See Capric Acid and Glycol.

CAPRYLYL HYDROXYETHYL IMIDAZOLINE • See Imidazoline.

CAPSANTHIN/CAPSORUBIN • A hair coloring that is used in European products but is banned from American colors. It is a coal tar color.

CAPSELLA BURSA • **Shepherd's Heart. Shepherds Purse.** Extract of the herb, *Capsella bursa-pastoris,* a member of the mustard family. Pungent and bitter, it was valued for its astringent properties by early American settlers. Cotton moistened with its juice was used to stop nosebleed. In an oil-in-water emulsion, it is used as a base for skin preparations. Among its constituents are saponins, choline, acetylcholine, and tyramine *(see all)*. These preparations are used in modern medicine to stimulate neuromuscular function. The herb also reduces urinary tract irritation, and has been shown to contract the uterus and lower blood pressure.

CAPSICUM • The dried, ripe fruit of the capsicum or African chili plant used in hair tonics to stimulate the scalp, medicinally to soothe irritated skin and as an internal gastric stimulant. May cause skin irritation and allergic reaction.

CAPTAN • A preservative used in cosmetics. It is a fungicide of low toxicity, but in large doses can cause diarrhea and weight loss. No human poisonings are known. It is mutagenic and has produced cancer in mice following oral administration. The CIR Expert Panel *(see)* concludes that the avaiable data are insufficient to support the safety of captan as used in cosmetics.

CARAMEL • Used as a coloring in cosmetics and a soothing ingredient in skin lotions. Burnt sugar with a pleasant, slightly bitter taste. Made by heating sugar or glucose and adding small quantities or alkali or a trace mineral acid during heating. Used in food as a flavoring and coloring. The FDA permanently listed caramel in 1981.

CARAPA GUAIANENSIS OIL • A denaturant *(see)*.

CARAWAY SEED AND OIL • The dried ripe seeds of a plant common to Europe and Asia and cultivated in England, Russia, and the United States. A volatile, colorless to pale yellow liquid, it is used in liquor flavorings for beverages, ice cream, baked goods, and condiments; also used as a spice in baking. The oil is used in grape licorice, anisette, kummell, liver, sausage, mint, caraway, and rye flavorings for beverages, ice cream, ices, candy, baked goods, chewing gum, meats, condiments, and liquors. The oil is used to perfume soap. Can cause contact dermatitis.

CARBAMATE • A compound based on carbamic acid, which is used only in the form of its numerous derivatives and salts. Carbamates are used in pesticides. Among the carbamate pesticides are aldicarb, 4-benzothienyl-N-methyl carbamate, bufencarb (BUX), carbaryl, carbofuran, isolan, 2-isopropyl phenyl-N-methyl carbamate, 3-isopropyl phenylmethyl carbamate, maneb, propoxur, thiram, Zectran, zineb and ziram. Carbamic acid, which is colorless and odorless, causes depression of bone marrow and degeneration of the brain, nausea, and vomiting. It is moderately toxic by many routes.

CARBAMIDE • See Urea.

CARBENIA BENEDICTA • *Cnicus benedictus.* **Blessed Thistle. Holy Thistle.** The thistle contains tannin *(see),* lactone, mucilage *(see),* and essential oil. Used by herbalists to treat stomach and liver complaints. It increases appetite, lowers fevers, and reputedly breaks up blood clots, relieves jaundice and hepatitis, and stops bleeding. In 1992, the FDA issued a notice that blessed thistle had not been shown to be safe and effective as claimed in OTC digestive-aid products or oral menstrual drugs.

CARBITOL® • **Carbide. Carbon.** A solvent for nail lacquers and enamels. Absorbs water from the air and is mixable with acetone, benzene, alcohol, water, and ether. More toxic than polyethylene glycol *(see)*.

CARBOCYSTEINE • See carbon and cysteine.

CARBOMER -934, -940, -941 • **Carbopol. Carboxypolymethylene.** A white powder, slightly acidic, that reacts with fat particles to form thick, stable emulsions of oils in water. Used as thickening, suspending, dispersing, and emulsifying ingredients in the cosmetic field. No known toxicity. The CIR Expert Panel *(see)* concludes this is a safe ingredient.

CARBON • A nonmetallic element occurring as diamond and graphite and forming a constituent of coal, petroleum, and asphalt, of limestone and other carbonates, and of all organic compounds and also obtained artificially in varying degrees of purity such as carbon black, charcoal, and coke.

CARBON BLACK • Several forms of artificially prepared carbon or charcoal, including animal charcoal, furnace black, channel (gas) black, lamp black, activated charcoal. Animal charcoal is used as a black coloring in confectionery. Activated charcoal is used as an antidote for ingested poisons, and as an adsorbent in diarrhea. The others have industrial uses. Carbon black, which was not subject to certification *(see)* by the FDA was reevaluated and then banned in 1976. It was found in tests to contain a cancer-causing by-product that was released during dye manufacture. It can no longer be used in candies such as licorice and in jelly beans or in drugs or cosmetics.

CARBON DIOXIDE • Colorless, odorless, noncombustible gas with a faint acid taste. Used as a pressure-dispensing ingredient in gassed creams. Also used in the carbonation of beverages and as dry ice for refrigeration in the frozen food industry. Used onstage to produce harmless smoke or fumes. May cause shortness of breath, vomiting, high blood pressure, and disorientation if inhaled in sufficient amounts.

CARBOPOL • See Carbomer.

CARBOWAX® • Solid polyethylene glycols used in cosmetics and pharmaceuticals. May cause an allergic reaction. See Polyethylene Glycol.

CARBOXYBUTYL CHITOSAN • A film-former and hair and skin-conditioning ingredient. See Chitin.

CARBOXYLIC ACID • A broad group of organic acids which include the fatty acids as well as the amino acids, benzoic acids and salicylic acids.

CARBOXYMETHYL CELLULOSE • **Sodium.** A synthetic gum used in bath preparations, beauty masks, dentifrices, hair-grooming aids, hand creams, rouge, shampoos, and shaving creams. As an emulsifier, stabilizer, and foaming ingredient, it is a barrier ingredient *(see)* made from cotton by-products, and occurs as a white powder or in granules. Employed as a stabilizer in ice cream, beverages, and other foods; and medicinally as a laxative or antacid. It has been shown to cause cancer in animals when ingested. Its toxicity on the skin is unknown.

CARBOXYMETHYL CHITIN • See Chitin.

s-CARBOXYMETHYL CYSTEINE • Used in astringents and lotions. See Cysteine.

CARBOXYMETHYL DEXTRAN • A film-former and thickener. See Dextran.

CARBOXYMETHYL HYDROXETHYLCELLULOSE • A binder and emulsifier. See Cellulose and Ethylene Glycol.

CARBOXYMETHYL HYDROXYPROPYL GUAR • A gum used as a binder and stabilizer. See Guar Gum.

CARBOXYPOLYMETHYLENE • See Carbomer.

CARCINOGEN • A cancer-causing agent.

CARCINOGENIC • A substance that is capable of causing cancer.

CARDAMON OIL • **Grains of Paradise.** A natural flavoring and aromatic ingredient from the dried, ripe seeds of trees common to India, Ceylon, and

Guatemala. Used in perfumes and soaps, in butter, chocolate, and other food flavorings. As a medicine, it breaks up intestinal gas. No known toxicity.

CARMINE • *Cochineal.* A crimson pigment derived from a Mexican and Central American species of a scaly female insect that feeds on various cacti. The dye is used in cosmetic colors, red applesauce, and other food. The FDA permanently listed carmine for use in food in 1977. Cochineal, itself, is no longer permitted for use in foods or cosmetics but its extracts are permitted.

CARMINIC ACID • **Natural Red No. 4.** Used in mascaras, liquid rouge, paste rouge, and red eye shadows. It is the glucosidal coloring matter from a scaly insect (see Carmine). Color is deep red in water and violet to yellow in acids. May cause allergic reactions. See Colors. Banned by the FDA.

CARNATION • The essential oil of the double-flowered variety of clove pink. Pale green solid that does not have the characteristic odor of carnations until diluted. Used in fragrances. No known toxicity.

CARNAUBA WAX • The exudate from the leaves of the Brazilian wax palm tree used as a texturizer in foundation makeups, mascara, cream rouge, lipsticks, liquid powders, depilatories, and deodorant sticks. It comes in a hard, greenish to brownish solid and rarely causes allergic reactions. The CIR Expert Panel *(see)* concludes this is a safe ingredient.

CARNITINE • Vitamin B_T. A thyroid inhibitor found in muscle, liver, and meat extracts. It stimulates fatty-acid oxidation and manufacture. Muscles which contain approximately 98 percent of carnitine must take it up from the blood. When carnitine is deficient, muscles become weak, and the person is intolerant of exercise. Used in skin creams.

CAROB EXTRACT • See Locust Bean Gum.

CAROTENE • See Beta-Carotene.

CAROTENOIDS • Found in parsley, carrots, sweet potatoes, and most green, red, and yellow vegetables and fruits, these are vitamin A precursors that are antioxidants and cell-differentiation agents (cancer cells are undifferentiated). There are hundreds of carotenoids in nature.

CARRAGEENAN • **Irish Moss.** A stabilizer and emulsifier, seaweedlike in odor, derived from Irish Moss, used in oils in cosmetics and foods. It is completely soluble in hot water and not coagulated by acids. Used medicinally to soothe the skin. Nontoxic. The use of Irish moss in food and medicine has been known in India for hundreds of years. Its use in the United States began in 1935 but really became common during World War II as a replacement for agar-agar. Sodium carrageenan is on the FDA list for further study. Carrageenan stimulated the formation of fibrous tissue when subcutaneously injected into the guinea pig. When a single dose of it dissolved in saline was injected under the skin of the rat, it caused sarcomas after approximately two years. Its cancer-causing ability may be that of a foreign body irritant, because upon administration to rats and mice at high levels in their diet, it did not appear to induce tumors, although survival of the animals for this period was not good. Its use as a food additive is being studied.

CARRIBEAN SEA-WHIP EXTRACT • Used in "antiaging" products, it is said to soothe inflammation, and is used in "natural sunscreens" based upon the adaptations of shallow-water marine life.

CARROT JUICE POWDER • See Carrot Oil.

CARROT OIL • Either of two oils from the seeds of carrots *Daucus carota sativa*. A light yellow essential oil, which has a spicy odor, and is used in liqueurs, flavorings, and perfumes. Rich in Vitamin A, it is also used as a coloring. No known toxicity.

CARROT SEED EXTRACT • Extract of the seeds of *Daucus carota sativa*.

CARUM CARVI • See Caraway.

CARVEOL • A synthetic mint, spearmint, spice, and caraway flavoring ingredient for beverages, ice cream, ices, candy, and baked goods. Found naturally in caraway and grape, and baked fruit. No known toxicity.

CARVONE (D or L) • **Oil of Caraway.** D-Carvone is usually prepared by distillation from caraway seed and dill seed oil. It is colorless to light yellow with an odor of caraway. L-Carvone occurs in several essential oils. It may be isolated from spearmint oil or synthesized commercially from d-limonene. It is colorless to pale yellow with the odor of spearmint. D-Carvone is a synthetic liquor, mint, and spice flavoring ingredient for beverages, ice cream, ices, candy, and baked goods. Used also in perfumery and soaps. It breaks up intestinal gas and is used as a stimulant. No known toxicity. GRAS.

CARVYL ACETATE • A synthetic mint flavoring for beverages, ice cream, ices, candy, and baked goods. No known toxicity.

CARVYL PROPIONATE • A synthetic mint flavoring for beverages, ice cream, ices, candy, and baked goods. No known toxicity.

CARVYLOPHYLLENE ACETATE • A general fixative that occurs in many essential oils, especially in clove oil. Colorless, oily, with a clovelike odor. Used for beverages, ice cream, ices, candy, baked goods, and chewing gum. Practically insoluble in alcohol. No known toxicity.

CARYA ILLINOENSIS • **Pecan.** A coloring ingredient used in cosmetics. Employed medicinally by the American Indians. It is the nut from a hickory of the southern central United States with rough bark and hard but brittle wood. Edible. No known toxicity.

CASCARA • A natural flavoring derived from the dried bark of a plant grown from northern Idaho to northern California. Cathartic. Used in butter, caramel, and vanilla flavoring. Formerly used to treat skin diseases. Used to soothe skin in lotions and creams. No known toxicity.

CASCARILLA BARK • A natural flavoring ingredient obtained from the bark of a tree grown in Haiti, the Bahamas, and Cuba. The dried extract is added to smoking tobacco for flavoring and is used in bitters and spice flavorings for beverages. The oil, obtained by distillation, is light yellow to amber with a spicy odor. It is used in cola, fruit, root beer, and spice flavorings for beverages, ice cream, ices, candy, baked goods, and condiments. No known toxicity. GRAS.

CASEARIA SYLVESTRIS • A plant that contains analgesics, antiacids, anti-inflammatory, and styptic properties. Herbalists use it to treat burns, wounds, and small skin injuries. It is also used in South America in dental-care products as an antiseptic.

CASEIN • The principal protein of cow's milk used in protective cream and as the "protein" in hair preparations to make the hair thicker and more manageable. It is a white, water-absorbing powder without noticeable odor and is used to make depilatories less irritating and as a film-former in beauty masks. It is also used as an emulsifier in many cosmetics and in special diet preparations. Nontoxic.

CASHEW NUT OIL • Oil expressed from the seeds of *Anacardium occidentale.*

CASSIA OIL • **Cloves. Chinese Oil of Cinnamon.** Darker, less agreeable, and heavier than true cinnamon. Obtained from a tropical Asian tree and used in perfumes, poultices, and as a laxative. It can cause irritation and allergy such as a stuffy nose.

CASTANEA SATIVA • *Castanea vulgaris.* **Chestnut. Spanish Chestnut. Sweet Chestnut. Horse Chestnut.** Nut from a tree of the beech family, used as a remedy for piles, backaches, and for coughs. An astringent, the bark and leaves were used to make a tonic, which also was useful, reportedly, in the treatment of upper respiratory ailments such as coughs, particularly whooping cough. The bark of Spanish chestnut contains tannin *(see).*

CASTILE SOAP • A fine, hard, bland soap, usually white or cream-colored, but sometimes green, named for the region of Spain where it was originally made. Made from olive oil and sodium hydroxide *(see).* No known toxicity.

CASTOR • See Castoreum.

CASTOR OIL • **Palm Christi Oil.** The seed of the castor-oil plant. After the oil is expressed from the beans, a residual castor pomace remains, which contains a potent allergen. This may be incorporated in fertilizer, which is the main source of exposure, but people who live near a castor-bean processing factory may also be sensitized. Used in bath oils, nail polish removers, solid perfumes, face masks, shaving creams, lipsticks, and many men's hairdressings. It is also used as a plasticizer in nail polish. It forms a tough shiny film when dried. More than 50 percent of the lipsticks in the United States use a substantial amount of castor oil. Ingestion of large amounts may cause pelvic congestion. Soothing to the skin.

CASTOREUM • **Castor.** Used in perfumes as a fixative *(see).* A creamy, orange-brown substance with strong, penetrating odor and bitter taste that consists of the dried perineal glands of the beaver and their secretion. The glands and secretions are taken from the area between the vulva and the anus in the female beaver and from the scrotum and the anus in the male beaver. Professional trappers use castor to scent bait.

CATALASE • An enzyme from bovine liver used in milk, for making cheese, and for the elimination of peroxide. It is used also in combination with glucose oxidase for treatment of food wrappers to prevent oxidative deterioration of food and cosmetics.

CATALYST • A substance that causes or speeds up a chemical reaction but does not itself change.

CATECHOL • **Catechin.** A modifier in hair colorings used as a drabber. It is phenol alcohol found in catechu black *(see)*.

CATECHU BLACK • A preparation from the heartwood of the acacia catechu, used in toilet preparations and for brown and black colorings. Used as an astringent. May cause allergic reactions.

CATIONIC • A group of synthetic compounds employed as emulsifiers, wetting ingredients, and antiseptics in special hand creams. Their positively charged ions (cations) repel water. Any class of synthetic detergents usually consisting almost entirely of quaternary ammonium compounds *(see)* with carbon and nitrogen. Used also as wetting and emulsifying ingredients in acid to neutralize solutions or as a germicide or fungicide. Toxicity depends upon ingredients used.

CATNIP • *Nepeta cataria.* **Catnep. Catnip.** An aromatic plant of the mint family common to North America and Europe, it was said in folk medicine that the root, when chewed, made the quietest person fierce and quarrelsome. In modern medicine it is used as a digestive herb, prescribed for stomach pains and flatulence. The leaves contain essential oils and tannins. Herbalists use it in a tea as a sedative, for insomnia, fever, colds, and diarrhea. It has been reported effective in treating iron-deficiency anemia, menstrual and uterine disorders, and dyspepsia. The FDA issued a notice in 1992 that catnip has not been shown to be safe and effective as claimed in OTC digestive aid products.

CAULERPA TAXIFOLIA • See Quercitin.

CAULIFLOWER UNSAPONIFIABLES • The portion of cauliflower oil which is not saponified *(see)* during the refining recovery of cauliflower fatty acids.

CAUSTIC SODA • See Sodium Hydroxide.

CAVIAR EXTRACT • The extract of eggs of the fish, sturgeon.

CD • The abbreviation for Completely Denatured alcohol, meaning a poison was added so that it would not be drinkable.

CD ALCOHOL 19 • A denatured alcohol used as a solvent. See Denaturant.

CEANOTHUS EXTRACT • The extract of the herb *Ceanothus americanus.* Also called New Jersey Tea.

CEDAR • *Cedrus* (or *Cedrys*) *Atlantica.* **Cedar Wood Oil.** The oil from white, red, or various cedars obtained by distillation from fresh leaves and branches. It is often used in perfumes, soaps, and sachets for its warm woodsy scent. Used frequently as a substitute for oil of lavender. There is usually a strong camphor odor that repels insects. Cedar oil can be a photosensitizer, causing skin reactions when the skin is exposed to light.

CEDRENOL • See Cedar.

CEDRO OIL • See Lemon Oil.

CEDROL • See Cedar.

CEDRYL ACETATE • See Cedar.

CEDRYS ATLANTICA • See Cedar.

CELANDINE EXTRACT • *Chelidonium majus.* **Swallowwort.** This tall herb contains alkaloids, choline, histamine, tyramine, saponins, chelidoniol, chelidonic acid, carotene, and Vitamin C. Herbalists use it for the treatment of hepatitis, jaundice, cancer, psoriasis, eczema, corns, and warts. Used for more than 2000 years to soothe the eyes, it also reputedly detoxifies the liver and relieves muscle spasms and bronchospasms.

CELERY • *Apium graveolens.* The root, leaves, and seed are used for medicinal purposes. It grows wild in ditches and salt marshes and has a coarse texture. The seed was one of the first condiments to reach the country of the Gauls and Franks. It was introduced into Europe by military men upon returning home from Roman conquests. Celery seed is used by herbalists as a diuretic, blood cleanser, and to treat arthritis. It is used in "organic" cosmetics. Celery seed may cause a sensitivity to light, and some people are allergic to it.

CELLULAR MEMBRANE COMPLEX • A fluid in the shaft that binds the hair. The difference between coarse and fine hair has a physiochemical basis: All hairs have a tough, shell-like casing (the cuticle) and a soft, fibrous inner cortex. In coarse hair, the cuticle makes up 10 percent of the volume and the cortex 90 percent. In fine hair, the proportion is 40 percent cuticle and 60 percent cortex. Hair product manufacturers claim cellular membrane complex can benefit from a "conditioner." Hair is dead. Active growth of the hair is only within the bulb.

CELLULOID® • A nail finish composed essentially of cellulose nitrate and camphor (see) or other plasticizers. Also used for brushes and combs as well as for photographic films and various household products. No known toxicity.

CELLULOSE • Chief constituent of the fiber of plants. Cotton contains about 90 percent. It is the basic material for cellulose gums *(see).* Used as an emulsifier in cosmetic creams. No known toxicity.

CELLULOSE GUMS • Any of several fibrous substances consisting of the chief part of the cell walls of plants. Ethylcellulose is a film-former in lipstick. Methylcellulose (Methocel®) and hydroxy ethylcellulose (Cellosize®) are used as emulsifiers in hand creams and lotions. They are resistant to bacterial decomposition and give uniform viscosity to products. On the basis of the available animal and human data, the CIR Expert Panel *(see)* concludes that this ingredient is safe as used in cosmetics.

CENTAUREA CYANUS • **Cornflower.** European plant with blue, pink, or white flowers.

CENTAURY • *Erythraea centaureum.* A small, pretty annual native to the United Kingdom, it is used by herbalists for jaundice. A tisane *(see)* made as a tonic, to stimulate appetite and digestion. It is a strong antiseptic and good for cuts and scratches, and is also used as a mouthwash. Legend has it that its medicinal properties were discovered by a centaur. Used in "organic" cosmetics.

CENTELLA • **Asiaticoside.** A member of the *Umbelliferae* family like celery, the active principle is asiaticoside. It has wound healing properties.

CENTURY EXTRACT • **Agave American.** A succulent perennial native to tropical America. The leaves and juice contain saponins, volatile oil, gums, and proteins. It is used by herbalists as a diuretic, laxative, antiseptic, and to induce menstrual flow. It is used internally for digestive disorders, liver ailments, pulmonary tuberculosis, and venereal disease. It is also used for skin diseases and to treat burns and cuts. Agave may be toxic in large doses. It can cause irritation of the mucous membranes of the stomach, nausea, vomiting, and hemorrhage. Large and frequent doses can lead to liver damage.

CEPHALINS • Central nervous system tissue used in skin conditioners and "anti-aging" creams.

CERA ALBA • See Beeswax.

CERA MICROCRISTALLINA • See Microcrystalline Wax.

CERAMIDES • Synthetic fatty alcohols used in hair conditioners and skin conditioners.

CEREBROSIDES • Fatty acids and sugars found in the covering of nerves.

CERESIN • **Ceresine® Earth Wax.** Used in protective creams. It is a white or yellow, hard, brittle wax made by purifying ozokerite *(see),* found in the Ukraine, Utah, and Texas. It is used as a substitute for beeswax and paraffin *(see both);* also used to wax paper and cloth, as a polish, wax, and paraffin *(see both);* also used to wax paper and cloth, as a polish, and in dentistry for taking wax impressions. May cause allergic reactions.

CEREUS GRANDIFLORUS • See Cactus.

CERIA/SILICA • An ultraviolet light absorber. See Silica.

CERIA/SILICA TALC • Ultraviolet light absorber. See Talc.

CERIUM OXIDE • An opacifying ingredient.

CEROTIC ACID • **Hexacosanoic Acid.** A fatty acid obtained from beeswax, carnauba wax, or Chinese wax. White, odorless crystals or powder soluble in alcohol, benzene, ether, and acetone. See Beeswax.

CERTIFIED • Each batch of coal tar or petrochemical colors, with the exception of those used in hair dyes, must be certified by the FDA as "harmless and suitable for use." The manufacturer must submit samples of every batch for testing and the lot test number accompanies the colors thorough all subsequent packaging.

CETALKONIUM CHLORIDE • Derived from ammonium, it is an antibacterial ingredient used in cosmetics. Soluble in water, alcohol, acetone, and ethyl acetate. See Quaternary Ammonium Compounds.

CETEARALKONIUM BROMIDE • The quaternary ammonium salt that is a blend of cetyl and stearyl radicals.

CETEARETH-3 • **Cetyl/Stearyl Ether.** An oily liquid distilled from a combination of cetyl alcohol made from spermaceti *(see)* and stearyl alcohol made from sperm whale oil. The compound is used as an emollient, an emulsifier, an antifoam ingredient, and a lubricant in cosmetics. Nontoxic.

CETEARETH-4,-6,-8,-10,-12,-15,17,-27,-30 • See Ceteareth-3.

CETEARETH-5 • Emollient and emulsifier from cetyl alcohol and ethylene oxide. See Cetyl Alcohol and Ceteareth-3.

CETEARETH-20 • Widely used polyethylene glycol ether of Cetearyl Alcohol *(see)* as a surfactant, cleansing ingredient, and solubilizer. Used in hair conditioners and dyes, body and hand preparations, moisturizers, indoor tanning and suntan products, and mudpacks. The CIR Expert Panel *(see)* cautioned that this ingredient enhances skin absorption of drugs and that care should be taken when creating formulations, especially those products intended for use on infants.

CETEARETH-25 • Widely used polyethylene glycol ether of Cetearyl Alcohol that is used as a surface-active ingredient, cleansing ingredient, and a solubilizer.

CETEARYL ALCOHOL • **Cetostearyl Alcohol.** Emulsifying wax. A mixture chiefly of the fatty alcohols—cetyl and stearyl *(see both)*—and used primarily in ointments as an emulsifier. Very widely used in hair tints, cleansing lotions, skin care preparations, night skin care, shampoos, hair straighteners, suntan preparations, lipsticks, permanent waves, eye makeup, makeup bases, foot powders and sprays. The CIR Expert Panel *(see)* concludes this is a safe ingredient.

CETEARYL GLUCOSIDE • Made from cetearyl alcohol and glucose *(see both)* and used as an emulsifier in fragrances, cleansers, body and hand preparations.

CETEARYL OCTANOATE • See Caprylic Acid.

CETEARYL STEARATE • A skin-conditioning ingredient.

CETETH-1 • See Ceteth-2.

CETETH-2 • **Polyethylene (2) Cetyl Ether.** A compound of derivatives of cetyl, lauryl, stearyl, and oleyl alcohols *(see all)* mixed with ethylene oxide, a gas used as a fungicide and a starting material for detergents. Oily liquids or waxy solids. Used as surface-active ingredients *(see)* and an emulsifier to allow oil and water to mix to form a smooth cosmetic lotion or cream. See individual alcohols for toxicity.

CETETH-4, -6, -10, -2, -30 • The CIR Expert Panel *(see)* concludes this is a safe ingredient. See Ceteth-2.

CETETH-20 • Polyethylene glycol ether of Cetyl Alcohol *(see)* widely used in hair products, skin-care preparations, cleansing products, and moisturizers. Also used in shaving preparations and depilatories.

CETETHYL MORPHOLINIUM ETHOSULFATE • The CIR Expert Panel *(see)* concludes there is insufficient data to support the safety of this ingredient for use in cosmetics.

CETRARIA ISLANDICA • **Iceland Moss. Iceland Lichen.** So named because Icelanders reputedly were the first to discover its benefits. It is high in mucilage, with some iodine, traces of Vitamin A, and usnic acid. Herbalists use the lichen as a gentle laxative and to relieve upper respiratory problems associated with degenerative wasting.

CETRIMONIUM BROMIDE • A cationic *(see)* detergent and antiseptic, disinfectant, and cleansing ingredient in skin-cleaning products and shampoos. It masks or decreases perspiration odors. Can be fatal if swallowed. Toxic to mice embryos given intravenously and in food. Can be irritating to the skin and eyes. The CIR Expert Panel *(see)* concludes on the basis of animal studies this ingredient is safe for use in "rinse-off" products, and for use at concentrations of up to 0.25 percent in "leave-on" products.

CETRIMONIUM CHLORIDE • The CIR Expert Panel *(see)* concludes on the basis of animal studies this ingredient is safe for use in "rinse-off" products, and for use at concentrations of up to 0.25 percent in "leave-on" products. See Quaternary Ammonium Compounds.

CETRIMONIUM TOSYLATE • A quaternary ammonium compound *(see)*.

CETYL- • Means derived from cetyl alcohol *(see)*.

CETYL ACETATE • The ester *(see)* of cetyl alcohol and acetic acid *(see both)*. Used in hand lotions.

CETYL ACETYL RICINOLEATE • See Oleic Acid and Cetyl Acetate.

CETYL ALCOHOL • An emollient and emulsion stabilizer used in many cosmetic preparations including baby lotion, brilliantine hairdressings, deodorants and antiperspirants, cream depilatories, eyelash creams and oils, foundation creams, hair lacquers, hair straighteners, hand lotions, lipsticks, liquid powders, mascaras, nail polish removers, nail whiteners, cream rouges, and shampoos. Cetyl alcohol is waxy, crystalline, and solid, and found in spermaceti *(see)*. It has a low toxicity for both skin and ingestion and is sometimes used as a laxative. Can cause hives.

CETYL AMMONIUM • An ammonium compound, germicide, and fungicide used in cuticle softeners, deodorants, and baby creams. Medicinally an antibacterial ingredient. See Quaternary Ammonium Compounds for toxicity.

CETYL ARACHIDATE • An ester produced by the reaction of cetyl alcohol and arachidic acid. The acid is found in fish oils and vegetables, particularly peanut oil. A fatty compound used as an emulsifier and emollient in cosmetic creams. Nontoxic.

CETYL BETAINE • Occurs in the common beet and many vegetable and animal substances. Colorless, deliquescent crystals with a sweet taste. See Quaternary Ammonium Compounds.

CETYL ESTERS • The CIR Expert Panel *(see)* concludes on the basis of animal studies this ingredient is safe for use in "rinse-off" products, and for use at concentrations of up to 0.25 percent in "leave-on" products. See Synthetic Spermaceti.

CETYL HYDROXYETHYLCELLULOSE • An emulsifier and stabilizer. See Methylcellulose and Cetyl Alcohol.

CETYL LACTATE • An emollient to improve the feel and texture of cosmetic and pharmaceutical preparations. Produced by the reaction of cetyl alcohol and lactic acid *(see both)*. No known toxicity.

CETYL MYRISTATE • Produced by the reaction of cetyl alcohol and myristic acid *(see both)*.

CETYL OCTANOATE • The ester of cetyl alcohol and 2-ethylhexamonic acid. A moisturizer used in creams and lipsticks. See Cetyl Alcohol and Caproic Acid.

CETYL OLEATE • The ester of cetyl alcohol and oleic acid *(see both)*.

CETYL PALMITATE • Produced by the reaction of cetyl alcohol and palmitic acid. Used in the manufacture of soaps and lubricants. Widely used in skin care preparations, eye shadows, foundations, mud packs, after-shave lotions, and eye lotions. Nontoxic. The CIR Expert Panel *(see)* concludes that this ingredient is safe for use in cosmetic products.

CETYL PHOSPHATE • A mixture of esters of phosphoric acid and cetyl alcohol *(see both)*.

CETYL PYRROLIDONYLMETHYL DIMONIUM CHLORIDE • A quaternary ammonium *(see)* product.

CETYL RICINOLEATE • Salt derivative of castor oil used in tanning preparations. See Ricinoleic Acid.

CETYL STEARATE • An emollient used as a skin conditioning ingredient. On the basis of the available animal and human data, the CIR Expert Panel *(see)* concludes that this ingredient is safe as used in cosmetics.

CETYL STEARYL GLYCOL • A mixture of cetyl glycol and stearyl glycol fatty alcohols that are used as emulsifiers and emollients in cosmetic creams. Nontoxic.

CETYLAMINE HYDROFLUORIDE • An organic salt of fluoride. See Fluoride.

CETYLARACHIDOL • A suds and foam stabilizer that is used in hair and body shampoos and in various types of household detergents. It also has mild conditioning properties, and in some instances it may be used as an emulsifier. See Quaternary Ammonium Compounds for toxicity.

CETYLPYRIDINIUM CHLORIDE • A white powder soluble in water and alcohol. The quaternary salt of pyridine *(see)* and cetyl chloride. A white powder used as an antiseptic and disinfectant in mouthwashes and topical antiseptics and as a deodorant. See Quaternary Ammonium Compounds for toxicity.

CETYLTRYMETHYLAMMONIUM BROMIDE • An antimicrobial preservative that helps destroy and prevent growth of germs. See Quaternary Ammonium Compounds.

CGAENOMELES JAPONICA • See Quince Seed.

CHALK • Purified calcium carbonate *(see)* used in nail whiteners, powders, and liquid makeup to assist in spreading and to give characteristic smooth feeling. A grayish white, amorphous powder usually molded into cones for the cosmetic industry. Used medicinally as a mild astringent and antacid. Nontoxic.

CHAMAECYPARIS OBTUSA • **Cypress.** An essential oil used in fragrances.

CHAMAZULENE • A hydrocarbon used in skin conditioners.

CHAMOMILE • **Roman, German, and Hungarian Chamomile.** The daisylike white and yellow heads of these flowers provide a coloring ingredient known as apigenin. The essential oil distilled from the flower heads is pale blue and is added to shampoos to impart the odor of chamomile. Powdered flowers are used to bring out a bright yellow color in the hair. Also used in rinses and skin fresheners. Roman chamomile is used in berry, fruit, vermouth, maple, spice, and vanilla flavorings. English chamomile is used as a flavoring in chocolate, fruit, and liquor flavorings for beverages, ice cream, ices, candy, and baked goods. Roman chamomile oil is used in chocolate, fruit, vermouth, and spice flavorings for beverages, ice cream, ices, candy, baked goods, gelatin desserts, and liquors. Hungarian chamomile oil is used in chocolate, fruit, and liquor flavorings for beverages, ice cream, ices, candy, baked goods, chewing gum, and liquors. Chamomile contains sesquiterpene lactones, which may cause allergic contact dermatitis and stomach upsets.

CHAMOMILLA RECUTITA • Camomile Oil. Wild Chamomile Extract. The volatile oil distilled from the dried flower heads or extract of the flower heads of *Matricaria chamomilla*. Used internally as a soothing tea and tonic and externally as a soothing medication for contusions and other inflammation. See Tannic Acid and Chamomile.

CHAPARRAL EXTRACT • The extract of the desert plant chaparral, *Larrea mexicana*. The leaves of this dwarf evergreen contain antioxidants and are considered by herbalists as an antibiotic. The leaves are ground and may be used in a tea or in capsules. It is used for blood purification, cancer and tumors, antioxidants, arthritis, colds and flu, diarrhea, and urinary tract infections. The American Indians used it to treat arthritis. A modern Argentine study showed that the primary constituent of chaparral, NDGA (nordihydroguaiaretic acid), an antioxidant, possesses pain-relieving properties and blood-pressure lowering properties. Two cases of chaparral-induced toxic hepatitis were reported in 1992 by the FDA.

CHAULMOOGRA OIL • *Taraktogenos Kurzil.* An East Indian tree, the oil has long been used to treat leprosy and skin diseases. The soft fat from the seeds are composed chiefly of glycerides *(see)*.

CHEILITIS • Dermatitis of the lips attributed to lipsticks. The symptoms are dryness, chapping, cracked and peeling lips. Sometimes this is accompanied by swelling and blistering. About 95 percent of the symptoms have been found to be caused by the indelible dyes used in most lipsticks. The lips are more susceptible to irritation and allergic problems than other parts of the body due to the absence of the horny or dead layer of skin that protects the rest of the body. Even minute amounts of lipstick can cause gastrointestinal problems such as gastritis, enteritis, and colitis in susceptible women. Many allergic women are able to solve the problem of cheilitis merely by changing brands of lipsticks. Others may be able to use hypoallergenic brands that do not contain the most common sensitizers—lanolin and perfumes or the staining dye, dibromofluorescein *(see)*.

CHELATING INGREDIENT • Any compound, usually that binds and precipitates metals, such as ethylenediamine tetraacetic acid (EDTA), which removes trace metals. See Sequestering Ingredient.

CHELIDONIUM MAJUS • Swallowwort. Devil's Milk. Rock poppy. This tall herb contains alkaloids, choline, histamine, tyramine, saponins, chelidoniol, chelidonic acid, carotene, and Vitamin C. Herbalists use it for the treatment of hepatitis, jaundice, cancer, psoriasis, eczema, corns, and warts. Used for more than two thousand years to soothe the eyes, it also reputedly detoxifies the liver, and relieves muscle spasms and bronchospasms. It is used to treat gallbladder problems. The plant can cause a miscarriage when ingested and therefore should not be used during pregnancy. Sanguinarine found in this plant produces glaucoma in experimental animals and also cancer.

CHENOPODIUM • See Quince Seed.

CHERIMOYA • A small, widely cultivated American tree, *Annona cherimols* with three-petalled, yellowish flower. Used in "organic" cosmetics.

CHERRY PIT OIL • A natural lipstick flavoring and fragrance extracted from the pits of sweet and sour cherries. Also a cherry flavoring for beverages, ice cream, and condiments. No known toxicity.

CHESTNUT • *Castanea Vulgaris.* **Spanish Chestnut. Sweet Chestnut. Horse Chestnut.** Nuts from European tree used as a remedy for piles, backaches, and for coughs. An astringent, the bark and leaves were used to make a tonic, which was also reportedly useful in the treatment of upper respiratory ailments such as coughs, and particularly whooping cough.

CHIA OIL • Oil expressed from the seed of *Salvia hispanica.* Fats and oils used in skin conditioners.

CHICKWEED • *Stellaria media.* **Starweed. Herbal Slim.** The herb contains saponins, which exert an anti-inflammatory action similar to cortisone but according to herbalists, it is much milder and without the side effects. Chickweed is also used for weight loss, for skin irritations, itches, and rashes and to soothe sore throat and lungs.

CHICORY EXTRACT • *Cichorium Intybus.* **Wild Succory.** Related to dandelion, in ancient times it was used as a narcotic, sometimes administered before operations. It is used by herbalists to treat liver problems, constipation, and arthritis.

CHIMYL ALCOHOL • Obtained from shark liver oil and other fish oils. Used as skin conditioners and emollients.

CHINA CLAY • See Kaolin.

CHINESE ANGELICA ROOT • *Aralia Chinensia.* An Asiatic shrub with prickly skin and a long inflorescence. Used in "organic" cosmetics.

CHINESE HIBISCUS EXTRACT • From the leaves and flowers of *Hibiscus rosasinensis.*

CHINESE MAGNOLIA EXTRACT • From the flowers and buds of *Magnolia biondii* or other species of magnolia.

CHINESE TEA EXTRACT • From the leaves of *Thea sinensis* or the seeds of *Camelia oleifera abal.* Contains tannin, which is soothing to the skin.

CHITIN • A white powder similar in structure to cellulose *(see),* it is the principal constituent of the shells of crabs, lobsters, and beetles. It is also found in some fungi, algae, and yeasts. It is used in wound-healing emulsions and in tanning products.

CHITOSAN • A derivative of chitin *(see)* used to aid coloring.

CHLORACETAMIDE • See Quaternary Ammonium Compounds.

CHLORAL HYDRATE • **Knockout Drops.** Transparent, colorless crystals with a slightly acrid odor and bitter taste, it is used in hypnotic drugs, in the manufacture of liniments and in hair tonic. It may cause contact dermatitis, gastric disturbances, and when ingested it is narcotic. The lethal human dose is 10 grams.

CHLORAMINE-T • **Sodium p-Toluenesulfonchloramide.** A preservative and antiseptic used in nail bleaches, dental preparations, and mouthwashes. White crystals fairly soluble in water, which lose moisture at 100 degrees F. It is a powerful antiseptic and is used for washing wounds. May be irritating to the skin and cause allergic reactions.

CHLORELLA • Green Algae. A cheap source of Vitamin B complex and used in "antiaging" products.

CHLORELLA FERMENT • An extract of the rust of the fermentation of chlorella *(see)* by yeast. Used for astringents, hair tonics, and moisturizers.

CHLORHEXIDINE • A white, crystalline powder used as a topical antiseptic and skin sterilizing ingredient in liquid cosmetics and in European feminine hygiene sprays. May cause contact dermatitis. Strongly alkaline. The CIR Expert Panel *(see)* concludes on the basis of present data, chlorhexidine and its salts are safe for use in cosmetic products at concentration of up to 0.14 percent as chlorhexidine; 0.19 percent as chlorhexidine diacetate *(see);* 0.20 percent as chlorhexidine digluconate and 0.16 percent as chlorhexidine dihydrochloride.

CHLORHEXIDINE DIACETATE • The salt of chlorhexidine and acetic acid. Derived from methanol and acetic acid *(see),* which are derived from fruits. It is used as an antiseptic. See Chlorhexidine.

CHLORHEXIDINE DI GLUCONATE • See Chlorhexidine.

CHLORHEXIDINE DIHYDROCHLORIDE • Salt of chlorhexidine and hydrochloric acid. Derived from methanol. Used as a solvent. See Chlorhexidine.

CHLORINATED HYDROCARBONS • Hydrocarbons in which one or more of the hydrogen atoms have been replaced by chlorine *(see).* Many members of the group have been shown to cause cancer in animals and some of them to cause cancer in humans. Among the designated carcinogens: chloroform, vinyl chloride, trichloroethylene, and carbon tetrachloride *(see all).* Concern about the potential hazard of certain chlorinated hydrocarbons is based on their ubiquity; their persistence in the environment; their capacity to accumulate in living organisms including humans and the human fetus; and the experimental evidence of a potential carcinogenic effect.

CHLORINE • A nonmetallic element, a diatomic gas that is heavy, noncombustible, and greenish yellow, it is found in the earth's crust and has a pungent suffocating odor. In liquid form it is a clear amber color with an irritating odor. It does not occur in a free state but as a component of the mineral halite (rock salt). Toxic and irritating to the skin and lungs, it has a tolerance level of one part per million in air. It is used in the manufacture of carbon tetrachloride and in flame retardant compounds; and in processing fish, vegetables, and fruit. It is used in the manufacture of carbon tetrachloride, trichloroethylene, shrinkproofing wool, in special batteries, and in the manufacture of ethylene dichloride (see). The chlorine used to kill bacteria in drinking water may contain carcinogenic carbon tetrachloride, a contaminant formed during the production process. Chlorination has also been found to sometimes form undesirable "ring" compounds in water, such as toluene, xylene, and the suspected carcinogen styrene—they have been observed in both the drinking water and waste-water plants in the Midwest. Chlorine is a powerful irritant, and can be fatal upon inhalation. In fact it is in military arsenals as a poison gas. A National Cancer Institute study published in 1987 linked bladder cancer to people who had been drinking chlorinated surface water for 40 or more years.

CHLORACETAMIDE • A preservative used in cold cream, cleansing lotions, body and hand preparations, mud packs, shampoos, and hair preparations. See Acetamide.

CHLOROACETIC ACID • Made by the chlorination of acetic acid *(see)* in the presence of sulfur or iodine. Used in the manufacture of soaps and creams. It is irritating to the skin and mucous membranes and can be toxic and corrosive when swallowed.

4-CHLORO2-AMINOPHENOL • A coal tar and an amine color. See Coal Tar.

CHLOROBUTANOL • A white, crystalline alcohol used as a preservative in eye lotions and as an antioxidant in baby oils. It has a camphor odor and taste. Formerly used medicinally as a hypnotic and sedative; today it is employed as an anesthetic and antiseptic. A central nervous system depressant, it is used as a hypnotic drug. No known skin toxicity.

p-CHLORO-m-CRESOL • A preservative in skin care and suntan cosmetic formulations. Prohibited for use in products in contact with mucous membranes. A solution as low as 0.05 percent caused eye irritation in rabbits. A chronic feeding study caused kidney damage in male rats and an increase in adrenal tumors. Some evidence of skin irritation and sensitization was found in animal studies. The CIR Expert Panel *(see)* concludes that the available data are insufficient to support the safety of this ingredient in cosmetic products. See Cresols.

CHLOROFORM • Used in products to clean wool or synthetic fabrics, and as a solvent for fats, oils, waxes, resins, and as a cleaning ingredient. It has many serious side effects and is considered a carcinogen. Exposure to it may also cause respiratory and skin allergies. Complaints received by the FDA about blisters and inflammation of the gums caused by toothpaste were found to be due to the amount of chloroform in the product. The manufacturer was asked to reduce the amount of the substance. Large doses may cause low blood pressure, heart stoppage, and death. In April 1976, the FDA determined that chloroform may cause cancer and asked drug and cosmetic manufacturers who have not already done so to discontinue using it immediately, even before it was officially banned. The National Cancer Institute made public in June 1976, the finding that chloroform was found to cause liver and kidney cancers in test animals. It is no longer permitted in cosmetics.

CHLOROGENIC ACIDS • Isolated from coffee beans, used as an antioxidant.

5-CHLORO-8-HYDROXYQUINOLONE • See Oxyquinoline Sulfate.

CHLOROMETHOXYPROPYLMERCURIC ACETATE • A preservative. See Mercury Compounds.

2-CHLORO-5-NITRO-N-HYDROXYETHYL-p-PHENYLENEDIAMINE • A coal tar hair coloring. See Coal Tar and Phenylenediamine.

CHLOROPHENE o-BENZYL-p-CHLOROPHENOL • Prepared from benzyl chloride and phenoxide followed by chlorination. Used in Lysol® Disinfectant. See Phenol for toxicity.

p-CHLOROPHENOL • A bacteria killer. Can cause ear, nose, and throat irritations, skin rashes, and reproductive problems. Chlorophenol compounds are on the Community Right to Know List *(see)*. Caused tumors and birth defects in laboratory animals.

2-CHLORO-p-PHENYLENEDIAMINE • See p-Phenylenediamine.

2-CHLORO-p-PHENYLENEDIAMINE SULFATE • See p-Phenylenediamine.

CHLOROPHYLL • The green coloring matter of plants, which plays an essential part in the plant's photosynthesis process. Used in antiperspirants, dentifrices, deodorants, and mouthwashes as a deodorizing ingredient. It imparts a greenish color to certain fats and oils, notably olive oil and soybean. Can cause a sensitivity to light.

CHLOROPHYLLIN • Copper derivative, used as a deodorant ingredient in mouthwashes, breath fresheners, and body deodorants. Derived from chlorophyll, the green coloring matter of plants. See Chlorophyll. Banned by the FDA.

CHLOROPHYLLIN COPPER COMPLEX • See Chlorophyllin. Banned by the FDA as a coloring.

CHLOROPROPIONIC ACID AND SALTS • Prepared from cyanohydrin and hydrochloric acid. It absorbs water.

4-CHLORORESORCINOL • See Resorcinol.

CHLOROTHYMOL • A chloro derivative of thymol *(see)* and a powerful germicide used in mouthwashes, hair tonics, and baby oils. It kills staph germs and is used topically as an antibacterial. Can be irritating to the mucous membranes and can possibly be absorbed through the skin.

CHLOROXYLENOL • A white, crystalline solid used as an antiseptic, germicide, and fungicide in hair tonics, shampoos, contraceptive douches, deodorants, bath salts, vaginal deodorants, and brushless shaving creams. Penetrates the skin but has no apparent irritating effects when diluted at 5 percent. May cause greenish discoloration of the hair when swimming in chlorinated water. Active ingredient in germicides, antiseptics, and antifungal preparations. Toxic by ingestion. May be irritating to and absorbed by the skin. The CIR Expert Panel *(see)* concludes, on the basis of animal studies, this ingredient is safe. See p-Chloro-m-Xylenol.

CHLORPHENESIN • An alcohol used as a germicide.

CHLORPHENIRAMINE • An antihistamine re-categorized first in low dosage from RX to OTC in 1976 and in stronger strengths in 1981. It is used to treat stuffy nose and other allergy symptoms. The Food and Drug Administration issued a notice in 1992 that chlorpheniramine maleate has not been shown to be safe and effective for stated claims in OTC products for poison ivy, poison oak, and poison sumac drug products.

CHLORZOXAZONE • Crystals from acetone *(see)*. Used as a skeletal muscle-relaxant.

CHOLESTEROL • A fat-soluble, crystalline steroid alcohol *(see)* occurring in all animal fats and oils, nervous tissue, egg yolk, and blood. Used as an emulsifier and lubricant in brilliantine hairdressing, eye creams, shampoos, and other cosmetic products. It is important in metabolism but has been implicated as contributing to hardening of the arteries and subsequently heart attacks. Nontoxic to the skin.

CHOLESTERYL ACETATE • An ester *(see)* of cholesterol *(see)* used as a skin conditioner.

CHOLESTERYL ISOSTEARATE • A skin conditioning ingredient. See Cholesterol.

CHOLESTERYL MACADAMIATE • Fatty acids obtained from macadamia nuts and used as a skin conditioning ingredient.

CHOLESTERYL OLEYL CARBONATE • A skin conditioning ingredient used in "antiaging" products. See Cholesterol and Oleic Acid.

CHOLESTERYL/BEHENYLOCTYL-DODECYL LUROYL GLUTAMATE • A skin conditioning ingredient. See Cholesterol.

CHOLESTERYL/OCTYLDODECYL LAUROYL GLUTAMATE • A skin conditioning ingredient. See Cholesterol and Glutamate.

CHOLETH-10–20 • The polyethylene glycol ether *(see)* of cholesterol *(see)*. Used in hand creams.

CHOLIC ACID • A colorless or white, crystalline powder that occurs in the bile of most vertebrates and is used as an emulsifying ingredient in dried egg whites and as a choleretic to regulate the secretion of bile. Bitter taste, sweetish aftertaste. No known toxicity. The final report to the FDA of the Select Committee on GRAS Substances stated in 1980 that it should continue its GRAS status with no limitations other than good manufacturing practices.

CHOLINE • A syrupy liquid included in the B complex vitamins. It is a base widely distributed among plant and animal products. It is either free or in combination with lecithin. It is essential to the metabolism of fat, especially in the liver, and it is used in the form of salts to treat liver disease. It is also used to feed animals, especially poultry.

CHOLINE BITARTRATE • A dietary supplement included in the B complex vitamins and found in the form of a thick syrupy liquid in most animal tissue. It is necessary to nerve function and fat metabolism and can be manufactured in the body but not at a sufficient rate to meet health requirements. Dietary choline protects against poor growth, fatty liver, and renal damage in many animals. Choline deficiency has not been demonstrated in man but the National Academy of Sciences lists 500 to 900 milligrams per day as sufficient for the average man. The final report to the FDA of the Select Committee on GRAS Substances stated in 1980 that it should continue its GRAS status with no limitations other than good manufacturing practices.

CHOLINE CHLORIDE • **Ferric Choline Citrate.** A dietary supplement with the same function as choline bitartrate *(see)*. The final report to the FDA of the Select Committee on GRAS Substances stated in 1980 that it should continue its GRAS status with no limitations other than good manufacturing practices.

CHOLINE HYDROCHLORIDE • Colorless to white, water-absorbing crystals used as a fungicide on various feeds. In the Community Right to Know List *(see)*. Moderately toxic to humans by ingestion. May be mutagenic.

CHONDROITIN • A major constituent of cartilage in the body.

CHONDRUS • See Carrageenan.

CHROMIC ACID • See Chromium Compounds.

CHROMIUM COMPOUNDS • **Oxides.** Chromium occurs in the earth's crust. Chromic oxide is used for green eye shadow and chromium oxide for greenish mascara. Inhalation of chromium dust can cause irritation and ulceration. Ingestion results in violent gastrointestinal irritation. Application to the skin may result in allergic reaction. The most serious effect of chromium is lung cancer, which may develop 20 to 30 years after exposure. One study showed that the death rate from lung cancer among exposed chromium workers is twenty-nine times that of the normal population.

CHROMIUM HYDROXIDE GREEN • Coloring, permanently listed for use as a cosmetic coloring in 1977. See Chromium Compounds.

CHROMIUM OXIDE GREENS • Widely used coloring in eyeliners, mascara, eyebrow pencils, eye makeup, face powders, makeup bases, dusting powders, and cleansing products. See Chromium Compounds.

CHROMIUM SULFATE • Violet or red powder used in the textile industries, in green paints and varnishes, green ice, ceramics, in tanning, and in green eye shadows. Can cause contact dermatitis.

CHRYSANTHELLUM INDICUM • See Chrysanthemum.

CHRYSANTHEMUM • *Chrysanthemum sinense.* **Ye Ju. Corn Marigold.** A large family of perennial herbs thought to originate in Asia. A tea made from this flower is used to treat conjunctivitis and skin diseases. Taken internally, it is used to lower blood pressure. A number of medicines and the insecticidal pyrethrins *(see)* are derived from this family.

CHYMOTRYPSIN • **Catarase. Chymar. Zolyse.** A pancreatic enzyme. See Enzyme.

CHYPRE • A nonalcoholic type of perfume containing oils and resins.

CI 10006-CI 77947 • Inorganic colors used mostly in hair dyes. They are listed by number in the European Union but are not permitted to be listed that way on U.S. labels. Most of them are designated D & C colors or by ingredient name such as Manganese Violet instead of CI 77742 if they are permitted in U.S. products.

CIBOTIUM BAROMETZ • **Pengawar.** A genus of oriental tree ferns with gracefully drooping flowers. Used in fragrances.

CICHORIUM INTYBUS • **Chicory. Wild Succory.** Related to dandelion, in ancient times it was used as a narcotic, sometimes administered before operations. Used by herbalists to treat liver problems, constipation, and arthritis.

CICLOPIROX OLAMINE • A germicide. See Pyridine.

CIMICIFUGA RACEMOSA • **Black Cohosh. Snakeroot. Bugbane. Black Snakeroot. Rattleroot.** Used in astringents, perennial herb with a flower that is supposedly distasteful to insects. Grown from Canada to North Carolina and Kansas. It has a reputation for curing snakebites. It is used in ginger ale flavoring. A tonic and antispasmodic. No known toxicity. The root contains various glycosides *(see)* including estrogenic substances and tannins. Herbalists have used it to relieve nerve pains, menstrual pains, and the pain of childbirth. Also used to speed delivery and to reduce blood pressure. Black cohosh is also believed to have sedative properties. In 1992, the FDA proposed a ban on black cohosh in oral menstrual drug products because it had not been shown to be safe and effective as claimed.

CINCHONA EXTRACT • The extract of the bark of various species of *Cinchona* cultivated in Java, India, and South American. Quinine is derived from it.

CINNAMAL • **Cinnamaldehyde. Cinnamic Aldehyde.** A synthetic, yellowish, oily liquid with a strong odor of cinnamon isolated from a wood-rotting fungus. Occurs naturally in cassia bark extract, cinnamon bark, and root oils. Used for its aroma in perfume and for flavoring in mouthwash and toothpaste. Also to scent powder and hair tonic. It is irritating to the skin and mucous membranes, especially if undiluted. One of the most common allergens.

CINNAMATE • Salt or ester of Cinnamic Acid *(see)*.

CINNAMIC ACID • Used in suntan lotions and perfumes. Occurs in storax, Balsam Peru, cinnamon leaves, and coca leaves. Usually isolated from wood-rotting fungus. It may cause allergic skin rashes.

CINNAMIC ALCOHOL • Fragrance ingredient. One of the most common allergens in fragrances and flavorings. Used in mouthwashes, toilet soaps, toothpastes, and sanitary napkins. See Cinnamal.

CINNAMIC ALDEHYDE • Found in cinnamon oil, cassia oil, cinnamon powder, patchouli oil, flavoring ingredients, toilet soaps and perfumes. It cross-reacts with Balsam Peru and benzoin. May cause depigmentation and hives. It is used in synthetic jasmine and may be the cause of a reaction to that compound.

CINNAMOMUM CASSIA • See Cinnamon Oil.

CINNAMOMUM ZEYLANICUM • See Cinnamon.

CINNAMON • Used to flavor toothpaste and mouthwash and to scent hair tonic and powder. Obtained from the dried bark of cultivated trees. See Cinnamal for toxicity. Extracts have been used to break up intestinal gas and to treat diarrhea, but can be irritating to the gastrointestinal system. When used as a flavoring in toothpaste, it can cause mouth irritation if patients are sensitive to cinnamon.

CINNAMON BARK • Extract and Oil. From the dried bark of cultivated trees, the extract is used in cola, eggnog, root beer, cinnamon, and ginger ale for beverages, ice cream, baked goods, condiments, and meats. The oil is used in berry, cola, cherry, rum, root beer, cinnamon, and ginger ale flavorings for beverages, condiments, and meats. Can be a skin sensitizer in humans and cause mild sensitivity to light.

CINNAMON LEAF OIL • See Cinnamon Oil.

CINNAMON OIL • **Oil of Cassia. Chinese Cinnamon.** Yellowish to brown, volatile oil from the leaves and twigs of cultivated trees. About 80 to 90 percent cinnamal. It has the characteristic odor and taste of cassia cinnamon and darkens and thickens upon aging or exposure to air. Cinnamon oil is used to scent perfumes and as a flavoring in dentifrices. Can cause contact dermatitis.

CINNAMYL ACETATE • A flavoring agent. See Cinnamyl Alcohol and Acetic Acid.

CINNAMYL ALCOHOL • Occurs in storax, Balsam Peru, cinnamon leaves, and hyacinth oil. A crystalline alcohol with a strong hyacinth odor used in synthetic perfumes and in deodorants for flavoring and scent. Can cause allergic reactions.

CINNAMYL ANTHRANILATE • A synthetic flavoring ingredient and fragrance ingredient used since the 1940s as an imitation grape or cherry flavor. It is used as a fragrance in soaps, detergents, creams, lotions, and perfumes. United States sales equaled more than 2000 pounds in 1976. The National Cancer Institute reported, December 20, 1980, that it caused liver cancer in male and female mice and caused both kidney and pancreatic cancers in male rats in feeding studies. Earlier studies showed it increased lung tumors in mice. The FDA banned the use of it in food in 1982. Most companies voluntarily stopped using it in cosmetics after publication of the NCI information.

CINNAMYL ESTERS • Used in perfumery. See Cinnamic Acid and Esters.

CINOXATE • See Cinnamic Acid.

CIR • Abbreviation for the Cosmetic Ingredient Review.

CIR EXPERT PANEL • Established in 1976 by the Cosmetic, Toiletry, and Fragrance Association (CTFA), the CIR Expert Panel reviews in a public forum the safety of ingredients used in cosmetics. The CIR Expert Panel's formal decision regarding the safety of an ingredient, and the basis for that decision, is made publicly available in its Final Reports. In addition to making reports directly available to the public, CIR submits its safety assessments for publication in the *International Journal of Toxicology*.

CIS- • Latin meaning "on the side." When a certain atom is positioned on one side of a group of carbons, it is called cis- as in cis-jasmone.

CIS-3-HEXEN-1-OL • See Cis- and Hexanol.

CIS-3-HEXENYL ACETATE • See Cis- and Hexanol.

CIS-3-HEXENYL SALICYLATE • See Salicylates and Hexanol.

CIS-JASMONE • A substance found in jasmine *(see)*. Used in perfumery.

CISTUS INANUS • **Rockrose.** Widely distributed woody herb in the Mediterranean region.

CITRAL • A flavoring used in foods and beverages. Used in perfumes, soaps, and colognes for its lemon and verbena scents. Found also in detergents and furniture polish. Occurs naturally in grapefruit, orange, peach, ginger, grapefruit oil, oil of lemon, and oil of lime. A light oily liquid isolated from citral oils or made synthetically. The compound has been reported to inhibit wound healing and tumor rejection in animals. Vitamin A counteracts its toxicity but in commercial products to which pure citral has been added, Vitamin A may not be present.

CITRAL DIMETHYL ACETAL • See Citric Acid and Acetic Acid.

CITRATES • The salts or esters of Citric Acid *(see)* used as softening ingredients. Citrates may interfere with the results of laboratory tests including tests for pancreatic function, abnormal liver function, and blood alkalinity and acidity.

CITRIC ACID • One of the most widely used acids in the cosmetic industry, it is derived from citrus fruit by fermentation of crude sugars. Employed as a preservative and sequestering ingredient *(see)* to adjust acid-alkali balance, as a foam inhibitor and plasticizer. It is also used as an astringent alone or in astringent compounds. Among the cosmetic products in which it is frequently found are freckle and nail bleaches, bath preparations, skin fresheners, cleansing creams, depilatories, eye lotions, hair colorings, hair rinses, and hair-waving preparations. The clear, crystalline, water-absorbing chemicals are also used to prevent scurvy, a deficiency disease, and as a refreshing drink with water and sugar added. No known toxicity. See Alpha-Hydroxy Acids.

CITRONELLA OIL • A natural food flavoring extract from fresh grass grown in Asia. Used in perfumes, toilet waters, and perfumed cosmetics; also an insect repellent. May cause allergic reactions such as stuffy nose, hay fever, asthma, and skin rash when used in cosmetics.

CITRONELLAL • A fragrance ingredient. See Citronella Oil.

CITRONELLOL • Used in perfumes. It has a roselike odor. Occurs naturally in citronella oil, lemon oil, lemon grass oil, tea, rose oil, and geranium oil. A mild irritant.

CITRONELLYL ESTERS • See Citronella Oil and Esters.

CITRULLINE • An amino acid used as a skin conditioning agent.

CITRULLUS COLOCYNTHIS • **Coloc.** From the family of *Cucurbitaceae,* colocynthis is a trailing plant that grows in sandy places. Homeopaths mix the powdered, dried fruit with alcohol and allow the compound to sit for a week. This is one of the main colic remedies used by homeopaths. See Colocynth.

CITRULLUS VULGARIS • Watermelon.

CITRUS GRANDIS • Grapefruit.

CITRUS LIMONUM • Lemon.

CITRUS NOBILIS • Mandarin Orange.

CITRUS OILS • **Eugenol. Eucalyptol.** Anethole, iron, orris, and menthol *(see all).*

CITRUS PARADISI • Grapefruit.

CITRUS TANGERINA • Tangerine.

CITRUS UNSHIU • Japanese Orange Peel.

CIVET • A fixative in perfumery. It is the civet cat's unctuous secretion from between the anus and genitalia of both male and female. Semisolid, yellowish to brown mass, with an unpleasant odor. No known toxicity.

CLARIFYING INGREDIENT • A substance that removes from liquids small amounts of suspended matter. Butyl alcohol, for instance, is a clarifying ingredient for clear shampoos.

CLARY • **Clary Sage.** A fixative *(see)* for perfumes. A natural extract of an aromatic herb grown in southern Europe and cultivated widely in England. A well-known spice in food and beverages. No known toxicity.

CLAY PACK • See Face Masks and Packs.

CLAYS • **Bentonite. Veegum®. China Clay. Kaolin.** Used for color in cosmetics as a clarifying ingredient *(see)* in liquids, as an emollient, and as a poultice. Nontoxic.

CLEANSING CREAMS AND LOTIONS • Used to dissolve sebum, loosen particles of grim, and to facilitate the removal of dirt. They usually contain mineral oil, triethanolamine stearate, and water. Among other ingredients commonly used are alcohol, alkanolamines, allantoins, antibacterials, and preservatives, methyl and propyl parabens, fatty alcohols, lanolin, perfumes, glycerol, propylene glycol, fatty oils, thickeners, and waxes. A well-known hypoallergenic cold cream contains water, mineral oil, waxes, borax, and depollenized beeswax. The American Medical Association and dermatologists say that soap and water will serve the same purpose as cleansing creams and lotions, is less expensive and offers less risk of allergy. (However, soap can be more drying to the skin.) Antibacterials, preservatives, parabens, lanolin, thickeners and perfumes are all common causes of allergic contact dermatitis *(see all)*.

CLEAVERS • *Galium aparine.* **Catchweed. Goosegrass. Clives.** A native of Europe, Asia, and North America, the Greeks called it *philantropon* because they considered its clinging habit showed a love of mankind. In rural medicine it was used for jaundice, scarlet fever, and measles. The crushed herb was folded into a cloth and applied hot in cases of earache and toothache. A cooling drink was given every spring as a tonic. It was also used by dieters to keep them lean and lank. In homeopathic medicine for skin diseases such as psoriasis and scurvy. The whole herb is used by herbalists to treat kidney and bladder problems and gallstones. It has diuretic properties. It is used in "organic" cosmetics.

CLEMATIS EXTRACT • **Old Man's Beard Extract.** The extract obtained from the leaves of *Clematis vitalba.* A red or violet herb or woody vine. It is used in "organic" cosmetics.

CLIMBAZOLE • Germicide.

CLINTONIA BOREALIS • **Lily of the Valley. May Blossom.** The wildflower, which grows in woodlands, causes vomiting. The powdered root is used to slow heartbeat. Also used by herbalists to reduce fluid retention. It has long been used to expel worms from the intestinal tract. The flower was believed to stimulate secretions of the nasal mucous membranes and was employed in the treatment of apoplexy, epilepsy, coma, and dizziness. Contains certain cardiac glycosides similar to those of digitalis. It is used in cosmetics as an anti-irritant and there is some research to show that it increases cell proliferation.

CLOFLUCARBAN • See Aniline Dyes.

CLORTRIMAZOLE • A germicide.

CLOVE OIL • **Eugemoa Caryophyllus.** Used as an antiseptic and flavoring in tooth powders and as a scent in hair tonics and to flavor postage stamp glue, as a toothache treatment, as a condiment, and as a flavoring in chewing gum. It is 82 to 87 percent eugenol *(see)* and has the characteristic clove oil odor and taste. It is strongly irritating to the skin and can cause allergic skin rashes. Its use in perfumes and cosmetics is frowned upon, although in very diluted forms it is allegedly innocuous. In 1992, the FDA proposed a ban on clove oil in astringent *(see)* drug products because it has not been shown to be safe and effective for its stated claims.

CLOVER • An herb, a natural flavoring extract from a plant characterized by three leaves and flowers in dense heads. Used in fruit flavorings for beverages, ice cream, ices, candy, and baked goods. May cause sensitivity to light.

CLOVER BLOSSOM EXTRACT • **Trifolium Extract.** The extract of the flowers of *Trifolium pratense.* Used in fruit flavorings. May cause sensitivity to light.

CLOVERLEAF OIL • **Eugenia Caryophyllus Leaf Oil.** The volatile oil obtained by steam distillation of the leaves of *Eugenia caryophyllus.* It consists mostly of eugenol *(see).*

CLUB MOSS • *Lycopodium clavatum.* American Indians sprinkled a powder made from this herb on wounds to stop bleeding. The powder is used today for minor skin wounds. Both the spores and the whole herb were considered diuretic and antispasmodic, and decoctions were used in rheumatism and diseases of the lungs and kidneys.

CNIDIUM OFFICINALE • A Chinese herb long used for kidney problems, impotence, vaginal infections, and fungus. Used in cosmetics as a fragrance ingredient and skin conditioner.

COAL TAR • Used in adhesives, creosotes, insecticides, phenols, woodworking, preservation of food, and dyes to makes colors used in cosmetics, including hair dyes. Thick liquid or semisolid tar obtained from bituminous coal, it contains many constituents including benzene, xylenes, naphthalene, pyridine, quinoline, phenol, and creosol. The main concern about coal tar derivatives is that they cause cancer in animals but they are also frequent sources of allergic reactions, particularly skin rashes and hives. It is a substance included in many topical preparations for the treatment of psoriasis and dandruff. Coal tar over-the-counter products for dandruff, seborrheic dermatitis, and psoriasis have to state the concentrations of coal tar contained in any coal tar solution, derivative or fraction used in the source of the coal tar product, the FDA ruled in 1992. The FDA then issued a notice in 1992 that coal tar has not been shown to be safe and effective for stated claims in OTC products.

COBALT ACETYLMETHIONATE • The metal cobalt mixed with methionine *(see).*

COBALT CHLORIDE • A metal used in hair dye. Occurs in the earth's crust; gray, hard, and magnetic. Excess administration can produce an over-production of red blood cells and gastrointestinal upset. See Metallic Hair Dyes.

COBALT NAPHTHTHENATE • See Cobalt Chloride.

COCAINE AND SALTS • From the leaves of *Erythroxylon Erythroylacecoca* and other species of *Erythroxylon,* it is a controlled substance. It is used in cosmetics as a topical anesthetic.

COCAMIDE (DEA, MEA) • Widely used fatty acid of coconut oil. Used as a thickener and foam booster. Formation of nitrosamines *(see)* are a problem with these ingredients. Based on the available data, the CIR Expert Panel *(see)* concludes that cocamide DEA is safe as a cosmetic ingredient in concentrations up to 10 percent; however, it should not be used in cosmetic products containing nitrosating agents. See Coconut Oil.

COCAMIDE BETAINE • May form nitrosamines *(see).* Based on the available data, the CIR Expert Panel *(see)* concludes that this ingredient is safe as a cosmetic ingredient. However, it should not be used in cosmetic products containing nitrosating agents. See Quaternary Ammonium Compounds and Coconut Oil.

COCAMIDE MIPA • See Coconut Oil.

COCAMIDOPROPYL BETAINE • Widely used salt of fatty acids, it is used in hair conditioners. It is antistatic and a cleanser. It is also a foam booster and a thickener. See Coconut Oil.

COCAMIDOPROPYL DIMETHYLAMINE • See Coconut Oil.

COCAMIDOPROPYL OXIDE • See Coconut Oil.

COCAMIDOPROPYL SULTAMINE • See Coconut Oil.

COCAMIDOPROPYLAMINE OXIDE • See Coconut Oil.

COCAMINE OXIDE • See Coconut Oil.

COCAMINOBUTYRIC ACID • See Coconut Oil and Butyric acid.

COCAMINOPROPIONIC ACID • See Coconut Oil.

COCAMPHODIPRIOPIONATE • See Coconut Oil.

COCAMPHODIPROPIONIC ACID • See Coconut Oil.

COCETH-6 • See Coconut Oil.

COCETH-10 • A derivative of coconut alcohol, it is used as an emulsifying agent.

COCHINEAL • Banned by the FDA. See Carmine.

COCHLEARIA ARMORACIA AND OFFICINALIS • *Armoracia lapathifolia gilib.* **Horseradish. Scurvy Grass.** A condiment ingredient utilizing the grated root from the tall, coarse, white-flowered herb native to Europe. Often combined with vinegar or other ingredients. Contains ascorbic acid *(see)* and acts as an antiseptic in cosmetics. It contains Vitamin C and is used by herbalists to treat arthritis pain by stimulating blood flow to inflamed joints. Potential adverse reactions include diarrhea and sweating if taken internally in large amounts. GRAS.

COCILLANA BARK • Dried bark of *Guarea rusbyi,* grown in Bolivia. Contains resins, fat, and tannin. Used in emollients. Has been used medicinally as an expectorant.

COCKSCOMB EXTRACT • Obtained by enzyme treatment of roosters' cockscombs.

COCOA • A powder prepared from the roasted and cured kernels of ripe seeds of *Theobroma cacao* and other species of *Theobroma.* A brownish powder with a chocolate odor, it is used as a flavoring. May cause wheezing, rash, and other symptoms of allergy, particularly in children.

COCOA BUTTER • **Theobroma Oil.** Softens and lubricates the skin. A solid fat expressed from the roasted seeds of the cocoa plant that is used in eyelash creams, lipsticks, nail whiteners, rouge, pastes, soaps, and emollient creams as a lubricant and skin softener. Frequently used in massage creams and in suppositories because it softens and melts at body temperature. May cause allergic skin reactions.

COCOA EXTRACT • Extract of *Theobroma cacao.* See Cocoa Butter.

COCOALKONIUM CHLORIDE • A Quaternary Ammonium Compound *(see).*

COCOAMIDOETHYL BETAINE • A surfactant, cleansing ingredient, and foam booster. See Betaines and Coconut Oil.

COCOAMIDOPROPYL BETAINE • Made from coconut oil and beets, it is used in eye makeup remover. May cause an eyelid rash.

COCOAMINDOPROPYL AMINE OXIDE • Widely used hair conditioner, bath ingredient, lotion, and tonic ingredient in hair grooming products. Based on the available data, the CIR Expert Panel *(see)* concludes that there is insufficient data to support the safety of this ingredient in cosmetic products. See Quaternary Ammonium Compounds and Coconut Oil.

COCOAMPHOACTATE • See Coconut Oil.

COCOAMPHOCARBOXYMETHYLHYDROXYPROPYLSULFONATE • See Coconut Oil.

COCOAMPHOCARBOXYPROPIONIC ACID • See Coconut Oil.

COCOAMPHODIACETATE • Widely used in cosmetics in the manufacture of toilet soaps, creams, lubricants, chocolate, and suppositories. See Coconut Oil.

COCOAMPHOHYDROXYPROPYLSULFONATE • See Coconut Oil.

COCO-BETAINE • See Coconut Oil.

COCO-CAPRYLATECAPRATE • An emollient. See Coconut Oil.

COCODIMONIUM-HYDROXYPROPYL HYDROLYZED COLLAGEN • See Quaternary Ammonium Compound.

COCODIMONIUM HYDROXYPROPYL HYDROLYZED HAIR KERATIN • Hydrolyzed *(see)* hair keratin. Used as an antistatic ingredient and as a skin conditioner.

COCOMORPHOLINE OXIDE • See Coconut Oil.

COCONUT ACIDS • Surfactants and cleansing agents used in bath soaps and detergents, shaving creams, cold creams, and shampoos. See Coconut Oil.

COCONUT ALCOHOLS • See Coconut Oil.

COCONUT FATTY ACIDS • See Coconut Oil and Fatty Acids.

COCONUT OIL • *Cocos Nuciferal.* The white, semisolid, highly saturated fat expressed from the kernels of the coconut. Widely used in the manufacture of baby soaps, shampoos, shaving lathers, cuticle removers, preshaving lotions, hairdressings, soaps, ointment bases, and massage creams. Stable when exposed to air. Lathers readily and is a fine skin cleanser. Usually blended with other fats. May cause allergic skin rashes.

COCO-RAPESEEDATE • An ester of coconut oil and rapeseed oil *(see both)* used as an emollient ingredient.

COCOS NUCIFERA • See Coconut Oil.

COCO-SULTAINE • An antistatic ingrdient in hair products and a skin conditioning ingredient. Also a foam booster. See Coconut Oil and Betaines.

COCOTRIMONIUM CHLORIDE • Coconut Trimethyl Ammonium Chloride. See Quaternary Ammonium Compounds.

COCOYL HYDROLYZED COLLAGEN • Formerly called Cocoyl Hydrolyzed Animal Protein. See Hydrolyzed and Proteins.

COCOYL HYDROLYZED SOY PROTEIN • Used as a hair and skin conditioning ingredient. See Coconut Oil and Soy Acid.

COCOYL HYDROXYETHYL IMIDAZOLINE • See Coconut Oil and Imidazoline.

COCOYL IMIDAZOLINE • Heterocyclic compound used as a detergent emulsifier. See Cocoa Butter and Ethylenediamine.

COCOYL SARCOSINAMIDE DEA • **Diethanolamine Cocoyl Sarcosinamide.** Used as a detergent emulsifier. See Cocoa Butter.

COCOYL SARCOSINE • Formed from caffeine by decomposition with barium hydroxide. Used to make antienzyme ingredients for toothpastes that help to prevent decay. No known toxicity.

COCOYLDIMONIUM HYDROXYPROPYL HYDROLYZED COLLAGEN • A hydrolyzed animal protein used in emollients. See Coconut Oil and Proteins.

COCYOL-POLYCLYCERYL-4-HYDROXYPROPYL DIHYDROXYETHYL-AMINE • See Coconut Oil and Surfactants.

COD-LIVER OIL • The fixed oil expressed from fresh livers used in skin ointments and special skin creams to promote healing. Pale yellow, with a bland, slightly fishy odor. Contains Vitamin A and D, which promote healing of wounds and abscesses. No known toxicity.

COENZYME A • Used in skin conditioners. Biotin is an example. See Ubiquinones.

COFFEA ARABICA • Extract of coffee.

COFFEA ROBUSTA EXTRACT • Extract of green coffee.

COFFEE OIL • Used as a flavoring.

COGNAC OIL • **Wine Yeast Oil.** The volatile oil obtained from distillation of wine, with the characteristic aroma of cognac. Green cognac oil is used as a flavoring for beverages, ice cream, ices, candy, baked goods, chewing gum, liquors, and condiments. White cognac oil, which has the same constituents as green oil, is used in berry, cherry, grape, brandy, and rum flavorings for beverages, ice cream, ices, candy, baked goods, and gelatin desserts. It is used in cosmetics as a flavoring and for its aroma. No known toxicity. GRAS.

COHOSH ROOT, BLACK AND BLUE • **Black Cohosh** is *Cimicifuga racemosa*. **Black Snakeroot. Bugbane. Rattleroot.** The root contains various glycosides *(see)* including estrogenic substances and tannins. Herbalists use it to relieve nerve pains, to relieve menstrual pains and the pain of childbirth. It is also used to speed delivery to reduce blood pressure. Black cohosh is also believed to have sedative properties. In 1992, the FDA proposed a ban on black cohosh in oral menstrual drug products because it has not been shown to be safe and effective for its stated claims. Blue cohosh is *Caulophyllum thalictroides*. **Papoose root. Squaw root.** The rhizome contains fungicidal saponin, glycosides *(see)*, gum, starch, salts, phosphoric acid, and a soluble resin. Herbalists use it for menstrual irregularities and pain and to ease the pain of childbirth. It is also used to treat worms.

COIX LACRYMA JOBI • **Extract of Job's Tears.** Asiatic flowers and seeds.

COLA ACUMINATA • **Kola nut extract. Guru Nut.** A natural extract from the brownish seed, about the size of a chestnut, produced by trees in Africa, the West Indies, and Brazil. Contains caffeine *(see)*. Used in butter, caramel, chocolate, cocoa, coffee, cola, walnut, and root beer flavorings for beverages, ice cream, ices, candy, and baked goods. Has been used to treat epilepsy. GRAS.

COLA NITIDA • See Cola Acuminata.

COLCHICINE • **Colabid. ColBenemid. Colsalide. Novo colchicine.** A drug introduced in 1763 prepared from roots of the meadow saffron *(see)* which is specific in relieving gout but why it works is unclear. Potential adverse reactions include nausea, vomiting, abdominal pain, anemia, diarrhea, hives, skin rash, and hair loss. Alcohol and diuretics may make it less effective. It impairs the absorption of Vitamin B_{12}.

COLD CREAM • Originally developed by the Greek physician Galen, the original formula consisted of a mixture of olive oil, beeswax, water, and rose petals. The product was called cold cream because after it was applied to the skin, the water evaporated and gave a feeling of coolness. Cold cream is still used, although the olive oil has been replaced with mineral or other oils that do not so easily become rancid. Beeswax *(see)* can cause allergic contact dermatitis, as can rose petals, perfume, or other additives added to the original formula. See also Cleansing Creams and Lotions.

C20-48 OLEFIN • Hydrocarbons used as skin conditioning ingredients. See Oleic Acid.

COLETH-24 • Emulsifier and emollient derived from cholesterol and ethylene oxide. No known toxicity.

COLEUS BARBATUS EXTRACT • An extract of the roots of an herb with large blue flowers.

COLLAGEN • Protein substance found in connective tissue. In cosmetics, it is usually derived from animal tissue. The collagen fibers in connective tissues of the skin undergo changes from aging and overexposure to the sun that contribute to the appearance of wrinkles and other outward signs of aging. Cosmetic manufacturers have heralded it as a new wonder ingredient but according to medical experts, it cannot affect the skin's own collagen when applied topically. However, it is being used to fill out acne scars and other depressions, including wrinkles, by injection. Allergic reactions are not infrequent and test spots are supposed to be done first to see whether an allergic response is provoked.

COLLAGEN AMINO ACIDS • Formerly called Animal Collagen Amino Acids. The major protein of the white fibers of connective tissue, cartilage, and bone, that is insoluble in water, but easily altered to gelatins by boiling in water, dilute acids, or alkalies. See Collagen and Amino Acids.

COLLODION • A mixture of nitrocellulose, alcohol, and ether in a syrupy liquid, colorless or slightly yellow. It is used as a skin protectant, in clear nail polish, as a corn remover, in the manufacture of lacquers, artificial pearls, and cement. May cause allergic skin reactions.

COLLOIDAL OATMEAL • **Aveeno Bath Products.** Meal obtained by grinding oats. Soothing to the skin. In 1992, the FDA proposed a ban on colloidal oatmeal in astringent *(see)* drug products because it had not been shown to be safe and effective as claimed.

COLLOIDAL SULFUR • A pale yellow mixture of sulfur and acacia *(see)* used as an emulsifier. See Sulfur.

COLLYRIUM • A commercial preparation for local application to the eye, usually a wash or lotion. See Boric Acid.

COLOCASIA ANTIQUORUM • A small family of Asiatic herbs. See Taro.

COLOCYNTH • **Bitter Apple.** A denaturant used in alcohols for cosmetics. Derived from the dried pulp of a fruit grown in the Mediterranean and Near East regions. It is a super cathartic if ingested and has caused deaths. Has also caused allergic problems in cosmeticians.

COLOGNE • Named originally after a town in Germany, it is usually limited to citrus and floral bases. It has a higher alcohol content than perfume, usually is applied more generously, and leaves a cooling, refreshing feeling on the skin. It is also made as a paste or semisolid stick. May cause allergic reactions depending on ingredients. Those allergic to citrus and floral bases should avoid colognes and try perfumes made of wood or animal scents. No known toxicity to the skin.

COLOGNE, SOLID • Solid colognes are used in sticks or in small containers. Such products consist of 80 percent alcohol, about 10 percent sodium stearate, some sorbitol, cologne essence, and water. Gel colognes consist of 60 to 70 percent alcohol, perfume oils, emulsifiers, and about 30 percent water.

COLOPHONY • See Rosin.

COLORS • Food colors of both natural and synthetic origin are extensively used in cosmetics. When the letters FD & C precede a color it means the color can be used in a food, drug, or cosmetic. When D & C precedes the color, it signifies that it can only be used in drugs or cosmetics, but not in food. Ext. D & C before a color means that it is certified for external use only in drugs and cosmetics and may not be used on the lips or mucous membranes. No coal tar colors are permitted for use around the eyes. In fact, the FDA does not allow any color additive to be applied around the area of the eye unless specifically approved for that purpose. There is still a great deal of controversy about the use of coal tar colors because almost all have been shown to cause cancer when injected into the skins of mice. Furthermore, many people are allergic to coal tar products. The bulk of the colors are derived from coal tar. Aniline, a coal tar derivative, is poisonous in its pure state. A provisional listing is a category that is supposed to be abolished. It consists of colors whose safety has not been proven or even studied; in some cases this dates back to when the list was enacted in 1960. Permanent listing means the FDA is convinced that the dye is safe to use as it is now employed in cosmetics. Batch-by-batch certification is used to determine how well the concoction matches the FDA standards—the chemical formula approved. The color additives for which certification is not required are mostly dyes or pigments of vegetable, animal, or mineral origin, and generally require less processing. Many of the colors are vegetable compounds—beet powder, caramel, beta-carotene, grape skin extract. A few are of animal origin—cochineal extract, taken from the dried bodies of certain insects.

Among the natural colors used are: annatto, carotene, chlorophyll, saffron, and turmeric. The big problem with coal tar colors, of course, is their potential as carcinogens but they are also potential sensitizers. Each batch of a coal tar color has to be certified as "safe." F & C Red No. 40 is one of the most widely used coal tar colorings. See also Yellow No. 5, Tartrazine, Coal Tar, Catechu Black, and Carmine. The word "pigment," however, usually means a colored or white chemical compound that is insoluble in a particular solvent. The word "dye" generally refers to a chemical compound, most often of coal tar origin, which is soluble. Cosmetic manufacturers have unique problems with coloring their products. They must choose a color substance that is not only safe and stable in a product, but one that will psychologically entice the customer into buying the product. For instance, most hand lotions are either white, pink, cream, or blue. Research sponsored by cosmetic companies has shown that women over twenty-five years of age want pink shades while teen-agers prefer blue hand lotions. Many natural colors derived from plants and animals have been in use since humans first started trying to make themselves look better with makeup. Examples of such naturally derived colors are annatto, saffron, chlorophyll, and beta-carotene *(see all)*. Inorganic colors used in cosmetics include iron oxides, bronze powder, ultramarines, chromium oxide greens, and a number of white products such as titanium dioxide, barium sulfate, and zinc oxide *(see all)*. However, widely used and under FDA scrutiny are the coal tar colors.

In 1900 there were more than 80 dyes in use in cosmetics, foods, and drugs. There were no regulations and the same dye used to color clothes could also be used to color candy or cosmetics. In 1906 the first comprehensive legislation for food colors was passed. There were only seven colors that, when tested, were shown to be composed of known ingredients that demonstrated no harmful effects. A voluntary system of certification for batches of color dyes was set up. In 1938 new legislation was passed, superseding the 1906 act. The colors were given numbers instead of chemical names and every batch had to be certified. The manufacturers must submit to the government samples from every batch of coal tar color. Each sample is analyzed for purity. The lot test number must then accompany the colors through all subsequent packaging. The manufacturer must pay 15 cents a pound and not less than $100 for each batch tested. Each petition for listing of a new color additive must be accompanied by a deposit of $2,600 for cosmetics. To amend a listing asking for a new use of a color, the government requires a check of $1,800. If you want to object or request public hearings on a color, it will cost you $250. What is considered a safe color? According to the FDA: "Safety for external color additives will normally be determined by tests for acute oral toxicity, primary irritation, sensitization, subacute skin toxicity on intact or abraded skin and carcinogenicity (cancer causing) by skin application." The FDA commissioner may waive any of such tests if data before him established otherwise that such a test is not required to determine safety. Here are the certified colors classified into the following categories according to their chemical ancestry:

1. Nitro Dyes. Containing one atom of nitrogen and two of oxygen, there are only a few certified because they can be absorbed through the skin and are toxic. Ext. D & C Yellow is one. See Nitro.

2. Azo (monoazo). This includes the largest number. They are all characterized by the presence of the azo bond. See Azo Dyes.

3. Triphenylmethane. FD & C Blue No. 1 is the most popular dye of this group and is widely used. See Triphenylmethane Group.

4. Xanthene. This group contains very brilliant, widely used lipstick colors. D & C Orange is one. See Xanthene.

5. Quinoline. There are only two certified in this category, D & C Yellow No. 10 and No. 11. They are bright greenish yellows. See Quinoline.

6. Anthraquinone. Widely used in cosmetics because it is not affected by light. Ext D & C Violet No. 2 is one. See Anthraquinone.

7. Indigo. These dyes have been in use a long time. D & C Blue No. 6 is an example. See Indigo. There are a few other miscellaneous dyes.

In 1950, children were made ill by certain coloring used in candy and popcorn. These incidents led to the delisting of FD & C Orange No. 1 and Orange No. 2 and FD & C Red No. 32. Since that time, because of experimental evidence of possible harm, Red 1, Yellow 1, 2, 3, and 4 have also been delisted. Violet 1 was removed in 1973. In 1976, one of the most widely used of all colors, FD & C Red No. 2, was removed because it was found to cause tumors in rats. In 1976 Red No. 4 was banned for coloring maraschino cherries (its last use) and carbon black was also banned at the same time because they contain cancer-causing ingredients.

Earlier, in 1960, scientific investigations were required by law to determine the suitability of all colors in use for permanent listing. Citrus Red No. 2 (limited to 2 ppm) for coloring orange skins has been permanently listed; Blue No. 1, Red No. 3, Yellow No. 5, and Red No. 40 are permanently listed but without any restrictions. In 1959, the Food and Drug Administration approved the use of "lakes," in which the dyes have been mixed with alumina hydrate to make them insoluble. See FD & C Lakes.

The other food, drug, and cosmetic coloring additives remained on the "temporary list." The provisional list permitted colors then in use to continue on a provisional, or interim, basis pending completion of studies to determine whether the colors should be permanently approved or terminated. FD & C Red No. 3 (Erythrosine) is permanently listed for use in food and ingested drugs and provisionally listed for cosmetics and externally applied drugs. It is used in foods such as gelatins, cake mixes, ice cream, fruit cocktail cherries, bakery goods, and sausage casings.

The FDA postponed the closing date for three provisionally listed color additives—FD & C Red No. 3, D & C Red No. 33 and D & C Red No. 36, May 2, 1988, to allow additional time to study "complex scientific and legal questions about the colors before deciding to approve or terminate their use in food, drugs and cosmetics." The Agency asked for 60 days to consider the impact of the October 1987 U.S. Court of Appeals ruling that there is no exception to the Delaney Amendment *(see)*, which says that cancer-causing ingredients may not be added to food. On July 13, 1988, the Public Citizens Health Research Group announced that the FDA agreed to revoke by July 15, 1988, the permanent listing of four color additives used in drugs and cosmetics—D & C Red No. 8, D & C Red No. 9, D & C Red No. 19, and D & C Orange No. 17. In a unanimous decision in October 1987, the U.S. Court of Appeals for the District of Columbia said the FDA lacked legal authority to approve two of the colors, D & C Orange No. 17 and D & C Red No. 19, since they had been found to induce cancer in laboratory animals. The Supreme Court ruled against an appeal on April 18, 1988. Meanwhile, Public Citizens Health Group also brought a similar suit, challenging the use of D & C Red No. 8 and D & C Red No. 9, which was before the U.S. Circuit Court of Appeals in Philadelphia. Under an agreement between the FDA and Public Citizens, the case was sent back to the FDA, and the agency delisted these colors as well as D & C Orange No. 17 and D & C Red No. 19. Other countries as well as the World Health Organization maintain there are inconsistencies in safety data and in the banning of some colors which, in turn, affects international commerce. As of this writing, there is still a great deal of confusion about the colors with the FDA maintaining that the cancer risk is minimal—as low as one in a billion—for the colors; and groups such as Ralph Nader's Public Citizens Health Group maintaining that any cancer risk for a food additive is unacceptable. In 1990, the lakes *(see)* of Red No. 3 were removed for all uses from the approved list. The color, itself, was also removed in 1990 for cosmetic and external drug use. It is still, as of this writing, approved for food and ingested drugs.

COLOSTRUM • A thin, white, opalescent fluid, the first milk secreted at the end of pregnancy. It differs from milk secreted later by containing more protein and alubmin. It is also rich in antibodies, which confer passive immunity to the newborn. Used in skin conditioning ingredients.

COLTSFOOT • **Wild Ginger.** Used for its soothing properties in shampoos and astringents. From an herb used historically to fight colds and asthma, it reputedly opens pores and allows sweating. It has been used as a soothing ointment. No known toxicity.

COMBRETUM MICRANTHUM • A tropical shrub rich in tannins *(see)*.

COMEDONES • Plugs of sebaceous (oil) matter that obstruct the hair follicle. They are called whiteheads if the top of the follicle remains narrow, and blackheads if the follicle is stretched wide.

COMFREY • *Symphytum officinale.* **Knitbone. Blackwort. Healing Herb.** The leaf and root contain allantoin, mucilage, tannins, starch, inulin *(see)*, steroidal saponins, and pyrrolizine alkaloids. It has been reported to be toxic when taken internally and to cause liver damage. Herbalists recommend comfrey for rapid wound and bone healing, and use a decoction for diarrhea, hemorrhage, and bleeding. Potential adverse reactions include liver dysfunction. Pyrrolizidine alkaloids have been found to cause cancer in laboratory rats. Formerly regarded as safe, reports of toxic effects surfaced when its use became popular. Symptoms of poisoning appear after a few months of use. It is a strong liver toxin. Comfrey was banned in Canada in 1989. Widely used in cosmetics in eye makeup, bath soaps, skin fresheners, foundations, cold creams, and cleansing lotions.

COMFREY EXTRACT • The extract of the roots and rhizomes of *Symphytum officinale*. Used for centuries by monks as a healer of bruises, a mouthwash and gargle, and as a compress for eye injuries.

COMMIPHORA ABYSSINICA • **Myrrh Gum. Commiphora molmol or myrrh or Guggul.** One of the gifts of the Magi, it is a yellowish to reddish brown, aromatic, bitter gum resin that is obtained from various myrrh trees, especially from East Africa and Arabia. The gum resin has been used to break up intestinal gas and as a topical stimulant. The Chinese, for centuries, used the herb to treat menstrual problems and bleeding. In Asia and Africa, it was used as an antiseptic for mucous membranes. It is also used as a stimulant tonic; there are constituents in myrrh that stimulate gastric secretions and relax smooth muscles. In modern studies, myrrh has been shown to inhibit gram-positive bacteria such as *Staphylococcus aureus*. The herb contains volatile oils, including limonene, eugenol, and pinene, which have been found helpful in easing breathing during colds, and increasing circulation. It also contains tannin, which is thought to be the reason that myrrh allays the pain and speeds the healing of mouth ulcers and sore gums. In 1992, the FDA issued a notice that myrrh fluid extract had not been shown to be safe and effective as claimed in OTC digestive aid products.

COMMUNITY RIGHT TO KNOW LIST • Manufacturers, who employ toxic chemicals while making products, must respond, under the law, to inquiries from employees and citizens in the area. Cyanide, which is used in the manufacture of pesticides and some food additives, is an example of a chemical on this list compiled by the U.S. Environmental Protection Agency.

CONCHIORIN POWDER • A protein found in the pearl oyster. Used as a skin conditioning ingredient.

CONCRETES • Waxlike substances prepared from natural raw materials, almost exclusively vegetable in origin, such as bark, flower, herb, leaf, and root and used in perfumes and stick deodorants. No known toxicity.

CONDITIONERS • See Hair Conditioners.

CONDITIONING CREAMS • See Emollients.

CONDURANGO EXTRACT • **Marsdenia Condurango.** An American vine. The dried bark contains glycosides, resin, tannin *(see all),* and oils. A bitter tasting herb, it is used to treat digestive and stomach problems, stimulate appetite, and relax nerves. Used in herbal makeups.

CONEFLOWER EXTRACT • See Echinacea.

CONEFLOWERS • See Echinacea.

CONIUM MACULATUM • **Hemlock. Poison Hemlock. Poison Parsley.** Found in many parts of Europe and the Americas, the hemlock is related to parsnip, carrot, celery, fennel, and parsley. It is famed as the poison used to execute Socrates and other ancient Greeks; it was mixed with opium and used as a suicide drink for old, frail Roman philosophers. The narcotic drug, conium, comes from the dried, unripe fruit of the hemlock. Herbalists once used it is a sedative, antispasmodic, and an antidote to other poisons. Hemlock is poisonous.

CONJUGATED GLYCOPROTEINS • A composition made up of carbohydrates and simple proteins. Used in tanning creams. No known toxicity.

CONJUNCTIVITIS • **Pink Eye.** An infection of the membrane that lines the eyelids and covers the white portion of the eye.

CONNECTIVE TISSUE • Extract of animal connective tissue used in "antiaging" products.

CONTACT DERMATITIS • See Allergic Contact Dermatitis.

CONTACT DERMATITIS OF THE EYELIDS • See Eyelids.

COPAIBA BALSAM • *Balsam capivi.* **Jesuit's balsam.** Oleoresin from South American species of *Copaifera Leguminosae* found in Brazil, Venezuela, Colombia, and the Amazon valley. A transparent, thick, yellowish liquid with a strange odor and bitter, acrid taste, it is used in the manufacture of paper and to remove oil.

COPAIFERA OFFICINALIS • See Copaiba Balsam.

COPAL • A resin obtained as a fossil or as an exudate from various species of tropical plants. Must be heated in alcohol or other solvents. Used in nail enamels. May cause allergic reactions, particularly skin rashes.

COPERNICIA CERIFERA • See Carnauba Wax.

COPOLYMER • Result of polymerization (*see* polymer), which includes at least two different molecules, each of which is capable of polymerizing alone. Together they form a new, distinct molecule. They are used in the manufacture of nail enamels and face masks.

COPPER, METALLIC POWDER, AND VERSENATE • Used as a coloring ingredient in cosmetics. One of the earliest known metals. An essential nutrient for all mammals. Naturally occurring or experimentally produced copper deficiency in animals leads to a variety of abnormalities including anemia, skeletal defects, and muscle degeneration. Copper itself is nontoxic, but soluble copper salts, notably copper sulfate, are highly irritating to the skin and mucous membranes and when ingested cause serious vomiting. Copper metallic powder was permanently listed as a cosmetic coloring in 1977.

COPPER GLUCONATE • An odorless, light blue, fine powder. Used as a feed additive, dietary supplement, and mouth deodorant. See Copper.

COPPER-8-HYDROXYQUINOLATE • See Copper and Oxyquinoline Sulfate.

COPPER PCA • A humectant. See Copper.

COPPER POWDER • A color additive that is exempt from certification (*see* Certified). See Copper.

COPTIS JAPONICA • A small herb with white flowers.

CORALLINA OFFICIALIS • A West Indian climbing plant with bright fruit.

CORCHORUS CAPSULARIS • A Japanese vegetable with large leaves and yellow flowers.

CORIANDER OIL • The volatile oil from the dried ripe fruit of a plant grown in Asia and Europe. Used as a flavoring ingredient in dentifrices. Colorless or pale yellow liquid with a taste and odor characteristic of coriander, which is also used as a condiment. Can cause allergic reactions, particularly of the skin.

CORIANDRUM SATIVUM • The colorless, or pale yellow, volatile oil from the dried ripe fruit of a plant grown in Asia and Europe, the name means "buglike odor." The ancient Egyptians used it for headaches. In the seventeenth century, it was used to dispel "wind." It still is used today as a laxative and to aid digestion. Coriander is used (up to 1 gram) to break up intestinal gas. It also is employed as a flavoring agent in dentifrices. Can cause allergic reactions, particularly of the skin.

CORN • **Corn Sugar. Dextrose.** Used in maple, nut, and root beer flavorings for beverages, ice cream, ices, candy, and baked goods. The oil is used in emollient creams and toothpastes. The syrup is used as a texturizer and carrying ingredient in cosmetics. It is also used for envelopes, stamps, sticker tapes, ale, aspirin, bacon, baking mixes, powders, beers, bourbon, breads, cheeses, cereals, chop suey, chow mein, confectioners' sugar, cream puffs, fish products, ginger ale, hams, jellies, processed meats, peanut butters, canned peas, plastic food wrappers, sherbets, whiskeys, and American wines. It may also be found in capsules, lozenges, ointments, suppositories, vitamins, fritters, Fritos, frostings, canned or frozen fruit, graham crackers, gravies, grits, gum, monosodium glutamate, Nescafé, oleomargarine, pablum, paper, tortillas, vinegar, yeasts, bologna, baking powders, bath powders, frying fats, fruit juices, laxatives. May cause allergic reactions including skin rashes and asthma.

CORN ACID • See Corn Oil.

CORN COB MEAL • The milled powder prepared from the cobs of *Zea mays*. Used as a thickener and an abrasive in cosmetics.

CORN FLOUR • A finely ground powder. Used in face and bath powder. See Corn Oil.

CORN GERM EXTRACT • The extract of the germ of *Zea mays*.

CORN OIL • Used in emollient creams and toothpastes. Obtained as a by-product by wet milling the grain for use in the manufacture of corn starch, dextrins, and yellow oil. It has a faint, characteristic odor and taste and thickens upon exposure to air. No known toxicity, but can cause skin reactions in the allergic.

CORN OIL PEG-6 ESTERS • See PEG and Esters.

CORN POPPY EXTRACT • The extract obtained from the petals of the *Papaver rhoeas*.

CORN SYRUP • **Corn Sugar. Dextrose.** A sweet syrup prepared from cornstarch. Used as a texturizer and carrying ingredient in cosmetics. Also used for envelopes, stamps, and sticking tapes, aspirin, and many food products. May cause allergic reactions.

CORNFLOWER • The dried flowers of *Centaurea cyanus*.

CORNFLOWER EXTRACT • The extract obtained from the flowers of *Centaurea cyanus*. Used as a blue dye.

CORNSTARCH • Many containers are powdered with cornstarch to prevent sticking. It is also used in dusting powder, and as demulcent for irritated colons. May cause allergic reactions, including skin rashes and asthma.

CORTHELLUS SHITAKE • A Japanese mushroom that has long been used for therapeutic purposes. May lower blood pressure and blood cholesterol, according to recent studies.

CORTICOSTEROIDS • A class of compounds comprising steroid hormones secreted by the adrenal cortex and their synthetic analogs. In pharmacologic doses introduced in 1948, corticosteroids are used primarily for their anti-inflammatory and/or immunosuppressive effects. Topical corticosteroids, such as betamethasone dipropionate, are effective in the treatment of corticosteroid-responsive skin problems primarily because of their anti-inflammatory, anti-itching, and vasoconstrictive actions. The absorption through the skin of topical corticosteroids involves many factors including the vehicle, the condition of the skin, and the use of covering dressings. Topical corticosteroids can be absorbed from normal, intact skin.

CORYLUS AMERICANA AND AVELLANNA AND ROSTRATA • Hazel Nut. An ornamental tree with a sweet gum. Used for brown coloring and as a skin conditioning ingredient.

COSMETICS • One of the most common causes, if not the most common cause, of Allergic Contact Dermatitis, and frequently the cause of nasal and lung symptoms, particularly scented products. Until fairly recently, it was believed that cosmetics could not be absorbed through the skin. It is now known that many things can be absorbed through the skin, some chemicals to a greater degree than others depending upon composition and upon the part of the anatomy to which they are applied. Many cosmetic manufacturers promote their products as "hypoallergenic." A non-allergenic product is impossible because there is always someone who will be allergic to something. There are sixty known ingredients in the past or present cosmetics known to cause allergic reactions in many people. Included in this list are such common substances as acacia, benzaldehyde, cornstarch, gum arabic, spearmint oil, and wheat starch *(see all)*. By leaving the sixty offenders out of cosmetics or by reducing the number of ingredients altogether, particularly perfumes, manufacturers then claim their products are "hypoallergenic." The FDA has wrestled for years with the claim and has asked manufacturers to prove that their products are unlikely to cause an allergic reaction. As the mandate stands now, it is up to the manufacturer to decide the testing method used to determine the hypoallergenicity of the product. Throughout this book there are ingredients that often cause allergic reactions when in cosmetics. If you read the labels and check the book, you will be able, in most instances, to avoid those products that may be causing you a problem.

COSTUS • A fixative in perfumes. The volatile oil is obtained by steam distillation from dried roots of an herb. Light yellow to brown viscous liquid, with a persistent violetlike odor. Used also as a food flavoring. No known toxicity.

COTTON • A soft, white, cellulosic substance composed of the fibers surrounding the seeds of various plants of the mallow family.

COTTONSEED • The water-soluble, protein material in cotton seed contains one of the most powerful allergens for humans. Occasionally it contaminates inexpensive cotton stuffing in upholstery, mattresses, and cushions. More often, exposures to the allergens arise from the use of cottonseed meal, which may be found in fertilizers and as a constituent of feed for cattle, hogs, poultry, and dogs. Symptoms usually result from inhalation but allergic reactions also can occur from ingesting cottonseed meal used in pan-greasing compounds and in foods such as some fried cakes, fig bars, and cookies.

COTTONSEED ACID • See Cottonseed Oil.

COTTONSEED FLOUR • Cooked, partly defatted, and toasted flour used for pale yellow color and to make gin. Can cause allergic skin reactions and asthma.

COTTONSEED OIL • The fixed oil from the seeds of the cultivated varieties of the plant. Pale yellow, oily, odorless liquid used in the manufacture of soaps, creams, baby creams, nail polish removers, and lubricants. The oil is used in most salad oils and oleomargarines and most mayonnaise and salad dressings. Lard compounds and lard substitutes are made with cottonseed oil. Sardines may be packed in it. Most commercial fried products such as potato chips and doughnuts are fried in cottonseed oil, and restaurants use it for cooking. Candies, particularly chocolates, often contain this oil; and it is used to polish fruits at stands. It is also used in cotton wadding or batting in cushions, comforters, mattresses, upholstery, varnishes, fertilizers, and in animal feeds. Known to cause many allergic reactions but because of its wide use in cosmetics, foods, and other products, it is hard to avoid.

COUCH GRASS ROOT EXTRACT • *Agropyron repens*. **Dog grass. Twitch Grass.** A weed that herbalists use to cool fevers and soothe and heat internal irritation or inflammation. Dogs and cats, when they have upset stomachs, will seek out and eat this plant. The roots possess both diuretic and demulcent properties, and have been used by herbalists for centuries to treat bladder problems in humans. Couch Grass contains high concentrations of mucilage, which gives the plant its soothing effect on mucous membranes. The plant is also reported to have antibiotic activity. In 1992, the FDA proposed a ban on couch grass in oral menstrual drug products because it has not been shown to be safe and effective for its stated claims.

COUMARINS • **Tonka Bean. Cumarin.** A fragrant ingredient of Tonka beans, Sweet Woodruff, Cramp Bark, and many other plants. It is made synthetically as well. Used in over 300 products in the United States including acne preparations, antiseptics, deodorants, "skin fresheners," hair dyes, and shampoos. It has been widely used as a fragrance in soaps, detergents, perfumes, and sunscreens. May produce allergic contact dermatitis *(see)* and photosensitivity *(see)*. It has anti–blood clotting effects and anticlotting ingredients are derived from it. Coumarin is prohibited in foods because it is toxic by ingestion and carcinogenic. No known toxicity on the skin.

COUNTERIRRITANT • An ingredient applied locally to produce superficial inflammation with the object of reducing existing inflammation in deeper adjacent structures. Iodine *(see)* is an example of a counterirritant.

C-PARETHS • Emulsifiers from Carboxylic Acid or Phosphoric Acid *(see both)*.

CRANBERRY • Several low, berry-bearing shrubs related to the blueberry, native to Northern Eurasia and North America. The American Cranberry, *Vaccinium macrocarpon,* is cultivated in Massachusetts, New Jersey, and Wisconsin. Used in "organic" cosmetics.

CRANE'S BILL EXTRACT • The extract of wild geranium, *Geranium maculatum,* or other native geranium species. See Geranium Oil.

CRATAEGUS • The extract of the berries, flowers, and/or leaves of the English Hawthorn, *Crataegus oxyacantha.* Used in dyes and skin tonics and to relieve inflammation and acne. Can cause dilation of blood vessels. See Hawthorn Berry.

CREAM • The thick, yellow part of cow's milk that contains 18 to 40 percent butterfat. Used as a skin conditioning ingredient.

CREAM OF TARTAR • A white, crystalline salt in tartars from winemaking, prepared especially from argols and also synthetically from tartaric acid *(see)*. Has a pleasant acid taste. Used as a thickening ingredient and in certain treatment of metals. No known toxicity.

CREAM RINSE • **Creme Rinse.** Hair Conditioners *(see)* that are poured on the hair after shampooing and then rinsed with water. A typical formula for a cream rinse: lanolin, 10 percent; mineral oil and lanolin esters, 5 percent; cholesterol, 0.25 percent; sorbitan stearate, 3 percent; preservative, 0.15 percent; distilled water, 78.60 percent; and perfume.

CREAMS • See Emollients, Hand Creams and Lotions, Cold Cream, and Hormone Creams.

CREATININE • A waste product of protein breakdown.

o-CRESOL • A phenol *(see)* used as a preservative.

p-CRESOL • Used as a preservative and as a synthetic nut and vanilla flavoring ingredient. Obtained from coal tar. It occurs naturally in tea, and is used in cosmetics, beverages, ice cream, ices, candy, and baked goods. It is more powerful than phenol *(see)* and less toxic.

P-CRESYL ACETATE • See P-Tolyl Acetate.

CRITHMUM MARITIMUM • **Sea Fennel Oil and Extract. Samphire.** A seacoast plant. A moisturizing ingredient.

CROCUS SATIVUS • **Saffron Crocus.** Used in perfumery and coloring in cosmetics. It is the dried stigma of the crocus cultivated in Spain, Greece, France, and Iran. Used also in bitters, liquors, and spice flavorings. Homeopathic physicians use it to induce menstruation, and as an antispasmodic. Excessive doses can cause miscarriage. Severe poisoning causes bleeding from the skin, a severe lowering of the heart rate and collapse. Fatal cases have been reported when 5 to 10 grams of saffron have been ingested.

CROSCARMELLOSE • The absorbent, cross-linked polymer of Cellulose Gum *(see)*.

CROSS-REACTIVITY • When the body mistakes one compound for another of similar chemical composition.

CROTON GLABELLUS • **Croton tiglium.** A small shrub or tree, the seeds of which are used in Chinese and homeopathic medicines as a strong cathartic, rubefacient, and vesicant. It is very toxic and is a potential cancer-promoter.

CROTONIC ACID • Found in the clay soil of Texas. It is used in the manufacture of Vitamin A and in lacquers.

CRUELTY-FREE • Implies that products have not been tested on animals. Most ingredients have been at some point tested on animals so you may want to look for "no new animal testing" to get a more accurate designation.

CRYPTOCARYA MASSOY • The bark of this East Indian tree yields a volatile oil.

CRYSTALLINS • The protein found in the fiber cells of vertebrate eye lenses. It is used as a hair and skin conditioning ingredient.

CTFA • Abbreviation for Cosmetic, Toiletry, and Fragrance Association.

CUBEB BERRIES • *Piper cubeba.* **Tailed Pepper. Java Pepper.** The mature, unripe dried fruit of a perennial vine grown in South Asia, Java, Sumatra, the Indies, and Sri Lanka. Java pepper was formerly used to stimulate healing of mucous membranes. The fruit has been used as a stimulant and diuretic and sometimes is smoked in cigarettes. The oil is used for chronic bladder troubles and is reputed to increase the flow of urine.

CUBEB OIL • See Cubeb Berries.

CUCUMBER • *Cucumis sativus.* The juice of the cucumber was reputedly used by Cleopatra to preserve her skin. It imparts a cool feeling to the skin. By ingestion, it is said by herbalists to be a good diuretic and to prevent constipation. Researchers are now studying its effect on cholesterol. The juice is soothing to the skin.

CUCUMIS MELO • Melon.

CUCUMIS SATIVUS • See Cucumber.

CUCURBITACEAE • **Gourd Extract.**

CUCURBITA PEPO • **Pumpkin Seed Oil.**

CUDWEED EXTRACT • *Gnaphalium ulginosum.* The plant is used by herbalists to treat upper-respiratory inflammation including laryngitis, tonsillitis, and bronchitis. Grown widely in North America.

CUMIN • *Cuminum cyminum.* A fragile plant cultivated in Asia and the Middle East, it contains cuminic aldehyde, which may have some antiviral properties, and cumene, which is narcotic in high doses and potentially toxic by ingestion. The seed was used in medicine in ancient times as a stimulant and remedy for stomach ailments. It is used by herbalists to treat sore eyes.

CUMINALDEHYDE • Used to make perfumes. Colorless to yellowish, oily, with a strong, lasting odor. It is a constituent of eucalyptus, myrrh, cassia, cumin, and other essential oils, but often is made synthetically for fragrances. No known toxicity.

CUPRESSUS SEMPERVIRENS • **Cypress.** See Cedrol.

CUPRIC ACETATE • The copper salt of acetic acid and copper *(see both).*

CUPRIC CHLORIDE • **Copper Chloride.** A copper salt used in hair dye. A yellow to brown, water-absorbing powder that is soluble in diluted acids. It is also used in pigments for glass and ceramics and as a feed additive, disinfectant, and wood preservative. Irritating to the skin and mucous membranes. Irritating when ingested, causing vomiting.

CUPRIC SULFATE • Copper sulfate occurs in nature as hydrocyanite. Grayish white to greenish white crystals. Used as an agricultural fungicide, herbicide, and in the preparation of azo dyes *(see).* Used in hair dyes as coloring. Very irritating if ingested. No known toxicity on the skin and is used medicinally as a skin fungicide.

CURCUMA LONGA • **Tumeric.** Derived from an East Indian herb, *Curcuma longa l.* An aromatic pepperlike, but somewhat bitter, taste. The cleaned, boiled, sun-dried, pulverized root is used in coconut, ginger ale, and curry flavorings for puddings, condiments, meats, soups, and pickles; also for yellow coloring used to color sausage casings, oleomargarine, shortening, and marking ink. The extract is used in fruit, meat, and cheese flavorings; for beverages, condiments, meats, soup bases, and pickles. The oleoresin *(see)* is obtained by extraction with one or more of the solvents acetone, ethyl alcohol, ethylene dichloride *(see all),* and others. It is used in spice flavorings for condiments, meats, pickles, and brine. Both turmeric and its oleoresin have been permanently listed for coloring food since 1966. It is exempt from certification. GRAS.

CURCUMA ZEDOARIA • **Zedoary Oil.** A bark extract from the East Indies, *Curcuma zeodaria,* used as bitters and ginger ale flavorings for beverages. GRAS.

CURLED DOCK • **Sour dock.** A weed with coarse leaves that is a member of the sorrel family and contains a sour juice. An extract of *Rumex crispus.*

CURRANT EXTRACT • From the berries of the red currant.

CURRY RED • A color classed as a monoazo, the name can be used only when applied to uncertified batches of color. The CTFA adopted name for certified *(see)* batches is FD & C Red No 40 *(see).*

CUTANEOUS • Pertaining to the skin.

CUTANEOUS LYSATE • The end product of the controlled bacterial degradation of animal skin. It consists of a complex mixture of proteins and amino acids.

CUTICLE REMOVERS • Cuticle is the dead skin that covers the base of the nail. Chemicals are used to either plasticize or dissolve the cuticle. Alkalies, such as lye, are used as cuticle softeners and removers. A typical cuticle remover contains coconut oil, potassium phosphate, potassium hydroxide, triethanolamine, and water. Contact dermatitis may occur. Potassium phosphate, potassium hydroxide, and triethanolamine can be irritants. Coconut oil *(see)* can cause allergic reactions.

CUTTLEFISH EXTRACT • An extract of the glands of *Sepia officinalis.*

CYANIDE • **Prussic Acid. Hydrocyanic Acid.** An inorganic salt that is one of the most rapid poisons known. Poisoning may occur when any compound releases cyanide. Cyanide is used as a fungistat, insecticide, and rodenticide and is used in metal polishes, especially for silver, and in electroplating solutions, art materials, photographic processes, and metallurgy. It has been reported to reduce oxygen availability in the blood even in low doses.

CYANO-, CYAN- • From the Greek *kaynos,* meaning a dark blue. The prefix is commonly used to signify compounds containing the cyanide group CN. If the cyanide is not released from the compound, its presence is presumed not harmful.

CYANOCOBALAMIN • Vitamin B_{12}.

CYANOPSIS TETRAGONOLOBA • See Guar Gum.

CYANOTIS ARACHNOIDEA • **Spider Plant.**

CYATHEACEAE • **Pengawar.** A family of tropical tree ferns.

CYCLAMATES • Artificial sweetening ingredient about 30 times as sweet as refined sugar, removed from the food market on September 1, 1969, because they were found to cause bladder cancer in rats.

CYCLAMEN • A small genus of widely cultivated Eurasian plants of the family *Primulaceae.* Cyclamens have nodding white or pink flowers.

CYCLAMEN ALDEHYDE • A colorless liquid aldehyde *(see)* having a lily-of-the-valley odor, made synthetically, and used in perfumes, especially for soap.

CYCLAMIC ACID • Fairly strong acid with a sweet taste. It is the acid from which cyclamates *(see)* were derived.

CYCLOCARBOXYPROPYLOLEIC ACID • **Acrylinoleic Acid. C 29-70 Carboxylic Acid.** Thickening, suspending, dispersing, and emulsifying ingredient in cosmetics. No known toxicity.

CYCLODEXTRIN • A sweet compound. See Dextrin.

CYCLOETHOXYMETHICONE • A solvent used in skin conditioners.

CYCLOHEXANOL • Obtained from phenol, it is used as a solvent for resins. It has a narcoticlike action and has caused severe kidney problems in experimental animals.

CYCLOHEXANONE • Obtained from cyclohexanol *(see),* it has a combination peppermint and acetone odor. The vapor is harmful. It is used as a solvent for cellulose and in the preparation of resins.

CYCLOHEXYLAMINE • A buffering agent used in hairsprays.

CYCLOMETHICONE • A widely used silicone *(see)* in hair and skin conditioners. It is also used in deodorants, after-shave lotions, suntan gels, eye-makeup removers, lipsticks, dusting powders, skin freshener, and blushers.

CYCLOPENTANE • A colorless liquid derived from benzene and used as a solvent and in distillation.

N-CYCLOPENTYL-m-AMINOPHENOL • Coal tar hair coloring. See Coal Tar.

CYMBIDIUM GRANDIFLORM • Orchid extract used in fragrances.

CYMBOPOGON MARTINI • *Palmarosa.* **Geranium Oil.** The volatile oil obtained by steam distillation from a variety of partially dried grass, grown in East India and Java. Used in rose, fruit, and spice flavorings for ice cream, ices, candy, and baked goods. Believed as toxic as other essential oils, causing illness after ingestion of a teaspoonful and death after ingestion of an ounce. A skin irritant. GRAS.

CYMBOPOGON NARDUS • See Citronella.

CYMBOPOGON SCHOENANTHUS • See Lemongrass Oil.

p-CYMENE • A synthetic flavoring, a volatile hydrocarbon solvent that occurs naturally in star anise, coriander, cumin, mace oil, oil of mandarin, and origanum oil. Used in fragrance, also in citrus and spice flavorings for beverages, ice cream, candies, and baked goods. Its ingestion in pure form may cause a burning sensation in the mouth, and nausea, salivation, headache, giddiness, vertigo, confusion, and coma. Contact with the pure liquid may cause blisters of the skin and inflammation of mucous membranes.

o-CYMEN-3-OL • See p-Cymene.

o-CYMEN-5-OL • Based on the available data, the CIR Expert Panel *(see)* concludes that the safety of this ingredient has not been documented for use in cosmetics. See Quaternary Ammonium Compounds.

CYNARA SCOLYMUS • **Artichoke.** A tall herb that resembles a thistle. Used as a flavoring.

CYPERUS • **Sedge Root.** A common wayside weed, it is closely related to the Egyptian papyrus plant. The root contains essential oils *(see),* including pinene and sesquiterpenes. It is used by herbalists to treat stomach cramps, colds, flu, menstrual irregularities, and depression. Used in cosmetics as a fragrance ingredient.

CYPRESS EXTRACT • An extract derived from the leaves and twigs of the cypress tree, *Cupressus sempervirens.* The oil has been used in folk medicine to treat whooping cough.

CYPRIPEDIUM PUBESCENS • **Lady's Slipper.** Herbalists use it to treat anxiety, stress, insomnia, neurosis, restlessness, tremors, epilepsy, and palpitations. It contains volatile oils, resins, glucosides, and tannin *(see all).*

CYSTEAMINE • **MEA. Mercamine. 2-Aminoethanethiol.** A compound with an unpleasant odor that has many biological effects. It is used as an antidote to acetaminophen and experimentally as a radioprotective ingredient.

CYSTAMINE BIS-LACTAMIDE • An amide *(see)* that is used as a skin conditioning ingredient.

CYSTEINE, L-FORM • An essential amino acid *(see),* it is derived from hair and used in hair products and creams. soluble in water, it is used in bakery products as a nutrient. It has been used to promote wound healing. On the list of FDA additives to be studied.

CYSTINE • A nonessential amino acid *(see)* found in urine and in horsehair. Colorless, practically odorless, white crystals, it is used as a nutrient supplement and in emollients and hair products.

CYTOCHROME C • A protein found in animal cells. It is used as a skin conditioning ingredient.

D

D & C • Abbreviation for Drug and Cosmetic.

D & C BLUE NO. 1 ALUMINUM LAKE • **Brilliant Blue Lake.** Insoluble pigment prepared from FD & C Blue No. 1 *(see).* A coal tar derivative, this brilliant blue is used as a coloring in hair dyes and powders, among other cosmetics; also used in soft drinks, gelatin desserts, and candy. May cause allergic reactions. It will produce malignant tumors at the site of injection in rats. On the FDA permanent list of color additives. Rated 1A for toxicology by the World Health Organization, meaning it is completely acceptable for use in foods and cosmetics. See Colors.

D & C BLUE NO. 2 ALUMINUM LAKE • Acid Blue 74. Indigotine 1A, Indigo Carmine. An Indigo *(see)* dye Acid Blue No. 1 is the uncertified counterpart of FD & C Blue No. 1.

D & C BLUE NO. 4 • Acid Blue 9 (Ammonium Salt). Bright, greenish blue. A coal tar, triphenylmethane color used primarily in hair rinses. Permanently listed by the FDA, January 3, 1977. The name Acid Blue No. 4 can be used only when applied to batches of color that have been certified. The CTFA Adopted Name for noncertified batches of this color is Acid Blue 9 Ammonium Salt. See Colors.

D & C BROWN NO. 1 • Resorcin Brown. Capracyl Brown®. Acid Orange 24. Light orange-brown. A diazo color *(see* Colors) permitted for use only in preformed hair colors. The cosmetic industry has petitioned the FDA to allow wider use. Resorcin is irritating to the skin and mucous membranes. Absorption can cause depletion of oxygen in the body and death. Also used as an antiseptic and fungicide. Permanently listed for external use only in 1976. D & C Brown No. 1 can be used only when applied to certified colors. The CTFA name for noncertified batches of this color is Acid Orange 24.

D & C GREEN NO. 3 ALUMINUM LAKE • Food Green 3. The aluminum salt of FD & C Green No. 3. A brilliant, but not fast, dye. Fast Green FCF is the name for uncertified batches of this color. See Aniline Dyes for toxicity.

D & C GREEN NO. 5 • Acid Green 25. Dullish blue-green. Classed chemically as an anthraquinone color *(See* Colors). Used in suntan oils, bath salts, shampoos, hair rinses, toothpastes, soaps, and hair-waving fluids. Low skin toxicity but may cause skin irritation and sensitivity. Permanently listed by the FDA in 1982. The CTFA adopted name for uncertified batches of this color is Acid Green 25.

D & C GREEN NO. 6 • Solvent Green 3. Dull blue-green. Classified chemically as an anthraquinone color. Used in hair oils and pomades. Permanently listed by the FDA in 1982. The name for uncertified batches of this color is Solvent Green 3. See Colors.

D & C GREEN NO. 8 • Solvent Green 7. Yellowish green. Classed chemically as a pyrene color. Permanently listed by the FDA in 1976. The name for uncertified batches of this color is Solvent Green 7. See Colors.

D & C ORANGE NO. 4 • Acid Orange 7. Bright orange. Transparent orange used in lipsticks and face powders. Classed chemically as a monoazo color. Permanently listed in 1977. The name for uncertified batches of this color is Acid Orange 7. See Colors.

D & C ORANGE NO. 4 ALUMINUM LAKE • Persian Orange. Insoluble pigment prepared from D & C Orange No. 4 *(see)*. See Colors and Lakes.

D & C ORANGE NO. 5 • Acid Orange 11. Solvent Red 72. Dibromofluorescein *(see)*. Reddish orange. An orange stain used in lipsticks, face powders, and talcums. Permanently listed for use in lipsticks, mouthwashes, and dentifrices in 1982. Permanently listed for externally applied drugs and cosmetics in 1984. The name for uncertified batches of this color is Acid Orange 11.

D & C ORANGE NO. 5 ALUMINUM LAKE • Dawn Orange. Manchu Orange. Insoluble pigment prepared from D & C Orange No. 5 *(see)*. See Colors and Lakes.

D & C ORANGE NO. 5 ZIRCONIUM LAKE • Petite Orange. Dawn Orange. Acid Red 26. Ponceau R. See Lake and Zirconium. A monoazo dye. See Azo Dyes.

D & C ORANGE NO. 10 • Solvent 73. Diiodofluorescein. Reddish orange. Classed chemically as a fluoran color. Orange-red powder used in lipsticks and other cosmetics. The name for uncertified batches of this color is Solvent Red 73. See Colors.

D & C ORANGE NO. 10 ALUMINUM LAKE • Solvent Red 73. Erythrosine G. A xanthene color *(see)*.

D & C ORANGE NO. 11 • Acid Red 95. Clear red. Classed chemically as a xanthene color. It is the conversion product of D & C Orange No. 10 *(see)* to the sodium or potassium salt. The name for uncertified batches of this color is Acid Red 95. See Colors.

D & C ORANGE NO. 17 • Permanent Orange. Pigment Orange 5. Bright orange. Classed chemically as a monoazo color. The FDA permanently listed Orange No. 17, but its ruling was reversed by the U.S. Court of Appeals in 1987 for the District of Columbia, which said the FDA lacked legal authority to approve it since it was found to induce cancer. The court's ruling was in response to a lawsuit by Public Citizens Health Research Group, a consumer advocacy group. The color is no longer authorized for use. See Colors.

D & C RED NO. 4 ALUMINUM LAKE • Food Red 1. A monoazo color. The aluminum salt of FD & C Red No. 4 or Ponceau SX, the uncertified counterpart of FD & C Red No. 4 may be used to prepare this lake. See Azo Dyes.

D & C RED NO. 6 • Lithol Rubin B. Medium red. Classed chemically as a monoazo color. It is the calcium salt of D & C Red No. 7 *(see)*. Lithol is a topical antiseptic. Permanently listed in 1983. Nontoxic. The CTFA adopted name for uncertified batches of this color is Pigment Red 57. See Colors.

D & C RED NO. 6 ALUMINUM LAKE • Pigment Red 57. Lithol Rubine. A monoazo color. See Azo Dyes.

D & C RED NO. 6 BARIUM LAKE • Rubine Lake. Pigment Red 57. Lithol Rubine B. A monoazo dye. An insoluble pigment prepared from D & C Red No. 6 *(see)* and barium. The CTFA name for uncertified batches of this color is Pigment Red 57:2 Barium Lake. See Colors and Azo Dyes.

D & C RED NO. 6 BARIUM/STRONTIUM LAKE • An insoluble pigment prepared by mixing barium and strontium salts of D & C Red No. 6.

D & C RED NO. 6 POTASSIUM LAKE • An insoluble pigment composed of the potassium salt of D & C Red No. 6. See D & C Red No. 6.

D & C RED NO. 6 STRONTIUM LAKE • An insoluble pigment prepared by mixing strontium with D & C Red No. 6.

D & C RED NO. 7 • Lithol Rubin B Ca. Bluish red. Classed chemically as a monoazo color. Used in nail lacquers and lipsticks. Lithol is a topical antiseptic. Permanently listed in 1987 for ingested drug and cosmetic lip products, amount not to exceed 5 mg. per daily dose of drug. For general cosmetic use according to good manufacturing practices. This color is the salt of D & C Red No. 6. Uncertified batches of this color must be called Pigment Red 57. See Colors.

D & C RED NO. 7 ALUMINUM LAKE • Pigment Red 57. See Azo Dyes.

D & C RED NO. 7 BARIUM LAKE • Insoluble pigment prepared from D & C Red No. 7 *(see)*. See also Colors and Lakes.

D & C RED NO. 7 CALCIUM LAKE • Pigment Red 57. Lithol Rubine B. A monoazo dye. An insoluble pigment prepared from D & C Red No. 7 *(see)* and calcium. See Colors and Azo Dyes.

D & C RED NO. 7 ZIRCONIUM LAKE • Pigment Red 57. Lithol Rubine B. A monoazo color. Carcinogenic in animals. See Colors. Ruling postponed.

D & C RED NO. 8 • Lake Red C. Pigment Red 53. Orange. Classed chemically as a monoazo color. Carcinogenic in animals. Permanently listed in 1987 for ingested drug and cosmetic lip products, amount not to exceed 0.1 percent by weight of finished product. The FDA permanent listing of D & C Red No. 8 has been challenged by a lawsuit by Public Citizens Health Research Group, a consumer advocacy group. This color is no longer authorized for use. See D & C Red No. 19 and Colors.

D & C RED NO. 9 • Lake Red C Ba. Scarlet coloring. It is the barium salt of D & C Red No. 8 *(see)*. Used in face powders. Carcinogenic in animals. Permanently listed in 1987 for ingested drug and cosmetic lip products, amount not to exceed 0.1 percent of finished product. The permanent listing of this color, which has shown to be carcinogenic in animals, was challenged in 1988 by the Public Citizens Health Research Group, a consumer advocacy organization. This color is no longer authorized for use. See D & C Red No. 19 and Colors.

D & C RED NO. 10 • Litho Red. Yellowish red. No longer authorized for use.

D & C RED NO. 17 • Toney Red. Classed chemically as a diazo color. It is used in soaps, suntan oils, hair oils, and pomades. Carcinogenic in animals. No longer used much in lipsticks because of reports of ill-effects. The FDA permanently listed D & C Red No. 17 in 1988, but its ruling was reversed by the U.S. Court of Appeals for the District of Columbia, which said the FDA lacked legal authority to approve it since D & C Red No. 17 was found to induce cancer. The court's ruling was in response to a lawsuit by Public Citizens Health Research Group, a consumer advocacy group. The uncertified name of this color is Solvent Red 23. See Colors.

D & C RED NO. 19 • Rhodamine B. Mingredienta. Classed chemically as a xanthene color. Its greenish crystals or yellow powder turns violet in solution. Used in lipsticks, rouges, soaps, bath salts, nail enamel, toothpaste, hair-waving fluids, and face powders. The FDA permanently listed D & C Red No. 19 in 1988, but its ruling was reversed by the U.S. Court of Appeals for the District of Columbia, which said the FDA lacked legal authority to approve D & C Red No.

19 since it was found to induce cancer. The court's ruling was in response to a lawsuit by Public Citizens Health Research Group, a consumer advocacy group. No longer authorized for use. See Colors.

D & C RED NO. 21 • Solvent Red 43. Tetrabromofluorescein *(see)*. Classed chemically as a fluoran color. A bluish pink stain used in lipsticks, rouges, and nail enamels. Insoluble in water but used to color oils, resins, and lacquers. Permanently listed, 1982. The uncertified name for batches of this color is Solvent Red 43. See Colors.

D & C RED NO. 21 ALUMINUM LAKE • Insoluble pigment prepared from D & C Red No. 21 *(see)* and aluminum. The uncertified name for this color is Pigment Red 90:1 Aluminum Lake. See Colors and Lakes.

D & C RED NO. 21 ZIRCONIUM LAKE • Solvent Red 43. Merry Pink. A xanthene dye *(see)*.

D & C RED NO. 22 • Eosine YS. Yellowish pink. Classed chemically as a xanthene color. It is used in soaps, hair rinses, lipsticks, and nail polishes. Red crystals with bluish tinge or brownish red powder. Freely soluble in water. Lethal dose in animals is quite small. Permanently listed in 1982. The CTFA name for uncertified batches of this color is Acid Red 87. See Colors.

D & C RED NO. 27 • Solvent Red 48. Philoxine B. Veri Pink. A xanthene *(see)* dye. Classed chemically as a fluoran color. A deep, bluish red stain used in lipsticks and rouges. Permanently listed, 1982. The uncertified name for this color is Solvent Red 48. See Colors.

D & C RED NO. 27 ALUMINUM LAKE • Tetrabromo Tertrachloro Fluorescein Lake. Insoluble pigment prepared from D & C Red No. 27 *(see)* and aluminum. See Color.

D & C RED NO. 27 BARIUM LAKE • Solvent Red 48. Petite Pink. A xanthene *(see)* dye.

D & C RED NO. 27 CALCIUM LAKE • An insoluble pigment composed of the calcium salt of D & C Red No. 27.

D & C RED NO. 27 ZIRCONIUM LAKE • Solvent Red 48. A xanthene *(see)* dye, deep, bluish red. Used in lipsticks and rouges.

D & C RED NO. 28 • Phloxine B. Acid Red 92. Classed chemically as a xanthene color. It is the conversion product of D & C Red No. 27 *(see)* to the sodium salt. Permanently listed, 1982. The name for uncertified batches of this color is Acid Red 92. See Colors.

D & C RED NO. 30 • Helindone Pink CN. Vat Red 1. Bluish pink. Classed chemically as an indigoid color. It is used in face powders, talcums, lipsticks, rouges, and soaps. The uncertified name for this color is Vat Red 1. See Colors.

D & C RED NO. 30 ALUMINUM LAKE • Vat Red 1. Thioindigoid Pink R. A thioindigoid color. A red vat dye made from indigo and sulfur. See Vat Dyes and Indigo.

D & C RED NO. 30 CALCIUM LAKE • Permanent Pink. Vat Red 1. Thioindigo Pink R. A thioindigo dye. See Vat Dyes and Indigo.

D & C RED NO. 30 LAKE • Insoluble pigment prepared from D & C Red No. 30 *(see)* with an approved metal. See Colors and Lakes.

D & C RED NO. 31 • **Brilliant Lake Red R.** Classed chemically as a monoazo color. It is used in lipsticks and nail enamels. See Colors.

D & C RED NO. 31 CALCIUM LAKE • **Brilliant Lake Red R.** Monoazo color used in lipsticks and nail enamels. See Azo Dyes.

D & C RED NO. 33 • **Acid Red 33.** Dull, bluish red. Classed chemically as a monoazo color. It is used in lipsticks, rouges, soaps, bath salts, and hair rinses. Was to be permanently listed in 1988, but the ruling has been postponed to allow the FDA "additional time to study complex scientific and legal questions about it." The uncertified name for this color is Acid Red 33. See Azo Dyes and Colors.

D & C RED NO. 34 • **Fanchon Maroon. Deep Maroon.** Classed chemically as a monoazo color. It is used in face powders, talcums, nail lacquers, lipsticks, rouges, toothpastes, and soaps. The uncertified name for this color is Pigment Red 63:1. See Colors.

D & C RED NO. 34 CALCIUM LAKE • Insoluble pigment prepared from D & C Red No. 34 *(see)*. See Colors and Lakes.

D & C RED NO. 36 • **Pigment Red 4. Tiger Orange.** A monoazo dye. It is a bright orange used in lipsticks, rouges, face powders, and talcums. Was to be permanently listed in 1988, but the ruling has been postponed to allow the FDA "additional time to study complex scientific and legal questions about it." The uncertified name for this color is Pigment Red 4. See Colors and Azo Dyes.

D & C RED NO. 36 BARIUM LAKE • **Pigment Red 4. Permanent Red 12.** Orange hue. A monoazo color. See Azo Dyes.

D & C RED NO. 36 LAKE • **Chlorinated Para Lake. Tang Orange.** Insoluble pigment prepared from D & C Red No. 36 *(see)*. See Colors and Lakes.

D & C RED NO. 36 ZIRCONIUM LAKE • **Pigment Red 4.** See D & C Red No. 36 Barium Lake.

D & C RED NO. 37 • **Rhodamine B-Stearate Solvent.** Banned in 1988. See Colors.

D & C RED NO. 40 ALUMINUM LAKE • Bluish pink. Classed chemically as a xanthene *(see)* color. Used in soaps. An insoluble color prepared from FD & C Red No. 40 *(see)*.

D & C VIOLET NO. 2 • **Alizurol Purple SS. Solvent Violet 13.** Classed chemically as an anthraquine color. It is a dull, bluish violet used in suntan oils, pomades, and hair colors. The uncertified batch of this color must be called Solvent Violet 13.

D & C YELLOW NO. 5 ALUMINUM LAKE • Greenish yellow. Insoluble pigment prepared from FD & C Yellow No. 5 *(see)* and aluminum. See Colors and Lakes.

D & C YELLOW NO. 5 ZIRCONIUM LAKE • An insoluble pigment prepared from FD & C Yellow No. 5 *(see)* and zirconium. See Colors and Lakes.

D & C YELLOW NO. 6 ALUMINUM LAKE • Insoluble pigment prepared from FD & C Yellow No. 6 *(see)* and aluminum. See Colors and Lakes.

D & C YELLOW NO. 7 • Acid Yellow 73. Fluorescein. Classed chemically as a fluoran color. It is a water-absorbing, yellowish red powder freely soluble in water. The fluorescence disappears when the solution is made acid and reappears when it is made neutral. No toxic action on fish, and believed to be nontoxic to humans. An uncertified batch of this color must be called Acid Yellow 73. See Colors.

D & C YELLOW NO. 8 • Uranine. Sodium fluorescein. Naphthol Yellow S. Classed chemically as a xanthene color. It is the sodium salt of D & C Yellow No. 7 *(see)*. Light yellow or orange-yellow powder soluble in water. The uncertified color is called Acid Yellow 73 Sodium Salt. See Colors.

D & C YELLOW NO. 10 • Acid Yellow 3. Quinoline Yellow. Classed chemically as a quinoline color. It is a bright, greenish yellow used in hair-waving fluids, toothpastes, bath salts, soaps, and shampoos. It is a potential allergen. It is present in yellow Irish Spring®, pink Dove®, and Caress Bath Soap®. It may cross-react with other quinoline colors used in drugs. The uncertified color is called Acid Yellow 3.

D & C YELLOW NO. 10 ALUMINUM LAKE • Insoluble pigment prepared from D & C Yellow No. 10 *(see)* and aluminum. The uncertified version of this color is Pigment Yellow 115. See Colors and Lakes.

D & C YELLOW NO. 11 • Solvent Yellow 33. Classed chemically as a quinoline color. It is a bright, greenish yellow used in soaps, shampoos, suntan oils, hair oils, and pomades. The uncertified version of this color is Solvent Yellow 33. See Colors.

DAFFODIL EXTRACT • Narcissis Pseudo. Narcissus Extract. A brilliant yellow, trumpetlike flowered plant of the family Narcissus.

DAISY EXTRACT • Extract of Daisy. Extract of the flowers of the English Daisy, *Bellis perennis*. Certain plants of the daisy family may cause blisterlike eruptions when crushed on the skin. Used in sachets. Also included in love potions by ancient herbalists.

DALEA SPINOSA • Indigo Bush Oil. Probably the oldest known dye. Prepared from various *Indigofera* plants native to Bengal, Java, and Guatemala. Dark blue powder with a coppery luster. No known skin irritation.

DAMAR • Resin used to produce a gloss and adhesion in nail lacquer. It is a yellowish white, semitransparent exudate from a plant grown in the East Indies and the Philippines. Comes in varying degrees of hardness. It has a bitter taste. Also used for preserving animal and vegetable specimens for science laboratories. May cause allergic contact dermatitis.

a-DAMASCONE • A fragrance ingredient.

DAMIANA LEAVES • The dried leaves of a plant of California and Texas used as a flavoring. Formerly used as a tonic and aphrodisiac. No known toxicity.

DANDELION LEAF AND ROOT • Lion's Tooth. Taraxacum Officinale. Used as a skin-refreshing bath additive. Obtained from *Taraxacum* plants, which grow abundantly in the United States. The common dandelion weed eaten as a salad green was used by the Indians for heartburn. Rich in Vitamins A and C, it is also used as a flavoring. No known toxicity.

DANDRUFF, HUMAN • The allergen in human skin flakes has been recognized for a long time and has been used as a test to determine a general tendency toward allergy. In one study, more than 90 percent of asthma patients had a positive skin test reaction in contrast to normals, who showed no reaction to the test. The reaction rate is even higher in those with allergic contact dermatitis or eczema. The subject of dandruff is a matter of controversy among allergists. Some point out that it is a self-produced antigen; others say it is part of the allergenic house-dust antigen; and still others say it is not a true allergen.

DANDRUFF SHAMPOOS • Usually shampoos that combine detergents with dry skin dissolvers. They contain sulfur, salicylic acid, resorcinol, and hexachlorophene. There are also after-shampoo dandruff rinses that contain quaternary ammonium compounds. And there are scalp lotions with antiseptics and stimulants such as resorcinol and/or chloral hydrate or tincture of capsicum. Hairdressings with zinc and cetalkonium chloride are also used to treat dandruff. Among other ingredients in dandruff products are allantoin for its healing properties and salicylanilide. A typical antidandruff formulation contains zinc pyrithione and a detergent. Another contains salicylic acid, sulfur, lanolin, cholesterol, and petrolatum. Certain ingredients such as sulfur, tar, lanolin, and salicylic acid are common allergens and may cause allergic contact dermatitis.

DASHEEN EXTRACT • See Taro.

DATE • *Phoenix dactylifera.* The fruit from a tall palm tree cultivated in Asia and Africa. Used in organic cosmetics.

DATEM • A hair and skin conditioning ingredient as well as an emollient and emulsifying agent. See fatty acids.

DATURA STRAMONIUM • See Stramonium.

DAUCUS CAROTA • See Carrot Oil.

DAVANA OIL • A plant extract used in fruit flavoring for cosmetics, beverages, ice cream, ices, candy, baked goods, and chewing gum. No known toxicity.

DEA • The abbreviation for diethanolamine *(see)*.

DEA-C12-15 ALKYL SULFATE • See Alcohol and Sulfate.

DEA-COCOAMPHODIPROPIONATE • See Coconut Oil and Quaternary Ammonium Compounds.

DEA-CYCLOCARBOXYPROPYLOLEATE • The diethanolamine *(see)* salt of acrylinoleic acid.

DEA-DODECYLBENZENESULFONATE • See Quaternary Ammonium Compounds.

DEA-HYDROLYZED LECITHIN • See Hydrolyzed and Lecithin.

DEA-ISOSTEARATE • See Diethanolamine and Isostearic Acid.

DEA-LAURAMINOPROPIONATE • The diethanolamine salt of propionic acid *(see both)*.

DEA-LAURETH SULFATE • See Quaternary Ammonium Compounds.

DEA-LAURYL SULFATE • See Quaternary Ammonium Compounds.

DEA-LINOLEATE • See Linoleic Acid.

DEA-METHOXYCINNAMATE • The diethanolamine salt of methoxycinnamic acid. See Diethanolamine and Cinnamic Acid.

DEA-METHYL MYRISTATE SULFONATE • **Biterge.** See Quaternary Ammonium Compounds.

DEA-MYRETH SULFATE • The diethanolamine salt of ethyoxylated myristyl sulfate. See Quaternary Ammonium Compounds.

DEA-MYRISTATE • The diethanolamine salt of myristic acid. Also called diethanolamine myristate. See Quaternary Ammonium Compounds.

DEA-OLETH-3 • See Oleth-20.

DEA-OLETH-10 PHOSPHATE • The diethanolamine salt of a mixture of esters of phosphoric acid and Oleth-10. See Quaternary Ammonium Compounds.

DEA-STYRENE/ACRYLATES/DVB COPOLYMER • The diethanolamine salt of a polymer of styrene, divinylbenzene, and two or more monomers consisting of acrylic acid, methacrylic acid, or their esters. Used as an opacifier. See Acrylates, Styrene, Vinyl, and Benzene.

DECANAL • An aldehyde *(see)* used as a fragrance ingredient.

DECANOIC ACID • A synthetic flavoring ingredient that occurs naturally in anise, butter acids, oil of lemon, and oil of lime, and is used in cosmetic fragrances. Also used to flavor butter, coconut, fruit, liquor, and cheese. No known toxicity.

DECENAL • An aldehyde *(see)* used as a fragrance ingredient.

DECENE/BUTENE COPOLYMER • A synthetic polymer *(see)* used as a thickening ingredient.

9-DECEN-1-OL • See Decylene.

DECETH-4 • See Polyglycol and Decyl Alcohol.

DECETH-6 • The polyethylene glycol ether of decyl alcohol *(see)*.

DECETH-7-CARBOXYLIC ACID • See Myristic Acid.

DECETH-4-PHOSPHATE • A mixture of polyethylene glycol, phosphoric acid esters, and decyl alcohol *(see all)*.

DECETH-6-PHOSPHATE • A mixture of polyethylene glycol, phosphoric acid esters, and polyoxyethylene *(see all)*.

DECYL ALCOHOL • An intermediate *(see)* for surface-active ingredients, an antifoam ingredient, and a fixative in perfumes. Occurs naturally in sweet orange and ambrette seed. Derived commercially from liquid paraffin *(see)*. Colorless to light yellow liquid. Used also for synthetic lubricants and as a synthetic fruit flavoring. Low toxicity in animals. No known toxicity for the skin.

DECYL BETAINE • See Betaine.

DECYL GLUCOSIDE • See Decyl Alcohol and Glucose.

DECYL ISOSTEARATE • See Decyl Alcohol and Isostearic Acid.

DECYL MERCAPTOMETHYLIMIDAZOLE • See Imidazole.

DECYL MYRISTATE • An ester of myristic acid *(see)* used as a skin conditioning ingredient. It is opaque.

DECYL OLEATE • Used in skin conditioners. See Decyl Alcohol.

DECYL POLYGLUCOSE • See Decyl Alcohol and Glucose.

DECYL SUCCINATE • Decyl Hydrogen Succinate. Produced by the reaction of decyl alcohol and succinic acid *(see both).* Used in the manufacture of perfumes and in cosmetic creams as a buffer and neutralizing ingredient. No known toxicity.

DECYL TETRADECANOL • See Decanoic Acid.

DECYLAMINE OXIDE • Capric Dimethylamine Oxide. See Capric Acid.

DECYLENE • A colorless liquid used in the manufacture of flavors, perfumes, pharmaceuticals, and dyes.

DECYLTETRADECETH-30 • See Polyethylene Glycol and Decanoic Acid.

DEDM • Abbreviation for diethylol dimethyl.

DEDM HYDANTOIN • A preservative. See Hydantoin.

DEDM HYDANTOIN DILAURATE • A preservative. See Hydantoin and Lauric Acid.

DEER'S TONGUE LEAVES • Liatris. Vanilla Plant. Leaves of *Trilisa odoratissima,* found from Virginia to Florida and Louisiana. Contains the volatile oil coumarin *(see).* Used in perfumery and to make tobacco smell better.

DEHYDRATED • With the water removed.

DEHYDROACETIC ACID DHA • Sodium Dehydroacetate. A weak acid that forms a white, odorless powder with an acrid taste. Used as an antienzyme ingredient in toothpastes to prevent tooth decay and as a preservative for shampoos. Also used as a fungi and bacteria-destroying ingredient in cosmetics. The presence of organic matter decreases its effectiveness. Not irritating or allergy-causing, but it is a kidney-blocking ingredient and can cause impaired kidney function. Large doses can cause vomiting, imbalance, and convulsions.

7-DEHYDROCHOLESTEROL • See Cholesterol.

DELANEY AMENDMENT • Written by Congressman James Delaney, the amendment was part of a 1958 law requested by the Food and Drug Administration. The law stated that food and chemical manufacturers had to test additives before they were put on the market and the results had to be submitted to the FDA. Delaney's amendment specifically states that "no additive may be permitted in any amount if the tests show that it produces cancer when fed to man or animals or by other appropriate tests."

DELAYED HYPERSENSITIVITY • Manifested primarily as contact dermatitis due to drugs such as neomycin or to parabens *(see both),* a common preservative in topical medications. Certain multiple allergic reactions to drugs such as penicillin, nitrofurantoin, and hydantoin may also fall into this category.

DELESSERIA SANGUINEA • See Sanguinaria.

DELTA CADINENE • A sesquiterpenes occurring in essential oils from Juniper species and cedars (oil of cade). Used in perfumery. See Sesquiterpene Lactones.

DEMULCENT • A soothing, usually thick, oily, or creamy substance used to relieve pain in inflamed or irritated mucous surfaces. The gum acacia, for instance, is used as a demulcent.

DENATONIUM BENZOATE • A denaturant for alcohol that is to be used in cosmetics. It is intended to make alcohol unpalatable for drinking purposes and, therefore, is unpleasant to smell and taste. No known toxicity. See Denatured Alcohol.

DENATONIUM SACCHARIDE • A denaturant for alcohol. See Denatonium Benzoate.

DENATURANT • A poisonous or unpleasant substance added to alcoholic cosmetics to make them undrinkable. It is also considered a substance that changes another substance's natural qualities or characteristics.

DENATURED ALCOHOL • Ethyl alcohol must be made unfit for drinking before it can be used in cosmetics. Various substances such as denatonium benzoate *(see)* are added to alcohol to make it malodorous and obnoxious in order to completely prevent its use or recovery for drinking purposes.

DENTIFRICES • Their primary purpose is to clean accessible surfaces of the teeth with a toothbrush. Such cleansing is important to the appearance of teeth and to gum health, and it prevents mouth odor. Dentifrices usually come in the form of a paste or powder. Despite the brand claims, most dentifrices contain similar ingredients: binders, abrasives, sudsers, humectants, flavors, unique additives, and liquids. Binders include karaya gum, bentonite, sodium alginate, methylcellulose, carrageenan, and magnesium aluminum silicate. Among the abrasives are calcium carbonate, dibasic calcium phosphate, calcium sulfate, tricalcium phosphate, and sodium metaphosphate hydrated alumina. Sudsers include hard soap and the detergents sodium lauryl sulfate, sodium lauryl sulfoacetate, dioctyl sodium sulfosuccinate, sulfolaurate, and sodium lauryol sarcosinate. Humectants include glycerin, propylene glycol, and sorbitol. The most popular flavors are spearmint, peppermint, wintergreen, and cinnamon, but there are also such odd ones as bourbon, rye, anise, clove, caraway, coriander, eucalyptus, nutmeg, and thyme. Fluorides are added to reduce decay; also added are antienzyme ingredients (sodium dehydroacetate) and tooth whiteners (sodium perborate). Still other ingredients in dentifrices are sodium benzoate, ammonium antiseptics, sodium coconut monoglyceride sulfonate, sodium copper chlorophyllin, chloroform, starch, sodium chloride, calcium sulfate, strontium chloride, p-hydroxybenzoate as a preservative, and sodium dehydroacetate. Toothpastes promoted for sensitive teeth are questionable, according to the American Dental Association. The most popular toothpaste contains sodium fluoride, calcium pyrophosphate, glycerin, sorbitol, and a blend of anionic surfactants *(see);* its competitor contains sodium n-lauryol sarcosinate and sodium monofluorophosphate. Complaints to the FDA about dentifrices include sore mouth and gums, tooth enamel worn away, sore tongue, and sloughing of mucous membranes. Some toothpastes contained too much chloroform, which was reduced by the manufacturer upon the FDA's request. Tartar control became the "buzz word" in the 1980s, and most toothpastes promoted it. In the 1990s, as the population is growing older, manufacturers are promoting toothpastes for sensitive teeth and bicarbonate of soda and other ingredients for healthy gums as well as tartar removal.

DEODORANTS • Includes antiperspirants. It is not the normal secretions of the skin that produce an objectionable odor but the action of bacteria and chemicals on sweat that creates the unpleasant smell. The difference between deodorants and antiperspirants is in sequence. Deodorants control perspiration odors, but antiperspirants retard the flow of perspiration. Deodorants inhibit the growth of microorganisms, which produce the malodors; antiperspirants, which contain a hydrolyzing metal salt, develop a low pH (increased acidity) and inhibit moisture. The inhibiting action may be enhanced by antiseptics that deodorize. Aluminum salts are the most widely used for inhibiting perspiration; urea *(see)* may be added to neutralize the fabric-damaging acidity of the metal. Antiseptics may be incorporated into deodorant soaps. Deodorants, formerly called "unscented toilet waters" and "sanitary liquid preparations," once contained formaldehyde or benzoic acid, which have been replaced with quaternary ammonium compounds *(see)*. Deodorant-action, liquid antiperspirants today usually contain aluminum chloride, urea, propylene glycol, and about 75 percent water. Deodorant-action, cream antiperspirants contain aluminum chlorhydroxide, sorbitan monostearate, poloxamers, stearic acid, boric acid, petrolatum, perfume, propylene glycol, and water. Spray deodorants have the same ingredients as liquid ones but are mixed with a propellant. The aluminum, alcohol, and zinc salts in deodorants and antiperspirants can cause skin and gastrointestinal irritations. Deaths from intentional inhalation of deodorant sprays have been reported. Vision has been affected by spray in the eyes. With all deodorants there can be stinging and burning, itching, sebaceous cysts, enlarged sweat glands, pimples under the arms, and lung and throat irritation. Seven cases of lung tumors attributed to underarm deodorant sprays were reported at the 1971 American Thoracic Society meeting in Los Angeles. See Vaginal Deodorants.

DEODORIZED KEROSENE • Deo-Base. Derived from petroleum, it is a mobile, water-white transparent liquid that has been deodorized and decolorized by washing kerosene with fuming sulfuric acid. It is a solvent used in brilliantines and emulsified lotions and creams, and as a constituent of hand lotions. It is a skin irritant, and dermatitis often occurs. Because of its solvent action on fats, it can cause a defatting and drying of the skin. In cosmetics, however, when it is used with fatty substances, its fat-solvent action is minimized and it is considered innocuous.

DEOXYRIBONUCLEASE • An enzyme that hydrolyzes *(see)* DNA *(see)*.

DEPILATORIES • The most effective chemical hair removers yet discovered are the sulfides *(see)*, particularly hydrogen sulfide, but they have an unpleasant odor that is hard to mask. Most sulfides have been replaced with salts of thioglycolic acid *(see)*, which take more time to act but smell better and are not as irritating as sulfides. However, persons who have difficulty with detergent hands, ammonia, or strong soaps often have difficulty with thioglycolic depilatories. Also, ingestion of thioglycolic depilatories may cause severe gastrointestinal irritation. Cream depilatories that act by dissolving the hair usually contain calcium thioglycolate, calcium carbonate, calcium hydroxide, cetyl alcohol, sodium lauryl sulfate (a detergent), water, and a strong perfume (so as to remain stable in an alkali medium). Another type of depilatory made of wax acts by hardening around the hair and pulling it out. Such products usually contain rosin, beeswax, paraffin, and petrolatum. (See above ingredients under separate listings.) Among injuries recently reported to the FDA concerning depilatories were skin irritation, headaches, scars on the legs, skin burns, and rash. It can cause allergic reactions. See Flaxseed.

DEPROTEINATED YEAST • See Protein and Yeast.

DEPROTEINIZED SERUM • The fluid portion of the blood from which protein has been removed.

DEQUALINIUM CHLORIDE • See Quaternary Ammonium Compounds.

DEQUALIUM ACETATE • See Quaternary Ammonium Compounds.

DERMATAN SULFATE • **Chondroitin Sulfate.** Chondroitin Sulfuric Acid. Occurs in both skeletal and soft connective tissue. It is abundant in skin, arterial walls, and heart valves.

DERMATITIS • Inflammation of the skin.

DERMIS • The lower layer of skin, overlying subcutaneous fat and composed of blood vessels, lymph sacs, sensory nerve endings, hair follicles, and oil and sweat glands.

DERMOLECTINE • New ingredient that at this writing was being developed. It is from potatoes and acts similar to a hormone. It is a cellular growth promoter. Whether it will be accepted as a cosmetic ingredient or a drug is yet to be determined.

DESAMIDO COLLAGEN • Animal collagen that has been modified to change the amide group into carboxylic acid groups to change its texture and odor for use in "youth creams." The word "animal" was removed from the label.

DESOXYCHOLIC ACID • An emulsifying ingredient, white, crystalline powder, almost insoluble in water. Used in dried egg whites up to 0.1 percent. No known toxicity. The final report to the FDA of the Select Committee on GRAS Substances stated in 1980 that it should continue its GRAS status with no limitations other than good manufacturing practices. Moderately toxic by ingestion. Has caused tumors in animals.

DESOXYEPHEDRINE HYDROCHLORIDE • **Epinine. Desoxyephedrine.** Obtained from laudanosine, or papaverine, which are both derived from the poppy. It is a blood vessel constrictor.

DESOXYRIBONUCLEIC ACID • **DNA.** A chain of molecules that contains the genetic code (blueprint) of cells.

DETERGENT • Any of a group of synthetic, organic, liquid, or water-soluble cleansing ingredients that, unlike soap, are not prepared from fats and oils and are not inactivated by hard water. Most of them are made from petroleum derivatives but vary widely in composition. The major advantage of detergents is that they do not leave a hard water scum. They also have wetting ingredient and emulsifying ingredient properties. Quaternary ammonium compounds *(see)*, for instance, through surface action, exert cleansing and antibacterial effects. PHisoDerm is an example of a liquid detergent, and Dove is an example of a solid detergent. Toxicity of detergents depends upon alkalinity. Dishwasher detergents, for instance, can be dangerously alkaline while detergents used in cosmetic products have an acidity-alkalinity ratio near normal skin, 5 to 6.5 pH.

DEXTRAN • A term applied to polysaccharides produced by bacteria growing on sugar. Used as a thickening ingredient in cuticle removers, it is also employed as a foam stabilizer in beer. Injection into the skin has caused cancer in rats.

DEXTRAN SULFATE • The sulfuric acid ester of dextran *(see)*.

DEXTRIN • **British Gum. Starch Gum.** White or yellow powder produced from starch and used as a diluting ingredient for dry extracts and emulsions and as a thickener in cream and liquid cosmetics. May cause an allergic reaction.

DIACETIN • A mixture of the diesters *(see)* of glycerin *(see)* and acetic acid *(see)*, used as a plasticizer, softening ingredient, or as a solvent for cellulose derivatives, resins, and shellacs. No known toxicity.

DIACETONE ALCOHOL • Used as a solvent for nail enamels, fats, oils, waxes, and resins. Also used as a preservative. Prepared by the action of an alkali such as calcium hydroxide on acetone *(see)*. Highly flammable with a pleasant odor, it mixes easily with other solvents. May be narcotic in high concentrations and has caused kidney and liver damage, as well as anemia, in experimental animals when given orally.

DIACETYL • A catalyst *(see)* in the manufacture of fake nails. It occurs naturally in cheese, cocoa, pears, coffee, raspberries, strawberries, and cooked chicken but is usually prepared by a special fermentation of glucose. It is a yellowish green liquid. Also used as a carrier of aroma of butter, vinegar, and coffee, and to flavor oleomargarine. Diacetyl compounds have been associated with cancer when ingested by experimental animals.

DIAMINO • A prefix meaning two amine atoms from ammonia.

3,4-DIAMINOBENZOIC ACID • See Benzoic Acid.

4,5-DIAMINO-1-((4-CHLOROPHENYL)METHYL)-1H-PYRAZOLE-SULFATE • A hair coloring. See Coal Tar colors.

2,4-DIAMINODIPHENYLAMINE • A hair coloring. See Coal Tar Colors, Phenylamine, and Ammonia.

2,4-DIAMINO-5-METHYLETHIOXYPHENOL HCL • See Phenol and Ammonia.

4,5-DIAMINO-1-METHYLPYROZOLE HCL • See Ammonia and Pyrazole.

DIAMINONAPHTHALINE • A black dye. See Coal Tar.

DIAMINOPHENOL • A brown dye. See Phenol.

2,4-DIAMINOPHENOL • Manufactured from aniline *(see)* and used in hair dye. The CIR Expert Panel *(see)* concluded that its use in hair dyes at concentrations up to 0.2 percent was safe. For toxicity, see *p*-Phenylenediamine.

DIAMINOPHENOL HYDROCHLORIDE • A black-brown dye. The CIR Expert Panel *(see)* concluded that its use in hair dyes at concentrations up to 0.2 percent was safe. See Phenol.

2,4-DIAMINOPHENOXYETHANOL HCL • An aromatic amine salt used as a fixative, bactericide, and insect repellent. Slightly irritating to the skin. See Quaternary Ammonium Compounds.

4,4-DIAMINOPHENYLAMINE • See Ammonia and Phenylamine.

2,6-DIAMINOPYRIDINE • See Pyridine.

DIAMMONIUM CITRATE • Ammonium Salt of Citric Acid, Dibasic. See Citric Acid.

DIAMMONIUM DIMETHICONE COPOLYOL SULFOSUCCINATE • See Dimethicone and Surfactants.

DIAMMONIUM DITHIODIGLYCOLATE • Acetic acid, 2,2'-dithiobis-diammonium salt used in hair removal and hair waving. See Thioglycolic Acid Compounds.

DIAMMONIUM LAURYL SULFOSUCCINATE • The ammonium salt of lauryl alcohol. See Quaternary Ammonium Compounds.

DIAMMONIUM OLEAMIDO-PEG-2-SULFOSUCCINATE • An ammonium soap used as an emulsifying ingredient. See Quaternary Ammonium Compounds.

DIAMMONIUM PHOSPHATE • See Phosphate, Ammonia, and Surfactants.

DIAMMONIUM SODIUM SULFOSUCCINATE • The sodium salt of the diester of amyl alcohol and sulfosuccinic acid. A wetting ingredient and emulsifier. See Surfactants.

DIAMOND POWDER • A crystallized carbon used as an abrasive.

DIAMYLHYDROQUINONE • Santovar A®. An antioxidant for resins and oils and a polymerization inhibitor. See Hydroquinone.

DIAPER RASH • Ammonia Dermatitis. Skin irritation caused by urine and feces, and also by soap or detergents left in diapers if they are not thoroughly rinsed. The skin becomes red, spotty, sore, and moist.

DIAPER RASH PRODUCTS • The FDA issued a notice in 1992 that any diaper rash products with ingredients labeled with claims or directions for the use in the treatment or prevention of diaper rash have not been shown to be safe and effective as claimed in OTC products.

DIASTASE • A mixture of enzymes from malt. It converts at least 50 times its weight of potato starch into sugars in 30 minutes. Used to convert starch into sugar. In 1992, the FDA ruled that diastase and diastase malt aluminum hydroxide have not been shown to be safe and effective as claimed in OTC digestive aid products.

DIATALLOWETHYL HYDROXYETHYLMONIUM METHOSULFATE • See Quaternary Ammonium Compounds.

DIATOMACEOUS EARTH • Kieselguhr. A porous and relatively pure form of silica formed from fossil remains of diatoms—one-celled algae with shells. Inert when ingested. Used in pomades, dentifrices, nail polishes, face powders, as a clarifying ingredient, and as an absorbent for liquids because it can absorb about four times its weight in water. The dust can cause lung damage after long exposure to high concentrations. Not recommended for use on teeth or skin because of its abrasiveness.

DIAZO • A compound containing two nitrogen atoms, such as diazolidinyl urea (see), one of the newer preservatives, or diazepam, a tranquilizer and popular muscle relaxant.

DIAZO DYES • Coloring ingredients that contain two linked nitrogen atoms united to an aromatic group and to an acid radical. See Heliotropin.

DIAZOLIDINYL UREA • Oxymethurea. 1,3-Bis(hydroxymethyl) Urea. Germall II®. One of the newer cosmetic preservatives, not much has been reported about it except that it may be a sensitizer. Crystals from alcohol, very soluble in water. Used in the textile industry in cotton; as a pesticide and in cosmetics as an antiseptic. May release formaldehyde *(see)*. At concentrations up to 0.4 percent it was a mild cumulative skin irritant in humans. The CIR Expert Panel *(see)* concluded that on the basis of animal and clinical data, it is safe as a cosmetic ingredient up to a maximum concentration of 0.5 percent. See also Urea.

DIBA • The abbreviation for dihydroxyisobutylamine.

DIBEHENYL METHYLAMINE • Methyl Dibenehenylamine. See Behenic Acid.

DIBEHENYL/DIARACHIDYL DIMONIUM CHLORIDE • See Quaternary Ammonium Compounds.

DIBEHENYLDIMONIUM CHLORIDE • See Quaternary Ammonium Compounds.

DIBEHENYLDIMONIUM METHOSULFATE • See Quaternary Ammonium Compounds.

DIBENZOTHIOPHENE • Thioxanthene. Diphenylene Sulfide. Prepared from thioxanthrone, it gives a green fluorescence. Used in dandruff treatment shampoos and products. Colorless crystals made from alcohol, chloroform, and sulfur. Used as a psychopharmaceutical to treat mental disorders. When ingested can affect central nervous system, the blood, and blood pressure. However, no known toxicity when applied to the skin.

DIBENZOXAZOYL NAPHTHALENE • An ultraviolet light absorber. See Benzoic Acid and Naphthalene.

DIBENZYL ETHER • A synthetic fruit and spice flavoring ingredient for beverages, ice cream, ices, candy, baked goods, and chewing gum. The Flavor and Extract Manufacturer's Association evaluated the safety of this additive. High-dose female rats had increased liver weights. A no-effect level was achieved at 196 mg/kg/day. In a 60-kg human (about 132 pounds), this would be equivalent to approximately 11.8 grams a day.

DIBENZYLIDENE SORBITOL • See Sorbitol.

DIBROMOFLUORESCEIN • Used in indelible lipsticks, it is made by heating resorcinol and phthalic anhydride *(see both)* to produce fluorescent orange-red crystals. Ingestion can cause gastrointestinal symptoms. Skin application can cause skin sensitivity to light, inflamed eyes, skin rash, and even respiratory symptoms. See Colors.

DIBROMOPROPAMIDINE DIISETHIONATE • The salt of isethionic acid mixed with propane. Almost insoluble in alcohol and water and fixed oils, it is used as an antiseptic and antimicrobial. May be irritating to the skin.

DIBROMOSALAN • 4,5-Dibromosalicylanilide. An antibacterial ingredient used as an antiseptic and fungicide in detergents, toilet soaps, creams, lotions, and powders. No oral toxicity reported in man but has caused skin sensitivity to light, causing rash and swelling.

DIBUCAINE • Nupercaine. Bitter, water-absorbing crystals. Used as a local anesthetic for the skin, particularly in wax depilatories to prevent pain. Similar to cocaine when applied to the skin. Highly toxic when injected into the abdomens of rats; only one part per kilogram of body weight is lethal. No known toxicity is reported in humans.

DIBUTYL ADIPATE • The diester of butyl alcohol and adipic acid *(see both)*. A thickener in cosmetic products. A reduction in weight gain occurred in rabbits whose skin was painted with this substance. It was also mildly irritating to their skin and eyes. A significant increase in fetal abnormalities also occurred. The CIR Expert Panel *(see)* concludes that the available data are insufficient to support the safety of this ingredient in cosmetics.

DIBUTYL LAUROYL GLUTAMIDE • A gelling ingredient. See Lauric Acid and Glutamic Acid.

DIBUTYL OXALATE • A plasticizer and solvent. See Butyl Alcohol and Oxalic Acid.

DIBUTYL PHTHALATE • The ester of the salt of phthalic acid *(see),* which is isolated from a fungus. The colorless liquid is used as a plasticizer in nail polish and as a perfume solvent, fixative, and antifoam ingredient. It is also an insect repellent. Has a low toxicity but if ingested can cause gastrointestinal upset. The vapor is irritating to the eyes and mucous membranes. It also produced testicular atrophy in various test rodents. On the basis of available data, the CIR Expert Panel *(see)* concludes that this ingredient is safe for topical application in the present practices of use and concentration as a cosmetic.

DIBUTYL SEBACATE • Sebacic Acid. A synthetic fruit flavoring usually obtained from castor oil and used for beverages, ice cream, and baked goods. Used in fruit-fragrance cosmetics. No known toxicity.

DIBUTYLENE TETRAFURFURAL • Derived from bran, rice hulls, or corncobs, it is used in the manufacture of medicinals and as a solvent and flavoring in cosmetics and food. Toxic when absorbed by the skin. Irritating to the eye.

DI-t-BUTYLHYDROQUINONE • A yellow powder used as an antioxidant. Animal studies show that this ingredient as low as 10 percent can cause redness of the skin and in feeding, it caused the deaths of all rats in the study within two weeks. The CIR Expert Panel *(see)* concluded that the available data for this ingredient are insufficient to support its safety as a cosmetic ingredient. See Hydroquinone.

DICALCIUM PHOSPHATE • Tooth polisher for dentifrices. See Calcium Phosphate.

DICALCIUM PHOSPHATE DIHYDRATE • Dicalcium phosphate *(see)* in powder form.

DI-C-12-15 ALKYL ADIPATE • See Alcohol and Adipic Acid.

DI-C12 ALKYL FUMARATE • An ester *(see)* of alcohol and fumaric acid *(see)*. Used as a skin conditioning ingredient.

DICAPRYL ADIPATE • The diester of capryl alcohol and adipic acid *(see both)*.

DICAPRYL/DICAPRYLYL DIMONIUM CHLORIDE • See Quaternary Ammonium Compounds.

DICAPRYL ETHER • A skin conditioning ingredient. See Caproic Acid.

DICAPRYLOYL CYSTINE • See Caprylic Acid and Cystine.

DICAPRYLSODIUM SULFOSUCCINATE • The sodium salt of the diester of capryl alcohol and sulfosuccinic acid. See Quaternary Ammonium Compounds.

DICETEARETH-10 PHOSPHATE • See Phosphoric Acid and Stearic Acid.

DICETYL ADIPATE • The diester of cetyl alcohol and adipic acid *(see both)*.

DICETYL PHOSPHATE • A mixture of cetyl alcohol and phosphoric acid *(see both)*.

DICETYL THIODIPROPIONATE • The diester of cetyl alcohol and thiodipropionic acid *(see both)*.

DICETYLDIMONIUM CHLORIDE • See Quaternary Ammonium Compounds.

DICHLOROBENZYL ALCOHOL • An insecticide. See Benzyl Alcohol.

DICHLORODIMETHYL HYDANTOIN • See Hydantoin.

5,7-DICHLORO-8-HYDROXYQUINOLINE • See Chlorine and Oxyquinoline.

DICHLOROPHENE • **Dichlorophen. Antiphen. Hyosan.** Crystals from toluene *(see)*. A fungicide and bactericide used in dentrifrices, shampoos, antiperspirants, deodorant creams, powder, and toilet waters. It is a potent allergen and is closely related to hexachlorophene *(see)*.

DICHLOROPHENYL IMIDAZOLDIOXOLAN • A preservative. See Imidazole.

DICHLORO-m-XLENOL • A phenol used as a bactericide in soaps and as a mold inhibitor and preservative. See Phenol.

DICOCAMINE • See Coconut Acid.

DICOCODIMETHYLAMINE DILINOLEATE • The diamine salt of dimer acid and dimethyl cocamine *(see both)* used as a plasticizer. See Coconut Acid.

DICOCODIMETHYLAMINE DIMERATE • See Dicocodimethylamine Dilinoleate.

DICOCODIMONIUM CHLORIDE • See Quaternary Ammonium Compounds.

DICOCOYL PENTAERYTHRITYL DISTEARYL CITRATE • Fatty acids derived from coconut oil *(see)*.

DICOCOYLETHYL HYDROXYETHYLMONIUM METHOSULFATE • See Quaternary Ammonium Compounds.

DI-C12-15-PARETH-2-PHOSPHATE • A surfactant and emulsifying ingredient. See Phosphoric Acid.

DICYCLOHEXYL SODIUM SULFOSUCCINATE • See Quaternary Ammonium Compounds.

DICYCLOPENTADIENE • **Cyclopentadiene.** Obtained from coal, it is used in the manufacture of resins and in camphors.

DIDECENE • A hydrocarbon *(see)* used as a skin conditioning ingredient.

DIDECYLDIMONIUM CHLORIDE • See Quaternary Ammonium Compounds.

DIERUCIC ACID • A skin conditioning ingredient and cover-up. See Erucic Acid.

DIESTER- • A compound containing two ester groupings. An ester is formed from an alcohol and an acid by eliminating water. Usually employed in fragrant liquids for artificial fruit perfumes and flavors.

DIETHANOLAMIDOOLEAMIDE DEA • See Quaternary Ammonium Compounds.

DIETHANOLAMINE • **Abbreviated as DEA.** Colorless liquid or crystalline fatty acids from soybeans or coconut oils. It is used as a solvent, emulsifying agent, and detergent. Also employed in emollients for its softening properties and as a dispersing agent and humectant in other cosmetic products. It may be irritating to the skin and mucous membranes. The FDA became aware of a National Toxicology Program (NTP) study showing an association between the topical application of diethanolamine and certain DEA-related ingredients and cancer in laboratory animals. For the DEA-related ingredients, the NTP study suggests that the cancer response is linked to possible residual levels of DEA. Although DEA itself may be used in few products, DEA-related ingredients such as oleamide DEA, lauramide DEA, cocamide DEA, are widely used as emulsifiers or foaming agents and generally used at levels of one to 5 percent. The FDA is studying the problem and is going to consider legal options at this writing. See Ethanolamines.

DIETHANOLAMINE BISULFATE • See Ethanolamines.

DIETHOXYETHYL SUCCINATE • See Succinic Acid.

DIETHYL ASPARTATE • The diester of ethyl alcohol and aspartic acid *(see both)*.

DIETHYL GLUTAMATE • See Glutamate.

DIETHYL KETONE • **3-Pentanone.** Liquid with an acetone odor used as an emulsifier.

DIETHYL MALONATE • 2-Butanedioic acid, diethyl ester. Used in the manufacture of chemicals. See Malic Acid.

DIETHYL PALMITOYL ASPARTATE • See Aspartic Acid.

DIETHYL PHTHALATE • Made from ethanol and phthalic acid *(see both)*. Used as a solvent, a fixative for perfume, and a denaturant *(see)* for alcohol. It has a bitter and unpleasant taste. Irritating to mucous membranes. Produces central nervous system depression when absorbed through the skin.

DIETHYL SEBACATE • See Sebacic Acid.

DIETHYL SUCCINATE • The diester of ethyl alcohol and succinic acid *(see both)*.

DIETHYL TOLUAMIDE • Made from *m*-toluoyl chloride and diethylamine in benzene or ether. A liquid soluble in water, it is used as an insect repellent. Irritating to the eyes and mucous membranes but not to the skin. Ingestion can cause central nervous system disturbances.

DIETHYLAMINE LAURETH SULFATE • See Surfactants.

DIETHYLAMINOETHYL COCOATE • Derived from coconut oil. See Surfactants.

DIETHYLAMINOETHYL METHYLCRYLATE • See Acrylates.

DIETHYLAMINOETHYL PEG-5 COCOATE • Derived from coconut oil *(see)*. See Surfactants and Polyethylene Glycol.

DIETHYLAMINOETHYL PEG-5-LAURATE • See Polyethylene Glycol and Lauric Acid.

DIETHYLAMINOETHYL STEARAMIDE • See Diethylamine.

DIETHYLAMINOETHYL STEARATE • See Stearic Acid and Amines.

DIETHYLAMINOMETHYL COUMARIN • See Coumarin.

N,N-DIETHYL-m-AMINOPHENOL • See Phenol.

N,N-DIETHYL-m-AMINOPHENOL SULFATE • See Phenol.

DIETHYLENE GLYCOL • Made by heating ethylene oxide and glycol. A clear, water-absorbing, almost colorless liquid; it is mixable with water, alcohol, and acetone. Used as a solvent, humectant, and plasticizer in cosmetic creams and hairsprays. A wetting ingredient *(see)* that enhances skin absorption. Can be fatal if swallowed. Not usually irritating to the skin, but can be absorbed through the skin and the use of glycols on extensive areas of the body is considered hazardous.

DIETHYLENE GLYCOL DIBENZOATE • The polyethylene glycol diester of benzoic acid *(see)*.

DIETHYLENE GLYCOL DIOCTANOATE/DIISONONANOATE • A complex mixture of acids used as a texturizer *(see)*.

DIETHYLENE GLYCOLAMINE/EPICHLOROHYDRIN PIPERAZINE CO-POLYMER • A polymer formed by the reaction of a mixture of diethylene glycolamine and piperazine with epichlorohydrin, used as a solvent. See Epichlorohydrin.

DIETHYLENE TRICASEINAMIDE • Made from the milk protein and casein *(see)*.

DIETHYLSTILBESTROL (DES) • **Stilbestrol.** A synthetic estrogen fed to cattle and poultry to "fatten them." A proven carcinogen, hormonal in nature, according to the FDA, which has given top priority to the study of the safety of DES. The FDA stipulates a zero tolerance for the compound after a proper withdrawal period. In 1971, three Harvard scientists linked DES to a rare form of vaginal cancer in the daughters of women who had taken DES during pregnancy. An estimated 100,000 to 150,000 head of cattle containing residues of the hormone are apparently getting to market. The European Common Market, Italy, and Sweden have forbidden the use of DES in cattle. Can be absorbed through the skin. It is offered for sale to cosmetic manufacturers, so presumably some are using it as a hormone in creams.

DIFFUSIVE • A term used to describe a perfume compound odor that spreads quickly and widely. This quality is good in perfumes but may be disliked in other products, such as hairsprays and deodorants.

DIGALLOYL TRIOLEATE • From digallic acid and oleic acid. An oily sunscreen ingredient devoid of anesthetic properties and stable under long periods of ultraviolet radiation. It may cause the skin to break out and redden when exposed to light.

DIGENEA SIMPLEX • **Kainic Acid.** Dried red algae that is used as a preservative. It is used to combat worms.

DIGITOXIN • **Crystodigin. Purodigin.** The main ingredient in digitalis, digitoxin is found in the leaves of the foxglove plant. It is used to treat congestive heart failure and irregular heartbeat and flutter. It works by strengthening the force of the heart's contractions and by regulating abnormal heart rhythms, especially fast irregular heartbeats. It is used in cosmetics.

DIGLYCERIN • A humectant *(see)* derived from glycerin *(see)*.

DIGLYCERYL STEARATE MALATE • The mixed ester of stearic acid and malic acid and glycerin polymer *(see all)*.

DIHEPTYL SODIUM SULFOSUCCINATE • Available as a waxlike solid. Used as a wetting ingredient in bath oil preparation. No known toxicity to the skin.

DIHEPTYLUNDECYL ADIPATE • See Adipic Acid.

DIHEXYL ADIPATE • A low-temperature plasticizer. See Adipic Acid.

DIHEXYL SODIUM SULFOSUCCINATE • See Quaternary Ammonium Compounds.

DIHEXYLDECYL LAUROYL GLUTAMATE • An amino acid used as an emollient ingredient. See Glutamate.

DIHYDROABIETYL ALCOHOL • See Abietic Acid and Abietyl Alcohol.

DIHYDROABIETYL METHACRYLATE • See Abietyl Alcohol.

DIHYDROACETIC ACID • Used in tanning creams. See Acetic Acid.

DIHYDROANISOLE • See Anisole.

DIHYDROCHALCONES • **Abbreviated DHC.** A new class of intensely sweet compounds obtained by a simple chemical modification of naturally occurring bioflavonoids.

DIHYDROCHOLESTEROL • See Cholesterol.

DIHYDROCHOLESTERYL MACADAMIATE • Fatty acids *(see)* derived from Macadamia nuts. See Macadamia Nut Oil.

DIHYDROCHOLESTERYL OCTYLDECAOATE • See Cholesterol and Octyldecanoic Acid.

DIHYDROCHOLETH-15 • The polyethylene glycol *(see)* ether of dihydrocholesterol. See Cholesterol.

DIHYDROCHOLETH-30 • The polyethylene glycol *(see)* ether of dihydrocholesterol. See Cholesterol.

DIHYDROCOUMARIN • See Coumarin.

DIHYDROGENATED TALLOW BENZYLMONIUMCHLORIDE • See Quaternary Ammonium Compounds.

DIHYDROGENATED TALLOWAMIDOETHYL HYDROXYETHYLMONIUM METHOSULFATE • Fatty acids *(see)* derived from hydrogenated tallow. See Tallow.

DIHYDROGENATED TALLOWETHYL HYDROXYETHYLMONIUM METHOSULFATE • A quaternary ammonium compound made from tallow *(see)*.

DIHYDROGENATED TALLOW METHYLAMINE • See Tallow and Hydrogenated.

DIHYDROGENATED TALLOW PHTHALATE • A surfactant made from tallow alcohol and phthalic acid *(see)*. See Tallow.

DIHYDRO-JASOMONE • See Jasomone.

DIHYDROPHYTOSTERYL OCTYLDECANOATE • See Octyldecanoic Acid.

DIHYDROSTREPTOMYCIN • An antibiotic active against streptococcal bacteria. Used as a preservative.

DIHYDROXYACETONE • Permanently listed in 1973. Also used as an emulsifier, humectant, and fungicide. No known toxicity. The Food and Drug Administration declared in 1973 that this color additive is safe and suitable for use in cosmetics or drugs that are applied to color the skin (suntan). A white powder that turns colorless in liquid form, it colors the skin an orange-brown shade, giving it a suntanned appearance. It is an ingredient in some suntan lotions for use indoors without sunlight. Obtained by the action of certain bacteria on glycerol, it has a sweet taste and characteristic odor. It is a strong reducing ingredient (see). It is converted by alkali to the fruit sugar fructose. Lethal when injected in large doses into rats. No known skin toxicity, and the FDA has exempted it from color additive certification, which means there is no need to test each batch as a means of protecting consumers as there is with coal tar colors. However, it can cause allergic contact dermatitis (see).

2,6,DIHYDROXY-3,4-DIMETHYLPYRIDINE • A hair coloring. See Coal Tar Colors.

DIHYDROXYETHYL C9-11 ALKOXYPROPYLAMINE OXIDE • See Quaternary Ammonium Compounds.

DIHYDROXYETHYL C12-15 ALKOXYPROPYLAMINE OXIDE • See Thioglycolic Acid Compounds.

DIHYDROXYETHYL COCAMINE OXIDE • See Coconut Oil.

DIHYDROXYETHYL SOYA GLYCINATE • See Quaternary Ammonium Compounds.

DIHYDROXYETHYL SOYAMINE DIOLEATE • The diester of oleic acid and dihydroxyethyl soyamine. See Thioglycolic Acid Compounds.

DIHYDROXYETHYL STEARAMINE OXIDE • See Stearic Acid.

DIHYDROXYETHYL STEARYL GLYCINATE • See Quaternary Ammonium Compounds.

DIHYDROXYETHYL TALLOWAMINE OLEATE • See Oleic Acid and Tallow.

DIHYDROXYETHYL TALLOWAMINE OXIDE • See Tallow.

2,5-DIHYDROXYETHYLAMINOTOLUENE • An amine hair coloring. See Coal Tar Colors.

DIHYDROXYETHYLOLEYL GLYCINATE • See Glycine.

DIHYDROXYINDOLE • See Indole and Hydroxylation.

DIHYDROXYINDOLINE • A hair coloring. See Coal Tar Colors.

DIIODOMETHYLTOLYLSULFONE • A preservative. See Toluene.

DIISOBUTYL SODIUM SULFOSUCCINATE • The sodium salt of the diester of isobutyl alcohol and sulfosuccinic acid, used as an alkalizer. See Succinic Acid.

DIISOCETYL ADIPATE • The diester of hexadecyl alcohol and adipic acid. See Adipic Acid.

DIISODECYL ADIPATE • Made from adipic acid and decyl alcohol (see both).

DIISOPROPANOLAMINE • Widely used ingredient in fragrances, tonics, hair grooming aids, permanent waves, hair dyes, and colors. Requires a patch test. Corrosion inhibitor and acid-alkali adjuster in cosmetic compounds. The CIR Expert Panel *(see)* concludes that this ingredient is safe in the present practices of use and concentrations in cosmetics. However, it should not be used in products containing nitrosating agents lest it form nitrosamines *(see)*. See Isopropanolamine.

DIISOPROPYL ADIPATE • Widely used ingredient. An emollient that helps prevent dryness and protect the skin by softening and lubricating it to minimize moisture loss. Used in bath products, colognes, and toilet waters, after-shave lotions, skin fresheners, and suntan gels. On the basis of available data, the CIR Expert Panel concludes that this igredient is safe as presently used in cosmetics. See Adipic Acid.

DIISOPROPYL DIMER DILINOLEATE • Skin conditioning agent. The CIR Expert Panel *(see)* concludes that there is insufficient data available to support the safety of this ingredient in cosmetics. See Dilinoleate.

DIISOPROPYL DIMERATE • See Dilinoleate.

DIISOPROPYL SEBACATE • See Isopropyl Alcohol and Sebacic Acid.

DIISOPSTEARYL ADIPATE • Made from stearic acid and adipic acid *(see both)*.

DIKETENE • Colorless, non–water absorbing liquid with a pungent odor. Obtained from acetone *(see)*, it is used in the production of pigments, toners, pesticides, and food preservatives.

DILAURETH-4 DIMONIUM CHLORIDE • See Quaternary Ammonium Compounds.

DILAURYL CITRATE • See Lauryl Alcohol and Citric Acid.

DILAURYL THIODIPROPIONATE • An antioxidant. White, crystalline flakes with a sweet odor. No known toxicity. The CIR Expert Panel *(see)* concludes that based upon data available, this ingredient is safe for use in cosmetic products at concentrations not to exceed 0.05 percent.

DILAURYLDIMONIUM CHLORIDE • See Quaternary Ammonium Compounds.

DILINOLEAMIDOPROPYL DIMETHYLAMINE • An antistatic ingredient in hair preparations. See Linoleic Acid.

DILINOLEATE • Dimer Acid. Widely used as an emulsifier, it is derived from linoleic acid *(see)*.

DILINOLEIC ACID • See Linoleic Acid.

DILINOLEIC ACID/ETHYLENEDIAMINE COPOLYMER • Made from dilinoleic acid and ethylenediamine *(see both)*.

DILL • *Anethum graveolens*. A hardy herb native to southern Europe and western Asia as well as the Americas, it was said by the ancient Greek physician Galen that it "procureth sleep." The name dill is derived from a Saxon word meaning "to lull." It is used by herbalists to treat symptoms of colic in children and insomnia in adults caused by indigestion. Used in "organic" cosmetics. Chewing dill seeds supposedly cures bad breath, and drinking dill tea calms upset stomachs and hiccups. It contains a volatile oil that includes carvone, used by herbalists to break up intestinal gas, and limonene, used in foods as a flavoring. Dill in hot milk is recommended by herbalists as a drink that calms the nerves. Herbalists say that it increases milk production when taken by nursing mothers. Limonene can be a skin irritant and sensitizer.

DILUENT • Any component of a color additive mixture that is not of itself a color additive and has been intentionally mixed therein to facilitate the uses of the mixture in coloring cosmetics or in coloring the human body, food, and drugs. The diluent may service another functional purpose in cosmetics, as, for example, emulsifying or stabilizing. Ethylcellulose is an example.

DIMER ACID • See Dilinoleate.

DIMETHICONE • **Dimethicone Copolyol.** A silicone *(see)* oil, white, viscous, used as an ointment base ingredient, as a topical drug vehicle, and as a skin protectant. Very low toxicity.

DIMETHICONE COPOLYOL • Hair conditioner and emollient. The CIR Expert Panel *(see)* concludes that this ingredient is safe in cosmetics. See Dimethicone.

DIMETHICONOL • See Dimethicone.

DIMETHOXY BENZENE • **Veratrole.** Colorless crystals or liquid derived from methanol. It is used as an antiseptic.

p-DIMETHOXY BENZENE • A synthetic raspberry, fruit, nut, hazelnut, root beer, and vanilla flavoring ingredient for beverages, ice cream, ices, candy, and baked goods. See above for toxicity.

DIMETHOXY METHANE • **Methylal.** A solvent for cosmetic aerosols and pump formulations and a perfume solvent. Has a formaldehydelike odor and is toxic by ingestion and inhalation.

m-DIMETHOXYBENZENE • **Resorcinol.** A synthetic fruit, nut, and vanilla flavoring for beverages, ice cream, ices, candy, and baked goods. Used on the skin as a bactericidal and fungicidal ointment. Has the same toxicity as phenol (extremely toxic), but causes more severe convulsions.

DIMETHOXYDICGLYCOL • A solvent. See Glycols.

2,6-DIMETHOXY-3,5-PYRIDINEDIAMINE • A hair coloring. See Coal Tar Colors.

DIMETHYL ANTHRANILATE • Colorless, pale yellow liquid with a grapelike odor. Used in perfumes and flavorings. See Benzoic Acid.

DIMETHYL ASPARTIC ACID • See Aspartic Acid.

DIMETHYL BEHENAMINE • See Behenic Acid.

DIMETHYL BENZYL CARBINOL • A flavoring ingredient. See Diphenolic Acid.

DIMETHYL BENZYL CARBINYL ACETATE • See Dimethyl Benzyl Carbinol and Acetic Acid.

DIMETHYL BRASSYLATE • Used in polyethylene films and water-resistant products.

DIMETHYL COCAMINE • See Coconut Oil.

DIMETHYL ETHER • Methyl Ether. Colorless gas with an ethereal odor. Used in refrigeration.

DIMETHYL ETHER RESORCINOL • A benzene derivative originally obtained from certain resins but now usually synthesized. See Dimethoxybenzene.

DIMETHYL GLUTAMIC ACID • See Glutamic Acid.

DIMETHYL GLUTARATE • Nail polish remover ingredient. See Glutamic Acid.

DIMETHYL HEXAHYDRONAPHTHYL DIHYDROXYMETHYL ACETAL • Used as a fragrance ingredient.

DIMETHYL HYDANTOIN • See Hydantoin.

DIMETHYL HYDROGENATED TALLOWAMINE • See Tallow.

DIMETHYL HYDROQUINONE • See Hydroquinone.

N,N, DIMETHYL-N-HYDROXYETHYL-3-NITRO-p-PHENYLENE DIAMINE • See *p*-Phenylenediamine.

DIMETHYL IMIDAZOLIDINONE • A skin conditioning agent. See Imidazolidinone.

DIMETHYL ISOSORBIDE • See Sorbitol.

DIMETHYL LAURAMINE • An antistatic ingredient. It has antifungal and antimicrobial properties. The CIR Expert Panel *(see)* concludes that there is insufficient data available to support the safety of this ingredient in cosmetics. See Lauric Acid.

DIMETHYL LAURAMINE OLEATE • See Lauric Acid and Oleic Acid.

DIMETHYL LAUROYL LYSINE • Amino acids used in skin conditioners. See Amino Acids.

DIMETHYL MALEATE • A solvent. See Maleic Acid and Methyl Alcohol.

DIMETHYL MYRISTAMINE • See Myristic Acid.

DIMETHYL OCTANOL • A synthetic flavoring, colorless, with a sweet, roselike odor. No known toxicity.

DIMETHYL OCTANYL ACETATE • A synthetic roselike scent.

DIMETHYL OCTYNEDIOL • See Citronellol.

DIMETHYL OXAZOLIDINE • A fragrance ingredient. See Oxazoline.

DIMETHYL PABA ETHYL CETEARYLDIMONIUM TOSYLATE • See Quaternary Ammonium Compounds.

DIMETHYL PALMITAMINE • See Palmitic Acid.

N,N-DIMETHYL-p-PHENYLENE DIAMINE SULFATE • See *p*-Phenylenediamine.

DIMETHYL PHTHALATE • Phthalic Esters. A colorless, aromatic oil insoluble in water. A solvent, especially for musk *(see)*. Used to compound calamine lotion and as an insect repellent. Absorbed through the skin. Irritating to the eyes and mucous membranes.

N,N-DIMETHYL 2,6-PYRIDINEDIAMINE HCL • Used in hair coloring. See Pyridine.

DIMETHYL SOYAMINE • See Soy Acid.

DIMETHYL STEARAMINE • An antistatic agent in hair products. The CIR

Expert Panel *(see)* concludes that there is insufficient data available to support the safety of this ingredient in cosmetics. See Stearic Acid.

DIMETHYL SULFATE • **Sulfuric Acid. Dimethyl Ester.** Colorless, oily liquid used as a methylating ingredient (to add methyl) in the manufacture of cosmetic dyes, perfumes, and flavorings. Methyl salicylate is an example *(see)*. Extremely hazardous, dimethyl sulfate has delayed lethal qualities. Liquid produces severe blistering, necrosis of the skin. Sufficient skin absorption can result in serious poisoning. Vapors hurt the eyes. Ingestion can cause paralysis, coma, prostration, kidney damage, and death.

DIMETHYL SULFONE • An organic compound that is used as an emulsifier. See Sulfonated Oils.

DIMETHYL SULFOXIDE • A water-absorbing liquid used as a solvent. It readily penetrates the skin and other tissues. It is approved by the FDA for humans but must comply with FDA regulations. It is used to help anti-inflammatory medicines to penetrate the skin.

DIMETHYL TALLOWAMINE • See Tallow.

DIMETHYLAMINE • Prepared from methanol *(see)* and ammonia *(see)*, it is very soluble in water and in alcohol. Used in the manufacture of soaps and detergents. It also promotes hardening of plastic nails. Irritating to the skin and mucous membranes.

DIMETHYLHYDROXYMETHYLPYRAZOLE • A broad spectrum bactericide and fungicide compatible with proteins. See Pyrazole.

DIMETHYLADIPATE • A solvent that is used as a nail polish remover ingredient. See Adipic Acid.

DIMETHYLAMINOETHYL METHACRYLATE • See Acrylates.

DIMETHYLAMINOPROPYL OLEAMIDE • See Oleic Acid.

DIMETHYLAMINOPROPYL STEARAMIDE • See Stearic Acid.

DIMETHYLOCTAHYDRO-2-NAPHTHALDEHYDE • A fragrance ingredient.

DIMETHYLOL ETHYLENE THIOUREA • A preservative.

DIMETHYLOL UREA • A preservative. May release formaldehyde *(see)*.

DIMETHYLSILANOL HYALURONATE • See Hyaluronic Acid.

DIMYRISTYL THIODIPROPIONATE • The diester of myristyl alcohol and thiodipropionic acid *(see both)*.

DINKUM OIL • See Eucalyptus Oil.

DINONOXYNOL-9-CITRATE • The diester of citric acid and nonoxynol-9. See Citric Acid and Nonoxynol-2.

DINONYL PHENOL • See Phenol.

DINOXYNOL-4 PHOSPHATE • See Nonoxynol and Surfactants.

DIOCTYL- • Containing two octyl groups. Octyl is obtained from octane, a liquid paraffin found in petroleum.

DIOCTYL ADIPATE • An emollient made from octyl aclohol and adipic acid *(see both)*. On the basis of available data, the CIR Expert Panel concludes that it is safe as presently used in cosmetics. See Adipic Acid.

DIOCTYL DIMER DILINOLEATE • A skin conditioning ingredient. The CIR Expert Panel *(see)* concludes that there is insufficient data available to support the safety of this ingredient in cosmetics. See Dilinoleic Acid.

DIOCTYL MALEATE • See Malic Acid.

DIOCTYL PHTHALATE • An oily ester *(see)* used chiefly as a plasticizer, solvent, and fixative in perfumes and nail enamels. Because of its bitter taste, also used as a denaturant for alcohol *(see)*. Irritating to mucous membranes, and a central nervous system depressant if absorbed through the skin.

DIOCTYL SODIUM SULFOSUCCINATE • **Docustae Sodium.** A waxlike solid that is very soluble in water. It is used as a dispersing and solubilizing ingredient in foods and cosmetics. On the basis of available data, the CIR Expert Panel concludes that this ingredient is safe as presently used in cosmetics.

DIOCTYL SUCCINATE • A white wax, soluble in water, it is a wetting ingredient used in compounding calamine lotion. No known skin toxicity.

DIOCTYLAMINE • Di-2-Ethylhexyl-Amine. See Amines.

DIOCTYLDODECYL FLUOROHEPTYL CITRATE • A skin conditioning ingredient. See Citric Acid.

DIOCTYLDODECYL LAUROYL GLUTAMATE • A hair and skin conditioning ingredient. See Lauric Acid and Glutamic Acid.

DIOLEOYL EDETOLMONIUM METHOSULFATE • A pH *(see)* adjuster and emulsifier.

DIOLEOYLISOPROPYL DIMONIUM METHOSULFATE • See Quaternary Ammonium Compounds.

DIOLETH-8-PHOSPHATE • The mixture of diesters of phosphoric acid and oleth-8 *(see both)*.

DIOLEYL TOCOPHERYL METHYLSILANOL • A fatty compound used in creams. See Tocopherol.

DIOSCOREA VILLOSA • *Dioscorea mexicana. Dioscorea paniculata.* **Wild Yam. Colicroot. Rheumatism Root. Chinese Yam.** Japanese researchers in 1936 discovered glycoside saponins of several Mexican yam species from which steroid saponin *(see)*, primarily diosgenin, could be derived. These derivatives were then converted to progesterone, an intermediate in cortisone production. Steroid drugs derived from diosgenin include corticosteroids, oral contraceptives, androgens, and estrogens. For more than two centuries, American herbalists used wild yam roots to treat painful menstruation, ovarian pain, cramps, and problems of childbirth. Wild yam root also has been used to treat gallbladder pain, and ease the passage of gallstones. Wild yam root also reputedly can lower blood cholesterol and blood pressure. The most widely prescribed birth control pill in the world, Desogen, is made from the wild yam, confirming what the ancient Mexican women knew all along. They used wild yam as a contraceptive. Long-term use may cool libido. Contraindicated in pregnancy and kidney impairment. Used in "antiaging" cosmetics.

DIOSMINE • An antioxidant. See Phenol.

DIOSPYROS KAKI • **Persimmon.** American Indians used the fruit from this tree grown in the southern and eastern United States. Used as a wax in cosmetics.

DIPA • The abbreviation for diisopropanolamine.

DIPALMETHYL HYDROXYETHYLMONIUM METHOSULFATE • See Quaternary Ammonium Compounds.

DIPALMITAMINE • An antistatic ingredient in hair products. See Palmitic Acid.

DIPALMITOYL CYSTINE • A fatty compound with cystine *(see)* and used in creams.

DIPALMITOYL HYDROXYPROLINE • A fatty compound made with amino acids and used in creams.

DIPENTAERYTHRITYL HEXACAPRYLATE/HEXACAPRATE • A mixture of caprylic and capric acids and pentaerythritol *(see all)*. Used in cosmetic creams and oils.

DIPENTENE • See Limonene.

DIPERODON HYDROCHLORIDE • Obtained by condensing a piperdine and glycerol chlorohydrin with an alkali. Bitter taste. Soluble in alcohol. Used as an anesthetic in solution. No known toxicity.

DIPHENOLIC ACID • Prepared by condensing phenol *(see)* with another acid. Soluble in hot water. It is an intermediate for lubricating oil additives. Used in cosmetics as a surfactant and plasticizer. See Phenol for toxicity.

DIPHENYL ACETONITRILE • **Diphenatrile.** Yellow crystalline powder used in the preparation of antispasmodics and herbicides.

DIPHENYL DIMETHICONE • See Dimethicone.

DIPHENYL METHANE • **Benzyl Benzene.** Used chiefly as a perfume in soaps. Prepared from methylene chloride and benzene, with aluminum chloride as a catalyst. Smells like oranges and geraniums. A petroleum distillate and like all such substances can, when imposed, produce local skin irritation and more rarely a skin reaction to sunlight, which includes prickling, swelling, and sometimes pigmentation. Methylene Chloride is no longer permitted in cosmetics.

DIPHENYL OXIDE • Colorless crystals or liquid with a geraniumlike odor. Derived from benzene, it is used in perfumery, particularly soaps. Toxic by inhalation of vapor.

DIPHENYLENE SULFIDE • See Dibenzothiophene.

DIPOTASSIUM AZELATE • The salt of azelic acid. Used as a plasticizer. No known toxicity.

DIPOTASSIUM EDTA • See Ethylenediamine Tetraacetic Acid.

DIPOTASSIUM GLYCYRRHIZATE • The dipotassium salt of glycyrrhizic acid *(see)*.

DIPOTASSIUM PHOSPHATE • A sequestrant. A white grain, very soluble in water. Used as a buffering ingredient to control the degree of acidity in solutions. It is used medicinally as a saline cathartic. No known toxicity.

DIPROPYLENE GLYCOL • See Propylene Glycol.

DIPROPYLENE GLYCOL DIBENZOATE • Light colored liquid that is used as a plasticizer. See Propylene Glycol and Benzoic Acid.

DIPROPYLENE GLYCOL SALICYLATE • Insoluble in water, it is used as a plasticizer and in sunscreen lotions. See Propylene Glycol and Salicylates.

DIRECT BLACK 51 • Classed as a diazo dye *(see)*.

DIRECT BLUE 86 • A phthalocyanine color (*see* Phthalic Acid). See also Direct Dyes.

DIRECT DYES • These compounds need salts to be effective. When combined with aniline, they improve in fastness. They are used in hair dyes and in some pigments. See Aniline Dyes for toxicity.

DIRECT RED 23 • **Fast Scarlet 4BSA.** Classed chemically as a diazo color. See Colors.

DIRECT RED 80 • Classed chemically as a diazo color, it is a brilliant red. See Coal Tar.

DIRECT RED 81 • **Benzo Fast. Red 8 BL.** A diazo dye. See Azo Dyes and Direct Dyes.

DIRECT VIOLET 48 • A diazo dye. See Azo Dyes and Direct Dyes.

DIRECT YELLOW 12 • **Chrysophenine G.** A diazo dye. See Azo Dyes and Direct Dyes.

DISELENIUM SULFIDE • An antidandruff ingredient used in prescription items and OTC brands. See Selenium Sulfide.

DISODIUM ADENOSINE TRIPHOSPHATE • A preservative derived from adenylic acid. See Adenosine Triphosphate.

DISODIUM ASCORBYL SULFATE • Used in skin care products. See Ascorbic Acid.

DISODIUM CAPROAMPHODIACETATE • See Quaternary Ammonium Compounds and Surfactants.

DISODIUM CAPROAMPHODIPROPIONATE • See Surfactants.

DISODIUM CAPRYLOAMPHODIACETATE • See Surfactants.

DISODIUM CAPRYLOAMPHODIPROPIONATE • See Surfactants.

DISODIUM CETEARYL SULFOSUCCINATE • The disodium salt of cetearyl alcohol and sulfosuccinic acid *(see both)*.

DISODIUM COCAMIDO MIPA-SULFOSUCCINATE • See Coconut Oil and Surfactants.

DISODIUM COCAMPHODIACETATE • See Coconut Oil and Surfactants.

DISODIUM COCOAMPHOCARBOXYMETHYLHYDROXYPROPYLSULFONATE • See Coconut Oil and Surfactants.

DISODIUM C12-15 PARETH SULFOSUCCINATE • The sodium salt of sulfosuccinic acid *(see)*. See surfactants.

DISODIUM DECETH-6 SULFOSUCCINATE • See Sulfonated Oils.

DISODIUM DIMETHICONE COPOLYOL SULFOSUCCINATE • See Dimethicone and Succinic Acid.

DISODIUM DISTRYLBIPHENYL DISULFONATE • Use of this colorant in cosmetic products is prohibited in the United States and may be restricted in other countries.

DISODIUM EDTA-COPPER • **Copper Versenate.** Used as a sequestering ingredient. Permanently listed as a coloring for shampoos in 1974. See Ethylenediamine Tetraacetic Acid for toxicity.

DISODIUM HYDROGENATED COTTONSEED GLYCERIDE SULFOSUC-CINATE • See Sulfonated Oils.

DISODIUM HYDROGENATED TALLOW GLUTAMATE • See Hydrogenated Tallow.

DISODIUM ISODECYL SULFOSUCCINATE • See Sulfonated Oils.

DISODIUM ISOSTEARAMINO MEA-SULFOSUCCINATE • See Surfactants.

DISODIUM ISOSTEAROAMPHODIPROPIONATE • See Surfactants.

DISODIUM LANETH-5-SULFOSUCCINATE • See Sulfonated Oils.

DISODIUM LAURAMIDE PEG-2 SULFOSUCCINATE • See Surfactants.

DISODIUM LAURAMIDO MEA-SULFOSUCCINATE • See Surfactants.

DISODIUM LAURETH SULFOSUCCINATE • See Surfactants.

DISODIUM LAURIMINIDIPROPIONATE • See Surfactants.

DISODIUM LAUROAMPHODIPROPIONATE • An ingredient used in hair products as a conditioner and foam booster.

DISODIUM LAURYL SULFOSUCCINATE • See Surfactants.

DISODIUM MONOCOCAMIDOSULFOSUCCINATE • See Dioctyl Sodium Sulfosuccinate.

DISODIUM MONOLAURETHSULFOSUCCINATE • See Dioctyl Sodium Sulfosuccinate.

DISODIUM MONOLAURYLAMIDOSULFOSUCCINATE • See Dioctyl Sodium Sulfosuccinate.

DISODIUM MONOLAURYLSULFOSUCCINATE • See Dioctyl Sodium Sulfosuccinate.

DISODIUM MONOMYRISTAMIDOSULFOSUCCINATE • See Dioctyl Sodium Sulfosuccinate.

DISODIUM MONOOLEAMIDOSULFOSUCCINATE • See Dioctyl Sodium Sulfosuccinate.

DISODIUM MONORICINOLEAMIDO MEA-SULFOSUCCINATE • See Sulfonated Oils.

DISODIUM MYRISTAMIDO MEA-SULFOSUCCINATE • See Dioctyl Sodium Sulfosuccinate.

DISODIUM NONOXYNOL-10 SULFOSUCCINATE • See Surfactants.

DISODIUM OLEOAMPHODIPROPIONATE • An ingredient used in hair products as a conditioner and foam booster. See Oleic Acid.

DISODIUM OLEYL SULFOSUCCINATE • See Surfactants.

DISODIUM PALMITOLEAMIDO PEG-2 SULFOSUCCINATE • See Succinic Acid and Surfactants.

DISODIUM PARETH-25 SULFOSUCCINATE • See Surfactants.

DISODIUM PEG-4-COCAMIDO MIPA-SULFOSUCCINATE • See Surfactants.

DISODIUM PHOSPHATE • See Sodium Phosphate.

DISODIUM PPG-2-ISODECETH-7 CARBOXYAMOPHODIACETATE • An organic salt that is used in hair products as a conditioning and foam booster.

DISODIUM PYROPHOSPHATE • **Sodium Pyrophosphate.** An emulsifier and texturizer used to decrease the loss of fluid from a compound. It is GRAS for use in foods as a sequestrant. See Sodium Pyrophosphate Peroxide.

DISODIUM RICINOLEAMIDO MEA-SULFOSUCCINATE • Widely used as a surfactant, it is the disodium salt of ethanolamide and sulfosuccinic acid *(see)*.

DISODIUM STEARMIDO MEA-SULFOSUCCINATE • See Surfactants.

DISODIUM STEARMINODIPROPIONATE • See Steareth-2.

DISODIUM STEARYL SULFOSUCCINATE • See Sulfonated Oils.

DISODIUM SUCCINATE • See Succinic Acid.

DISODIUM SUCCINOYL GLYCYRRHETINATE • A flavoring agent. See Licorice.

DISODIUM TALLAMIDO MEA-SULFOSUCCINATE • See Surfactants.

DISODIUM TALLOW SULFOSUCCINAMATE • See Succinic Acid and Tallow.

DISODIUM TALLOWAMINODIPROPIONATE • See Surfactants.

DISODIUM TRIDECYLSULFOSUCCINATE • See Succinic Acid.

DISODIUM UNDECYLENAMIDO MEA-SULFOSUCCINATE • See Surfactants.

DISODIUM WHEAT GERMAMIDO MEA-SULFOSUCCINATE • See Surfactants.

DISODIUM WHEAT GERMAMIDO PEG-2-SULFOSUCCINATE • See Wheat Germ Oil and Surfactants.

DISOYADIMONIUM CHLORIDE • See Quaternary Ammonium Compounds.

DISOYAMINE • See Soybean Oil.

DISPERSANT • A dispersing ingredient, such as polyphosphate, for promoting the formation and stabilization of a dispersion of one substance in another. An emulsion, for instance, would consist of a dispersed substance and the medium in which it is dispersed.

DISPERSE BLACK 9 • **Nacelan Diazine Black JS.** Classed chemically as an azo dye *(see)*. This was not found to be carcinogenic or tetratogenic in rats or rabbits and was not cancer-causing when applied to the skin of mice. At 3 percent suspension it did not irritate or sensitize the skin of human subjects. On the basis of available data, the CIR Expert Panel concludes that this ingredient is safe as presently used in cosmetics.

DISPERSE BLUE 1 • **1, 4, 5, 8-Tetraaminoanthraquinone.** Classed chemically as an anthraquinone *(see)* color. A skin cancer study in mice was negative. There was questionable urinary bladder tumors in mice but due to calculi rather than arising from toxicity to the genes. Such bladder calculi, it is reported, do not form in humans. The ingredient is also poorly absorbed so that exposure to hair dyes is brief. On the basis of available data, the CIR Expert Panel concludes that this ingredient is safe as presently used in cosmetics.

DISPERSE BLUE 3 • **Disperse Fast Blue.** An anthraquinone *(see)* dye. See also Disperse Dyes.

DISPERSE BLUE 3:1 • **Nacelan Brilliant Blue NR.** Classed chemically as an anthraquinone *(see)* color.

DISPERSE DYES • These compounds are only slightly soluble in water but are readily dispersed with the aid of sulfated oils. Used on nylon knit goods, sheepskins, and furs, they are in human hair dyes as well as resins, oils, fats, and waxes. Not permanently listed as safe.

DISPERSE ORANGE 3 • A monoazo *(see)* color.

DISPERSE RED 11 • An anthraquinone *(see)* color.

DISPERSE RED 15 • An anthraquinone *(see)* color.

DISPERSE VIOLET 1 • Classed as an anthraquinone *(see)* color. Although there are limited human studies, on the basis of available data, the CIR Expert Panel concludes that this ingredient is safe as presently used in cosmetics.

DISPERSE VIOLET 4 • **Solvent Violet 12.** Classed chemically as an anthraquinone color. See Colors.

DISPERSE VIOLET 15 • A hair coloring. See Coal Tar Colors.

DISTARCH GLYCERYL ETHER • An anticaking ingredient. See Starch and Glycerin.

DISTARCH PHOSPHATE • A combination of starch and sodium metaphosphate. It is a water softener, sequestering ingredient, and texturizer. It is used in dandruff shampoos. No known toxicity.

DISTEARETH-6 DIMONIUM CHLORIDE • See Quaternary Ammonium Compounds.

DISTEARETH-2-LAUROYL GLUTAMATE • See Surfactants.

DISTEARETH-5 LAUROYL GLUTAMATE • See Surfactants.

DISTEARYL ETHER • A skin conditioning ingredient. See Stearic Acid.

DISTEARYL EXPOXYPROPYLMONIUM CHLORIDE • See Quaternary Ammonium Compounds.

DISTEARYL PHTHALIC ACID AMIDE • An emollient. See Stearic Acid and Phthalic Acid.

DISTEARYL THIODIPROPIONATE • The diester of stearyl alcohol and thiodipropionic acid used as a stabilizer *(see all)*.

DISTEARYLDIMETHYLAMINE DILINOLEATE • Used as a hair conditioning ingredient. See Dilinoleic Acid and Dimer Acid.

DISTEARYLDIMETHYLAMINE DIMERATE • See Dimer Acid.

DISTEARYLDIMONIUM CHLORIDE • See Quaternary Ammonium Compounds.

DISTILLATE • The volatile material recovered by condensing the vapors of an extract, or material from fruits that is heated to its boiling point in a still.

DISTILLATION • The physical process of heating a product to the boiling point in a still and collecting the vapors by condensing them through cooling.

DISTILLED • The result of evaporation and subsequent condensation of a liquid, as when water is boiled and steam is condensed.

DISTILLED OIL • An essential oil obtained by the distillation of the portion of a botanical material, such as peel, leaves, and stem, containing the essential oil.

DITALLOWDIMONIUM CHLORIDE • See Quaternary Ammonium Compounds and Tallow.

DI-TEA-OLEAMIDO PEG-2-SULFOSUCCINATE • See Quaternary Ammonium Compounds.

DI-TEA-PALMITOYL ASPARTATE • See Aspartic Acid.

DITHIODIGLYCOLIC ACID • See Thioglycolic Acid Compounds.

DITRIDECYL ADIPATE • The diester of tridecyl alcohol and adipic acid *(see both)*.

DITRIDECYL DILINOLEATE • The diester of tridecyl alcohol and dilinoleic acid. See Dimer Acid.

DITRIDECYL DIMER DILINOLEATE • A skin conditioning agent. The CIR Expert Panel *(see)* concludes that there is insufficient data available to support the safety of this ingredient in cosmetics. See Tridecyl Alcohol and Dilinoleic Acid.

DITRIDECYL SODIUM SULFOSUCCINATE • See Sulfonated Oils.

DITRIDECYL THIODIPROPIONATE • The diester of tridecyl alcohol and thiodipropionic acid *(see both)*.

DM HYDANTOIN • See Hydantoin.

DMDM • The abbreviation for Dimethylol Dimethyl. See Methyl Alcohol and Imidazolidinone.

DMDM HYDANTOIN • A preservative. May release formaldehyde *(see)*. Can be a skin irritant. On the basis of available data, the CIR Expert Panel concludes that this ingredient is safe as presently used in cosmetics. See also Hydantoin.

DMHF • The abbreviation for the resin formed by heating hydantoin and formaldehyde *(see both)*.

DNA • **Deoxyribonucleic acid.** The complex substance that makes up genes; it contains the genetic information for all organisms.

DOCOSAHEXAENOIC ACID • See Behenic Acid.

DODECANEDIOIC ACID/CETEARYL ALCOHOL/GLYCOL COPOLYMER • The coconut oil, cetearyl alcohol, and ethylene glycol monomers, used to form a wax *(see all)*.

DODECYL GALLATE • The ester of gallic acid derived from tannin and used in ink.

DODECYLBENZENE SULFONIC ACID • A sulfonic acid anionic *(see)* detergent. Made from petroleum. May cause skin irritation. If swallowed, will cause vomiting.

DODECYLBENZYLTRIMONIUM CHLORIDE • See Quaternary Ammonium Compounds.

DODECYLHEXADECANOL • An alcohol used as an emollient and emulsion stabilizer. See Hexanol.

DODECYLHEXADECYLTRIMONIUM CHLORIDE • An antistatic ingredient in hair conditioners and an emulsifier. See Quaternary Ammonium Compounds.

DODECYLTETRADECANOL • See Myristic Acid.

DODECYLXYLDITRIMONIUM CHLORIDE • See Quaternary Ammonium Compounds.

DODOXYNOL-5, -6, -7, -9, -12 • See Phenol.

DOG ROSE EXTRACT • Extract of the fruit of *Rosa canina,* a wild rose. Used as a skin conditioner.

DOLOMITE • A common mineral, colorless to white or yellowish gray, containing calcium, phosphorous, and magnesium. It is one of the most important raw materials for magnesium and its salts. It is used in toothpaste as a whitener. No known toxicity.

DOLLOF • See *Filipendula rubra.*

DOMIPHEN BROMIDE • Clear, colorless, odorless crystalline powder with a slightly bitter taste. Soluble in water, but incompatible with soap, it is used as an antiseptic and detergent in cosmetics. No known toxicity.

DONG QUAI • *Angelica sinensis.* **Tang Kwei.** The root of the herb is used for the treatment of female gynecological ailments, particularly menstrual cramps, irregularity, and malaise during the menstrual period. It is also used to relieve the symptoms of menopause. Dong quai is used by herbalists as an antispasmodic for treating insomnia, high blood pressure, and cramps. It is reputedly useful in treating anemia and constipation. Used in "organic" cosmetics. See also Angelica.

DRAIZE TEST • An animal test used to determine the effects of different substances on the eye. Animal rights advocates oppose the use of animals—usually rabbits—for this purpose. Replacements include laboratory techniques that use freshly isolated tissues, tissue-cultured cells, or nonliving systems. According to studies at the Medical College of Georgia, each of the nonanimal tests has at least one drawback relative to tests in living animals. See pages 14–15.

DRIED BUTTERMILK • The dehydration of the liquid recovered from churning cow's milk. Used as an emollient.

DRIED EGG YOLK • Used for coloring and protein in cosmetics. Particularly associated with eczema in children. May also cause reactions ranging from hives to anaphylaxis. Egg yolk may also be found in root beer, soups, sausage, and coffee.

DROMETRIZOLE • A derivative of benzene used as a solvent in nail polish and as an ultraviolet light absorber to make cosmetics less susceptible to light. On the basis of available data, the CIR Expert Panel concludes that this ingredient is not safe for use in cosmetics until such time as appropriate safety data has been obtained. See Benzene.

DROMICEIUS • See Emu Oil.

DROSERA • **Common Sundew.** A dried flowering plant that grows in Europe, Asia, and in North America as far south as Florida. Formerly used to treat chest disorders. Used as a mild astringent in skin lotions and perfumes. No known toxicity.

DRY SHAMPOOS • Usually consist of a water-absorbent powder such as talc *(see)* and a mild alkali. The product is placed in the hair and then brushed out, carrying with it any oil or dirt. Many women use baby powder or bath powder to "dry" wash their hair. See Shampoos.

DRYING INGREDIENTS • See Rosin.

DRYOPTERIS FILIX-MAS • **Shield fern.** A fern that grows in Bermuda.

DRY-OUT • Just as the top-note *(see)* is the first impression of a perfume, this is the last impression. It may begin to become apparent after an hour or several hours or even the next day. The dry-out notes show the fixative *(see)* effects of the components and will reveal the body-note *(see)*. The dry-out depicts the tenacity of the composition and the fixative's ability to hold the scent. The better the perfume, usually the better the dry-out.

DULCAMARA EXTRACT • **Bitter Sweet Nightshade.** Extract of the dried stems of *Solanum dulcamara*. Belonging to the nightshade family, it is used as a preservative. The ripe berries are used for pies and jams. The unripened berries are deadly. It is made into an ointment by herbalists to treat skin cancers and burns. It induces sweating. See also Horse Nettle.

DURVILLEA ANTARTICA EXTRACT • An algae *(see)* extract used in "antiaging" products.

DUSTING POWDER • See Powder.

E

EAR ALLERGY • The condition, *Serous otitis,* which is fullness in the ears associated with the formation of thick mucus behind the eardrum, is sometimes an allergic phenomenon. The first symptom may be hearing loss, and allergies of the nose contribute to the problem. Allergic contact dermatitis in and around the ear is not uncommon. Nickel in earrings, eyeglasses, hair dye, cologne or perfume, and otic drops and ointments applied to the ear are among the most common offenders.

EAR LOBE • Frequently a site of allergic contact dermatitis from earrings containing nickel. May also be affected by hair products.

EARTH WAX • General name for ozocerite, ceresin, and montan waxes. See Waxes.

EASTERN PINE EXTRACT • An extract of *Pinus strobus*. Pine preparations are used for their scent and for "healing" properties.

ECBALLIUM ELATERIUM • **Squirting Cucumber.** See Cucumber.

ECHINACEA • *Echinacea angustifolia*. **Snakeroot. Stone Flower. Cone Flower.** The roots and leaves of this herb served as a medicine for the Plains Indians. It is said by herbalists to be a natural antibiotic and immune enhancer. It contains a volatile oil that is antiseptic and glycosides *(see)* as well as phenol, which is an antiseptic. It was widely used by Dr. Wooster Beach, who in the mid-1800s founded Eclectic Medicine, a blending of homeopathic and North American herbalism. It has been found that it increases the ability of white blood cells to fight, digest, and destroy toxic organisms that invade the body. Echinacea is taken to combat colds, infections, and inflammations. The herb produces a numbing sensation when held in the mouth for a few minutes.

ECHINACIN • See Echinacea.

ECZEMA • Inflammation of the skin.

EDC • See Ethylene Dichloride.

EDETATE DISODIUM • **Disodium EDTA. Disotate. Endrate Versenate. Edathamil Disodium. EDTA. Sodium Edetate.** A chelating ingredient *(see)* used to reduce minerals in compounds.

EDTA SALTS • See Edetate Disodium.

EGG • Particularly associated with eczema in children. May also cause reactions ranging from hives to anaphylaxis. Eggs may also be found in root beer, soups, sausage, coffee, and cosmetics.

EGG OIL • A mixture of the fat-soluble emollients and emulsifiers extracted from the whole egg. Provides protection against dehydration and has lubricating and antifriction properties when rubbed on the skin.

EGG POWDER • Used in many cosmetics, including shampoos, ointments, creams, face masks, and bath preparations. Dehydrated egg powder is often incorporated into shampoos on the theory that protein is beneficial to damaged hair. There is little scientific evidence to substantiate this, but the egg coating does make the hair more cohesive and more manageable. The oil of egg yolk, which mixes easily with other oils, is used in ointment bases and cosmetic creams. Egg albumen is used in facial masks to give a tight feeling. For a homemade egg treatment, four beaten eggs are required, with a jigger of rum mixed in. Then the solution is massaged into the scalp, followed by a rinse with cold (never hot) water; the hot water would make the egg sticky. For persons not allergic to egg products, the ingredient is harmless.

EGG YOLK • The yellow matter of chicken eggs.

EGG YOLK EXTRACT • The extract of egg yolk. See Egg Oil.

EGGPLANT • **Aubergine.** A tender perennial plant, *Solanum melongena,* of the nightshade family, closely allied to the potato. The fruit is a large, egg-shaped berry, varying in color from dark purple to red, yellowish, or white. Used in "organic" cosmetics.

EICOSANE • A white, crystalline solid that is a mixture of hydrocarbons. It is used as a lubricant or plasticizer in cosmetic preparations.

EICOSAPENTAENOIC ACID • **EPA** Found in fish oil *(see),* it is used in creams. In the human body, it reduces production of thromboxane, a clotting ingredient, in the blood, thus making the platelets less "sticky."

ELAEISIS GUINEENSIS • See Palm-Kernel Oil.

ELASTASE • A term used for an enzyme that dissolves elastin.

ELASTIN • A protein in connective tissue.

ELASTOMERS • Used for face masks. Rubberlike substances that can be stretched from twice to many times their length. Upon their release, they return rapidly to almost their original length. Synthetic elastomers have similar properties and are actually superior to the natural ones. They have been in use since 1930. Thiokol was the first commercial synthetic elastomer. It is a condensation polymer *(see);* for example, neoprene, and silicone rubber.

ELDER FLOWERS • *Sambucus nigra. S. canadensis.* **Sambucus. Black Elder. Bourtree. Judas Tree.** Extracted from the honey-scented flowers of the elder tree. Herbal additive to China tea, it contains essential oil, terpenes, glycosides *(see),* rutin, quercitrin *(see),* mucilage, and tannin *(see).* The fruits are high in Vitamin C. Used in skin and eye lotions and bath preparations. Mildly astringent, it supposedly keeps the skin soft and clean. Old-time herb doctors used it. Elder flowers increase perspiration and therefore reduce body water. Used to scent perfumes and lotions. Elder flower is used to treat colds and flu; in salves to treat burns, rashes, and minor skin ailments; and to diminish wrinkles. It was used by herbalists to soothe the nerves. Hippocrates mentioned its use as a purgative. The inner bark and the young leaf buds, as well as the juice root, are all considered cathartics. The berries induce sweating and act as a diuretic. Only the black elder is safe to use internally. Red elder is toxic.

ELDERBERRY JUICE POWDER • Dried powder from the juice of the edible berry of a North American elder tree. Used for red coloring. Nontoxic.

ELECAMPANE EXTRACT • An extract of *Enula helenium,* a large, coarse European herb now grown in the United States.

ELEMI • A soft, yellowish, fragrant plastic resin from several Asiatic and Philippine trees. Slightly soluble in water but readily soluble in alcohol. Used for gloss and adhesion in nail lacquer and to scent soaps and colognes. No known toxicity.

ELEOCHARIS DULCIS • **Water Chestnut.** See Cyperus.

ELETTARIA CARDAMOMUM • See Cardamom Oil.

ELEUTHRERO GINSENG • See Gingseng.

ELM BARK • Extract of *Ulmus campestris.* Elm derivatives have been widely used in herbal medicine. The inner bark contains a lot of mucilage and is used in cosmetics, in baby products, and in herbal products to soothe the skin.

EMBRYO EXTRACT • An oil extracted from fetal calves, often promoted in "youth-restoring" creams and lotions.

EMETINE CHLORIDE • A preservative. Made from ipecac *(see),* it is used in medicine to treat amebic dysentery. Acute toxicity can occur at any dose.

EMOLLIENTS • Creams, Lotions, Skin Softeners, and Moisturizers. An emollient by whatever designation—night cream, hand cream, eye cream, skin softener, moisturizer, and so on—remains an emollient. The selection of a cream, spray, or lotion is really a matter of taste and the influence of advertising and packaging. The AMA's Committee on Cutaneous Health finds little difference between liquid, cream, lotion, drop, or dew emollients, since they all perform the same function. These preparations do help to make the skin feel softer and smoother and to reduce the roughness, cracking, and irritation of the skin; they may possibly help retard the fine wrinkles of aging. However, in any application of oil to the skin, what happens is that the roughened, scaly surface is coated with a smooth film, cementing down the dry flakes. And although the oil retards the evaporation of water, as far as the oil penetrating the skin, dermatologists say this has been overemphasized.

Any dryness would be in the layer known as the stratum corneum, and it is due to insufficient water in the skin. Exposure to low humidities in artificially heated or cooled rooms, aging, and heredity may all contribute to dry skin. The ancient Greek physician Galen is credited with making the first emollient of beeswax, spermaceti, almond oil, borax, and rose water *(see all)*. Most emollients today are still a mixture of oils. If the oils have a low melting point, the emollient will feel greasy; with a high melting point, it disappears from the skin. Because emollients are usually colorless, and seem to be absorbed rapidly, they are called vanishing creams. But, according to the AMA, it is the water in such creams, and not the oil, that benefits dry skin. Experiments with a specimen of calloused skin placed in oils for three years could not make it flexible again. However, when a brittle piece of callus is placed in water, it soon becomes flexible. Most emollients are intended to remain on the skin for a significant period of time, including overnight. Petrolatum (Vaseline) is one of the least expensive and one of the most efficient emollients. It tends to keep the loss of natural moisture from the skin at a minimum. Next in efficiency and also inexpensive is zinc oxide *(see)*. Mineral oil, vegetable oil, and shortening also work well. All may be found on your supermarket shelf. Vitamin A and hormone creams *(see both)* are added to keep the skin moist and supple. However effective they are in doing so is a matter of medical controversy. Glycerin *(see)* is widely used in emollients and has been found to work best in humid air because it draws moisture from the air. (When the humidity is high, most people do not need emollients.) A simple conditioner or emollient cream may contain lanolin, petrolatum, and oil of sweet almond. A moisturizing cream may contain mineral oil, stearic acid, lanolin, beeswax, sorbitol, and polysorbates *(see all)*. Among other ingredients in emollients and lotions are natural fatty oils such as olive, coconut, corn, peach kernel, peanut, and sesame oils in hydrogenated form; natural fats such as cocoa butter and lard; synthetic fatty oils such as paraffin; alcohols such as cetyl, stearyl, and oleyl; emulsifiers, preservatives, and antioxidants, including Vitamin E and parabens *(see all);* and antibacterials and perfumes, especially menthol and camphor *(see both)*. Among the problems with creams and lotions reported to the FDA were body and hand rashes, swelling of the eyes and face, blood vessels on the surface of the nose, red and painful eyes, burning of the face, and skin eruptions and irritations.

EMU OIL • The emu is a large, flightless bird. The cosmetic and moisturizing properties of its oil were studied at the University of Sydney, Australia. It was found to have anti-inflammatory and skin penetrating properties. It reportedly has better moisturizing properties than mineral oil and lower incidence of pore clogging.

EMULSIFIERS • Ingredients used to assist in the production of an emulsion. Among common emulsifiers in cosmetics are stearic acid soaps such as potassium and sodium stearates; sulfated alcohols such as sodium lauryl sulfate, polysorbates, poloxamers, and pegs; and sterols such as cholesterol. (See all under separate listings.)

EMULSIFYING OIL • **Soluble Oil.** Jan oil, when mixed with water, produces a milky emulsion. Sodium sulfonate is an example.

EMULSIFYING WAX • Waxes that are treated so that they mix more easily.

EMULSION • What is formed when two or more nonmixable liquids are shaken so thoroughly together that the mixture continues to appear to be homogenized. Most oils form emulsions with water.

ENCAPSULATION • Scents can be encapsulated in gelatin and are released when a fragrance product is placed in hot water. Some microencapsulated products contain coated perfume granules that are so small they give the impression of free-flowing powder.

ENFLEURAGE • The technique of making perfumes from flowers that cannot be subjected to steam distillation, such as roses and orange blossoms. It includes the use of glass trays that are lined with lard, on which flowers picked early in the morning are scattered. The trays are stacked on one another. The next day the flowers are removed from the fat and replaced with fresh ones. The cycle is repeated for several weeks. The lard is then scraped from the trays and mixed with alcohol. The alcohol in turn is removed by distillation, leaving behind the flower-scented essential oil, or "absolute." The process usually takes 36 days and is therefore expensive and done only for fine perfumes.

ENGLISH OAK EXTRACT • Extract of the bark of *Quercus robur*. The wood is used for cabinetmaking. The extract is used in chestnut brown dye.

ENTERIC COATING • Coating on a compound allowing the slow release of the active ingredients.

ENTEROMORPHA COMPRESSA • Green algae. See Algae.

ENZYME • Any of a unique class of proteins that catalyze a broad spectrum of biochemical reactions. Enzymes are formed in living cells. One enzyme can cause a chemical process that no other enzyme can. Among the enzymes used in cosmetics are amylase and chymotrypsin *(see both)*.

EOSIN • Red crystalline powder soluble in alcohol and acetic acid. It is used as a coloring in cosmetic products. See Fluorescein.

EOSIN YELLOW • See Tetrabromofluorescein.

EPA GENETIC TOXICOLOGY PROGRAM • The U.S. Environmental Protection Agency has certain chemicals under study to determine their effects on genes, the parts of the cell that carry inherited characteristics. Damage to the mechanisms of genes can lead to birth defects and cancer, as well as other illnesses.

EPHEDRA • *Ephedra gerardiana. E. trifurca. E. sinica. E. equisetina. E. helvetica.* **Ma Huang. Morman Tea.** There are about 40 species of this herb mentioned in ancient scriptures of India and used by the Chinese for more than 5,000 years. The stems contain alkaloids *(see),* including ephedrine *(see).* Herbalists use the herb to treat arthritis, asthma, emphysema, bronchitis, hay fever, and hives. See also Ephedrine.

EPHEDRINE • The alkaloid ephedrine is derived from the plant *Ephedra equisetina* and others of the 40 species of ephedra or produced synthetically. Ephedra has been used for more than 5,000 years in Chinese medicine and has become more and more popular in Western medicine. It acts like epinephrine *(see)* and is used as a bronchodilator, nasal decongestant, to raise blood pressure, and topically to constrict blood vessels.

EPICHLOROHYDRIN • A colorless liquid with an odor resembling chloroform. It is soluble in water but mixes readily with alcohol and ether. Used as a solvent for cosmetic resins and nitrocellulose *(see)* and in the manufacture of varnishes, lacquers, and cements for celluloid articles; also a modifier for food starch. A strong skin irritant and sensitizer. Daily administration of 1 milligram per kilogram of body weight to skin killed all of a group of rats in four days, indicating a cumulative potential. Chronic exposure is known to cause kidney damage. A 30-minute exposure to air concentrations of 8,300 parts per million was lethal to mice. Poisoned animals showed cyanosis, muscular relaxation or paralysis, convulsions, and death.

EPIDERMIS • Four to five layers of cells covering the skin *(dermis)*.

EPIGAEA REPENS • See Arbutus Extract.

EPILATORIES • Waxlike products that are softened by heat and applied when cool and then "yanked" off, taking embedded hair with them. (Some epilatories do not have to be heated.) They may be formulated from roses, paraffin, beeswax, ceresin, carnauba wax, mineral and linseed oils, and petrolatum. (See ingredients under separate listings.) Sometimes benzocaine is added in low concentrations for its local anesthetic effect. Nontoxic. See Depilatories.

EPILOBIUM ANGUSTIFOLIUM • A widely grown herb.

EPINEPHRINE • **Adrenalin. Adrenaline Chloride.** The major hormone of the adrenal gland, epinephrine increases heart rate and contractions (vasoconstriction or vasodilation), relaxation of the muscles in the lungs and smooth muscles in the intestines, and the processing of sugar and fat. It is the hormone that readies us for "fight or flight" in stressful situations. Introduced as a medication in 1900 to treat bronchospasm, hypersensitivity reactions, and anaphylaxis, a life-threatening allergic reaction. It is also used to restore heart rhythm in cardiac arrest. In eye solutions, it is used to dilate the pupil in the treatment of glaucoma and during surgery. In nose drops, it is used to relieve stuffy nose and local superficial bleeding. Potential adverse reactions include nervousness, tremor, euphoria, anxiety, coldness, vertigo, headache, sweating, disorientation, agitation, and, in patients with Parkinson's disease, increased rigidity and tremor. Other adverse reactions include palpitations, high blood pressure, rapid heartbeat, irregular heartbeat, stroke, angina, high blood sugar, fluid in the lungs, shortness of breath, and pallor. In eye medications, it may cause redness, fluid retention, rash, severe stinging, burning, and tearing upon instillation, palpitations, and rapid heartbeat.

EPITHELIAL • Refers to those cells that form the outer layer of the skin, those that line all the portions of the body that have contact with external air, and those that are specialized for secretion.

EPITHELIUM • A thin layer of cells forming a tissue that covers surfaces and lines hollow organs.

EPOXY- • Chemical prefix describing an oxygen atom bound to two linked carbon atoms. Epoxies are used as chemical intermediates and are widely employed in thickening resins.

EPOXY RESINS • The versatile epoxy resins are used widely in manufacturing electrical equipment, in automobile plants, in paints for surface coating, and in aircraft and other industries for adhesive purposes. Epoxy glues are used for household purposes. They are often made available in two parts, the hardener and the resin. Such products are advertised as being able to cement anything including metals, rubber, polyester resins, glass, and ceramics. Among the many other uses are beads in necklaces, model making, flame retardants, dental cement, flooring, plastic gloves, adhesive tapes, plastic panties, and handbags. They are used to coat household appliances, in wall panels, cements and mortars, in road surfaces, in rigid foams, as a matrix for stained glass windows, as a metal finish, in antirust paints, and as fillers for cracks in cement.

EPSOM SALTS • See Magnesium Sulfate.

EQUISETUM ARVENSE and HIEMALE • See Horsetail.

ERGOCALCIFEROL • Vitamin D_2.

ERGOSTEROL • **Provitamin D_2.** Derived from yeast or fungus ergot. It has Vitamin D and estrogen activity.

ERGOT • *Claviceps purpurea.* A fungus most frequently growing on rye. In the Middle Ages epidemics of ergotism from eating contaminated rye flour produced both gangrene and convulsions. The principal uses of ergot are as a uterine stimulant and a vasoconstrictor. Ergot was also used to check excessive menstrual bleeding. Ergot alkaloids are used widely today in the treatment of migraine and to stimulate the heart and other involuntary muscles. Ergot is known to contain a number of complex and potent alkaloids, some of which are very similar to lysergic acid (LSD). The two major indole alkaloids are ergonovine, which acts primarily to contract uterine muscles and to constrict blood vessels of the endometrium of the uterus, and ergotamine, which acts primarily on the blood vessels of the brain. Long-term use may cause constriction of the blood vessels of the extremities, the end result of which may be gangrene. The FDA proposed a ban in 1992 on the use of ergot fluid extract to treat insect bites and stings because it has not been shown to be safe and effective for stated claims in OTC products.

ERICA CINEREA • **Purple Heath.** A shrub that yields a red coloring.

ERIGERON OIL • **Horseweed. Fleabane Oil.** Derived from the leaves and tops of a plant grown in the northern and central United States. Use in fruit and spice flavorings for beverages, ice cream, ices, candy, baked goods, and sauces. No known toxicity.

ERIOBOTRYA JAPONICA • **Loquat.** A plant whose leaves and fruit are used by herbalists to treat coughs and lung inflammations. Loquats contain amygdalin, which is also found in cherry bark and apricot kernel, both of which are used to treat coughs.

ERIODICTYON CALIFORNIUM • See Yerba Santa Fluid Extract.

ERUCA SATIVA • Garden Rocket Extract. From a small shrub that is related to broccoli. See Erucic Acid.

ERUCALKONIUM CHLORIDE • See Quaternary Ammonium Compounds.

ERUCAMIDE • Erucylamide. An aliphatic amide slightly soluble in alcohol and acetone. Used as a foam stabilizer; s solvent for waxes, resins, and emulsions; and an antiblock ingredient for polyethylene.

ERUCAMIDOPROPYL HYDROXYSULTAINE • An antistatic ingredient for hair products. See Erucic Acid and Betaines.

ERUCIC ACID • Cis-13-Docosenoic Acid. A fatty acid derived from mustard seed, rapeseed, and carambe seed. Used in polyethylene film, lipsticks, and water-resistant nylon.

ERUCYL ARACHIDATE • The ester of erucyl alcohol and arachidic acid. See Arachidic Acid.

ERYCYL ERUCATE • The ester of erucyl alcohol and erucic acid. A fatty alcohol derived from erucic acid that is used as a lubricant and surfactant, and in plastics and textiles.

ERYNGIUM MARITIMUM • Sea Holly. This European plant is found on sandy shores and is used by herbalists to treat many urinary ailments. A diuretic, it is often used to treat kidney stones and gravel, especially if there is urinary retention. Herbalists maintain it will ease colic due to urinary problems, as well as reduce hemorrhage. It can help, they say, in cystitis, urethritis, and enlarged and inflamed prostate gland.

ERYTHORBIC ACID • Isoascorbic Acid. Antioxidant. White, slightly yellow crystals, which darken on exposure to light. Isoascorbic acid contains one-twentieth the vitamin capacity of ascorbic acid *(see)*. Nontoxic. It is used in pickling brine at a rate of 7.5 ounces per 100 gallons; in meat products at the rate of 0.75 ounce per 100 pounds; in beverages; in baked goods; and in cured cuts and cured pulverized products to accelerate color fixing in curing at 0.75 ounce per 100 pounds. Nontoxic. The final report to the FDA of the Select Committee on GRAS Substances stated in 1980 that it should continue its GRAS status, with no limitations other than good manufacturing practices.

ERYTHRITOL • Isolated from algae, lichens, and grasses, it is about twice as sweet as sugar. It is used as a humectant *(see)* and a conditioning ingredient in moisturizing creams and lotions.

ERYTHROSINE • Sodium or potassium salt of tetraiodofluorescein, a coal tar derivative. A brown powder that becomes red in solution. FD & C Red No. 3 is an example. It is used in rouge. See Coal Tar for toxicity.

ESCIN • A saponin occurring in the seeds of the horse chestnut tree, *Aesculus hippocastanum.* Practically insoluble in water, it is used as a sunburn protective.

ESCULIN • Occurs in the bark and leaves of the horse chestnut tree. It has been used as a skin protectant in ointments and creams. No known toxicity.

ESERINE ALKALOID AND SALTS • See Physostigmine.

ESSENCE • An extract of a substance that retains its fundamental or most desirable properties in concentrated form, such as a fragrance or flavoring.

ESSENCE OF MIRBANE • Used to scent cheap soap. See Nitrobenzene.

ESSENTIAL OIL • The oily liquid obtained from plants through a variety of processes. The essential oil usually has the taste and smell of the original plant. Essential oils are called volatile because most of them are easily vaporized. The only theories for calling such oils essential are (1) the oils were believed essential to life and (2) they were the "essence" of the plant. The use of essential oils as preservatives is ancient. A large number of oils have antiseptic, germicidal, and preservative action; however, they are used primarily for fragrances and flavorings. No known toxicity when used on the skin. A teaspoon may cause illness in an adult, and less than an ounce may kill.

ESTER • A compound formed from an alcohol and an acid by elimination of water, as ethyl acetate *(see)*. Usually, fragrant liquids used for artificial fruit perfumes and flavors. Esterification of rosin, for example, reduces its allergy-causing properties. Toxicity depends on the ester.

ESTERIFICATION • The process of forming an ester, as in the reaction of ethyl alcohol and acetic acid to form ethyl acetate.

ESTRADIOL • Most potent of the natural estrogenic female hormones. See Hormone Creams and Lotions. Also used in perfumes.

ESTRADIOL BENZOATE • See Estradiol.

ESTRAGON OIL • **Tarragon.** A flavoring ingredient from the oil of leaves of a plant native to Eurasia, used in fruit, licorice, liquor, root beer, and spice flavorings for beverages, ice cream, ices, candy, baked goods, meats, liquor, and condiments. GRAS.

ESTROGEN • A female hormone. See Hormone Creams and Lotions.

ESTRONE • A follicular hormone that occurs in the urine of pregnant women and mares, in human placenta, and in palm-kernel oil *(see)*. Used in creams and lotions as a "hormone" to improve the skin. Usually, there is not enough in the creams to have an effect. It can have harmful systemic effects if used by children.

ETHANE • Colorless, odorless gas used as a source of ethylene *(see)*.

ETHANOL • **Ethyl Alcohol. Rubbing Alcohol. Ordinary Alcohol.** An antibacterial used in mouthwashes, nail enamel, astringents, liquid lip rouge, and many other cosmetic products. Clear, colorless, and very flammable, it is made by the fermentation of starch, sugar, and other carbohydrates. Used medicinally as a topical antiseptic, sedative, and blood vessel dilator. Ingestion of large amounts may cause nausea, vomiting, impaired perception, stupor, coma, and death. When it is deliberately denatured *(see),* it is poisonous.

ETHANOLAMINE DITHIODIGLYCOATE • See Ethanolamines.

ETHANOLAMINE THIOGLYCOLATE • See Ethanolamines.

ETHANOLAMINES • Three compounds—monoethanolamine, diethanolamine, and triethanolamine—with low melting points, colorless, and solid, that readily absorb water and form viscous liquids; soluble in both water and alcohol. They have an ammonia smell and are strong bases. Used in cold permanent-wave lotions as a preservative. Also form soaps with fatty acids *(see),* and are widely used as detergents and emulsifying ingredients. Very large quantities are required for a lethal oral dose in mice (2,140 milligrams per kilogram of body weight). They have been used medicinally as sclerosal ingredients for varicose veins. Can be irritating to skin if very alkaline. See Diethanolamine.

ETHER • An organic compound. Acetic ether (see Ethyl Acetate) is used in nail polishes as a solvent. Water-insoluble, fat-insoluble liquid with a characteristic odor. It is obtained chiefly by the distillation of alcohol with sulfuric acid and is used chiefly as a solvent. A mild skin irritant. Inhalation or ingestion causes central nervous system depression.

ETHIODIZED OIL • The ethyl ester of the fatty acids derived from poppy seeds with iodine. It is used as an antiseptic. See Iodine.

ETHOXYDIGLYCOL • A liquid solvent prepared from ethylene oxide, a petroleum product. It is used as a solvent and thinner in nail enamels. Absorbs water. More toxic orally in animals than polyethylene glycol *(see).* No specific human data is available. It is nonirritating and nonpenetrating when applied to human skin.

ETHOXYDIGLYCOL ACETATE • **Carbitol Acetate.** Used as a solvent and plasticizer for nail enamels and resins and gums. Less toxic than ethoxydiglycol alone by ingestion but is more toxic when applied to the skin. See Butylene Glycol.

ETHOXYETHANOL • **Cellosolve. Ethylene Glycol Monoethyl Ether.** A solvent for nail enamels and a stabilizer in cosmetic emulsions. Obtained by heating ethylene chloride with alcohol and sodium acetate. Colorless and practically odorless. Acute toxicity is several times greater than polyethylene glycol *(see)* in animals. Produces central nervous system depression and kidney damage. Can penetrate the intact skin.

ETHOXYETHANOL ACETATE • **Cellosolve Acetate.** Used to give high gloss to nail polish and to retard evaporation. A colorless liquid with a pleasant odor. Somewhat less toxic than ethoxyethanol alone, it is a central nervous system depressant but does not cause as much kidney damage. It can be readily absorbed through the skin.

2-ETHOXYETHYL-p-METHOXYCINNAMATE • Slightly yellow, viscous liquid, practically odorless, almost insoluble in water. UV absorber in suntan preparations.

ETHOXYHEPTYL BICYCLOOCTANONE • **Ethocyn.** A skin conditioning ingredient.

ETHOXYLATE • Ethyl (from the gas ethane) and oxygen are mixed and added to an additive to make it less or more soluble in water, depending upon the mixture. Ethoxylate acts as an emulsifier.

ETHOXYLATED FATTY ACIDS • See Ethoxylate and Fatty Acids.

ETHOXYLATED FATTY ALCOHOLS • See Ethoxylate and Fatty Alcohols.

ETHOXYLATED SURFACTANTS • Detergents, wetting ingredients, and emulsifiers that have been treated with ethane gas and oxygen to make them more or less soluble, depending upon the mixture. The FDA is studying these ingredients to determine their safety in cosmetics.

4-ETHOXY-m-PHENYLENEDIAMINE SULFATE • See Phenylenediamine.

ETHYL ACETATE • A colorless liquid with a pleasant fruity odor that occurs naturally in apples, bananas, grape juice, pineapple, raspberries, and strawberries. A very useful solvent in nail enamels and nail polish removers. Also an artificial fruit essence for perfumes. It is a mild local irritant and central nervous system depressant. The vapors are irritating, and prolonged inhalation may cause kidney and liver damage. Irritating to the skin. Its fat solvent action produces drying and cracking, and sets the stage for secondary infections. On the basis of available data, the CIR Expert Panel concludes that this ingredient is safe as presently used in cosmetics.

ETHYL ACETOACETATE • **Acetoacetic Ester.** A synthetic flavoring that occurs naturally in strawberries. Pleasant odor. Used in loganberry, strawberry, apple, apricot, cherry, peach, liquor, and muscatel flavorings for beverages, ice cream, ices, candy, baked goods, chewing gum, and gelatin desserts. Moderately irritating to skin and mucous membranes.

ETHYL ACRYLATE • Used for testing for acrylate allergy, which is common. See Acrylates. According to Dr. Frances Storrs, professor of dermatology at Oregon Health Sciences University, in 1997, more than 90 percent of patients who are allergic to acrylates found in artifical nails will test positive to ethyl acrylate, making it a good screener.

ETHYL ALCOHOL • See Ethanol.

ETHYL ALMONDATE • An ester of fatty acids derived from sweet almond oil, it is used in hair and skin conditioners.

ETHYL AMINOBENZOATE • See Ethyl Anthranilate.

ETHYL ANTHRANILATE • Colorless liquid, fruity odor, soluble in alcohol and propylene glycol. A synthetic flavoring ingredient, clear, colorless-to-amber liquid with an odor of orange blossoms. Used in berry, mandarin orange, floral, jasmine, neroli, fruit, grape, peach, and raisin flavorings for beverages, ice cream, ices, candy, baked goods, gelatin desserts, and chewing gum. Used in perfumery. No known toxicity.

ETHYL APRICOT KERNELATE • Derived from apricot kernel oil *(see)* and used as an emollient.

ETHYL ARACHIDONATE • The ester of ethyl alcohol and arachidonic acid *(see both).*

ETHYL ASPARTATE • The ester of ethyl alcohol and aspartic acid *(see both).*

ETHYL AVOCADATE • See Avocado.

ETHYL BENZOATE • **Essence de Niobe.** An artificial fruit essence used in perfumes. Almost insoluble in water. Also used in strawberry and raspberry flavorings. No known toxicity.

ETHYL BIOTINATE • Used in hair and skin conditioners. See Biotin.

ETHYL BROMIDE • Colorless liquid from ethanol or ethylene and hydrobromic acid. Used as a solvent, anesthetic, and fumigant. Toxic by ingestion, inhalation, and skin absorption. It is a strong irritant.

ETHYL BUTYL VALEROLACTONE • A fragrance ingredient. See Valeric Acid.

ETHYL BUTYLACETYLAMINO PROPIONATE • An insect repellent.

ETHYL BUTYRATE • **Pineapple Oil.** An ingredient in perfumes; colorless, with a pineapple odor. It occurs naturally in apples and strawberries. Also used in synthetic flavorings such as blueberry and raspberry. No known toxicity.

ETHYL CAPRATE • Colorless liquid with a fragrant odor used as a flavoring ingredient. See Capric Acid.

ETHYL CAPROATE • Colorless to yellowish liquid, pleasant odor, soluble in alcohol and ether. Used in artificial fruit essences.

ETHYL CARBONATE • **Carbonic Acid Diethyl Ester.** Pleasant odor, practically insoluble in water. Used as a solvent for nail enamels. No known toxicity.

ETHYL CELLULOSE • **Cellulose Ether.** Binding, dispersing, and emulsifying ingredient used in cosmetics, particularly nail polishes and liquid lip rouge. Prepared from wood pulp or chemical cotton by treatment with an alkali. Also used as a diluent (see). Not susceptible to bacterial or fungal decomposition. No known toxicity.

ETHYL CHLORIDE • **Chloroethane.** Prepared by the action of chlorine on ethylene in the presence of hydrochloric acid and light. Used as a topical anesthetic in minor operative procedures and to relieve pain caused by insect stings, burns, and irritation. Mildly irritating to mucous membranes. High concentrations of vapors cause unconsciousness.

ETHYL CINNAMATE • An almost colorless, oily liquid with a faint cinnamon odor. Used as a fixative for perfumes; also to scent heavy oriental and floral perfumes in soaps, toilet waters, face powders, and perfumes. Insoluble in water. Also used as a synthetic food flavoring. No known toxicity for the skin.

ETHYL CYANOACRYLATE • See Acrylates.

ETHYL DIHYDROXYPROPYL PABA • The ester of ethyl alcohol and p-dihydroxypropyl aminobenzoic acid. See Ethyl Alcohol and PABA.

ETHYL DIISOPROPYLCINNAMATE • See Cinnamic Acid.

ETHYL 2,2-DIMETHYLHYDROCINNAMAL. • A fragrance ingredient. See Cinnamal.

ETHYL ESTER OF HYDROLYZED ANIMAL PROTEIN • The ester of ethyl alcohol and the hydrolysate of collagen (see).

ETHYL ESTER OF PVM/MA COPOLYMER • Used for its setting properties, it yields a nontacky film and is water-resistant. It is used in hair setting and bodying preparations. On the basis of available data, the CIR Expert Panel concludes that this ingredient is safe as presently used in cosmetics. See Vinyl Polymers.

ETHYL FORMATE • **Formic Acid.** A colorless, flammable liquid with a distinct odor occurring naturally in apples and coffee extract. Used as a yeast and mold inhibitor and as a fumigant for bulk and packaged raisins and dried currants; also as a fungicide for cashew nuts, cereals, tobacco, and dried fruits. Also used as a synthetic flavoring ingredient for blueberry, raspberry, strawberry, butter, butterscotch, apple, apricot, banana, cherry, grape, peach, plum, pineapple, tutti-frutti, brandy, rum, sherry, and whiskey flavorings for beverages, ice cream, ices, candy, baked goods, liquor, gelatin, and chewing gum. Irritating to the skin and mucous membranes, and narcotic in high concentrations. The final report to the FDA of the Select Committee on GRAS Substances stated in 1980 that it should continue its GRAS status with no limitations other than good manufacturing practices. See Formic Acid for further toxicity.

ETHYL GLUTAMATE • The ester of ethyl alcohol and glutamic acid. See Glutamate.

ETHYL HEPTANOATE • A synthetic flavoring ingredient, colorless, with a fruity, winelike odor and taste, and a burning aftertaste. Used in blueberry, strawberry, butter, butterscotch, coconut, apple, cherry, grape, melon, peach, pineapple, plum, vanilla, cheese, nut, rum, brandy, and cognac flavorings for beverages, ice cream, ices, candy, baked goods, gelatin desserts, chewing gum, and liqueurs. No known toxicity.

ETHYL HEXANEDIOL • A solvent. It is absorbed through the skin and is metabolized and eliminated in the urine. It affected the growth and liver of test animals. Skin application also affected birth defects in female rats. In humans studies, it was a weak sensitizer. On the basis of available data, the CIR Expert Panel concludes that this ingredient is safe as presently used in cosmetics. The Panel, however, did express concern about the birth defects caused in some rats following skin exposure to undiluted ethyl hexanediol.

ETHYL HEXYL-p-METHOXYCINNAMATE • Used as a sunscreen in hypoallergenic cosmetics. See Cinnamic Acid.

ETHYL-p-HYDROXYBENZOATE • See Benzoic Acid.

ETHYL HYDROXYMETHYL OLEYL OXAZOLINE • A synthetic wax. No known toxicity.

ETHYL ISOVALERATE • Colorless, oily liquid with a fruity odor derived from ethanol and valerate. Used in essential oils, perfumery, artificial fruit essences, and flavoring. See Valeric Acid.

ETHYL LACTATE • Colorless liquid with a mild odor. Derived from lactic acid with ethanol. Used as a solvent for nitrocellulose, lacquers, resins, enamels, and flavorings. See Lactic Acid.

ETHYL LAURATE • The ester of ethyl alcohol and lauric acid used as a synthetic flavoring. It is a colorless oil with a light, fruity odor. It is also used as a solvent. No known toxicity.

ETHYL LEVULINATE • Colorless liquid soluble in water. Used as a solvent for cellulose acetate and starch and flavorings. See Levulinic Acid.

ETHYL LINALOOL • See Linalool.

ETHYL LINOLEATE • The ester of ethyl alcohol and linoleic acid. Vitamin F. See Fatty Acids and Linoleic Acid.

ETHYL LINOLENATE • See Linoleic Acid.

ETHYL MALONATE • Colorless liquid, sweet ester odor. Insoluble in water. Used in certain pigments and flavorings. No known toxicity.

ETHYL MALTOL • See Maltose.

ETHYL MENTHANE CARBOXAMIDE • See Menthol.

ETHYL METHACRYLATE • The ester of ethyl alcohol and methacrylic acid. Birth defects were seen in rats injected with this ingredient. Positive evidence of mutagenicity were also observed in mouse cancers. Reports of human sensitivity to this ingredient have been made. On the basis of available data, the CIR Expert Panel concludes that this ingredient is safe as presently used in cosmetics but that skin contact should be avoided. See Acrylates.

ETHYL METHOXYCINNAMATE • Used as a sunscreen in hypoallergenic cosmetics. See Cinnamic Acid.

ETHYL METHYLPHENYLGLYCIDATE • **Strawberry Aldehyde.** Colorless to yellowish liquid having a strong odor suggestive of strawberry. Used in perfumery and flavors.

ETHYL MINKATE • Fatty acids from mink oil *(see)*.

ETHYL MORRHUATE • **Lipinate.** Salt of morrhuic acid, a fatty acid obtained from cod liver oil. Used in creams and lotions. No known toxicity.

ETHYL MYRISTATE • The ester of ethyl alcohol and myristic acid *(see both)*.

ETHYL NICOTINATE • Used as a skin conditioning ingredient. See Ethyl Alcohol and Nicotinic Acid.

N-ETHYL-3-NITRO PABA • Hair coloring. See Parabens.

ETHYL OLEATE • An ingredient in nail polish remover; yellowish, oily, insoluble in water. It is made from carbon, hydrogen, oxygen, and oleic acid *(see)* and used as a synthetic butter and fruit flavoring. No known toxicity.

ETHYL OLIVATE • Fatty acids derived from olive oil.

ETHYL PABA • An ultraviolet light absorber. See Parabens.

ETHYL PALMITATE • The ester of ethyl alcohol and palmitic acid *(see both)*.

ETHYL PEG-15 COCAMINE SULFATE • See Coconut Oil.

ETHYL PELARGONATE • The ester of ethyl alcohol and pelargonic acid *(see both)* used in the manufacture of lacquers and plastics, derived from rice bran. Pelargonic acid is a strong irritant.

ETHYL PERSATE • **Persic Oil Acid. Ethyl Ester.** The ethyl ester of the fatty acids derived from either apricot kernel oil or peach kernel oil. See Apricot Kernel Oil and Peach Kernel Oil.

ETHYL PHENETHYL ACETAL • Used in fragrances. See Benzene.

ETHYL PHENYLACETATE • A fixative for perfumes, colorless, or nearly colorless liquid, with a sweet honey rose odor. Also a synthetic flavoring ingredient in various foods. No known toxicity.

ETHYL SALICYLATE • Used in the manufacture of artificial perfumes. Occurs naturally in strawberries and has a pleasant odor. Also used as a synthetic flavoring ingredient in fruit drinks, baked goods, and so on. At one time it was used to treat rheumatics. It may cause allergic reactions, especially in those who are allergic to other salicylates, including those used in sunscreen lotions.

ETHYL SERINATE • The ester of ethyl alcohol and serine *(see both)*.

ETHYL STEARATE • The ester of ethyl alcohol and stearic acid *(see both)*.

ETHYL TOLUENESULFONAMIDE • Plasticizer for cellulose acetate and for ethylating. See Toluene.

ETHYL UNDECYLENATE • The ester of ethyl alcohol and undecylenic acid.

ETHYL UROCANATE • The ester of ethyl alcohol and urocanic acid. See Imidazoline.

ETHYL VALERATE • The ester of ethyl alcohol and valeric acid *(see both)*.

ETHYL VANILLIN • An ingredient in perfumes. Colorless flakes, with an odor and flavor stronger than vanilla. Also a synthetic food flavoring. No known toxicity.

ETHYLENE • The sixth highest volume chemical produced in the United States, it is a colorless gas with a sweet odor and taste. It is derived from heat-cracking hydrocarbon gases or from fluid removal from ethanol. It is used to make chemical compounds including those used to make plastics, refrigerants, anesthetics, and orchard sprays to accelerate fruit ripening. It is highly flammable and potentially explosive. It can asphyxiate.

ETHYLENE BRASSYLATE • See Behenic Acid.

ETHYLENE DEHYDROGENATED TALLOW AMIDE • See Tallow.

ETHYLENE DICHLORIDE • EDC. The halogenated aliphatic hydrocarbon derived from the action of chlorine on ethylene. It is used in the manufacture of vinyl chloride *(see);* as a solvent for fats, waxes, and resins; as a lead scavenger in antiknock gasolines; in paint, varnish, and finish removers; as a wetting ingredient; as a penetrating ingredient; in organic synthesis; and in the making of polyvinyl chloride (PVC) *(see)*. EDC is also used as an ingredient in cosmetics and as a food additive. It is one of the highest volume chemicals produced. It can be highly toxic whether taken into the body by ingestion, inhalation, or skin absorption. It is irritating to the mucous membranes. In cancer testing, the National Cancer Institute found this compound caused stomach cancer, vascularized cancers of multiple organs, and cancers beneath the skin in male rats. Female rats exposed to EDC developed mammary cancers—in some high-dose animals as early as the twentieth week of the study. The chemical also caused breast cancers as well as uterine cancers in female mice and respiratory tract cancers in both sexes.

ETHYLENE DIOLEAMIDE • See Fatty Acids.

ETHYLENE DISTEARAMIDE • See Fatty Acids.

ETHYLENE GLYCOL • A slightly viscous liquid with a sweet taste. Absorbs twice its weight in water. Used as an antifreeze and humectant *(see)*, also as a solvent. Toxic when ingested, causing central nervous system depression, vomiting, drowsiness, coma, respiratory failure, kidney damage, and possibly death. Polymers *(see)* of ethylene glycol are linked either with alcohols or fatty acids in many cosmetic ingredients. Some metabolites of ethylene glycol are reproductive and developmental toxins, according to the CIR Expert Panel *(see)*. For example, 2-butoxyethanol caused adverse reproductive and developmental effects in oral administration but not when applied to the skin. In general, the Panel concludes, these metabolites of concern are not expected to be formed in cosmetic formulations that contain polymers of ethylene glycol.

ETHYLENE OXIDE • See Polyethylene Oxide.

ETHYLENE UREA • See Urea.

ETHYLENE/ACRYLATE COPOLYMER • See Acrylates and Copolymers.

ETHYLENE/CALCIUM ACRYLATE COPOLYMER • See Acrylates.

ETHYLENEDIAMINE • Colorless, clear, thick, and strongly alkaline. A bacteria-killing component in processing sugarcane. Also used as a solvent for casein, albumen, and shellac. Has been used as a urinary acidifier. It can cause sensitization leading to asthma and allergic skin rashes.

ETHYLENEDIAMINE TETRAACETIC ACID EDTA • An important compound in cosmetics used primarily as a sequestering ingredient *(see)*, particularly in shampoos. It may be irritating to the skin and mucous membranes and cause allergies such as asthma and skin rashes. Also used as a sequestrant in carbonated beverages. When ingested, it may cause errors in a number of laboratory tests, including those for calcium, carbon dioxide, nitrogen, and muscular activity. It is on the FDA list of food additives to be studied for toxicity. It can cause kidney damage. The trisodium salt of EDTA was fed to rats and mice for nearly two years. According to a summary of the report: "Although a variety of tumors occurred among test and control animals of both species, the test did not indicate that any of the tumors observed in the test animals were attributed to EDTA. The tests were part of the National Cancer Institute's Carcinogenesis Bioassay Program."

ETHYLENE/MALEIC ANHYDRIDE COPOLYMER • Plastic material made from ethylene and maleic anhydride. Maleic anhydride is a powerful irritant causing burns. Contact with skin should be avoided. Ethylene is used in the manufacture of plastics and alcohols. High concentrations can cause unconsciousness.

ETHYLENE/VA COPOLYMER • Provides a continuous film for nail enamels or to control film in hairsprays.

2-ETHYLHEXOIC ACID • A mild-scented liquid, slightly soluble in water, it is used in paint and varnish driers and to convert some mineral oils to greases. Its esters *(see)* are used as plasticizers. No known toxicity.

ETHYLHEXYL PALMITATE • An emollient used in cosmetic creams. See Palmitic Acid.

ETHYLHEXYL PELARGONATE • Used in makeup. See Ethyl Pelargonate.

ETHYLPARABEN • Widely used preservative. See Propylparaben.

ETIDRONIC ACID • See Benzyl Alcohol.

ETOCRYLENE • The organic ester derived from acrylic acid widely used in nail polish. See Acrylates.

EU • Abbreviation for European Union.

EUCALYPTOL • A chief constituent of eucalyptus and cajeput oils. Occurs naturally in allspice, star anise, bay, calamus, and peppermint oil. An antiseptic, antispasmodic, and expectorant. Used to flavor toothpaste and mouthwash and to cover up malodors in depilatories. It is not used in hypoallergenic cosmetics. Fatalities followed ingestion of doses as small as 3 to 5 milliliters (about a teaspoon), and recovery has occurred after doses as large as 20 to 30 milliliters (about 4 to 5 teaspoons).

EUCALYPTUS CITRIODORA • See Eucalyptus Oil.

EUCALYPTUS EXTRACT • See Eucalyptus Oil.

EUCALYPTUS OIL • **Dinkum Oil.** Used in skin fresheners. The colorless to pale yellow, volatile liquid from the fresh leaves of the eucalyptus tree. It is 70 to 80 percent eucalyptol and has a spicy cool taste and a characteristic aromatic, somewhat camphorlike odor. Used as a local antiseptic. It can cause allergic reactions, and fatalities have followed ingestion of doses as small as 3 to 5 milliliters (about equal to a teaspoon); about 1 milliliter has caused coma.

EUCOMMIA ULMOIDES • **Kommi Gum.** A Chinese tree that yields rubber.

EUGENIA CARYOPHYLLUS • See Clove Oil.

EUGENIA CUMINI • **Jambul Extract.** Used as a flavoring.

EUGENOL • An ingredient in perfumes and dentifrices obtained from clove oil. Occurs naturally in allspice, basil, bay leaves, calamus, pimento, and laurel leaves. It has a spicy, pungent taste. Used as a fixative in perfumes and flavorings. Eugenol also acts as a local antiseptic. When ingested, it may cause vomiting and gastric irritation. Because of its potential as an allergen, it is left out of hypoallergenic cosmetics.

EUGLENA GRACILIS • A tropical tree. See Eugenol.

EUPATORIUM PURPUREUM • A perennial common to Europe, the eastern United States, and Canada, it grows in meadows. It was used to treat diarrhea and stomach upsets. Was also given for gout, arthritis, and flu. It is rich in Vitamin C and contains salicylic acid and citric acid *(see both)*.

EUPHORBIA EXTRACT • **Asthma Weed. Spurge Extract. Snake Weed Extract.** An extract of the herb *Euphorbia pilulifera*. A large genus of plants of greatly diverse appearance, some being fleshy and cactuslike, and others being leafy and herbaceous or shrubby, but all having milky juice and flowers. The plant yielding castor oil belongs to this family.

EUROPEAN ASH • A tall Eurasian tree, *Fraxinus excelsior,* with leaves that are dark green with prominent veins.

EUROPEAN HOLLY EXTRACT • The extract of *Ilex aquifolium.*

EURPHRASIA • **Eyebright Herbs.** A derivative from any of several herbs, regarded as a remedy for eye ailments. It is used to soothe the eye in a rinse. No known toxicity.

EUXYL K 400 • A newer preservative for cosmetics and toiletries rapidly increasing in use. It contains 1,2-dibromo-2,4-dicyanobutan and 2-phenoxyethanol. There are increasing reports of patients who are sensitive to it, and physicians are being encouraged to test for it in patients with allergic contact dermatitis *(see)*.

EVENING PRIMROSE • *Oenothera biennis*. **Sundrops.** The leaves and oil from the seed are used by herbalists to treat liver and kidney dysfunctions. The oil has a high content of linoleic acid (GLA), an essential polyunsaturated fatty acid that is converted into prostaglandins *(see)* and hormones. It is used as a tonic for inflammatory conditions. It is used in "organic" cosmetics. It is said to relieve premenstrual tension, high blood pressure, and anxiety associated with inflammatory conditions. It has been recommended for infantile eczema, painful breasts, arthritis, and neurosis. It reputedly lowers cholesterol.

EVERLASTING EXTRACT • An extract derived from the flowering plant *Helichrysum italicum* and related species.

EVERNIA PRUNASTRI • A lichen, *Evemia* species, that grows on oak trees and yields a resin for use as a fixative *(see)* in perfumery. Stable, green liquid with a long-lasting characteristic odor. Soluble in alcohol. Used in fruit, honey, and spice flavorings for beverages, ice cream, ices, candy, baked goods, gelatin desserts, condiments, and soups. A common allergen in after-shave lotions.

EXALTING FIXATIVES • A material that acts as an odor carrier, improving and fortifying transportation of the vapors of other perfume materials. Musk and civet are examples. See Fixatives.

EXCIPIENT • A more or less inert substance added to a prescription as a diluent or vehicle or to give form or consistency when the medication is in pill form. Not infrequently, excipients may be "hidden" allergens.

EXFOLIANT • Ingredient that causes skin to shed. See Exfoliation.

EXFOLIATION • Shedding of superficial cells of the skin. Many compounds containing acids are being used in products aimed at the older market as a means of peeling the skin to make it look younger. In the youth market, such products are sold to get rid of oily, blackhead-dotted top layers of skin. There is a question of whether such products are over-the-counter drugs or cosmetics. The cosmetic producers say they do not change the structure of the skin—just peel off the dead layers—and therefore, the products are cosmetics. Some early versions of the exfoliants were too strong and irritated the skin. The most recent versions are more gentle at peeling.

EXPOXIDIZED SOYBEAN OIL • A modified oil obtained from soybeans. See Epoxy and Soybean Oil.

EXT. D & C VIOLET NO. 2 • Classed chemically as an anthraquinone color. Bluish scarlet. Permitted only for use in preformed hair colors, but textbooks list use in bath salts, soaps, and hair-waving fluids as well. The cosmetics industry has petitioned the FDA to allow wider use. Permanently listed for external use, 1982. See Colors.

EXT. D & C YELLOW NO. 7 • Formerly FD & C Yellow No. 1. Greenish yellow. A coal tar color. Classed chemically as a nitro color. It is the disodium salt of 2, 4-dinitro-1-naphthol-7-sulfonic acid. Used in hair rinses and shampoos. See Colors.

EXT. D & C YELLOW NO. 7 ALUMINUM LAKE • **Naphthol Yellow Lake.** A coal tar color. Light yellow or orange-yellow powder. An insoluble pigment prepared from Ext. D & C Yellow No. 7 *(see)*. See Colors.

EXTENDER • A substance added to a product, especially a diluent or modifier *(see both)*. Petroleum jelly would be an example.

EXTENSIN • A protein that is a component of plant cell walls.

EXTRACT • The solution that results from passing alcohol or an alcohol-water mixture through a substance. Examples of extracts would be the alcohol-water mixture of vanillin, orange, or lemon extract found among the spices and flavorings on the supermarket shelf. Extracts are not as strong as essential oils *(see)*.

EYE ALLERGY • There are many forms of allergy of the eye. The mucous membranes of the eye may be involved in allergic rhinitis. Such allergic conjunctivitis may also occur by itself without irritation of the nose. Another form, spring "pinkeye," is probably due to allergens in the air. Dust, mold spores, foods, and eye medications may all cause conjunctivitis. There is also a less severe, chronic form of allergic conjunctivitis. Symptoms include prolonged photophobia, itching, burning, and a feeling of dryness. There may be a watery discharge, and finding the source of allergy is often difficult.

EYE BRIGHT • *Euphrasia officinalis.* **Euphrasy.** An annual herb native to Europe and western Asia and grown in the United States, it belongs to the foxglove family. It contains tannins, iridoid glycosides, phenolic acids, and volatile oil. It has been mentioned in medical literature since the early 1300s. It had the reputation of being able to restore eyesight in very old people and is still used today as an eyewash for inflamed and tired eyes and to treat sinus congestion. Used in "organic" cosmetics. Astringent infusions are made by herbalists for coughs, colds, and sore throats. It is also occasionally used to treat jaundice, loss of memory, and dizziness.

EYE CREAMS • **Eye Wrinkle Creams**. So-called eye creams are slightly modified emollient creams *(see)*, usually with the perfume omitted. There is less subcutaneous fat in the skin around the eyes, and it is likely for this reason that wrinkles first begin to develop there. According to the American Medical Association, eye creams will not prevent wrinkles but may make them less noticeable. Most eye creams contain essentially the same ingredients: lecithin, cholesterol, beeswax, lanolin, sodium benzoate, boric acid, mineral oil, ascorbyl palmitate, and almond oil *(see all)*.

EYE MAKEUP REMOVER • Pads saturated with ingredients to remove eye makeup. They may contain a solvent such as acetone *(see)*, an oil and/or lanolin *(see)*, and perfume. Hypoallergenic *(see)* cosmetic manufacturers use cotton pads saturated with pure mineral oil. Eye irritations from eye-makeup removers have been reported to the FDA within the past several years.

EYE MASCARA • Mascara is used to color and thicken eyelashes. Early mascara was composed of a pigment and soap. Today it still contains a salt of stearic acid *(see)* with pigments and/or lanolin, paraffin, and carnauba wax *(see all)*. Within the past few years there have been a number of complaints of itching, burning, and swelling of eyes and eye irritation due to mascara.

EYE SHADOW • Shades of blue, green, brown, red, yellow, and white are used to color the lid and area under the eyebrow to highlight the eyes. The waterless type of eye shadow uses colors mixed with a lightening ingredient such as titanium dioxide *(see)* and are then mixed with petrolatum *(see)* on a roller mill. Eye shadows may also contain lanolin, beeswax, ceresin, calcium carbonate, mineral oil, sorbitan oleate, and talc *(see all)*. The iridescent effect is achieved by adding very pure aluminum. There have been reports in recent years of eye irritation from eye shadow and one complaint of a package shattering in the eye and another of a sharp foreign article in the product applicator.

EYEBRIGHT HERBS • See Euphrasia.

EYEBROW DYES • No permanent dyes are approved for use around the eyes.

EYEBROW PENCILS • Usually contain lampblack, petrolatum, and paraffin *(see all)* and sometimes aluminum silicate and stearic acid *(see both)*. The use of eyeliner pencils applied to the upper and lower border of the eyelids inside the lashes rather than to the eyelid behind the lashes is not recommended by physicians. According to a report by an eye specialist quoted by the American Medical Association, this may lead to various problems, including permanent pigmentation of the mucous membrane lining of the inside of the eye, moderate redness and itching, tearing, and blurring of vision.

EYEBROW PLUCKING CREAM • Used to soften the skin to allow the hair to be pulled more easily and to alleviate the discomfort. Most eyebrow plucking creams contain benzocaine, a painkiller, and cold cream *(see both)*. Nontoxic if uncontaminated.

EYEDROPS, LOTIONS, AND WASHES • Soothe and clear eyes of redness. Work by constricting the blood vessels in the eyes, and by anesthetizing and soothing the eyes with anesthetics and emollients. Mild astringents such as boric acid or sodium chloride are used. Mild anesthetics used are antipyrine hydrastine hydrochloride and berberine hydrochloride. To contract the blood vessels tetrahydrozoline hydrochloride is used. Included for their pleasant smell are camphor, peppermint, or witch hazel. Among the preservatives used are phenols, cresol, and formaldehyde. A wetting ingredient such as benzalkonium is also usually included. Reports of eye irritations are infrequent from eye treatment products, but the largest danger is from contamination because eye solutions are good mediums for the growth of bacteria and molds; therefore, they must be kept sterile.

EYELASH CREAMS • Used to make the lashes soft and shiny. Such creams usually contain lanolin, cocoa butter, paraffin, cetyl alcohol, and peach kernel oil *(see all)*. Nontoxic if uncontaminated. However, ingredients may cause reactions in persons who are allergic to specific ingredients.

EYELASH DYES • Includes eyebrow dyes. Brown, black, and blue certified oil-soluble dyes are used. Because of possible damage to the eyes, only certain ingredients and colors may be used in these preparations *(see Colors)*. The U.S. Food and Drug Administration forbids the use of coal tar dyes *(see)* in the area of the eye. Highly purified inorganic pigments must be used; among them carbon black, charcoal black, black iron oxide, and ultramarine blue for black and blue shades. Iron oxides are used also for yellow and brown shades, carmine for red, chromic oxides for green, and titanium dioxide or zinc oxide for white. See Colors for toxicity.

EYELASH OILS • Used to make the lashes soft and shiny. Such oils usually contain lanolin, cocoa butter, cetyl alcohol, alcohol water, and olive oil. Nontoxic if uncontaminated. However, reactions may occur in persons allergic to specific ingredients.

EYELIDS • The skin of the eyelids is a common site of allergic contact dermatitis. The lesions, at first, may be swollen, red, and scaly, but as the victim tries to control the condition, the situation may become chronic and the skin of the lids thicken and roughen. Nail polish and perfume are among the most common allergens, but artificial eyelashes are also a source of trouble. See page 29 in introduction.

EYELINERS • Used to outline and accentuate the eyes, eyeliners may come in pencil or liquid form or in the newer pencil-brush container. Eyeliners usually contain an alkanolamine, a fatty alcohol, polyvinylpyrrolidone, cellulose ether, methylparaben, antioxidants, perfumes, and titanium dioxide *(see all)*. Waterproof eyeliners resist tears, moisture in the air, and perspiration. Some also resist ordinary soap and water. Most of the waterproof eyeliners are made of a pigment suspended in a gum or resin solution or a pigmented waxy base dissolved in a volatile solvent. Waterproof eyeliners must be removed with a solvent such as mineral oil or similar oils. Most facial cleansing lotions and creams contain such solvents. The FDA has found a persistent problem of bacterial contamination in some liquid eyeliners. Since bacterial infections around the eyes can lead to serious problems, it is probably better to purchase nonliquid eyeliners. There are also a significant number of persons allergic to eyeliners and other such products. The American Medical Association recommends that women stop using an eyeliner or eye makeup product if their skin becomes red, itchy, or swollen whenever an eye cosmetic is applied. The AMA also points out that because the eyelids are easily irritated, eye makeup, particularly eyeliner, should be removed with care. It also cautions against repeatedly applying eye makeup at one session because of the possibility of irritation. There have been a number of reports of swollen eyelids and eye irritation from well-known products.

EYEWASHES • See Eyedrops, Lotions, and Washes.

F

FABA BEAN EXTRACT • **Fava Bean. Common Bean.** The extract of the seeds of *Vicia faba.* Inhalation or ingestion of the pollen of its flower can cause fever and headache in certain sensitized individuals. Little is known about the toxicity of the seed extract.

FABIANA IMBRICATA • **Pichi extract.** A Peruvian shrub that yields a tonic and a diuretic.

FACE MASKS AND PACKS • Claims are made for face masks and for the thicker face packs that they shrink pores, remove wrinkles, and relieve tension. Only the last may be true. According to the American Medical Association, there is no evidence that any cosmetic can safely shrink pores, and only surgery removes wrinkles. However, the apparent cooling or tight feeling derived from their use may induce a clean feeling. Clay face masks usually contain purified siliceous earth, kaolin, glycerin, and water. Face packs usually contain zinc stearate, zinc oxide, tragacanth, alcohol, glycerin, and limewater. Both masks and packs may also contain acacia, Balsam Peru, glyceryl monostearate, magnesium carbonate, wax, salicylic acid, spermaceti, Turkey-red oil, talc, titanium oxide, and/or zinc sulfate. (See ingredients above under separate listings.) Complaints to the FDA about face masks and packs include burning sensation, swelling, blisters and lumps, eye ailments, skin irritation, and corneal ulcers.

FAEX • Compressed yeast. See Yeast.

FAGUS SYLVATICA • A member of the Beech family. Used as a coloring.

FAKE NAILS • See Artificial Nails.

FALSE EYELASHES • False eyelashes are made of real or synthetic hair on a thin stringlike base that is pasted over the natural eyelashes on the eyelid. There have been cases of eye irritation and one case of blindness reported to the FDA. Whether the problems were the result of the adhesive used, the dye on the eyelashes, or other materials is not clear.

FARNESOL • Used in perfumery to emphasize the odor of sweet floral perfumes such as lilac. Occurs naturally in ambrette seed, star anise, cassia, linden flowers, oils of muskseed, citronella, rose, and balsam. Also a food flavoring. No known toxicity.

FARNESYL • The ester of farnesol and acetic acid *(see both)*. Used as a fragrance ingredient.

FAST GREEN FCF • A name applied to uncertified FD & C Green No. 3 *(see)*.

FATIGUE • Everyone's nose becomes "fatigued" when smelling a certain odor. No matter how much you like a fragrance, you can only smell it for a short interval. It is nature's way of protecting humans from overstimulation of the olfactory sense.

FATTY ACID ESTERS • The fatty acid esters of low-molecular-weight alcohols are widely used in hand products because they are oily but nongreasy when applied to the skin. They are emollients and emulsifiers. No known toxicity. See Ester.

FATTY ACIDS • Fatty acids are used in bubble baths and lipsticks, but chiefly for making soap and detergents. One or any mixture of liquid and solid acids— capric, caprylic, lauric, myristic, oleic, palmitic, and stearic. In combination with glycerin, they form fat. Necessary for normal growth and healthy skin. In foods they are used as emulsifiers, binders, and lubricants. No known toxicity. See Stearic Acid.

FATTY ALCOHOLS • Cetyl, Stearyl, Lauryl, Myristyl. Solid alcohols made from acids and widely used in hand creams and lotions. Cetyl and stearyl alcohols form an occlusive film to keep skin moisture from evaporating, and they impart a velvety feel to the skin. Lauryl and myristyl are used in detergents and creams. Very low toxicity.

FD & C • Abbreviation for Food, Drug and Cosmetic.

FD & C BLUE NO. 1 • Brilliant Blue FD & C. A coal tar derivative, triphenylmethane, used for hair colorings, face powders, and other cosmetics. Also used as a coloring in bottled soft drinks, gelatin, desserts, cereals, and other foods. May cause allergic reactions. On the FDA permanent list of color additives. Rated 1A, that is, completely acceptable for nonfood use, by the World Health Organization. However, it produced malignant tumors at the site of injection and by ingestion in rats. See Colors.

FD & C BLUE NO. 2 • Moderate bright green. A coal tar derivative, triphenyl-methane, used in hair rinses and in mint-flavored jelly, frozen desserts, candy, confections, and cereals. It is a sensitizer in the allergic. Permanently listed for surgical sutures in 1971 and for food and ingested drug use in 1987. Produces malignant tumors at the site of injection when introduced under the skin of rats. See Colors.

FD & C BRILLIANT BLUE NO. 1 ALUMINUM LAKE • Aluminum salt of certified of Brilliant Blue No. 1 (see). See Colors and Lakes.

FD & C GREEN NO. 3 • Permanently listed by the FDA for use in food, drugs, and cosmetics in 1982, except in the area of the eye.

FD & C LAKES • **Aluminum or Calcium Lakes.** Lakes are pigments prepared by combining FD & C colors with a form of aluminum or calcium, which makes the colors insoluble. Aluminum and calcium lakes are used in confection and candy products and for dyeing eggshells and other products that are adversely affected by water.

FD & C RED NO. 2 • **Amaranth.** Formerly one of the most widely used cosmetic and food colorings. A dark, reddish brown powder that turns bright red when mixed with fluid. A monoazo color, it was used in lipsticks, rouges, and other cosmetics as well as in cereals, maraschino cherries, and desserts. The safety of this dye was questioned by American scientists for more than twenty years. Two Russian scientists found that FD & C Red No. 2 prevented some pregnancies and caused some stillbirths in rats. The FDA ordered manufacturers using the color to submit data on all food, drug, and cosmetic products containing it. Controversial tests at the FDA's National Center for Toxicological Research in Arkansas showed that in high doses FD & C Red No. 2 caused a statistically significant increase in a variety of cancers in female rats. The dye was banned by the FDA in January 1976.

FD & C RED NO. 3 • **Erythrosine.** Bluish pink. A coal tar derivative, a xanthene color, used in toothpaste and in canned fruit cocktail, fruit salad, and cherry pie mixes as well as maraschino cherries. Has been determined a carcinogen. FD & C Red No. 3 was permanently listed for use in food and ingested drugs, but only provisionally listed for cosmetics and externally applied drugs. In 1990, the lakes *(see)* of FD & C Red No. 3 were removed for all uses from the approved list. The color itself was also removed in 1990 for cosmetic and external drug use. It is still, as of this writing, approved for food and ingested drugs.

FD & C RED NO. 4 • A monoazo color and coal tar dye. Used in mouthwashes, bath salts, and hair rinses. It was banned in food by the FDA in 1964, when it was shown to damage the adrenal glands and bladders of dogs. The agency relented and gave it provisional license for use in maraschino cherries. It was banned in all food in 1976 because it was shown to cause urinary bladder polyps and atrophy of the adrenal glands in animals. It was also banned in orally taken drugs but is still permitted in cosmetics for external use only. The uncertified version is called Ponceau SX. See also Colors.

FD & C RED NO. 20 • Permanently listed by the FDA in 1983 for general use in drugs and cosmetics (except in areas around the eyes).

FD & C RED NO. 22 • Permanently listed by the FDA in 1983 for general use in drugs and cosmetics (except in areas around the eyes).

FD & C RED NO. 40 • **Allura Red AC.** Newest color. Used widely in the cosmetic industry. Approved in 1971, Allied Chemical has an exclusive patent on it. It is substituted for FD & C Red No. 4 in many cosmetics, food, and drug products. Permanently listed in 1971 because, unlike the producers of "temporary" colors, this producer supplied reproductive data. However, many American scientists feel that the safety of FD & C Red No. 40 is far from established, particularly because all the tests were conducted by the manufacturer. Therefore, the dye should not have received a permanent safety rating. The National Cancer Institute reported that p-credine, a chemical used in the preparation of FD & C Red No. 40, was carcinogenic in animals. See also Azo Dyes.

FD & C YELLOW NO. 5 • **Tartrazine.** A coal tar derivative, it is used as a coloring in hair rinses, hair-waving fluids, and bath salts. A pyrazole color, it is also found in prepared breakfast cereals, imitation strawberry jelly, bottled soft drinks, gelatin desserts, ice cream, sherbets, dry drink powders, candy, confections, bakery products, spaghetti, and puddings. Causes allergic reactions in persons sensitive to aspirin. The certified color industry petitioned for permanent listing of this color in February 1966, with no limitations other than good manufacturing practice. However, in February 1966, the FDA proposed the listing of this color with a maximum rate of use of 300 parts per million in food. The color industry had objected to the limitations. Yellow No. 5 was thereafter permanently listed as a color additive without restrictions. Rated 1A by the World Health Organization— acceptable in food. It is estimated that half the aspirin-sensitive people plus 47,000 to 94,000 others in the nation are sensitive to this dye. It is used in about 60 percent of both over-the-counter and prescription drugs. Efforts were made to ban this color in over-the-counter pain relievers, antihistamines, oral decongestants, and prescription anti-inflammatory drugs. Aspirin-sensitive patients have been reported to develop life-threatening asthmatic symptoms with ingestion of this yellow. Since 1981, it is supposed to be listed on the label if it is used. The uncertified version is Acid Yellow 23.

FD & C YELLOW NO. 5 ALUMINUM LAKE • The uncertified version is Pigment Yellow 100. See FD & C Yellow No. 5, Colors and Lakes.

FD & C YELLOW NO. 6 • **Sunset Yellow FCF.** A coal tar, monoazo color, used in hair rinses as well as other cosmetics, carbonated beverages, gelatin, desserts, and dry drink powders. It is not used in products that contain fats and oils. May cause allergic reactions. Permanently listed for food, drugs, and cosmetics in 1986. Labeling requirements began in 1989 because of its potentiality for causing allergic reactions. The uncertified version is Sunset Yellow. See Colors.

FD & C YELLOW NO. 6 ALUMINUM LAKE • The uncertified version is Pigment Yellow 104. See FD & C Yellow No. 6, Colors, and Aluminum Lakes.

FEMININE HYGIENE SPRAYS • See Vaginal Deodorants.

FENNEL OIL AND EXTRACT • One of the earliest known herbs from the tall, beautiful shrub. Used in astringents and perfumes. The fennel flowers appear in June and are bright yellow. Compresses of fennel tea are used by organic cosmeticians to soothe inflamed eyelids and watery eyes. May cause allergic reactions.

FENUGREEK SEED • **Greek Hay.** An annual herb grown in southern Europe, North Africa, and India, and used in hair tonics, supposedly to prevent baldness; also added to powders, poultices, and ointments. The seeds are used in making curry.

FERMENTED VEGETABLE • A mixture of cane sugar, molasses, and vegetable proteins. Used in "natural" cosmetics.

FERRIC AMMONIUM CHLORIDE • Brownish yellow, or orange, iron compound. Absorbs water readily. Used as a styptic and astringent. Irritating to the skin and not suitable for wide use.

FERRIC AMMONIUM FERROCYANIDE • **Iron Blue.** An inorganic salt used as a dark blue coloring for cosmetics. Permanently listed in 1977. See Iron Salts.

FERRIC FERROCYANIDE • **Iron Blue.** A coloring for externally applied cosmetics, including the eye area. Permanently listed in 1978. See Colors.

FERRIC NITRATE • Derived from the action of concentrated nitric acid on scrap iron or iron oxide. Used for dyeing and for tanning.

FERRIC PYROPHOSPHATE • Used as a nutrient source of iron *(see)*.

FERROUS AMMONIUM SULFATE • See Ammonia and Ferrous Sulfate.

FERROUS CHLORIDE • **Iron Chloride.** Greenish white crystals made from the action of hydrochloric acid on iron. Used in dyeing and in cosmetic and pharmaceutical preparations.

FERROUS FUMARATE • A salt of ferrous iron combined with fumaric acid. Odorless and tasteless, the reddish brown compound is used as a dietary supplement.

FERROUS LACTATE • **Lactic Acid. Iron Salt. Iron Lactate.** Greenish white crystals that have a slightly peculiar odor. It is derived from the interaction of calcium lactate with ferrous sulfate or the direct action of the lactic acid on iron fillings. It is used as a food additive and dietary supplement. Causes tumors when injected under the skin of mice. GRAS.

FERROUS SULFATE • **Green or Iron Vitriol.** Pale bluish green, odorless crystals, efflorescent in dry air. An astringent and deodorant. Used in hair dyes. A source of iron used medicinally. No known toxicity.

FERROUS SULFIDE • **Iron Sulfide.** Derived by fusing sulfide and iron. Employed in ceramics and pigments.

FERULA ASSA FOETIDA • **Asafetida.** See Asafoetida Extract.

FERULA FOETIDA • See Asafoetida Extract.

FERULA GALBANIFLUA • See Galbanum Oil.

FERULIC ACID • An antioxidant, preservative, and ultraviolet absorber. See Phenols.

FEVERFEW • *Chrysanthemum parthenium. Pyrethrum parthenium. Tanacetum parthenium.* **Flirtwort. Bachelor's Buttons. Maydes' Weed. Wild Quinine.** A small, hardy perennial herb, a member of the chamomile *(see)* family, it was introduced into Britain from Southeast Asia. Since ancient times it has been used by physicians for its action on the uterus. It was thought to promote menstrual evacuation and to aid in the expulsion of the placenta after childbirth. It was prescribed as an antidote against narcotic poisoning and was also considered a poultice herb with cooling and analgesic properties. Herbalists today use it as a laxative and to treat stings and bites. The name feverfew is derived from the word "febrifuge," which means "to lower fever," the most common use for the herb by Greek physicians. It is now being investigated as a preventative for migraines. Used in "organic" cosmetics.

FIBRONECTIN • A fibrous protein widely distributed in connective tissue and membranes and present on cell surfaces. Acts as an adhesive and as a defense mechanism.

FICIN • An enzyme occurring in the latex of tropical trees and usually isolated from figs. A buff-colored powder with an acrid odor. Absorbs water. Concentrated and used as a meat tenderizer. Ten to twenty times more powerful than papain tenderizers. Used to clot milk, as a protein digestant in the brewing industry, and as a chill-proofing ingredient in beer. Also in cheese as a substitute for rennet in the coagulation of milk, and for removing casings from sausages. Can cause irritation to the skin, eyes, and mucous membranes and in large doses can cause purging. Also used to combat worms and in cosmetics as a protein digestant.

FICUS CARICA • See Fig Extract.

FIELD POPPY EXTRACT • Extract of the petals of *Papaver rhoeas* used in coloring and as an odorant.

FIG EXTRACT • From *Opuntia ficus.* Any of several woody plants with oblong fruit.

FIGWORT • *Scrophularia nodosa.* A perennial plant native to Britain and the United States, it used to be hung in houses and barns to ward off witches. Herbalists used it as an ointment to treat eczema, rashes, bruises, scratches, and small wounds, and for removing freckles.

FILIPENDULA RUBRA • **Queen of the Prairie, Dollof, Bridewort.** Used by American Indians to treat burns and abrasions. It contains salicylides *(see)*. It was reported by researchers at Brooks Industries, South Plainfield, N.J., to increase cell respiration.

FINGERNAIL POLISH • See Nail Polish.

FINGERNAIL POLISH REMOVER • See Nail Polish Remover.

FINISHING RINSE • A product that coats only the surface fibers of the hair and is used to add sheen and to remove tangles.

FIR NEEDLE OIL • Fir Oil. An essential oil obtained by the steam distillation of needles and twigs of several varieties of pine trees native to both Canada and Siberia. Used as a scent in perfumes and as a flavoring ingredient.

FISH CARTILAGE EXTRACT • Used in "antiaging" products and moisturizers.

FISH GLYCERIDES • See Fish Oil and Glycerin.

FISH LIVER OIL • See Fish Oil.

FISH OIL • A fatty oil in soap manufacturing derived from fish or marine animals.

FIXATIVE • A chemical that reduces the tendency of an odor or flavor to vaporize by making the odor or flavor last longer. An example is musk *(see),* which is used in perfume.

FLAVONES • One of a group of plant pigments that produces ivory and yellow colors. They are reputed to have a wide range of activities, including reducing excess fluid and stimulating the heart. Some, such as rutin and hesperidin, are said to increase the strength of the capillaries and to lower blood pressure.

FLAVONOIDS • Flavonoids are a large group of compounds widely distributed throughout nature. They include quercetin, present in onion skins, and anthocyanins, the major commercially used group.

FLAVOR ENHANCERS • One of the newest and fastest growing categories of additives; potentiators, which enhance the total seasoning effect generally without contributing any taste or odor of their own. They are effective in minute doses— in parts per million or even less. A potentiator produces no identifiable effect itself but exaggerates one's response. They alter the response of the sensory nerve endings on the tongue and in the nose. The first true potentiators in the United States were the 5'-nucleotides, which are derived from a natural seasoning long in use in Japan: small flakes of dry bonito (a tunalike fish) are often added to modify and improve the flavor of soups. From bonito a 5'-nucleotide, disodium inosinate, has been isolated and identified as a flavor potentiator. Another 5'-nucleotide is disodium guanylate, one of the newer additives on the market, which gives one a sensation of "fullness" and "increased viscosity" when eating. The product is advertised as being able to give diners a sense of "full-bodied flavor" when ingesting a food containing it.

FLAXSEED • The seed of the flax plant may be "hidden" in cereals and in the milk of cows fed flaxseed. It is also in flaxseed tea and the laxative, flaxolyn. It is a frequent allergen when ingested, inhaled, or in direct contact. Flaxseeds are the source of linseed oil. Among other hidden sources are dog food, wave-setting preparations, shampoos, hair tonics, depilatories, patent leather, insulating materials, rugs and some cloths, Roman meal, cough remedies, and muffins.

FLEXIBLE COLLODION • A mixture of collodion *(see)* with camphor and castor oil to make collodion more malleable.

FLORAL BOUQUET • One of the basic perfume types, it is a blending of flower notes with no particular standouts. For balance and body, it may contain a medley of basic notes such as amber, musk, and vetiver, as well as a touch of the aromatic, but there is definitely the scent of a bouquet of flowers.

FLUORESCEIN • A yellow, granular or red, crystalline dye giving a brilliant yellow-green fluorescence in an alkaline solution. Very visible. See Tetrabromofluorescein for toxicity.

FLUORESCENT BRIGHTENERS • **(46, 47, 52).** Colorless, water- or solvent-soluble aromatic compounds with an affinity for fibers. They are usually violet, blue, or blue-green colors, and are capable of increasing both the blueness and the brightness of a substrate, with a resulting marked whitening effect. They improve the brightness of tints and are included in detergents of all kinds to enhance cleansing action.

FLUORIDE • An acid salt used in toothpaste to prevent tooth decay. See Sodium Fluoride and Stannous Fluoride.

FLUORINE COMPOUNDS • **Calcium Fluoride; Hydrofluorsillic Acid; Potassium Fluoride; Sodium Fluoride and Sodium Silicofluoride.** All have been used in the fluoridation of water. Fluorides cross the placental barrier and the effects on the fetus are unknown. New clinical evidence shows that kidney disturbance sometimes is due to the amount of fluoride it contributes to the blood. Fluorine containing compounds (sodium, potassium, or calcium fluoride) are illegal. A petition for extension in dietary supplements was terminated in 1973. Addition of fluorine compounds to food is limited to that from fluoridation of public water supplies and to that resulting from the fluoridation of bottled water within limits set by the FDA.

FLUORO C2-8 ALKKYLDIMETHICONE • An antifoaming ingredient. See Silicones.

FLUOROSALAN • A salicylide used as an antiseptic ingredient. See Salicylides.

FOAM STABILIZERS • Used in soft drinks and brewing. See Vegetable Gums.

FOENICULUM VULGARE • See Fennel.

FOLIC ACID • A yellowish orange compound and member of the Vitamin B complex, used as a nutrient. Used in cosmetic emollients. Occurs naturally in liver, kidney, mushrooms, and green leaves. Aids in cell formation, especially red blood cells. No known toxicity.

FOMES OFFICINALIS • See Mushroom Extract.

FOREST BLENDS • One of the basic perfume types, these blends are woody, mossy-leafy, or resinous. They either stand out alone with the aromatic notes of an individual nature, such as sandalwood, rosewood, the balsams, or cedar wood, or they have a combination of these notes. Quite often, the more pungent notes of geranium, lavender, fern, and herbs are used to give an earthy quality.

FORMALDEHYDE • A colorless gas obtained by the oxidation of methyl alcohol and generally used in watery solution. Vapors are intensely irritating to mucous membranes. It has been estimated that 4 to 8 percent of the general population may be sensitized to it. It is used in nail hardeners, nail polish, soap, and hair-growing products. It is widely used in cosmetics as a disinfectant, germicide, fungicide, defoamer, and preservative. Ingestion can cause severe abdominal pain, internal bleeding, loss of ability to urinate, vertigo, coma, and death. Skin reactions after exposure to it are very common because the chemical can be both irritating and allergy-producing. Physicians have reported severe reactions to nail hardeners containing formaldehyde. Its use in cosmetics is banned in Japan and Sweden. Some surfactants, such as the widely used lauryl sulfate, may contain formaldehyde as a preservative, and other surfactants may have it without listing it on the label. Formaldehyde is an inexpensive and effective preservative, but there are serious questions about its safety. It is a highly reactive chemical that is damaging to the hereditary substances in the cells of several species. It causes lung cancer in rats and has a number of other harmful biological consequences. Researchers from the Division of Cancer Cause and Prevention of the National Cancer Institute recommended in April 1983 that, since formaldehyde is involved in DNA damage and inhibits its repair, since it potentiates the toxicity of X rays in human lung cells, and since it may act in concert with other chemical ingredients to produce mutagenic and carcinogenic effects, it should be "further investigated." Some shampoos contain formaldehyde. Among them at this writing, Breck Shampoo and L'Oreal Ultra Rich Gentle Shampoo. The CIR Expert Panel *(see)* concludes that this ingredient is safe to the great majority of consumers. The Panel believes, however, that "because of skin sensitivity of some individuals to this agent, the formulation and manufacture of a cosmetic product should be such as to ensure use at the minimal effective concentration of formaldehyde, not to exceed 0.2 percent measured as free formaldehyde. It cannot be concluded that formaldehyde is safe in cosmetic products intended to be aerosolized," the Panel said.

FORMIC ACID • Used as a rubefacient *(see)* in hair tonics; also a synthetic food flavoring. Colorless, pungent, highly corrosive, it occurs naturally in apples and other fruits. Also used as a decalcifier and for dehairing hides. Chronic absorption is known to cause albuminuria—protein in the urine. It caused cancer when administered orally in rats, mice, and hamsters in doses from 31 to 49 milligrams per kilogram of body weight. On the basis of available data, the CIR Expert Panel concludes that this ingredient is safe as presently used in cosmetics as a pH adjuster with a 64 ppm limit for the free acid.

FO-TI • *Polygonum multiforum.* **Ho Shu Wu.** One of the most popular herbs in China. Employed to treat skin ulcers and stomach ulcers as well as abscesses. The Chinese claim this herb has rejuvenating properties and can prevent gray hair and other premature signs of aging. It is also believed to increase fertility and maintain strength and vigor. Modern animal tests using fo-ti extracts have demonstrated antitumor activity. This herb also shows heart-protecting possibilities. Studies in humans have shown fo-ti to reduce high blood pressure, high blood cholesterol, and the incidence of heart disease among people prone to these conditions. It is used by herbalists as a purgative and emetic. In India it is used against colic and stomach upsets. In Brazil it is used to treat hemorrhoids and gout.

FOUNDATION MAKEUP • Aimed at covering blemishes, protecting the skin from drying out, and giving a glowing, healthy look. There is a cream-type foundation that vanishes from the skin but leaves a smooth, protective base for the application of pigmented makeup. Such creams are usually about 75 percent water, 15 percent stearic acid, and the remainder either sorbitan stearate or sorbitol. The pigmented foundation creams, which are designed to tint and cover the skin, usually contain about 50 percent water, mineral oil, stearic acid, lanolin, cetyl alcohol, propylene glycol, triethanolamine, borax, and insoluble pigments. They may also contain emulsifiers and detergents; humectants such as propylene glycol, glycerin, and sorbitol to absorb and retain water; lanolin derivatives; perfume; preservatives such as paraben; special barrier ingredients such as zinc stearate; cellulose derivatives and silicone; synthetic esters; thickeners such as sodium alginate, gum tragacanth, quince seed, and mucilage; and such waxes as beeswax and spermaceti. Stick-type makeup is made from isopropyl myristate, beeswax, carnauba wax, mineral oil, perfume, and dry pigment. Cake makeup, which is used by applying a wet sponge to the material and then applying the sponge to the face, is usually made of finely ground pigment, talc, kaolin, zinc, titanium oxide, precipitated calcium carbonate, and such inorganic pigments as iron oxides. To these may be added sorbitol, propylene glycol, lanolin, mineral oil, and perfume. If you check the above ingredients against those listed in the book, you will see that many—such as lanolin, perfume, beeswax, and paraben—are quite common allergens. However, by the very nature of the allergic response, you may not be allergic to a common allergen but to an uncommon one. The more ingredients to which you are exposed, of course, the greater the chances of developing an allergic response.

FRAGARIA CHILOENSIS AND VESCA • Flavoring. See Strawberry Juice.

FRAGRANCE • Any natural or synthetic substance or substances used solely to impart an odor to a cosmetic product.

FRAGRANCE-FREE • Implies that a cosmetic so labeled has no perceptible odor. Products so labeled may still contain small amounts of fragrances to mask the fatty odor of soap or other unpleasant odors.

FRANGIPANI • *Plumeria alba.* A fragrance ingredient from the flowers of a small American shrub. See Jasmine.

FRANGULA ALNUS • See Buckthorn.

FRAXINUS EXCELSIOR • Ash tree extract.

FREESIA REFRACTA • Sweet African herb.

FRENCH ROSE • An extract of *Rosa gallica* used in fragrances.

FRESHENER • See Skin Freshener.

FRUCTOSE • A sugar occurring naturally in large numbers of fruits and honey. It is the sweetest of the foodstuffs. It is also used as a medicine and preservative. It caused tumors in mice when injected under the skin in 5,000 milligram doses per kilogram of body weight.

FRUITY BLENDS • One of the basic perfume types, fruity blends have other notes present but are noted for their clean, fresh citrus notes or a smooth, mellow, peachlike warmth.

FUCUS SERRATUS • **Sea Oak. Sea Wrack.** An abundant seaweed, found in the Atlantic and Pacific oceans, with little bladders on its fronds that contain a gel. Herbalists claim the gel strengthens weak limbs, and relieves arthritis, sprains, and strains. They use it as a diuretic and as an aid in losing weight.

FULLER'S EARTH • Used in dry shampoos, hair colorings, beauty masks, and as a dusting powder; also used for lubricants and soaps. A white or brown, naturally-occurring earthy substance. A nonplastic variety of kaolin *(see)* containing an aluminum magnesium silicate. Used as an absorbent and to decolorize fats and oils. No longer permitted in cosmetics.

FUMARIC ACID • White, odorless, derived from many plants and essential to vegetable and animal tissue respiration; prepared industrially. An acidulant used as a leavening ingredient and a dry acid for dessert powders and confections (up to 3 percent). Also as an apple, peach, and vanilla flavoring ingredient for beverages, baked goods (1,300 ppm), and gelatin desserts (3,600 ppm). Used in baked goods as an antioxidant and as a substitute for tartaric acid *(see)*. No known toxicity. GRAS.

FUMITORY EXTRACT • *Fumaria officinalis.* **Earth Smoke. Horned Poppy. Wax Dolls.** An abundant weed in fields, the extract of the leaves, twigs, and flowers are used by herbalists in drinks for clearing obstructions from the liver or kidneys and to cure many diseases of the skin. It may also be used as an eyewash to ease conjunctivitis *(see)*. Used as an odorant. No known toxicity.

FUNGICIDES • Any substances that kill or inhibit the growth of fungi. Older types include a mixture of lime and sulfur, copper oxychloride, and Bordeaux mixture. Copper naphthenate has been used to impregnate textile fabrics used for tenting and military clothing. Copper undecylenate with zinc undecylenate is used in foot powders and sprays.

FURFURAL • **Artificial Ant Oil.** Used as a solvent, insecticide, fungicide, to decolor resins, and as a synthetic flavoring in food. A colorless liquid with a peculiar odor. Occurs naturally in angelica root, apples, coffee, peaches, and skim milk. Darkens when exposed to air. It irritates mucous membranes and acts on the central nervous system. Causes tearing and inflammation of the eyes and throat. Ingestion or absorption of .06 grams produces persistent headache. Used continually, it leads to nervous disturbances and eye disorders.

FURZE EXTRACT • **Gorse.** Extract of *Ulex Europaeus,* a spiny evergreen shrub with yellow flowers. This common plant is often used for fuel and fodder.

G

GADI LECUR • The name is used only on EU *(see)* products. See Cod Liver Oil.

GALACTOARABINANAN • **Larch Tree Extract.** A polysaccharide extracted with water from larch wood used in the minimum quantity required to be effective as an emulsifier, stabilizer, binder, or bodying agent in essential oils. Also used in artificial sweeteners.

GALACTOSE • White crystals occurring in milk sugar or lactose. Used as a diagnostic aid.

GALACTURONIC ACID • Obtained from plant pectins by hydrolysis, it is used in combination with allantoin *(see)* in creams and lotions.

GALANGAL • *Alpinia officinarum.* An herb cultivated in China, the rhizomes are unearthed in late summer and early autumn, cut into segments, and dried. It is used by some Chinese herbalists to break up intestinal gas and to treat heartburn and nausea.

GALBANUM GUM • See Galbanum Oil.

GALBANUM OIL • A yellowish to green or brown, aromatic, bitter gum resin from an Asiatic plant used as an incense. The oil is a fruit, nut, and spice flavoring for beverages, ice cream, ices, candy, baked goods, and condiments. Has been used medicinally to break up intestinal gas and as an expectorant. No known toxicity.

GALEGA EXTRACT • **Goat's Rue.** Extract of the herb *Galega officinalis.* This plant contains alkaloids, saponins, flavone, glycosides, tannin *(see all),* and bitters. It is used to reduce blood sugar levels. It is also a powerful milk inducer in breast-feeding women.

GALIUM APARINE EXTRACT • From the herb *Gallium aparine.* See Cleavers.

GALLIC ACID • Obtained from tannins in nutgalls and also from broths of *Penicillin glaucum* or *Aspergillus niger.* Used as an astringent and antioxidant. See Propyl Gallate.

GAMBIR EXTRACT • *Uncaria Gambir.* A flavoring. See Catechu Extract.

GAMMA LINOLENIC ACID • See Linolenic Acid.

GAMMA-ORIZANOL • See Oryzanol.

GANODERMA LUCIDIUM • See Mushroom Extract.

GARCINIA GAMBOGIA EXTRACT • **Kokum Butter.** A large, Asiatic tree extract used in creams and lotions.

GARDEN BALSAM EXTRACT • From the flowers of *Impatiens balsamina.* See Impatiens.

GARDENIA • The white or yellow flowers used in fragrances. Obtained from a large genus of Old World tropical trees and shrubs. No known toxicity.

GARLIC EXTRACT • An extract from *Allium sativum,* a yellowish liquid with a strong odor used in fruit and garlic flavorings. It is being tested as an antibiotic and has been used to counteract intestinal worms.

GAULTHERIA PROCUMBENS • See Wintergreen Oil.

GEL • A semisolid, apparently homogeneous substance that may be elastic and jellylike (gelatin) or more or less rigid (silica gel), and that is formed in various ways, such as by coagulation or evaporation.

GELATIN • Used in protein shampoos because it sticks to the hair and gives it "more body," peelable face masks, and as a fingernail strengthener. Gelatin is a protein obtained by boiling skin, tendons, ligaments, or bones with water. It is colorless or slightly yellow, tasteless, and absorbs 5 to 10 times its weight of cold water. Also used as a food thickener and stabilizer and a base for fruit gelatins and puddings. Employed medicinally to treat malnutrition and brittle fingernails. No known toxicity.

GELATIN/KERATIN AMINOACIDS/LYSINE HYDROXYPROPLYTRIMONIUM CHLORIDE • A gelatin *(see)* made from a mixture of animal skins.

GELATIN/LYSINE/POLYACRYLAMIDE HYDROXYPROPLYTRIMONIUM CHLORIDE • A quaternary ammonium product made from gelatin and lysine *(see both).*

GELLAN GUM • A gum produced by the fermentation of a carbohydrate with *Pseudomonas elodea.*

GELLIDIELA ACEROSA AND EXTRACT • Algae Extract. Seaweederm. An extract derived from *Gellidiela acerosa*. Used in emollients.

GENTIAN • *Gentiana campestris. Gentiana lutea.* **Baldmony. Felwort. Field Gentian.** An annual plant that grows in dry, chalky soil in Great Britain, it is used in modern medicine. Herbalists make an infusion of the roots and herb as a digestive tonic for heartburn or gas after eating. They also use it to stimulate the appetite. In 1992, the FDA proposed a ban on *Gentiana lutea* in oral menstrual drug products because it has not been shown to be safe and effective for its stated claims. It is used in cosmetic creams and bath products to soothe the skin.

GERANIOL • Used in perfumery to compound artificial attar of roses and artificial orange blossom oil. Also used in depilatories to mask odors. Oily sweet, with a rose odor, it occurs naturally in apples, bay leaves, cherries, grapefruit, ginger, lavender, and a number of other essential oils. Geraniol is omitted from hypoallergenic cosmetics. Can cause allergic reactions.

GERANIUM OIL • Used in perfumery, dusting powder, tooth powder, and ointments. It is the light yellow to deep yellow oil of plants of the genus *Pelargonium* or of rose geranium leaves, with the characteristic odor of rose and geraniol. A teaspoon may cause illness in an adult, and less than an ounce may kill. May affect those allergic to geraniums.

GERANYL ACETATE • Geraniol Acetate. Clear, colorless liquid with the odor of lavender, it is a constituent of several essential oils. Used in perfumery and flavoring. See Geraniol.

GERANYL BUTYRATE • Geraniol Butyrate. Colorless liquid found in several essential oils, it is used in perfumes, soaps, and flavorings and as a synthetic attar of rose. See Geraniol.

GERANYL FORMATE • Geraniol Formate. Colorless liquid with a roselike odor, insoluble in alcohol, it occurs in several essential oils. Used in perfumes, soaps, and flavorings as a synthetic neroli bigarade oil *(see)*. See Geraniol.

GERANYL PHENYLACETATE • Phenylacetic Acid. A synthetic flavoring, yellow liquid, with a honey-rose odor. Used in fruit flavorings for beverages, ice cream, ices, candy, baked goods, and chewing gum. See Geraniol for toxicity.

GERANYL PROPIONATE • Geraniol Propionate. Colorless liquid with a roselike odor, it is soluble in most oils and is used in perfumery and flavoring. See Geraniol.

GERANYL TIGLATE • See Geraniol.

GERIANAL • See Citral.

GERIANALDEHYDE • See Citral.

GERMANDER EXTRACT • An extract of the herb *Teucrium scorodonia* or *T. chamaedrys.* **Wall Germander.** A member of the mint family, it has long been used by herbalists as far back as Hippocrates and Pliny. The Greeks used it as a tonic. In the mid-eighteenth century, herbalists used it to treat gout. It is an astringent, antiseptic, diuretic, and stimulant, and has been used in the treatment of jaundice, excess fluid due to heart failure, and ailments of the spleen. It continues to be used in folk medicine to heal ulcers and sores. Cases of its use in tea or capsules has been reported to the Centers for Disease Control as causing liver toxicity.

GERMANIUM • Suma. Occurs in the earth's crust, it is a naturally occurring isotope that is recovered from residues from refining of zinc and other sources. It is also present in some coals. It is used in infrared transmitting glass and electronic devices. It is used by Third World women as an eye makeup, a practice that is being discouraged because of its lead content. Also used as an intestinal astringent.

GERMANIUM MACULATUM • The roots of this plant were used by herbalists to treat canker sores, sunburn, and inflammation. It is being used in "antiaging" products.

GERMANIUM SESQUIOXIDE • See Germanium.

GEUM RIVALE • *Avena Geum Rivale.* See Avens and Clove.

GHATTI GUM • Indian Gum. The gummy exudate from the stems of a plant abundant in India and Ceylon. Used as an emulsifier and in butter, butterscotch, and fruit flavorings for beverages. Has caused an occasional allergy, but when ingested in large amounts, it has not caused obvious distress.

GIGARTINA STELLATA • Red algae mostly from the Pacific. See Algae.

GINGER • *Zingiber officinale.* **Gan Jiang.** Native to Asia but cultivated in many parts of the tropics, Hippocrates used ginger as a medicine. Ginger tea is soothing for colds and sore throats. It is an herb used to treat low blood sugar. It increases the availability of dietary nutrients for digestion and metabolism. Gingerroot is used by herbalists to treat headaches, diarrhea, and nausea, including motion sickness. Some studies have shown that gingerroot is a mild stimulant for the heart and brain and may even help ease learning. Ginger tea is widely used as a remedy for colds, producing perspiration, and for inducing menstruation if suppressed by a cold. Externally, ginger is a rubefacient *(see),* and has been credited with relieving toothache. Modern studies have shown that ginger inhibits prostaglandins, as do NSAIDs *(see both),* and thus reduces inflammation. Japanese scientists have found that extract of ginger inhibits stomach lesions. They concluded that the use of ginger in folk medicine was effective because of a constituent, zingiberone. Scientists have also found that ginger slows the formation of platelet clumping, and thus may help to prevent blood clots. In 1992, the FDA issued a notice that ginger had not been shown to be safe and effective as claimed in OTC digestive aid products. Contraindicated in persons with acute bowel disorder. It should also be avoided in individuals suffering from skin disease. An excessive dose can cause irritation of the mucous membrane lining of the stomach. It can also promote menstruation.

GINGER OIL • Obtained from the dried rhizomes of *Zingiber officinale,* it is used in flavorings. Also used in perfumes. Employed medicinally to break up intestinal gas. No known toxicity.

GINKGO EXTRACT • Maidenhair. An extract of *Ginkgo biloba.* A sacred tree of the Chinese, the fruit has an offensive odor but is resistant to smoke, disease, and insects. Used in perfumes and as an insecticide. No known toxicity.

GINSENG • Root of the ginseng plant grown in China, Korea, and the United States. It produces a resin, a sugar starch, glue, and volatile oil. Widely used in oriental medicine as an aromatic bitter. It is used in American cosmetics as a demulcent *(see)*. No known toxicity.

GLANDULAR SUBSTANCES • Extracts of animal glands widely used in the cosmetic industry for various purposes.

GLAUBER'S SALT • Crystalline sodium sulfate *(see)* used as an opacifier in shampoos and as a detergent in bath salts. Named for a German chemist, Johann R. Glauber, who died in 1668. Also used medicinally as a laxative. Skin irritations may occur.

GLECHOMA HEDERACEA • See Ground Ivy Extract.

GLEDITSIA AUSTRALIS • A thorny tree with green spikes of flowers. Sweet extract used as flavoring and as an emollient ingredient.

GLIADIN • A protein derived from wheat. See Wheat Germ Extract.

GLOSS WHITE • No longer permitted as a coloring in cosmetics.

GLUCAMINE • An organic compound prepared from glucose *(see)*.

GLUCARIC ACID • See Saccharin.

GLUCAROLACTONE • See Saccharin and Lactic Acid.

GLUCONIC ACID AND SALTS • A light, amber liquid with the faint odor of vinegar, produced from corn. It is water-soluble and used as a dietary supplement and a sequestrant *(see)*. The magnesium salt of gluconic acid has been used as an antispasmodic. No known toxicity. GRAS.

GLUCONIC LACTONE • Derived from the oxidation of glucose. See Gluconic Acid and Salts.

GLUCOSAMINE • Found in chitin *(see)*, it is used in medicine to treat arthritis.

GLUCOSE • Used as a flavoring, to soothe the skin, and as a filler in cosmetics. Occurs naturally in blood, grape, and corn sugars. A source of energy for plants and animals. Sweeter than sucrose *(see)*. No known toxicity in cosmetics, but confectioners frequently suffer erosions and fissures around their nails, and the nails loosen and sometimes fall off.

GLUCOSE GLUTAMATE • Used as a humectant in hand creams and lotions, it occurs naturally in animal blood, grape and corn sugars, and is a source of energy for plants and animals. It is sweeter than sucrose. Glucose syrup is used to flavor sausage, hamburger, and other processed meats. Also used as an extender in maple syrup and medicinally as a nutrient. Glutamate is the salt of glutamic acid and is used to enhance natural food flavors. The FDA has asked for further studies as to its potential mutagenic, teratogenic, subacute, and reproductive effects. The CIR Expert Panel *(see)* concludes that there is insufficient data to support the safety of this ingredient use in cosmetics.

GLUCOSIDES • Compounds with sugar and alcohol.

GLUCURONIC ACID • A carbohydrate widely distributed in the animal kingdom.

GLUCURONOLACTONE • See Glucuronic Acid and Lactic Acid.

GLUTAMATE • Ammonium and monopotassium salt of glutamic acid *(see)*. Used to enhance natural flavors and to improve the taste of tobacco. It is used as an antioxidant in cosmetics to prevent spoilage. It is being studied by the FDA for mutagenic, teratogenic, subacute, and reproductive effects.

GLUTAMIC ACID • A white, practically odorless, free-flowing crystalline powder, a nonessential amino acid *(see)* usually manufactured from vegetable protein. A salt substitute, it has been used to treat epilepsy and to correct stomach acids. It is used to enhance food flavors, as an antioxidant in cosmetics, and as a softener in permanent wave solutions to help protect against hair damage. It is being studied by the FDA for mutagenic, teratogenic, subacute, and reproductive effects.

GLUTAMINE • A nonessential amino acid *(see)* used as a medicine and as a culture medium. Nontoxic.

GLUTAMYL HISTAMINE • A hair conditioning ingredient. See Glutamic Acid.

GLUTARAL • **Glutaraldehyde.** An amino acid *(see)* that occurs in green sugar beets. Used in a wide variety of cosmetics such as creams and emollients as a germicide and preservative. It has a faint, agreeable odor. In a 2-year drinking test in rats, there was an increase in leukemia only in females. In humans, there is some evidence of skin irritation and sensitization. Occupational data and animal studies indicate that inhalation of this ingredient can cause respiratory irritation in addition to its skin effects. The CIR Expert Panel *(see)* is concerned about the carcinogenic potential of this ingredient when used in "leave-on" products. Based upon the animal and human data, the Panel concludes that glutaral is safe for use at concentrations up to 0.5 percent in "rinse-off" products. There is insufficient data to determine the safety of it in "leave-on" products. The Committee said it should not be used in aerosol products. See Glutaric Acid.

GLUTARALDEHYDE • A major allergen in the medical and dental workplace. It is used as a base in some waterless hand soaps. See Glutaral.

GLUTARIC ACID • **Pentanedioic Acid.** A crystalline fatty acid that is soluble in oil. Widely used in oriental medicine as an aromatic bitter. It is used in American cosmetics as a demulcent *(see)*. No known toxicity.

GLUTATHIONE • Cloves, caraway, dill weed, parsley, lemongrass oil, and celery have been found to have significant amounts of this protein. Acts to stimulate enzymes and is used in "antiaging" products and as an emulsifier.

GLUTEN • A mixture of proteins from wheat flour.

GLY- • The abbreviation for glycine *(see)*.

GLYCERETH-12-26 • Polyethylene glycols mixed with glycerin. The viscosity depends upon the number after glycereth. See Glycerin and Polyethylene Glycol.

GLYCERETH-7 TRIACETATE • A solvent used in emollients. See Polyethylene Glycol and Triacetic Acid.

GLYCERIDES • Any of a large class of compounds that are esters *(see)* of the sweet alcohol glycerin. They are also made synthetically. They are used in cosmetic creams as texturizers and emollients. No known toxicity.

GLYCERIN • Glycerol. Any by-product of soap manufacture, it is a sweet, warm-tasting, oily fluid obtained by adding alkalies *(see)* to fats and fixed oils. A solvent, humectant, and emollient in many cosmetics, it absorbs moisture from the air and, therefore, helps keep moisture in creams and other products, even if the consumer leaves the cap off the container. Also helps the products to spread better. A humectant in foods and a solvent for food colors and flavors. Among the many products containing glycerin are cream rouges, face packs and masks, freckle lotions, hand creams and lotions, hair lacquers, liquid face powder, mouthwashes, protective creams, skin fresheners, and toothpastes. In concentrated solutions it is irritating to the mucous membranes, but as used it is nontoxic, nonirritating, and nonallergenic. The FDA issued a notice in 1992 that glycerin has not been shown to be safe and effective as claimed in OTC poison ivy, poison oak, and poison sumac products as well as in diaper-rash drug products.

GLYCEROL • See Glycerin.

GLYCERYL ADIPATE • The ester of glycerin and adipic acid *(see both)*. See also Ester.

GLYCERYL ALGINATE • The ester of glycerin and alginic acid *(see both)*. See also Ester.

GLYCERYL-p-AMINOBENZOATE • A semisolid, waxy mass or syrup with a faint aromatic odor, liquefying and congealing very slowly, used in cosmetic sunscreen preparations. See Benzoic Acid.

GLYCERYL ARACHIDONATE • The ester of glycerin and arachidonic acid *(see both)*. See also Ester.

GLYCERYL BEHENATE • The ester of glycerin and behenic acid *(see both)*. See also Ester.

GLYCERYL CAPRATE • The monoester of glycerin and caprylic acid *(see both)*.

GLYCERYL CAPRYLATE • See Glycerin and Caprylic Acid.

GLYCERYL CAPRYLATE/CAPRATE • A mixture of caprylic acid and capric acid *(see both)*.

GLYCERYL COCONATE • See Glycerin and Coconut Oil.

GLYCERYL COLLAGENATE • The ester *(see)* of glycerin and collagen *(see both)*. Used as a hair-conditioning ingredient and as an emollient in skin creams.

GLYCERYL DIBEHENATE • A mixture of glycerin and beheneic acid *(see both)* used as an emollient ingredient.

GLYCERYL DILAURATE • See Glycerin and Lauric Acid.

GLYCERYL DIMYRISTATE • See Glycerin and Myristic Acid.

GLYCERYL DIOLEATE • The diester of glycerin and oleic acid *(see both)*.

GLYCERYL DIPALMITATE • See Glycerin and Palmitic Acid.

GLYCERYL DISTEARATE • The diester of glycerin and stearic acid *(see both)*.

GLYCERYL ERUCATE • See Glycerin and Erucic Acid.

GLYCERYL HYDROGENATED ROSINATE • A mixture of glycerin and rosin *(see both)*.

GLYCERYL HYDROSTEARATE • See Glyceryl Monostearate.

GLYCERYL HYDROXYSTEARATE • The monoester of glycerin and hydroxy-stearic acid *(see both)*.

GLYCERYL ISOSTEARATE • See Glyceryl Monostearate.

GLYCERYL LANOLATE • *See* Glycerin and Lanolin.

GLYCERYL LINOLEATE • *See* Glycerin and Linoleic Acid.

GLYCERYL MONOSTEARATE • An emulsifying and dispersing ingredient used in baby creams, face masks, foundation cake makeup, liquid powders, hair conditioners, hand lotions, mascara, and nail whiteners. It is a mixture of two glyceryls, a white, waxlike solid, or beads, and is soluble in hot organic solvents such as alcohol. Lethal when injected in large doses into mice. No known toxicity.

GLYCERYL MYRISTATE • See Glycerin and Myristic Acid.

GLYCERYL OLEATE • Used as an emulsifier in cosmetics up to 5 percent. Found to be nonirritating in humans. Based on human and animal studies, the CIR Expert Panel *(see)* concludes that this additive is safe as a cosmetic ingredient in the present practices of use and concentration. See Glycerin and Oleic Acid.

GLYCERYL PABA • The ester of glycine and p-aminobenzoic acid *(see both)*.

GLYCERYL PALMITATE LACTATE • The lactic acid ester *(see)* of glyceryl palmitate.

GLYCERYL PALMITATE/STEARATE • An ester of glycerin and a blend of palmitic and stearic acids *(see all)*.

GLYCERYL PHOSPHATES • See Glycerin and Phosphates.

GLYCERYL RICINOLEATE • An emollient. The CIR Expert Panel *(see)* concludes that there is insufficient data to determine the safety of this ingredient in cosmetics. See Glycerin.

GLYCERYL SESQUIOLEATE • See Glycerin.

GLYCERYL STARCH • See Starch and Glycerol.

GLYCERYL STEARATE • Widely used as an emulsifier and skin conditioning ingredient. It is in makeup, lotions, powders, and creams as well as foot powders and cuticile softeners. Based on available animal data and human experience, the CIR Expert Panel *(see)* concludes this ingredient is safe for use in applications to humans in the present practices of use and concentration. See Glycerin.

GLYCERYL STEARATE LACTATE • The lactic acid ester of glyceryl stearate. See Lactic Acid and Glycerin.

GLYCERYL STEARATE SE • A widely used emulsifier containing glyceryl stearate that contains some sodium and some potassium. Based on available animal data and human experience, the CIR Expert Panel *(see)* concludes this ingredient is safe for use in current concentrations. See Glycerin Monostearate.

GLYCERYL THIOGLYCOLATE • Found in permanent wave solutions, this is a common allergen among European hair stylists and is the second most common among U.S. beautificians. The CIR Expert Panel *(see)* concludes this ingredient is a potential sensitizer but can be safely used infrequently. Hairdressers who apply it to clients frequently are the most at risk for sensitization. See Glycerin and Thioglycolic Acid.

GLYCERYL TRIACETYL HYDROXYSTEARATE • See Glycerin and Octadecanoic Acid.

GLYCERYL TRIMYRISTATE • See Glycerin and Myristic Acid.

GLYCERYL TRIOCTANOATE • See Glycerin.

GLYCERYL TRIOLEATE • See Glycerin and Oleic Acid.

GLYCERYL TRIUNDECANOATE • The triester of glycerin and undecanoic acid *(see both)*.

GLYCERYL/SORBITAL OLEATE/HYDROXYSTEARATE • A mixed esterification product of glycerin and sorbitol with hydroxystearic acid and oleic acids *(see all)*.

GLYCINE • Used as a texturizer in cosmetics. An amino acid *(see)* classified as nonessential. Made up of sweet-tasting crystals, it is used as a dietary supplement and as a gastric antacid. No known toxicity.

GLYCO- • Prefix from the Greek meaning "sweetness."

GLYCOFUROL • The ethoxylated ether of tetrahydrofurfuryl alcohol. See Furfural.

GLYCOGEN • Distributed throughout cell protoplasm, it is an animal starch found especially in liver and muscle. Used as a violet dye and in biochemical research. No known toxicity.

GLYCOL DILAURATE • See Ethylene Glycol and Lauric Acid.

GLYCOL DIOCTANOATE • See Ethylene Glycol.

GLYCOL DISTEARATE • A widely used surfactant made from glycerin and stearic acid. It is also used as an opacifier *(see)*.

GLYCOL DITALLOWATE • The diester of ethylene glycol and tallow acid *(see both)*.

GLYCOL ESTERS • See Glycols and Ester.

GLYCOL ETHERS • Cellosolve®. Carbitol®. Dowanol®. Ektasolve®. EGME. EGMEA. EGEE. EGEEA. EGPE. EGDME. EGDEE. DEG. DEGME. DEGEE. DEGBE. DEGDME. TEGDME. PGME. DPG. DEPGME. 2-methoxyethanol. 2-methoxyethyl acetate. 2-ethoxyethanol. 2-ethoxyethyl acetate. 2-propoxyethanol. 1,2-dimethoxyethane. 2-(2-methoxyethoxy)ethanol. 2-(2-ethoxyethoxy)ethanol. 2-(2-butoxyethoxy)ethanol. bis(2-methoxyethl)-ether. Ethylene Glycol Monomethyl Ether. Ethylene Glycol Monopropyl Ether. Diethylene Glycol. Dipropylene Glycol. Dipropylene Glycol Monomethyl Ether. Glycol ether is the name for a large group of chemicals. Most glycol ether compounds are clear, colorless liquids. Some have mild, pleasant odors or no smell at all; others (mainly the acetates) have strong odors. The common belief that glycol ethers never evaporate fast enough to create harmful levels in the air is false, according to the Hazard Evaluation System and Information Service of California. Some evaporate quickly and can easily reach hazardous levels in the air; others evaporate very slowly and therefore are less hazardous by inhalation. EGME and EGEE are two that evaporate very quickly. The glycol ethers are widely used industrial solvents. Each may be used alone or as an ingredient in products such as paints, varnishes, dyes, stains, inks, deodorant sprays, and semiconductor chip coatings; as cleaners for degreasing, dry cleaning, film cleaning, and circuit board manufacture; as jet fuel deicing additives, brake fluids, perfumes, and cosmetics. Also widely used in metalworking fluids. Glycol ethers enter your body when they evaporate into the air you breathe, and they are rapidly absorbed into your body if the liquids contact your skin. Cases of poisoning have been reported where skin contact was the main route of exposure, even though there was no effect on the skin itself. The effects of overexposure can include anemia, mild intoxication, and irritation of the skin, eyes, nose, and throat. Some glycol ethers (EGPE, DEGBE, PGME, and DPGME) are hazardous to the male and female reproductive system. Within the class of glycol ethers, toxicity varies. All propylene glycol ethers are currently believed to be relatively safe, according to California's Hazard Evaluation System and Information Service. Most ethylene glycol ethers with "methyl" in their names are relatively toxic.

GLYCOL HYDROXYSTEARATE • The ester of ethylene glycol and hydroxy-stearic acid. See Ethylene Glycol and Stearic Acid.

GLYCOL MONTANATE • The ester *(see)* of glyol and montan wax *(see both)*. Used as emulsion stabilizers and opacifying ingredient in emollients.

GLYCOL RICINOLEATE • The ester of ethylene glycol and ricinoleic acid *(see both)*.

GLYCOL SALICYLATE • The ester of polyethylene glycol and salicylic acid.

GLYCOL STEARATE • One of the most widely used bases for cosmetic creams at concentrations ranging from less than 0.1 to 10 percent. Low toxicity. Based on available animal data and human experience, the CIR Expert Panel *(see)* concludes this ingredient is safe. See Glycols and Stearic Acid.

GLYCOL STEARATE SE • The self-emulsifying grade of glycol stearate that contains some sodium and/or potassium. See Glycols and Stearates.

GLYCOL/BUTYLENE GLYCOL MONTANATE • A mixture of esters of montan acid wax with ethyelene glycol and butylene glycol *(see all)*. Used as a surfactant *(see)*.

GLYCOLIC ACID • Contained in sugarcane juice and fruit, it is an odorless, slightly water-absorbing acid used to control the acid/alkali balance in cosmetics and whenever a cheap organic acid is needed. It is also used in copper brightening, decontamination procedures, and in dyeing. It is a mild irritant to the skin and mucous membranes. One of the more controversial services offered by skin care salons is the glycolic acid peel, a procedure that is also being performed by dermatologists. Glycolic acid is a compound related to alpha-hydroxy acids. As of this writing, glycolic acid is not considered a drug. Its marketers maintain it is a cosmetic because it does not change the structure of the skin. Has the potential of causing sun sensitivity and irritation. See Alpha Hydroxy Acids.

GLYCOLIPIDS • A mixture of fats, oils, and carbohydrates used in emollients.

GLYCOLS • **Propylene Glycol. Glycerin. Ethylene Glycol. Carbitol. Diethylene Glycol.** Literally it means "glycerin" plus "alcohol." A group of syrupy alcohols derived from hydrocarbons *(see)* that are widely used in cosmetics as humectants. The FDA cautions manufacturers that glycols may cause adverse reactions in users.

Propylene glycol and glycerin *(see both)* are considered safe. Other glycols in low concentrations may be harmless for external application but ethylene glycol, carbitol, and diethylene glycol are hazardous in concentrations exceeding 5 percent even in preparations for use on small areas of the body. Therefore, in sunscreen lotions and protective creams where the area of application is extensive, they should not be used at all. Wetting ingredients *(see)* increase the absorption of glycols and therefore their toxicity.

GLYCOPROTEINS • Sweet proteins from milk sugar.

GLYCOSAMINOGLYCANS • An ingredient in wrinkle creams. Derived from various animal tissues. See Mucopolysaccharides.

GLYCOSIDES • Many flowering plants contain cardiac glycosides. The best known are foxglove, lily-of-the-valley, and squill. Cardiac glycosides have the ability to increase the force and power of the heartbeat without increasing the amount of oxygen needed by the heart muscle. Among the glycosides in plants are cyanogens, goitrogens, estrogens, and saponins. They are found in lima beans, cassava, flax, legumes, broccoli, and other brassicas, most legumes and grasses.

GLYCOSPHINGOLIPIDS • GSL Sugary, fatty acid compounds, one of which was said to be developed by Christiaan Barnard, the pioneer heart surgeon, in Switzerland, to counteract wrinkles. Some companies, charging a great deal of money, claim their product contains Dr. Barnard's GSL, which can "accelerate cell renewal." If that were proven, it would have to be a drug, not a cosmetic.

GLYCYL GLYCINE • A combination of amides and amino acids *(see both)* used in hair conditioners and skin conditioners.

GLYCYRRHETINIC ACID • Used as a flavoring, to soothe skin, and as a vehicle for other chemicals. Prepared from licorice root, it is soluble in chloroform, alcohol, and acetic acid *(see)*. It has been used medicinally to treat a disease of the adrenal gland. No known toxicity when used in cosmetics.

GLYCYRRHETINYL STEARATE • The stearic acid ester of glycyrrhetinic acid *(see)*.

GLYCYRRHIZIC ACID • Used as a flavoring and coloring, and to soothe the skin in cosmetics. Extracted from licorice, the crystalline material is soluble in hot water and alcohol. See Glycyrrhetinic Acid.

GLYOXAL • **Oxaldehyde.** Prepared by the oxidation of acetaldehyde *(see)*, it consists of yellow prisms or irregular pieces that turn white when cooled. Used in the manufacture of cosmetics and as germicides and glues. Moderately irritating to the skin. Also may be a sensitizer. Based on available animal data and human experience, the CIR Expert Panel *(see)* concludes this ingredient is safe.

GLYOXYLIC ACID • Used as a coloring. Syrup or crystals that occur in unripe fruit, young leaves, and baby sugar beets. Malodorous and strong corrosive. Forms a thick syrup, very soluble in water, sparingly soluble in alcohol. It absorbs water from the air and condenses with urea to form allantoin *(see)*, and gives a nice blue color with sulfuric acid. It is a skin irritant and corrosive.

GNAPHALLIUM POLYCEPHALUM • See Cudweed Extract.

GOAT BUTTER • The fat from goat's milk used in emollients.

GOAT MILK • The whole milk obtained from goats used as a skin conditioning ingredient.

GOAT'S RUE • See Galega Extract.

GOATWEED EXTRACT • See Saint John's Wort.

GOLD • Used as a coloring and to give shine to cosmetics. The soft yellow metal is found in the earth's crust and used in jewelry, gold plating, and in medicine to treat arthritis. The pure metal is nontoxic, but the gold salts can cause allergic skin reactions.

GOLD OF PLEASURE • *Camelina Sativa.* A European false flax cultivated for its oil-rich seeds. Also grown in North America. Used as a skin conditioning ingredient.

GOLDEN SEAL • *Hydrastis canadensis.* **Puccoon Root. Yellow Root.** American Indians were the first to use it for sore eyes. Early pioneers, along with many Indian tribes, used it as a general tonic. The rhizome and root are used by herbalists to treat heartburn and acid indigestion, colitis, duodenal ulcers, heavy menstrual periods, and as a general tonic for the female reproductive tract. It is also used for penile discharge, eczema, and skin disorders. Herbalists claim it dries and cleanses the mucous membranes and is good for liver dysfunction and for all inflammations. It reputedly has potent antibiotic and antiseptic properties. It does contain berberine *(see).* It is contraindicated during pregnancy and for persons suffering from high blood pressure and ischemia (insufficient blood flow). The FDA issued a notice in 1992 that *H. canadensis* and hydrastis fluid extract have not been shown to be safe and effective as claimed in OTC digestive aid products and in oral menstrual products.

GOLDENROD • *Solidago virgauria* is a perennial that includes 125 species. It was valued for its medicinal properties by women in Elizabethan London. The name Solidago means "makes whole" and herbalists say it helps to heal wounds and, in fact, at one time it was called "woundwort." It is used by herbalists as an antiseptic. The pulped leaves, stalks, and flowers are good for staunching blood. American Indians used it to treat bee stings.

GOTU KOLA • *Centella asiastica.* **Thickleaved. Pennywort.** An herb grown in Pakistan, India, Malaysia, and parts of Eastern Europe, it is commonly used for diseases of the skin, blood, and nervous system. In homeopathy, it is used for psoriasis, cervicitis, pruritus vaginitis, blisters, and other skin conditions. Gotu kola is used in the Far East to treat leprosy and tuberculosis. It is also used as a sedative.

GOURD EXTRACT • The extract of various species of *Cucurbitaceae.*

GRAM • **g.** A metric unit of mass. One U.S. ounce equals 28.4 grams; one U.S. pound equals 454 grams. There are 1,000 milligrams (mg) in one gram.

GRAMICIDIN • **Cortisporin Cream. Mycolog II Cream. Neosporin Ophthalmic Solution. Spectrocin Ointment.** Introduced in 1949, it is a naturally occurring antibiotic produced by bacteria. Available only in combined preparations, it is used with other antibiotics to treat skin and eye infections. Some gramicidin medications contain corticosteroids *(see)* to relieve itching and inflammation. Gramicidin is also combined with antifungal drugs such as nystatin *(see)* to treat mixed fungal and bacterial infections. Potential adverse reactions include rash and irritation.

GRAPE EXTRACT • The extract of the pulp of *Vitis vinifera* used as a coloring.

GRAPE JUICE • The liquid expressed from fresh grapes used as a coloring.

GRAPE LEAF EXTRACT • The extract obtained from the leaves of *Vitis vinifera.*

GRAPEFRUIT EXTRACT • The extract of the seeds of the grapefruit, *Citrus paradisi.*

GRAPEFRUIT JUICE • The liquid expressed from the fresh pulp of *Citrus paradisi.*

GRAPEFRUIT OIL • An ingredient in fragrances obtained by expression from the fresh peel of the grapefruit. The yellow, sometimes reddish liquid is also used in fruit flavorings. No known toxicity.

GRAPEFRUIT PEEL EXTRACT • The extract of *Citrus decumana* or *C. paradisi.* See Grapefruit Oil.

GRAPE-SEED OIL • An ingredient in fragrances obtained by expression from the fresh peel of the grapefruit. The yellow, sometimes reddish liquid is also used in fruit flavorings. No known toxicity.

GRAPHITE • **Black Lead.** Obtained by mining, especially in Canada and Ceylon. Usually soft, black, lustrous scales. A pigment for cosmetics. Also used in lead pencils, stone polish, and as an explosive. The dust is mildly irritating to the lungs. No longer permitted in cosmetics.

GRAS • The Generally Recognized As Safe List was established in 1958 by Congress. Those substances that were being added to food over a long time, which under conditions of their intended use were generally recognized as safe by qualified scientists, would be exempt from premarket clearance. Congress had acted on a very marginal response—on the basis of returns from those scientists sent questionnaires. Approximately 355 out of 900 responded, and only about 100 of those responses had substantive comments. Three items were removed from the originally published list. Since then, developments in the scientific fields and in consumer awareness have brought to light the inadequacies of the testing of food additives and, ironically, the complete lack of testing of the Generally Recognized As Safe List. President Richard Nixon directed the FDA to reevaluate items on the GRAS list. The reevaluation was completed, and a number of items were removed from the list. A number were put on a priority list for further studies, but as of this writing, nothing new has been reported.

GRAVEOLENS SATIVA • See Oatmeal.

GRAY HAIR RINSES • To cover yellowish tinge that often appears in gray hair. Usually compounded with acids such as adipic or citric *(see both)* and color rinses such as Acid Violet 9 and Acid Black 52 *(see both).*

GREAT BURNET • *Sanguisorba officinalis. Poterium Officinale.* Used in medieval medicine as an astringent herb to stop hemorrhages. Also used in salves for ulcers and wounds.

GREAT PERIWINKLE • *Vinca major.* An everblooming perennial herb or small shrub, it is popular in gardens. The tropical periwinkle is an example of a folk medicine that made its way into modern medicine. In 1953, Dr. Faustino Garcia reported at the Pacific Science Congress that the plant, taken orally, is a folk medicine in the Philippines for the treatment of diabetes. Researchers at the Eli Lilly Company screened the plant and found that it showed good anticancer activity in test animals. The result was the discovery of two alkaloids that are useful in treating cancer. It has also been found useful in treating diabetes. Periwinkle has been found to stop external hemorrhages, apparently because it contains tannins *(see).* The effects of controlling menstrual hemorrhaging may be due to vincamine, which dilates blood vessels.

GREEN • Chrome oxide green used in face powders. See Colors.

GREEN BEAN EXTRACT • The extract of the unripe beans of the domesticated species of *Phaseolus.*

GREEN SOAP • A liquid soap made with potassium hydroxide and a vegetable oil other than coconut or palm-kernel oil.

GRINDELIA • A coarse, bumpy, or resinous herb grown in the western United States. It has flower heads with spreading tips. The dried leaves and stumps of these various gum weeds are used internally as a remedy in bronchitis and topically to soothe poison ivy rashes. Grindelia contains resin and an oil used in cosmetics. No known toxicity.

GROUND IVY EXTRACT • *Glechoma hederacea.* **Alehoof. Benth. Cat's Foot. Devil's Candlesticks. Hale House. Hay House. May House. Hay Maids. Hedge Maids. Thunder Vine. Tun-Hoof.** A common plant in wastelands, it is used by herbalists for coughs, headaches, and backaches caused by sluggishness of the liver or obstruction of the kidneys. It contains tannin, volatile oil, bitter principle, and saponin *(see all).* It is used to treat coughs and bronchitis. Mixed with yarrow, the herb makes a poultice that has been used by folk doctors for "gathering tumors" and to clear the head and relieve aching backs. The astringency of the herb helps in the treatment of diarrhea and hemorrhoids.

GROUNDSEL EXTRACT • Extract of *Senecio vulgaris,* a North American maritime shrub or tree.

GSL • See Glycosphingolipids.

GUAIACOL • Obtained from hardwood tar or made synthetically. White, or yellow, crystalline mass with a characteristic odor. Darkens when exposed to light. Used as an antiseptic both externally and internally. Ingestion causes irritation of the intestinal tract and heart failure. Penetrates the skin. Produces pain and burning and then loss of sensitivity when applied to mucous membranes. Causes the nose to run and the mouth to salivate. Deep irritant on the skin. Also used as a flavoring.

GUAIACWOOD OIL • Yellow to amber semisolid mass with a floral odor. Soluble in alcohol. Derived from steam distillation of guaiac wood. Used as a perfume fixative and modifier, soap odorant, and in fragrances.

GUAIAZULENE • A color additive also called azulene. Permanently listed as a cosmetic for external use only in 1978. See Azulene.

GUANIDINE CARBONATE • Used to adjust pH *(see)* and to keep cosmetics moist. Colorless crystals, soluble in water, found in turnip juice, mushrooms, corn germ, rice hulls, mussels, and earthworms. Occurs as water-absorbing crystals, which are very alkaline. Used in organic synthesis and as a rubber accelerator. It is a muscle poison if ingested. No known toxicity to the skin.

GUANINE • Pearl Essence. Obtained from scales of certain fish, such as alewives and herring, by scraping. It is mixed with water and used in nail polish. However, it has been largely replaced with either synthetic pearl (bismuth oxychloride; *see* Bismuth Compounds) or aluminum and bronze particles. Lethal when injected into the abdomens of mice but no known toxicity in humans. Permanently listed as a cosmetic coloring in 1977.

GUANOSINE • An organic compound that is found in the pancreas, clover, coffee plant, and pine pollen. Usually prepared from yeast. It is used in biochemical research. No known toxicity.

GUAR GUM • Used in emulsions, toothpastes, lotions, and creams. From the ground, nutritive, seed tissue of plants cultivated in India, it has 5 to 8 times the thickening power of starch. Employed also as a bulk laxative, appetite suppressant, and to treat peptic ulcers. A stabilizers in foods and beverages. No known toxicity.

GUARANA EXTRACT • *Paullina Cupana.* The dried paste consisting mainly of crushed seed from a plant grown in Brazil. Contains about 4 percent caffeine. Used in "antiaging" products. Used in cola flavorings for beverages and candy. See Caffeine for toxicity.

GUAR HYDROXYPROPYLTRIMONIUM CHLORIDE • See Quaternary Ammonium Compounds.

GUAVA • *Psidium guayava.* A small, shrubby, tropical tree that is widely cultivated for its yellow fruit. It is used in "organic" cosmetics.

GUM ARABIC • Acacia Gum. The exudate from acacia trees grown in the Sudan used in face masks, hairsprays, setting lotions, rouges, and powders for compacts. Serves as an emulsifier, stabilizer, and gelling ingredient. It may cause allergic reactions such as hay fever, dermatitis, gastrointestinal distress, and asthma.

GUM BENZOIN • Used as a preservative in creams and ointments and as a skin protective. It is the balsamic resin from benzoin grown in Thailand, Cambodia, Sumatra, and Cochin China. Also used to glaze and polish confections. No known toxicity.

GUM DAMMAR • See Damar.

GUM GUAIAC • Resin from the wood of the guaiacum used widely as an antioxidant in cosmetic creams and lotions. Brown or greenish brown. Formerly used in treatment of rheumatism. No known toxicity.

GUM KARAYA • Sterculia Gum. Used in hairsprays, beauty masks, setting lotions, depilatories, rouges, powder for compacts, shaving creams, denture adhesive powders, hand lotions, and toothpastes. It is the dried exudate of a tree native to India. Karaya came into wide use during World War I as a cheaper substitute for gum tragacanth *(see)*. Karaya swells in water and alcohol but does not dissolve. It is used in finger-wave lotions, which dry quickly and are not sticky. Because of its high viscosity at low concentrations, its ability to produce highly stable emulsions, and its resistance to acids, it is widely used in frozen food products. In 1971, however, the FDA put this additive on the list of chemicals to be studied for teratogenic, mutagenic, subacute, and reproductive effects. It can cause allergic reactions such as hay fever, dermatitis, gastrointestinal diseases, and asthma. It is omitted from hypoallergenic cosmetics.

GUM ROSIN • See Rosin.

GUM SUMATRA • See Gum Benzoin.

GUM TRAGACANTH • An emulsifier used in brilliantines, shaving creams, toothpastes, face packs, foundation creams, hairsprays, mascaras, depilatories, compact powders, rouges, dentifrices, setting lotions, eye makeup, and hand lotions. It is the gummy exudate from a plant grown in Iran and Asia Minor. Its acid forms a gel. It may cause allergic reactions such as hay fever, dermatitis, gastrointestinal distress, and asthma.

GUMS • The true plant gums are the dried exudates from various plants obtained when the bark is cut or otherwise injured. They are soluble in hot or cold water and sticky. Today, the term gum usually refers to water-soluble thickeners, either natural or synthetic; thickeners that are insoluble in water are called resins. Gums are used in perfumes, dentifrices, emollient creams, face powders, hair-grooming aids, hair straighteners, hand creams, rouges, shampoos, skin bleach creams, and wave sets. No known toxicity other than individual allergic reactions to specific gum.

GUTTA-PERCHA • **Gummi Plasticum.** The purified, coagulated, milky exudate of various trees grown in the Malay archipelago. Related to rubber; on exposure to air and sunlight, it becomes brittle. Used in dental cement, in fracture splints for broken bones, and to cover golf balls. No known toxicity.

GYPSOHILIA PANICULATA • See Saponaria Extract.

H

HAEMATOXYLIN CAMPECHIANUM • See Logwood.

HAIR • An outgrowth of skin, hair emanates from structures called follicles, of which the body has some 5 million—100,000 on the scalp alone, at least in youth. By the time a hair emerges into view from its follicle deep beneath the skin, it is dead; its cells are no longer capable of dividing to produce new hair. Hair texture depends on the diameter and shape of the hair's follicle and the proportion of hardshell cuticle in the hair's makeup. If the hair and its follicle are small in diameter, the hair will be fine. Whether it is straight or curly depends on how the cells in the follicle grow. An even growth pattern in the follicle produces straight hair, and an uneven pattern produces curly hair. See also Cellular Membrane Complex.

HAIR BLEACH • Among the most ancient of cosmetic preparations the Roman maidens used were various native minerals, such as quicklime mixed with lime, to produce reddish gold tresses. The most widely used bleach today is simply hydrogen peroxide. It has been employed to bleach hair since 1867. Reports of problems with hair bleach include nausea, burned scalp, severe life-threatening allergic reactions, and swelling of the face.

HAIR COLOR RINSE • This is a temporary hair color that covers the cuticle layer of the hair only and does not affect natural color pigment inside the hair shaft. Used after shampooing, it is usually washed out with the next shampooing. There are color shampoos formulated with a synthetic detergent and color, and there are powders, crayons, wave sets, and lacquers that are also used for temporary coloring. The most common color rinses today combine azo dyes *(see)*. Acids used in hair color rinses are usually citric and tartaric. The rinses may also contain fatty acids, alcohols or amides, borax, glycols, thickening ingredients, and isopropyl alcohol. Recent complaints to the FDA about hair rinses include ear numbness, headaches, and hair turning the wrong color. One of the problems with hair rinses is that when customers are allergic to permanent dyes, they become allergic to rinses, although the chemicals are not the same.

HAIR COLORING • Permanent hair-coloring products change the color of the hair. They cannot be shampooed away but remain until the hair grows out or is cut off. The root hair must be "retouched" as it grows in. There are basically three types: natural organics, synthetics, and metallics. Natural organics such as henna and chamomile have been used for centuries to color hair. Such dyes are placed on the hair and removed when the desired shade has been obtained. They are more difficult to apply, less reliable than manufactured dyes, and less predictable as far as color is concerned. They can cause allergic reactions to specific ingredients but are harmless otherwise. Synthetic dyes such as para- or amino derivatives work by oxidation—that is, they are applied cold and depend on the development of the shade by the action of a compound such as hydrogen peroxide to liberate oxygen. They frequently cause skin rashes and allergic skin reactions and the laws in most states require that patch testing be done before use. This means applying the dye to the skin 24 hours in advance to see if any irritation or reaction occurs. This precaution is rarely observed. Furthermore, there is evidence that p-phenylenediamine products may cause cancer. Semipermanent dyes, which also carry a warning to patch-test, require no mixing before use; there is a notice that they will last only for several shampoos. Metallic hair dyes offer no shade selection and directions indicate they develop gradually with each use. Recent reports of injuries from hair coloring to the FDA include scalp irritation, hair breakage and loss, contact dermatitis, swelling of the face, and itching.

In 1977, the National Cancer Institute reported that studies on laboratory animals showed those fed large amounts of hair dye developed thyroid and skin tumors. The agency warned that the studies indicated potential cancer danger to women who might absorb cancer-causing ingredients through their scalps. In 1978, a New York University Medical Center researcher reported that a study of

129 women with breast cancer and 193 without showed that the breast tumors were more likely to develop among hair-dye users who would otherwise be considered "at lower natural risks" for breast cancer. The cancers appeared about 10 years after dyes were in use. The cosmetic manufacturers voluntarily removed 4-MMPD, the dye ingredient known to be a cancer-causing ingredient. However, others in the phenylalanine group and other coal tar derivatives remain and women continue to dye their hair.

In 1979, the FDA attempted to force cosmetic manufacturers to include a cancer warning for coal tar hair dyes containing 4-methoxy-O-phenylenediamine, 2,4-diaminoanis. Japanese researchers showed that another hair dye intermediate, 2,4-diaminotoluene (2,4-DAT), caused cancer in animals. It was removed from most hair dyes in 1971 but was still a part of seven dyes in late 1977. The National Cancer Institute data shows that two other hair dye components cause cancer in laboratory animals: 2-nitro-p-phenylenediamine, contained in at least 354 hair dyes in 1979, and 4-amino-2-nitrophenol, contained in at least 90 hair dyes. Six other hair dye ingredients are positive on the AMES test, which shows 150 of 169 permanent hair dyes are mutagenic. The AMES test used genetic damage in bacteria as a signal that a chemical is potentially carcinogenic. Available evidence indicates that chemicals related to hair dyes can be absorbed through the skin and distributed throughout the body in small but significant amounts. The scalp is a good route for absorption of hair dyes into the system because it is a large surface with a large number of sebaceous glands. In 1998, an eight-year retrospective survey of 4,108 persons by a University of San Francisco researcher under a grant from the NIC found that hair coloring wasn't linked to any cancers in women. There was a "slightly higher non-Hodgkin's lymphoma" in men who used semipermanent hair dye frequently. The NCI and The American Cancer Society continue to study the dark hair dyes, and their research results are expected soon.

The FDA does not permit sale or distribution of a colorant that it has not approved. The exception to this ban concerns "coal-tar" hair dyes whose labels display the following:

"Caution: This product contains ingredients which may cause skin irritation on certain individuals and a preliminary test according to accompanying directions should first be made. This product must not be used for dyeing eyelashes or eyebrows; to do so many cause blindness."

Semipermanent dyes penetrate into the hair shaft and do not rinse off with water, as do temporary colorings. They do wash out of the hair after several shampoos. Semipermanent dyes usually come in liquid, gel, or aerosol foam forms. Temporary hair colors are applied in the form of rinses, gels, mousses, and sprays. These products merely sit on the surface of the hair and are usually washed out with the next shampoo, although some may last two to three washings. If the hair gets wet during a rainstorm, for example, the color can run from the hair onto the face or clothing. Gradual or progressive dyes are in the form of a rinse. They slightly darken the hair by binding to compounds on the hair's surface. Gradual dyes are usually applied daily until the desired shade is achieved. Unlike temporary dyes, gradual dyes don't wash off readily or run when the hair gets wet. Compounds suspected of causing cancer are found in temporary, semipermanent, and permanent dyes.

HAIR CONDITIONERS • Hair conditioners try to undo the damage from other hair preparations, particularly bleaches and dyes, and from the drying effects of the sun as well as the aging process. They include humectants, finishing ingredients, and emulsions. Hair is softened by water. Consequently, humectants bring moisture into the hair and reduce brittleness. Glycerin, propylene glycol, sorbitol, and urea *(see all)* help retain moisture and keep water from evaporating and consequently keep hair softer. Finishing ingredients, which include cream rinses, are added to shampoos or applied after shampooing. They leave a film on the hair to make it feel soft and look shiny. Isopropyl myristate and balsam are examples *(see both)*. Emulsions, including cream and protein conditioners, are applied before, during, or after shampooing and sometimes between shampoos. They should be nonsticking and, if rubbed between the hands, they should disappear. Such products usually contain lanolin, alcohols, sterols, glyceryl monostearate, spermaceti, glycerin, mineral oil, water, and perfume *(see all)*. The aerosol type of hair conditioner is made by preparing a "concentrate" from lanolin, isopropyl palmitate *(see)*, perfume oil, and some propellant. Protein conditioners contain a protein *(see)*, such as beer or egg, aimed at replacing lost protein. However, according to the American Medical Association, there is little, if any, evidence to substantiate this activity. There is no proof that protein from hair conditioners can penetrate the hair shaft and reconstruct healthy hair. If there is any effect, it is merely a coating similar to those of cream rinses *(see)*. Except for individual allergies, hair conditioners are nontoxic.

HAIR EXTRACT • An extract obtained from mammal hair. Used as a protein ingredient in hair products and emollients.

HAIR KERATIN AMINO ACIDS • Obtained by the hydrolysis *(see)* of human hair.

HAIR LACQUERS AND SPRAYS • These products "hold the set" and keep the hair looking as if it were just done at the beauty parlor. Once this was strictly a woman's product, but men now freely spray their hair. Hair lacquers usually come in either a plastic squeeze bottle or an aerosol. The early products contained shellac, and some still do. The shellac type is made by dissolving perfume in alcohol and adding shellac (the excretion of certain insects), and then adding a mixture of triethanolamine *(see)* and water. PEGs, lanolin, alcohols, and castor oil may also be included in the mixture *(see all)*. The early shellacs made hair shine but caused it to be brittle to the touch. The addition of lanolin, castor oil, and glycol counteract this effect. The newer hair lacquers contain a product used as a blood extender in medicine—polyvinylpyrrolidone (PVP). Related to plastics and similar to egg albumen in texture, it slightly stiffens the hair to keep it in place. PVP is dissolved in ether and then in glycerin, and perfume is added. The solution may also include polyethylene glycol, cetyl alcohol, and lanolin alcohols *(see all)*.

Pressurized hairsprays contain PVP, alcohol, sorbitol, and water. Additional ingredients may be lanolin, perfume, shellac, silicone, sodium alginate, or vegetable gums such as gum karaya, acacia, or gum tragacanth *(see all)*. The propellant is usually freon, the same one used as a coolant in air conditioners. Most sprays can cause eye and lung damage, and should be used with caution. The pump sprays are a better choice than aerosols because they are not as fine and, thus, not as easily inhaled. Complaints to the FDA about hairsprays include headache, hair loss, rash, change in hair color, throat irritation, suspected lung lesions, and death. In one case the hair ignited after a cigarette was lit. See Aerosols.

HAIR RELAXERS • See Hair Straighteners.

HAIR RINSES • Aimed at improving the feel and appearance of hair. Usually made of water-soluble material that can be dissolved and dispersed after application. When water has evaporated, a deposit is left behind, which forms a film. Among ingredients used are gums, certain protein derivatives, and synthetic polymers. A basic cream rinse contains glyceryl monostearate, 3 percent; benzalkonium chloride, 3 percent; water, about 94 percent; perfume; and coloring. The American Medical Association maintains that cream rinses cannot repair damaged hair as claimed in advertisements. See Hair Conditioners.

HAIR STRAIGHTENERS • Half the population wants curly hair and the other half wants straight hair. There are three methods, none perfect, for straightening hair: pomades that coat the hair and glue it straight; the much-advertised hot combs and irons; and chemical straighteners. Pomades, of course, are the least effective but the least damaging. The hair relaxers do their work by breaking about one-third of the chemical bonds that twist strands into curls, usually by hydrolyzing them with a 2 to 2.4 percent emulsion of sodium hydroxide. The emulsion reportedly not only coats the hair but invades it, causing it to swell up to 50 percent more than its original size. A water rinse then makes it swell even more. Heating the hair, when done properly at 300° to 500°F., does straighten the strands when tension is applied. Burns of the scalp are not uncommon, and the hair is dried out and may become very brittle. Chemical straighteners are effective but can cause burns, irritations, and hair damage. They usually contain either thioglycolic acid compounds *(see)* or alkalies such as sodium hydroxide, as well as polyethylene glycol, cetyl alcohol, stearyl alcohol, a triethanolamine, propylene glycol *(see all)*, perfume, and water. The glycols and alcohols may be caustic. The thioglycolate curl relaxers require the application of a neutralizer to the hair to stop the straightening process. Although there are home hair-straightening kits, there is a fine line between enough straightening and too much. If possible, the procedure should be done by a professional. The alkali curl relaxants, which are more effective for kinky hair, straighten the hair in about 5 to 10 minutes while a comb is run through. The hair is then rinsed with water to stop the chemical action. Again, there is a fine line between enough and too much, and the procedure should be done by a professional. Alkali straighteners contain strong burning ingredients, and first- to third-degree chemical burns can occur. They can also cause allergic reactions and swelling of the face and scalp. The greatest danger from these products is eye damage. Extreme caution must be used to avoid contact with the eyes. The hair will become fragile with any form of chemical or heat straightening. Bleached hair is particularly susceptible, and straightening of bleached hair is usually not recommended. Recent reports to the FDA of injuries include scalp irritation, loss of hair, and scalp burns.

HAIR THICKENERS • See Hair Tonics, Lotions, and Thickeners.

HAIR TONICS, LOTIONS, AND THICKENERS • Hair tonics and lotions are designed to keep the hair in place and looking healthy. There are three basic types: alcoholic, emulsion, and drug/tonic. Alcoholics may consist of an oil mixed with alcohol, glycerin *(see),* and perfume. Emulsions may be made by heating mineral oil and stearic acid *(see),* mixing it with hot water and triethanolamine *(see),* and adding perfume. The tonic or drug-type hairdressing usually contains antiseptics and may affect the function or structure of the human body or are designed to treat a diseased condition. They also contain low concentrations of rubefacients (these are products that cause a reddening and thus stimulation of the skin). Antiseptics employed may be creosols, phenols, chlorothymol, or resorcinol *(see all).* There is another type of hairdressing, used mostly by men, which is similar to a wave set common to women. It contains natural gums such as tragacanth, and karaya, or sodium alginate with alcohol, water, perfume, and glycerol. Among other chemicals in hair tonics and lotions are benzalkonium chloride, beta-naphthol, camphor, cantharides tincture, chloral hydrate, phosphoric acid, pilocarpine, glycols, quinine, sorbitan derivatives, salicylic acid, and tars *(see all).* Hair thickeners contain oils and proteins that coat the hair with an invisible film, thus giving it body. The thickeners make the hair feel smoother, and it is more manageable. A common hair tonic formula contains resorcinol, 0.8 percent; chloral hydrate, 1.5 percent; ethanol, 80 percent; beta-naphthol, 0.8 percent; Turkey-red oil, 16.9 percent; perfume; and color *(see all).* Complaints to the FDA about hair conditioners and dressings include hair loss, eye irritation, pimples, inflamed scalp, hair shrunk into knots, face irritation, dryness, and rash.

HAIRSPRAYS • See Hair Lacquers and Sprays.

HAMAMELIS WATER • See Witch Hazel.

HAND CREAMS AND LOTIONS • These are emollients, which apply easily and without stickiness. Most contain stearic acid, lanolin, and water. They may also contain cetyl alcohol, mineral oil, glycerin, potassium hydroxide, perfume, and glyceryl monostearate. The newer formulas may also contain healing ingredients such as allantoin *(see)* and water-repellent silicones *(see)* to protect the hands against further irritation from water, detergents, or wind. Most leading hand creams and lotions are uncolored, though surveys show that pink or blue hand creams are preferred; women over 25 years prefer pink and teenagers blue. The pH *(see)* level of most hand creams and lotions is between 5 and 8. A typical formula for hand cream contains cetyl alcohol, 2 percent; lanolin, 1 percent; mineral oil, 2 percent; stearic acid, 13 percent; glycerin, 12 percent; methylparaben, 0.15

percent; potassium hydroxide, 1 percent; water, 68 percent; and perfume in sufficient amounts *(see all)*. A typical hand lotion contains cetyl alcohol, 0.5 percent; lanolin, 1 percent; stearic acid, 3 percent; glycerin, 2 percent; methylparaben, 0.1 percent; triethanolamine, 0.75 percent; water, 85 percent; and perfume in sufficient amounts *(see all)*. Among problems reported to the FDA concerning hand preparations were rash, blisters, and swollen feet. Lanolin derivatives, colors, and perfumes, of course, are possible allergens.

HANDKERCHIEF PERFUMES • A woman's perfume in a retail shop. The name was derived from the practice of dabbing scent on a handkerchief to allow the sniffer to distinguish among perfume compounds.

HARPAGOPHYTUM EXTRACT • The extract of *Harpagophyton procumbens*. **Devil's Claw. Grapple Plant. Devil's Craw Root.** A perennial herb introduced into North America relatively recently, it has been used in South Africa for more than 250 years. It is used there by the natives as a tonic for arthritis. In cosmetics, it is used for hand and body lotions.

HASLEA OSTREARIA • **Blue Algae.** A rich source of Vitamin E, zinc, iron, and copper. It reportedly has a soothing effect on the skin. It is used in "antiaging" products.

HAWAIIAN WHITE GINGER • From the roots of *Hedychium coronarium*. Used in "organic" cosmetics. See Ginger Oil.

HAWKWEED EXTRACT • *Pilosella officinarum*. **Mouse Ear.** An extract of the various species of *Hieracium*, its ingredients include coumarin, flavones, and flavonoids. Used as an antispasmodic, expectorant, and astringent. It is used for respiratory problems where there is inflammation and a lot of mucus being formed. It is used by herbalists to treat bronchitis and bronchial asthma. It has been used in poultices for wound healing.

HAWTHORN BERRY • *Crataegus oxycantha*. **Mayblossom.** A spring-flowering shrub or tree. A number of scientific studies in Central Europe and the United States have found hawthorn berries can dilate the blood vessels and lower blood pressure. It has been used in Canada in poultices to reduce inflammation. They are used in "organic" cosmetics and in products to relieve acne. The berries reportedly can also increase the enzyme metabolism of the heart and make the heart's use of oxygen during exercise more efficient. Hawthorn extracts are also believed to have some diuretic properties. In the 1800s, the berries were used to treat digestive problems and insomnia. They do contain bioflavonoids, compounds that are necessary for Vitamin C function and that also help strengthen blood vessels.

HAYFLOWER EXTRACT • An extract of hayflowers used in bath salts.

HAZEL EXTRACT • The extract of the leaves of the European nut *Corylus avellana* or *C. americana*.

HAZELNUT OIL • The oil obtained from the various species of the hazelnut tree, genus *Corylus*.

HC • The abbreviation for hair color.

HC BLUE NO. 1 • Commercial hair coloring. Associated with fetal bone abnormalities in rats. In male rats, liver cancers occurred. Mice of both sexes also showed liver cancer in feeding studies. Based upon available data, the CIR Expert Panel *(see)* concludes that HC Blue No. 1 is not safe for use in cosmetics. See *p*-Phenylenediamine and Colors.

HC BLUE NO. 2 • Commercial hair coloring. Found in hair dyes at around 1.7 percent and in human volunteers, less than one-tenth of one percent was absorbed over a period of 30 days. A National Toxicology Program oral feeding study showed this to be nontoxic. It also was nonirritating in animals. On the basis of available data, the CIR Expert Panel *(see)* concludes this is safe for use in cosmetics. See p-Phenylenediamine and Colors.

HC BLUE NO. 4 • A reaction product of diaminoanthraquinone, epichlorohydrin, and diethanolamine. It contains benzenediamine. See p-Phenylenediamine.

HC BLUE NO. 5 • A reaction product of 2-nitro-p-phenylenediamine, epichlorohydrin, and diethanolamine. Contains benzenediamine. See p-Phenylenediamine.

HC BLUE NO. 6 • A commercial hair color. See Phenylenediamine.

HC BLUE NO. 7 • A commercial hair coloring. See Pyridinediamine.

HC BLUE NO. 8 • A commercial hair coloring. See Anthraquinone.

HC BLUE NO. 9 • A commercial hair coloring. See Nitrophenol.

HC BLUE NO. 10 • A commercial hair coloring. See Nitrophenol.

HC BLUE NO. 11 • A commercial hair coloring. See Nitrophenol.

HC BLUE NO. 12 • A commercial hair coloring. See Nitrophenol.

HC BROWN NO. 1 • Capracyl Brown 2R. Commercial hair coloring. See Colors.

HC BROWN NO. 2 • A commercial hair coloring. See Azo Dyes.

HC GREEN NO. 1 • A commercial hair coloring. See Aniline Dyes.

HC ORANGE NO. 1 • 2-Nitro-4-Hydroxydiphenylamine. Commercial semipermanent hair coloring. While it may be a mild eye irritation, it has not been shown to be a skin irritant or sensitizer in animals. In humans, the concentrations of 3 percent tested produced no significant sensitization, the CIR Expert Panel *(see)* concludes that this is safe for use in hair dye formulations at concentrations up to 3 percent. See Nitrophenol.

HC ORANGE NO. 2 • A commercial semipermanent hair coloring.

HC RED NO. 1 • 4-Amino-2-Nitrodiphenylamine. Commercial semipermanent hair coloring. Nonirritating. Approximately 1.6 percent was absorbed through the skin in laboratory tests. On the basis of the animal and clinical data, the CIR Expert Panel *(see)* concludes that this is safe for use in hair-dye formulations at concentrations less than 0.5 percent. See p-Phenylenediamine and Colors.

HC RED NO. 3 • N^1-(2-Hydroxyethyl)-2-Nitro-p-Phenylenediamine. Commercial semipermanent hair coloring. Was mutagenic in the AMES Test *(see)*. In a two-year feeding study, there was no evidence of cancer in either male or female rats. There was equivocal evidence in male mice and inadequate evidence to make a judgement of cancer-causing in female mice. On the basis of the available data, the CIR Expert Panel concludes that this dye is safe as a "coal tar" dye ingredient at the current concentrations of use, with the condition that it should not be used in products containing nitrosating agents *(see)*. See p-Phenylenediamine and Colors.

HC RED NO. 7 • A commercial hair coloring. See Nitrophenol.

HC RED NO. 8 • A commercial hair coloring. See Anthraquinone.

HC RED NO. 9 • A commercial hair coloring. See Nitrophenol.

HC RED NO. 10 • A commercial hair coloring. See Nitrophenol.

HC RED NO. 11 • A commercial hair coloring. See p-Phenylenediamine.

HC RED NO. 12 • A commercial hair coloring. See Nitrophenol.

HC RED NO. 13 • A commercial hair coloring. See Nitrophenol.

HC VIOLET NO. 1 • A commercial hair coloring. See Nitrobenzene.

HC VIOLET NO. 2 • A commercial hair coloring. See Benzene.

HC YELLOW NO. 2 • A commercial semipermanent hair coloring. Not a mutagen but can cause sensitivity. On the basis of the available data, the CIR Expert Panel *(see)* concludes that this dye is safe at concentrations up to 3 percent. The limitation on the concentration is based upon the available tests in humans. See Aniline Dyes.

HC YELLOW NO. 4 • Commercial hair coloring. Body weight decreases were found in animals given this ingredient by mouth. It did not produce irritation, sensitization, or photosensitization in animal tests. In some feeding studies, fetal toxicity was observed. It was mutagenic in several assays but no evidence of cancer-causing was found in oral or skin studies. No sensitization was found in patch tests on 200 human volunteers. Little HC Yellow No. 4 is absorbed through the scalp. On the basis of the available data, the CIR Expert Panel *(see)* concludes that this dye is safe. See p-Phenylenediamine and Colors.

HC YELLOW NO. 5 • N^1-2-(Hydroxyethyl)-4-Nitro-o-Phenylenediamine. Commercial hair coloring. See p-Phenylenediamine.

HC YELLOW NO. 6 • A commercial hair coloring. See p-Phenylenediamine and Coal Tar Colors.

HC YELLOW NO. 7 • A commercial hair coloring. See Coal Tar Colors.

HC YELLOW NO. 8 • A commercial hair coloring. See Coal Tar Colors.

HC YELLOW NO. 9 • A commercial hair coloring. See Nitrophenol.

HC YELLOW NO. 10 • A commercial hair coloring. See p-Phenylenediamine.

HC YELLOW NO. 11 • A commercial hair coloring. See p-Phenylenediamine.

HC YELLOW NO. 12 • A commercial hair coloring. See Nitrophenol.

HCL • The abbreviation for Hydrochloride.

HEALING INGREDIENTS • Medications added to hand creams and lotions *(see)* to treat chapped and irritated hands. Allantoin *(see)* is probably the most widely used healing ingredient in hand creams and lotions. Urea *(see)* has also been used.

HEART EXTRACT • The extract of animal heart tissue.

HEART HYDROLYSATE • The heart hydrolysate derived by acid, enzyme, or other method of hydrolysis.

HEATHER EXTRACT • An extract of *Calluna vulgaris,* also called Ling Extract.

HECTORITE • An emulsifier and extender. A clay consisting of silicate of magnesium and lithium, it is used in the chill-proofing of beer. The dust can be irritating to the lungs. No known toxicity of the skin.

HEDGE PARSLEY EXTRACT • Extract of the herb *Anthriscus sylvestris*.

HEDTA • **Hydroxyethyl Ethylenediamine Triacetic Acid.** A liquid with an ammonia odor, it is used in textile finishing compounds, antiquing ingredients, dyestuffs, cationic surfactants, resins, rubber products, insecticides, and medicines. Low toxicity.

HEDYCHIUM SPICATUM EXTRACT • **White Ginger.** See Ginger.

HELIANTHUS ANNUS • See Sunflower Oil.

HELICHRYSUM • See Everlasting Extract.

HELIOTROPE • **Desert Heliotrope.** Bluish purple flowers on a stem that coils in the shape of a fiddle neck. It grows through the southwestern United States and is a frequent cause of allergic contact dermatitis on the legs and ankles of persons walking through the desert.

HELIOTROPIN • **Heliotropine. Piperonal.** A purple diazo dye used in perfumery and soaps. Consists of colorless, lustrous crystals that have a heliotrope odor. Usually made from the oxidation of piperic acid. Ingestion of large amounts may cause central nervous system depression. Applications to the skin may cause allergic reactions and skin irritations. Not recommended for use in cosmetics or perfumes.

HEMATIN • The iron-containing portion of blood.

HEMLOCK OIL • **Spruce Oil.** A natural flavoring extract from North American or Asian nonpoisonous hemlock. Used in fruit, root beer, and spice flavorings for beverages, ice cream, ices, candy, baked goods, gelatin desserts, puddings, and chewing gum. No known toxicity.

HEMOGLOBIN • The red blood cells that carry oxygen from the lungs to the tissues where the oxygen is released.

HEMOLYMPH EXTRACT • An extract of crustacean blood.

HENNA • **Henna Leaves.** An ancient hair cosmetic obtained from the ground-up dried leaves and stems of a shrub found in North Africa and the Near East. A paste of henna and water is applied directly to the hair, and a reddish color is produced. There is no known toxicity, but allergic skin rashes may occur. However, those who are allergic to other dyes may be able to use henna without problems. Although it is rather messy and unpredictable to use, there is renewed interest in the dye because of the desire to return to "natural" products rather than using man-made cosmetics. The FDA ruled that henna is safe for coloring hair only. It may not be used for coloring eyelashes or eyebrows or in the area of the eyes. Permanently listed in 1965.

HEPARIN SALTS • An ingredient that prevents blood coagulation derived from beef lung or porcine intestinal mucosa. It is used to prevent lumping in cosmetics. In medicine, it is used to prevent and to treat deep vein blood clots, blood clots to the lung, and to treat heart attacks. It is used to flush and maintain indwelling catheters. Potential adverse reactions include hemorrhage, irritation, mild pain, and hypersensitivity reactions including chills, fever, itching, runny nose, burning of feet, red eyes, tearing, joint pain, and hives.

N-HEPTADECANOL • Colorless liquid, slightly soluble in water. Used in perfume fixatives, soaps, and cosmetics, and in the manufacture of wetting ingredients and detergents. May be irritating to the skin.

HEPTANAL • **Heptaldehyde.** Oily, colorless liquid with a penetrating fruit odor made from castor oil. Used in perfumery, pharmaceuticals, and flavoring.

HEPTANE • An aliphatic hydrocarbon. Volatile, colorless liquid derived from petroleum and used as an anesthetic and solvent. Highly flammable. Toxic by inhalation.

HEPTANOIC ACID • **Enanthic Acid.** Found in various fuel oils and in rancid oils, it has the faint odor of tallow. It is made from grapes and is a fatty acid used chiefly in making esters *(see)* for flavoring materials. No known toxicity.

2-HEPTANONE • Used in perfumery as a constituent of artificial carnation oils. Found in oil of cloves and in cinnamon bark oil. It has a peppery, fruity odor that is very penetrating. Heptanone is responsible for the peppery odor of Roquefort cheese. Can be irritating to human mucous membranes and is narcotic in high doses.

1-HEPTYL ACETATE • Liquid with fruit odor used in artificial fruit essences. See 2-Heptanone.

HEPTYL ALCOHOL • **1-Heptanol.** Colorless, fragrant liquid miscible with alcohol. Used in perfumery. See 2-Heptanone.

HEPTYL FORMATE • Used in artificial fruit essences. See 2-Heptanone.

HEPTYL HEPTOATE • Colorless liquid with fruity odor used in artificial fruit essences. See 2-Heptanone.

HEPTYL PELARGONATE • Liquid with pleasant odor used in flavors and perfumes. See 2-Heptanone.

n-HEPTYLIC ACID • See Heptanoic Acid.

HEPTYLUNDECANOL • Synthetic queen bee substance secreted by the jaw glands of queen bees to keep other bees from becoming rivals. See 2-Heptanone.

HERB ROBERT EXTRACT • Extract of the entire plant *Geranium robertianum*. See Geranium Oil.

HERBAL SHAMPOOS • Many contain saponins, a class of substances found in many plants. They possess the common properties of foaming, or making suds when agitated in water. They also hold resins and fatty substances in suspension in water. These products clean the scalp and reduce scaliness. Here is the typical formula for herbal shampoos: quillaja extract, powdered, 5 percent; ammonium carbonate, 1 percent; borax, 1 percent; bay oil, 1 percent *(see all);* and water, 9.2 percent. Saponins can be irritating when applied to the skin, and when given internally can cause nausea. Toxicity of herbal shampoos depends on ingredients and amounts used. The allergic potential of the shampoos also depends on sensitivity and the herbs used, as well as the other ingredients, such as quillaja bark and ammonium carbonate.

HERNIARIA GALABRA EXTRACT • **Rupture Wort.** A small herb with tiny green flowers.

HESPERIDIN • A natural bioflavonoid *(see)*. Fine needles from citrus fruit peel. Used as a synthetic sweetener.

HEXACHLOROPHENE • An antibacterial used in baby oil, baby powder, brilliantine hairdressings, cold creams, emollients, deodorants, antiperspirants, face masks, hair tonics, shampoos, and medicated cosmetics products. In 1969, scientists reported microscopically visible brain damage in rats from small concentrations of the antibacterial. The company that had the patent on hexachlorophene, Swiss-based Givaudan Corporation, sold the chemical only to those companies that could demonstrate a safe and effective use for it. Givaudan refused to sell hexachlorophene for use in toothpastes and mouthwashes. However, when the patents expired in the mid-1960s, the FDA allowed hexachlorophene to be used in toothpastes and mouthwashes. In 1971, the chemical was an ingredient of nearly 400 products ranging from fruit washes to baby lotion. Chloasma, a pigmenting of the face, was reported in 1961 in persons who had used hexachlorophene-containing products. Coma was reported in burn patients washed in hexachlorophene products in 1968. On March 29, 1971, August Curley and Robert E. Hawk of the U.S. Environmental Protection Agency (EPA) presented a paper in Los Angeles at the American Chemical Society meeting stating that hexachlorophene has been found toxic to experimental animals, capable of penetrating the skin, and present in the blood of some human beings. Tests on 13 human volunteers showed hexachlorophene levels of one part in a billion parts of blood to 89 ppb. Curley, chief research chemist at the EPA at the time, said that the agency thought the material was absorbed through the skin. He pointed out: "For over two decades, hexachlorophene has been widely used as a bactericide in the United States. However, relatively little quantitative data is available concerning its dermal absorption in either experimental animals or humans." On May 17, 1971, the American Academy of Pediatrics warned that products containing hexachlorophene that are intended for oral use, such as certain toothpastes or throat lozenges, may be poisonous to children. In December 1971, the FDA curbed the use of hexachlorophene-containing detergents and soaps for total body bathing. Winthrop, the makers of pHisoHex, which contained 3 percent hexachlorophene, sent out further information to doctors saying that the product should not be used as a lotion, left on the skin after use, used as a wet soak or compress, or transferred to another container that would allow for misuse. It should always be rinsed thoroughly from the skin after any use, should be used in strict accordance with directions, and should always be kept out of the reach of children. The FDA has limited it up to 0.75 percent. Products containing up to 0.75 percent will be able to continue on the market with a warning: "Contains hexachlorophene. For external use only. Rinse thoroughly." According to the summary of the report included in the Federal Register, the cancer-testing program showed that hexachlorophene did not cause tumors in rats under test conditions.

HEXADECANOIC ACID • See Palmitic Acid.

HEXADECANOLIDE • See Palmitic Acid.

HEXADECYL METHICONE • A silicone wax. See Silicones.

HEXADECYL STEARATE • See Stearic Acid.

HEXADIMETHRINE CHLORIDE • See Polymers.

HEXAMETHYLDISILOXANE • See Silicates.

HEXAMIDINE DIISETHIONATE • An organic salt derived from petroleum distillate *(see)* that is used as a topical antiseptic.

HEXANE • See Paraffin.

HEXANEDIOL DISTEARATE • The diester of hexanediol and stearic acid used as a wax and a plasticizer. It is derived from ethyl alcohol and stearic acid *(see both)*.

1, 2, 6-HEXANETRIOL • An alcohol used as a solvent. No known skin toxicity.

HEXANOL • Hexyl Alcohol. Used as an antiseptic and preservative in cosmetics, it occurs as the acetate *(see)* in seeds and fruits of *Heracleum sphondylium* and *Umbelliferae*. A colorless liquid, slightly soluble in water, it is miscible with alcohol. No known toxicity.

HEXENOL • Liquid with odor of green leaves. It occurs in grasses, leaves, herbs, and tea. Used in fragrances.

HEXETIDINE • An organic compound used as an antifungal ingredient.

HEXYL ALCOHOL • Used in antiseptics and in perfumery. See Hexanol.

HEXYL LAURATE • The ester of hexyl alcohol and lauric acid. Used as an emulsifier.

HEXYL NICOTINATE • The ester of hexyl alcohol and nicotinic acid *(see both)*.

HEXYLDECANOL • An alcohol of hexyldecanoic acid. Used as an exfoliant *(see)*.

HEXYLENE GLYCOL • A widely used aliphatic alcohol. See Glycols.

4-HEXYLRESORCINOL • Used in mouthwashes and sunburn creams. A pale yellow, heavy liquid that becomes solid upon standing at room temperature. It has a pungent odor and a sharp astringent taste, and has been used medicinally as an antiworm medicine and antiseptic. It can cause severe gastrointestinal irritation; bowel, liver, and heart damage has been reported. Concentrated solutions can cause burns of the skin and mucous membranes.

HIBISCUS • A widely distributed genus of herbs, shrubs, or small trees of the family *Malvaceae*, with lobed leaves and large showy flowers. The petals were used in folk medicine to soothe inflammation. Used today in "organic" cosmetics.

HIERACIUM PILOSELLA • See Hawkweed.

HIEROCHLOE OODORATA • See Sweet Grass Extract.

HIMANTHALIA ELONGATA • Seaweed containing Vitamins A, C, and E as well as amino acids. Used in "natural cosmetics."

HINOKITIOL • The organic compound distilled from the leaves of *Arborvitae*, it is a pale yellow oil with a camphor smell and is used in perfumery and flavoring. Low toxicity.

HIPPOPHAE RHAMINOIDES • **Seabuckthorn.** A seaweed containing high concentrations of Vitamins C, E, K, B_1, and B_2 as well as carotenes, flavinoids, and fatty acids. Used in "natural cosmetics."

HIRUDINEA EXTRACT • Obtained from leeches. Used in emollients.

HISTAMINE • A chemical released by mast cells and considered responsible for much of the swelling and itching characteristics of hay fever and other allergies.
HISTIDINE • A basic essential amino acid *(see)* used as a nutrient. It is a building block of protein and used in cosmetic creams.
HO LEAF OIL • See Fo-Ti.
HO SHOU WU • See Fo-Ti.
HOLLY • *Ilex Aquifolium* Extract. A small evergreen, the leaves were used to increase perspiration, to treat inflammations of the mucous membranes, pleurisy, gout, and smallpox. The leaves contain theobromine *(see)*. The berries were used to cause vomiting, and as a diuretic to remove excess fluid. The juice of the berries was used to treat jaundice.
HOMOSALATE • Heliphan. See Cresol.
HOMATRINE • See Homatropine.
HOMATROPINE • **Homatrine. Isopto Homatropine.** An eye solution that is used to dilate the pupils during diagnosis and to treat certain eye irritations. Potential adverse reactions include eye irritation, blurred vision, sensitivity to light, flushing, dry skin and mouth, fever, rapid heartbeat, awkward movements, irritability, confusion, and sleepiness. Should be used cautiously in infants and elderly people or debilitated patients; children with blond hair and blue eyes; patients with heart disease; or patients with increased pressure in the eyes. Patients who are hypersensitive to atropine will also be allergic to this drug. In 1992, the FDA proposed a ban on homatropine methylbromide in oral menstrual drug products because it has not been shown to be safe and effective for its stated claims.
HOMO SALICYLATE • See Salicylates.
HONEY • Used as a coloring, flavoring, and emollient in cosmetics. Formerly used in hair bleaches. The common, sweet, viscous material taken from the nectar of flowers and manufactured in the sacs of various kinds of bees. The flavor and color depend upon the plants from which it was taken.
HONEYDEW MELON JUICE • Liquid expressed from fresh honeydew. Used in "organic" cosmetics.
HONEYSUCKLE • The common fragrant tubular flowers, filled with honey, that are used in perfumes. No known toxicity.
HOPLOSTETHUS • **Orange Roughy Oil.** See Fish Oil.
HOPS • Used in perfumes and flavorings. Derived from the carefully dried pineconelike fruit of the hop plant grown in Europe, Asia, and North America. Light yellow or greenish, it is an oily liquid with a bitter taste and aromatic odor. Used also in beer brewing and for food flavorings. Hops at one time was used as a sedative. Can cause allergic reactions.
HOPS OIL • See Hops.
HORDEUM DISTICHON • See Barley Extract.
HOREHOUND • *Ballota nigra* (**Black Horehound**) and *Marrubium vulgare* (**White Horehound**). **Madweed.** Black horehound was used by the English

colonists as a medicine for gout and arthritis. White horehound, native to Europe and imported to the United States, was used in an herbal tea for sore throat and bronchitis. Black horehound is used occasionally by herbalists to get rid of lice, and when soaked in boiling water, it is applied to the skin to relieve gout and arthritis. It is also used by herbalists to treat chronic hepatitis, cancer, tuberculosis, leukemia, malaria, and hysteria. White horehound, used by ancient Egyptian doctors who dedicated it to the god Horus, and now native to Great Britain and the United States, is used in cough drops and cold medicines. Tops of young white horehound shoots are still gathered by herbalists to treat upset stomachs, jaundice, croup, asthma, and bronchitis.

HORMONE CREAMS • The cosmetic manufacturers claim that hormone creams containing estrogen or progesterone are cosmetics, and many dermatologists and some staff members of the U.S. Food and Drug Administration maintain they are drugs. Cosmetic manufacturers, ever aware of the human desire to stay young forever, have advertised the hormone creams as wrinkle preventatives and youthful skin restoratives. According to the American Medical Association, there is little scientific evidence that locally applied hormones can thicken the thinning skin of aging and that simple emollient creams may do a better job. In a review of the experimental data on the use of sex steroids in cosmetics, there was some evidence that topically applied steroidal hormones, both active and inactive biologically, do cause a slight thickening of aged skin. However, the effects are negligible, and in the amounts considered safe to use in cosmetics, topically applied hormones have no effect on human oil glands and oil secretion. Estrogen may be added at not more than 10,000 international units per ounce. Progesterone content may not exceed 5 mg per ounce. Enlargement of the breast in boys using an estrogen-containing hair lotion, La Cade®, was reported in *The American Journal of the Diseases of Childhood,* July 1982, p. 587, by Deborah Edidin, M.D., and Lynne Levitsky, M.D.

HORSE CHESTNUT • *Aesculus hippocastanum.* The seeds of *Aesculus hippocastanum.* A tonic, natural astringent for skin, and fever-reducing substance that contains tannic acid. Traditionally used by herbalists to reduce fever, it is also used by modern herbalists to treat varicose veins and hemorrhoids. The powdered kernel of the nut causes sneezing. The nuts reputedly contain narcotic properties. The seeds contain escin, which is used today as a sunburn protective. Escin is also widely used in Europe as an anti-inflammatory ingredient for a variety of conditions, including varicose veins. Escin has also been found to be a powerful diuretic to reduce excess fluid. No known toxicity.

HORSE NETTLE • **Solanum. Bull Nettle. Radical Weed.** Air-dried ripe fruit of *Solanum carolinense,* a South American nightshade plant. It is also grown in Florida. It is used as a skin treatment, sedative, and anticonvulsant.

HORSE TISSUE EXTRACT • An extract from the tissue near the horse's mane.

HORSEMINT OIL • *Monarda.* **Water Mint.** A tall, erect, perennial herb with hairy leaves and purple spotted creamy flowers. Used in flavorings.

HORSERADISH EXTRACT • *Amoracia lapathifolia.* **Scurvy Grass.** The grated root from the tall, coarse, white-flowered herb native to Europe. A condiment ingredient. It contains Vitamin C and acts as an antiseptic, particularly in cosmetics. It is applied by herbalists as a poultice to accelerate the healing of stubborn wounds. It is also reputed to be a good diuretic and expectorant. It is used for arthritis to relieve pain by stimulating blood flow to inflamed joints. Potential adverse reactions include diarrhea and sweating if taken internally in large amounts.

HORSETAIL • *Equisetum arvense.* **Shavegrass. Silica.** The American Indians and the Chinese have long used horsetail to accelerate the healing of bones and wounds. Horsetail is rich in minerals the body uses to rebuild injured tissue. It facilitates the absorption of calcium by the body, which nourishes nails, skin, hair, bones, and the body's connective tissue. The herb helps eliminate excess oil from skin and hair. It is a mild diuretic and was used to promote urination in heart failure and kidney dysfunction. The FDA issued a notice in 1992 that horsetail has not been shown to be safe and effective as claimed in OTC digestive aid products.

HOT OIL TREATMENT • Used to restore luster to bleach-damaged hair. The hair is completely doused with oil and then heated by a lamp or an electric cap. Oils include mineral and vegetable.

HOUSELEEK • *Sempervivum tectorium.* Native to the mountains of Europe and to the Greek Islands. Its longevity led to its being named "sempervivum," which means "ever alive." It has been used to treat shingles and gout, and to get rid of bugs. Its pulp was applied to the skin for rashes and inflammation, and to remove warts and calluses. The juice was used to reduce fever and to treat insect stings. Houseleek juice mixed with honey was prescribed for thrush, and an ointment made from the plant was used to treat ulcers, burns, scalds, and inflammation.

HOUSELEEK EXTRACT • Extract of the common houseleek *Sempervivum tectorium.* Old herbal remedy for soothing the skin.

HOUTTUYNIA CORDATA • A showy plant that grows in wet areas. A lily, it has heart-shaped leaves.

HUMAN PLACENTAL ENZYMES • Enzymes derived from human placentas obtained from normal afterbirth.

HUMAN PLACENTAL LIPIDS • The fats obtained from human placentas obtained from normal afterbirth.

HUMAN PLACENTAL PROTEIN • Protein derived from the sac that surrounds the fetus. Obtained from normal afterbirth. When placental materials were first used as cosmetic ingredients in the 1940s, manufacturers promoted the products as providing beneficial hormonal effects such as stimulating tissue growth and removing wrinkles although newborns emerge from the womb with wrinkled skin. The hormone content and tissue-growth and wrinkle-removing claims classified the placenta-containing products as drugs, and the FDA declared them to be ineffective and therefore misbranded. The FDA's challenge caused placenta suppliers to change marketing strategies by claiming that hormones in their placenta ingredients have been extracted and were no longer in the product. They then offered placental raw materials without medical claims—only as a source of protein. Placenta is used in some "antiaging" creams.

HUMAN UMBILICAL EXTRACT • Used in "antiaging" creams.

HUMECTANT • A substance used to preserve the moisture content of materials, especially in hand creams and lotions. The humectant of glycerin and rose water, in equal amounts, is the earliest known hand lotion. Glycerin, propylene, glycol, and sorbitol *(see all)* are widely used humectants in hand creams and lotions. Humectants are usually found in antiperspirants, baby preparations, beauty masks, dentifrices, depilatories, hair-grooming aids, and wave sets. See individual substances for toxicity.

HUMULUS LUPULUS • See Hops.

HYACINTH • Used in perfumes and soaps. It is the extract of the very common fragrant flower. Also used as a flavoring for chewing gum. Dark green liquid with a penetrating odor, the juice of hyacinth is very irritating to the skin and can cause allergic reactions.

HYALURONIC ACID • A natural protein found in umbilical cords, sperm, testes, and the fluids around the joints. Used as a cosmetic oil. If there is a lot of swelling, cosmetics containing this ingredient may help because it absorbs moisture, according to some dermatologists. No known toxicity.

HYBRID SAFFLOWER OIL • The oil derived from the seeds of a genetic strain that contains mostly oleic acid triglyceride, as distinct from safflower oil.

HYDANTOIN • Derived from methanol *(see)*, it is used as an intermediate in the synthesis of lubricants and resins. It caused cancer when injected into the abdomens of rats in doses of 1,370 mg per kg of body weight and when given orally to rats in doses of 1,500 mg per kilogram.

HYDRANGEA MACROPHYLLA • **Seven Barks.** Widely distributed shrubs with clusters of showy flowers. The roots contain glycosides, saponins, and resins *(see all)*. It is used by herbalists to treat inflamed or enlarged prostate gland, and for urinary stones or gravel associated with infections such as cystitis. In 1992, the FDA proposed a ban on hydrangea extract in OTC oral menstrual drug products because it had not been shown to be safe and effective as claimed.

HYDRASTINE • Found together with berberine *(see)*, it is used to stop uterine bleeding and as an antiseptic.

HYDRATED • Combined with water.

HYDRATED ALUMINA • See Aluminum Hydroxide.

HYDRATED SILICA • An anticaking ingredient to keep loose powders free-flowing. See Silica and Hydrated.

HYDRIODIC ACID • Strong acid similar to hydrochloric acid *(see)*.

HYDROABIETYL ALCOHOL • Used in eyebrow pencils. See Abietic Acid.

HYDROCARBONS • A large class of organic compounds containing only carbon and hydrogen. Petroleum, natural gas, coal, and bitumen are common hydrocarbon products. Hydrocarbons such as petrolatum, mineral oils, paraffin wax, and ozokerite have been used in sunscreens, hand creams, lotions, and nail polish. They are believed to work by forming a water-repellent film that keeps water from evaporating from the skin.

HYDROCHLORIC ACID • Acid used in hair bleaches to speed up oxidation in rinses and to remove color. Also a solvent. A clear, colorless, or slightly yellowish, corrosive liquid, it is a water solution of hydrogen chloride of varying concentrations. Inhalation of the fumes causes choking and inflammation of the respiratory tract. Ingestion may corrode the mucous membranes, esophagus, and stomach, and cause diarrhea.

HYDROCHLOROFLUOROCARBON, 22, 142B, 152a • Propellants and refrigerants derived from chlorofluorocarbon, any of several compounds composed of carbon, fluorine, chlorine, and hydrogen. Though they are safer than many propellant gases, their use has diminished because of suspected effects on stratospheric ozone.

HYDROCORTISONE • An adrenal gland *(see)* corticosteroid *(see)* hormone introduced in 1952, used to decrease severe inflammation, as an adjunctive treatment for ulcerative colitis and proctitis, for shock, and to treat adrenal insufficiency. Also suppresses the immune response, stimulates bone marrow, and influences protein, fat, and carbohydrate metabolism. Most adverse reactions are the result of dose or length of time of administration. Sudden withdrawal may be fatal. Contraindicated in systemic fungal infections. Potential adverse reactions include burning, itching, irritation, dryness, inflammation of the hair follicles, streaking, acne, rash around the mouth, spots of pigment loss, hairiness, allergic contact dermatitis and, if covered with a dressing, secondary infection, atrophy, streaks, and blisters. Should be used cautiously in skin problems caused by viruses such as herpes and in fungal or bacterial skin infections. Should not be applied near eyes or mucous membranes, under the arms, on the face or groin, or under the breast unless medically specified.

HYDROCOTYL EXTRACT • Extract from the leaves or roots of *Hydrocotyl asiatica.* Widely used in body and hand preparations, night skin care products, and face and neck creams.

HYDROGEN PEROXIDE • **Peroxyl.** A bleaching and oxidizing ingredient, detergent, and antiseptic. Used in skin bleaches, hair bleaches, cold creams, mouthwashes, toothpastes, and cold permanent waves. An unstable compound readily broken down into water and oxygen. It is made from barium peroxide and diluted phosphoric acid. Generally recognized as safe as a preservative and germ killer in cosmetics as well as in milk and cheese. A 3 percent solution is used medicinally as an antiseptic and germicide. A strong oxidizer, undiluted it can cause burns of the skin and mucous membranes. A skin antiseptic used to cleanse wounds, skin ulcers, and local infections, and used in the treatment of inflammatory conditions of the external ear canal. It is also used in mouthwash gargles. The FDA issued a notice in 1992 that hydrogen peroxide has not been shown to be safe and effective as claimed in OTC poison ivy, poison oak, and poison sumac products.

HYDROGENATED BUTYLENE/ETHYLENE/STYRENE COPOLYMER • Hydrogenated *(see)* butylene, ethylene, and styrene. Used as a thickener.

HYDROGENATED CANOLA OIL • See Hydrogenation and Canola Oil.

HYDROGENATED CASTOR OIL • Used as a wax. See Hydrogenation and Castor Oil.

HYDROGENATED COCO-GLYCERIDES • Widely used in makeup such as eyeliners, foundations, eye shadows, and blushers. See Hydrogenation, Coconut Oil, and Triglycerides.

HYDROGENATED COCONUT ACID • See Coconut Oil and Hydrogenation.

HYDROGENATED COCONUT OIL • See Hydrogenation and Coconut Oil.

HYDROGENATED C6-14 OLEFIN POLYMERS • Low-molecular-weight polymers of olefin monomers. Olefin is a class of unsaturated hydrocarbons obtained by "cracking" naphtha or other petroleum products, and they are used in the manufacture of surfactants *(see)*.

HYDROGENATED COTTONSEED GLYCERIDE • See Cottonseed Oil and Hydrogenation.

HYDROGENATED COTTONSEED OIL • See Hydrogenation and Cottonseed Oil.

HYDROGENATED DITALLOW AMINE • An amine derived from Hydrogenated Tallow Acid. See Tallow.

HYDROGENATED ETHOXYLATED LANOLIN • See Hydrogenation and Lanolin.

HYDROGENATED FATTY OILS • Used in baby creams and lipstick. See Fatty Acids and Hydrogenation.

HYDROGENATED HONEY • Controlled hydrogenation *(see)* of honey.

HYDROGENATED JOJOBA OIL, WAX • See Jojoba and Hydrogenation.

HYDROGENATED LANETH-5, -20, -25 • See Hydrogenated Lanolin.

HYDROGENATED LANOLIN • A light yellow to white, tacky solid that is soluble in ethyl ether but insoluble in water. It retains the emollient and adhering characteristics of lanolin but loses the latter's odor, taste, color, and tackiness. Used in eye makeup preparations; colognes and toilet water; manicuring preparations; waving preparations; skin care preparations such as creams, lotions, powders, and sprays; and suntan and sunscreen preparations. See Hydrogenation.

HYDROGENATED LANOLIN ALCOHOL • The CIR Expert Panel *(see)* found it safe. See Hydrogenated Lanolin.

HYDROGENATED LARD GLYCERIDE • See Lard and Hydrogenation.

HYDROGENATED LECITHIN • Widely used in skin conditioners, face powders, skin-care preparations, and eye shadows. See Lecithin and Hydrogenation.

HYDROGENATED MENHADEN ACID • The end product of hydrogenation of the fatty acids obtained from menhaden fish oil.

HYDROGENATED MENHADEN OIL • The hydrogenated oil from the fish menhaden.

HYDROGENATED MICROCRYSTALLINE WAX • Hydrogenated *(see)* crystalline wax.

HYDROGENATED MINK OIL • See Mink Oil and Hydrogenation.

HYDROGENATED OILS • Vegetable and animal and fish oils treated with hydrogen. The oil becomes partially converted from naturally polyunsaturated fats to saturated. Makes liquid oils partially solid.

HYDROGENATED ORANGE ROUGHY OIL • The hydrogenated oil *(see)* from the fish, orange roughy.

HYDROGENATED PALM GLYCERIDES • See Palm Oil and Hydrogenation.

HYDROGENATED PALM-KERNEL OIL • See Palm-Kernel Oil and Hydrogenation.

HYDROGENATED PALM-KERNEL OIL PEG-6 COMPLEX • See Palm-Kernel Oil, Hydrogenation, and Polyethylene Glycol.

HYDROGENATED PALM OIL • See Palm Oil and Hydrogenation.

HYDROGENATED PEANUT OIL • See Hydrogenation and Peanut Oil.

HYDROGENATED POLYISOBUTENE • See Isobutyric Acid and Hydrogenation.

HYDROGENATED RICE BRAN WAX • See Hydrogenation and Rice Bran Oil.

HYDROGENATED SHARK-LIVER OIL • See Shark-Liver Oil and Hydrogenation.

HYDROGENATED SOY GLYCERIDE • See Soybean Oil and Hydrogenation.

HYDROGENATED SOYBEAN OIL • See Soybean Oil and Hydrogenation.

HYDROGENATED STARCH HYDROLYSATE • The end product of the hydrogenation of corn syrup. See Hydrogenation and Corn Syrup.

HYDROGENATED TALLOW • A binder *(see)* in cosmetics. See Hydrogenation and Tallow.

HYDROGENATED TALLOW ACID • See Tallow and Hydrogenation.

HYDROGENATED TALLOW BETAINE • See Hydrogenation and Betaine.

HYDROGENATED TALLOW GLYCERIDE • See Tallow and Hydrogenation.

HYDROGENATED TALLOWAMIDE DEA • A mixture of fatty acids derived from Hydrogenated Tallow.

HYDROGENATED TALLOWETH-12-60 • Mixture of polyethylene glycol and hydrogenated tallow. The numbers signify the viscosity of the ingredient.

HYDROGENATED TALLOWTRIMONIUM CHLORIDE • See Quaternary Ammonium Compounds.

HYDROGENATED VEGETABLE GLYCERIDE • An emollient to prevent the skin from losing moisture. See Vegetable Oils and Hydrogenation.

HYDROGENATED VEGETABLE OIL • Widely used in moisturizing preparations, eye shadows, hair products, cold creams, night care preparations and cleansing lotions. See Vegetable Oils and Hydrogenation.

HYDROGENATION • The process of adding hydrogen gas under high pressure to liquid oils. It is the most widely used chemical process in the edible fat industry. Used in the manufacture of petrol from coal, and in the manufacture of margarine and shortening. Used primarily in the cosmetic and food industries to convert liquid oils to semisolid fats at room temperature. Reduces the amount of acid in the compound and improves color. Usually, the higher the amount of hydrogenation, the lower the unsaturation in the fat and the less possibility of flavor degradation or spoilage due to oxidation. Hydrogenated oils still contain some unsaturated components that are susceptible to rancidity. Therefore, the addition of antioxidants is still necessary.

HYDROLYSATE • A product of hydrolysis in which hydrogen is added to a compound.

HYDROLYSIS • Decomposition that changes a compound into other compounds by taking up the elements of water. For example, hydrolysis of salt into an acid and a base or hydrolysis of an ester into an alcohol and an acid.

HYDROLYZED • Subject to hydrolysis or turned partly into water. Hydrolysis is derived from the Greek *hydro,* meaning "water," and *lysis,* meaning "a setting free." It occurs as a chemical process in which the decomposition of a compound is brought about by water, resolving into a simpler compound. Hydrolysis also occurs in the digestion of foods. The proteins in the stomach react with water in an enzyme reaction to form peptones and amino acids *(see).*

HYDROLYZED ACTIN • A protein in skin that is treated with acid, enzymes, or some other method of hydrolysis. Used in hair and skin products as a conditioner.

HYDROLYZED ALBUMEN • Skin conditioning ingredient. See Hydrolyzed and Albumen.

HYDROLYZED CALF SKIN • Treated with enzymes, it is used in skin care products.

HYDROLYZED CASEIN • See Casein and Hydrolyzed.

HYDROLYZED COLLAGEN • The widely used hydrolysate of animal collagen derived by acid, enzyme, or other method of hydrolysis. It is used in many makeup products, and bath preparations, and cuticle softeners. On the basis of the available data, the CIR Expert Panel *(see)* concludes that this ingredient is safe.

HYDROLYZED DNA • The hydrolysate of DNA *(see).* Used in hair products and skin conditioners.

HYDROLYZED EGG PROTEIN • Used in hair conditioners. See Egg and Hydrolyzed.

HYDROLYZED ELASTIN • The hydrolysate of animal connective tissue, particularly the ligaments, used in "youth" creams.

HYDROLYZED FIBRONECTIN • The hydrolysate of fibronectin, a fibrous link in connective tissue derived by acid, enzyme, or other method of hydrolysis.

HYDROLYZED GADIDAE PROTEIN • See Hydrolyzed and Fish Oil.

HYDROLYZED GLYCOSAMINOGLYCANS • Formerly called hydrolyzed mucopolysaccharides, it is a sugary substance used in emollients.

HYDROLYZED HAIR KERATIN • The hydrolysate of human hair keratin derived by acid, enzyme, or other method of hydrolysis.

HYDROLYZED HEMOGLOBIN • The hydrolysate of hemoglobin derived by acid, enzyme, or other method of hydrolysis.

HYDROLYZED HUMAN PLACENTAL PROTEIN • See Human Placental Protein and Hydrolyzed.

HYDROLYZED KERATIN • The widely used hydrolysate of keratin derived by acid, enzyme, or other form of hydrolysis. The word "animal" was removed from this ingredient name. See Keratin.

HYDROLYZED MILK PROTEIN • The hydrolysate of milk protein derived by acid, enzyme, or other method of hydrolysis.

HYDROLYZED MUCOPOLYSACCHARIDES • A mixture of polysaccharides derived from the hydrolysis of animal connective tissue.

HYDROLYZED OAT PROTEIN • The hydrolysate of oat protein.

HYDROLYZED PEARL • Pearls from oysters that have been treated with acid, enzyme, or some other method of hydrolysis. Used in face powders and mascara.

HYDROLYZED PLACENTAL PROTEIN • The hydrolysate of placental protein derived by acid, enzyme, or other method of hydrolysis.

HYDROLYZED POTATO PROTEIN • The potato protein derived by acid, enzyme, or other method of hydrolysis.

HYDROLYZED PROTEIN • Improves the ability to comb hair. The word "animal" was removed from this ingredient's name. See Proteins and Hydrolyzed.

HYDROLYZED PRUNUS DOMESTICA • See Prunes and Hydrolyzed.

HYDROLYZED RETICULIN • The hydrolysate of the reticulin portion of animal connective tissue derived by acid, enzyme, or other form of hydrolysis.

HYDROLYZED RICE PROTEIN • The hydrolysate of rice protein derived by acid, enzyme, or other method of hydrolysis.

HYDROLYZED RNA • The hydrolysate of RNA *(see)* derived by acid, enzyme, or other method of hydrolysis.

HYDROLYZED SERUM PROTEIN • The hydrolysate of serum protein derived by acid, enzyme, or other method of hydrolysis.

HYDROLYZED SILK • The hydrolysate (turned partly into water) of silk protein derived by acid, alkaline, or enzymatic hydrolysis.

HYDROLYZED SOY PROTEIN • Widely used in hair and skin conditioning products. See Soybean and Hydrolyzed.

HYDROLYZED SPINAL PROTEIN • The hydrolysate of animal spinal cord protein derived by acid, enzyme, or other method of hydrolysis. Used in hair and skin conditioners.

HYDROLYZED SWEET ALMOND PROTEIN • See Almond and Hydrolyzed.

HYDROLYZED ULVA LACTUCA • See Algae and Hydrolyzed.

HYDROLYZED VEGETABLE PROTEIN • The hydrolysate (liquefaction) of vegetable protein derived by acid, enzyme, or other method of hydrolysis.

HYDROLYZED WHEAT GLUTEN • Widely used in hair and skin and bath preparations. The hydrolysate of wheat gluten derived by acid, enzyme, or other method of hydrolysis.

HYDROLYZED WHEAT PROTEIN • The hydrolysate of wheat protein derived by acid, enzyme, or other method of hydrolysis.

HYDROLYZED YEAST • The hydrolysate of yeast (liquefaction) derived from acid, enzyme, or other method of hydrolysis.

HYDROLYZED YEAST PROTEIN • See Hydrolyzed Yeast.

HYDROLYZED ZEIN • The hydrolysate of corn. See Zein and Hydrolyzed.

HYDROPHILIC OINTMENT • An oil-in-water emulsion used as a base for skin preparations.

HYDROQUINOL • An alkaline solution that turns brown in air and is made up of white leaflets that are soluble in water. Used as an antiseptic and reducing ingredient *(see)* in cosmetics. Has caused skin cancer in mice.

HYDROQUINONE • Antioxidant used in bleach and freckle creams and in suntan lotions. It is also used in hair colorings. A white, crystalline phenol *(see)* that occurs naturally but is usually manufactured in the laboratory. Hydroquinone combines with oxygen very rapidly and becomes brown when exposed to air. Death has occurred from the ingestion of as little as 5 grams. Ingestion of as little as one gram (1/30th of an ounce) has caused nausea, vomiting, ringing in the ears, delirium, a sense of suffocation, and collapse. Industrial workers exposed to the chemical have suffered clouding of the eye lens. Application to the skin may cause allergic reactions. It can cause depigmentation in a 2 percent solution. When injected into the abdomens of mice in 28-milligram doses per kilogram of body weight, it caused bladder cancers, but other studies in which animals were fed the chemical did not show it to induce cancer. However, it did cause atrophy of the liver and aplastic anemia. In 1990, a report from South Africa showed a link between ochronosis *(see)* and this ingredient. Toxic to livers and kidneys in rats when given orally. In rats' skin, it produced irritation. Oral administration also caused dose-dependent mortality, lethargy, tremors, and increased liver and kidney weights. It also causes mutations in laboratory tests. On the basis of the available data, the CIR Expert Panel *(see)* concludes that this ingredient is safe at concentrations of 1 percent and less for aqueous cosmetic formulations designed for discontinuous, brief use followed by rinsing from the skin and hair. Hydroquinone should not be used in "leave-on" non-drug cosmetic products.

HYDROQUINONE DIBENZYL ETHER • Tan powder insoluble in water. Used as a solvent and in perfumes, soap, plastics, and pharmaceuticals. See Hydroquinone.

HYDROQUINONE DIMETHYLETHER • White flakes with sweet clover odor used as a fixative in perfumes, dyes, cosmetics, and especially suntan preparations. See Hydroquinone.

HYDROTROPES • Water-soluble compounds used in cosmetics.

HYDROXY CETYLDIMONIUM CHLORIDE • A quaternary compound *(see)* used as an antistatic agent in hair products.

HYDROXY CITRONELLAL • Laurine®. Colorless liquid obtained by the addition of water to citronellol *(see)*. Used as a fixative *(see)* and a fragrance in perfumery for its sweet lilylike odor. It has been known to cause allergic reactions.

HYDROXYACETIC ACID • See Glycolic Acid.

p-HYDROXYANISOLE • Used as an antioxidant in cosmetic products up to 1 percent. Undiluted, it is a severe skin and eye irritant in rabbits but a minimal skin irritant. Because of the depigmenting action of this ingredient in black guinea pigs at reported concentrations approaching those used in cosmetics, it is concluded by the CIR Expert Panel *(see)* that its use in cosmetics is unsafe.

HYDROXYAPATITE • A mineral obtained from phosphate rock.

o-HYDROXYBENZOIC ACID • See Salicylic Acid.

p-HYDROXYBENZOIC ACID • Prepared from p-bromophenol. Used as a preservative and fungicide. See Benzoic Acid for toxicity.

HYDROXYBENZOMORPHOLINE • **4-Salicylomorpholine.** A hair coloring. Used medically to stimulate the liver. No satisfactory data were available on the possible presence of nitrosamines *(see)*. The CIR Expert Panel *(see)* advised that it should not be used in the presence of nitrosating *(see)* agents. On the basis of the available data, the Panel concludes that this ingredient is safe at current levels of use.

HYDROXYBUTYL METHYLCELLULOSE • See Methylcellulose.

HYDROXYCAPRIC ACID • Used in skin conditioners. See Capric Acid.

HYDROXYCAPRYLIC ACID • See Alpha-hydroxy Acids.

HYDROXYCETETH-60 • See Polyethylene Glycol and Hexadecanoic Acid.

HYDROXYCETYL PHOSPHATE • The esters of phosphoric acid and cetyl alcohol *(see both)*.

HYDROXYETHYL CARBOXYMETHYL COCAMINOPROPYLATE • See Coconut Oil.

HYDROXYETHYL CETYLDIMONIUM CHLORIDE • See Quaternary Ammonium Compounds.

HYDROXYETHYL CETYLDIMONIUM PHOSPHATE • See Quaternary Ammonium Compounds.

HYDROXYETHYL-2,6-DINITRO-p-ANISIDINE • See Nitrophenol.

HYDROXYETHYL ETHYLCELLULOSE • See Cellulose.

HYDROXYETHYL PEI-1000,-1500 • See PEI.

HYDROXYETHYL-p-PHENYLENEDIAMINE SULFATE • See p-Phenylenediamine.

HYDROXYETHYL PICRAMIC ACID • See Picramic Acid.

HYDROXYETHYL STEARAMIDE-MIPA • See Stearic Acid.

HYDROXYETHYLAMINO-5-NITROANISOLE • See Ethanol.

HYDROXYETHYLCELLULOSE • Widely used modified cellulose *(see)* used as a binder, emulsion stabilizer, and thickener. It is in tanning products, hair rinses, makeup foundations, shampoos, mascara, body and hand lotions, and many other products. On the basis of the available animal and human data, the CIR Expert Panel *(see)* concludes that this ingredient is safe as used in cosmetics.

HYDROXYLAMINE HCL • An antioxidant for fatty acids and soaps. May be slightly irritating to skin, eyes, and mucous membranes, and may cause a depletion of oxygen in the blood when ingested. In the body it is reportedly decomposed to sodium nitrite. See nitrite.

HYDROXYLAMINE SULFATE • A hair-waving component in permanent wave solutions, it is a crystalline ammonium sulfate compound. It is also used for dehairing hides, in photography, as a chemical reducing ingredient, and to purify aldehydes *(see)* and ketones *(see)*. No known toxicity to the skin. The lethal dose given in the abdomens of rats is small.

HYDROXYLATE • The process in which an atom of hydrogen and an atom of oxygen are introduced into a compound to make the compound more soluble.

HYDROXYLATED LANOLIN • It is better than plain lanolin because the hydroxylation *(see)* makes it mix better with water and be more absorbable on the skin. It is widely used in makeup and skin care preparations. The CIR Expert Panel *(see)* found it safe.

HYDROXLATED LECITHIN • The product obtained by the hydroxylation of lecithin. Used in skin products as an emulsifier. See Lecithin and Hydroxylation.

HYDROXYLATED MILK GLYCERIDES • Used as an emulsifying ingredient and in skin conditioners. See Milk and Hydroxylated.

HYDROXYLATION • The process in which an atom of hydrogen and an atom of oxygen are introduced into a compound to make that compound more soluble.

HYDROXYLAURIC ACID • A skin conditioner. See Lauric Acid and Hydroxylation.

HYDROXYLYCINE • Lycine that has been hydroxylated to make it more soluble and to supposedly increase the protein content of a product. Used in tanning products. See Lycine and Hydroxylation.

HYDROXYMETHYLCELLULOSE • Thickener and bodying ingredient derived from plants. Used to thicken cosmetics and as a setting aid in hair products. On the basis of the available data, the CIR Expert Panel *(see)* concludes that this ingredient is safe. See Carboxymethylcellulose.

HYDROXYOCTACOSANYL HYDROXYSTEARATE • See Stearic Acid and Hydroxylation.

HYDROXYPHENYL GLYCINAMIDE • Derived from the nonessential amino acid glycine *(see)* used as a buffering ingredient and as a violet scent.

HYDROXYPROLINE • A moisturizer used in face, neck, hand, and body preparations. It is also used in eye makeup. See Hydroxylation and Proline.

HYDROXYPROPYL BIS-OLEYL-DIMONIUM CHLORIDE • See Quaternary Ammonium Compounds.

HYDROXYPROLINE • L-Proline. The hydroxylated *(see)* amino acid used to add "protein" to cosmetics.

HYDROXYPROPYL GUAR • Guar Gum, 2-Hydroxypropyl Ether. See Guar Gum.

HYDROXYPROPYL METHYLCELLULOSE • Widely used ingredient in many hair and skin preparations as well as bubble bath and tanning preparations. On the basis of the available animal and human data, the CIR Expert Panel *(see)* concludes that this ingredient is safe as used in cosmetics. See Cellulose Gums.

HYDROXYPROPYLAMINE NITRITE • See Isopropanolamine and Nitrite.

4-HYDROXYPROPYLAMINE-2-NITROPHENOL • See Nitrophenol.

HYDROXYPROPYLCELLULOSE • A thickener. On the basis of the available animal and human data, the CIR Expert Panel *(see)* concludes that this ingredient is safe as used in cosmetics. See Hydroxymethylcellulose.

HYDROXYQUINOLINE • See Oxyquinoline Sulfate.

8-HYDROXYQUINOLINE SULFATE • Pale yellow powder with a slight saffron odor and burning taste. It is used as an antiseptic, antiperspirant, deodorant, and fungicide.

HYDROXYSTEARAMIDE MEA • A mixture of ethanolamide of hydroxystearic acid. See Stearic Acid.

HYDROXYSTEARIC ACID • A surfactant and cleansing agent in cosmetic products. Skin irritation has been produced by antiperspirant formulations in exaggerated conditions. On the basis of the available data, the CIR Expert Panel *(see)* concludes that this ingredient is safe. See Stearic Acid.

HYDROXYSTEARYL METHYLGLUCAMINE • An amino sugar. See Glucose.

HYOSCINE • See Scopolamine.

HYPERICUM • **Hypericin.** Blue-black needles obtained from pyridine *(see)*. The solutions are red or green with a red cast. Small amounts seem to be a tranquilizer and have been used as an antidepressant in medicine. It can produce a sensitivity to light.

HYPERSENSITIVITY • The condition in persons previously exposed to an antigen in which tissue damage results from an immune reaction to a further dose of the antigen. Classically, four types of hypersensitivity are recognized, but the term is often used to mean the type of allergy associated with hay fever and asthma.

HYPNEA • Red alga that inhibits yeast. See Algae.

HYPO- • Prefix from the Greek, meaning "under" or "below," as in hypoacidity—acidity in a lesser degree than is usual or normal.

HYPOALLERGENIC • A term for cosmetics supposedly devoid of common allergens that most frequently cause allergic reactions. However, spokesmen for both the FDA and the AMA find the claims of scientific proof for their efficacy to be insufficient. When first marketed in the 1930s, these cosmetics were called nonallergic, which implied they could not cause an allergic reaction. The term was abandoned because there are always people who will be allergic to almost any substance. The term "hypoallergenic" means "least likely to cause a reaction." Not only the user, but his or her companion may suffer an allergic reaction to cosmetics—for instance, a wife to her husband's shaving lotion or a child to its mother's hairspray.

HYPOPHOSPHORIC ACID • Crystals used in baking powder and sodium salt. No known toxicity.

HYPOPHOSPHOROUS ACID • Phosphorous treated with a resin. White, or yellow, crystalline mass used as a reducing ingredient and for phosphite salts.

HYPTIS SUAVEOLENS • A plant that yields an essential oil used in fragrances.

HYSSOP EXTRACT • Extract of *Hyssopus officinalis*. A synthetic flavoring from the aromatic herb. Used in bitters. The extract is a liquor flavoring for beverages, ice cream, and ice. The oil is a liquor and spice flavoring. No known toxicity.

I

ICELAND MOSS EXTRACT • The extract of *Lichen islandicus*. A water-soluble gum that gels on cooling. Used to flavor alcoholic beverages, as a food additive, and in cosmetic gels. No known toxicity.

ICHTHAMMOL • Pale yellow or brownish black, thick viscous liquid that smells like coal. It mixes with water, glycerol, fats, oils, and waxes, and is used medicinally as a topical antiseptic. It has slight bacteria-killing properties and is used in ointments for the treatment of skin disorders. It is also a feeble skin irritant. Formerly used medicinally as an expectorant. Large doses caused stomach upset and diarrhea.

IDOPROPYNYL BUTYLCARBAMATE • See Carbamate.

ILEX AQUIFOLIUM • *Ilex opaca.* **European Holly. American Holly.** A small evergreen, the leaves were used to increase perspiration, to treat inflammations of the mucous membranes, pleurisy, gout, and smallpox. The leaves contain theobromine *(see).* The berries were used to cause vomiting and as a diuretic to remove excess fluid. The juice of the berries was used to treat jaundice.

ILLIIPE BUTTER • Any of a number of vegetable fats. Used particularly in the chocolate industry.

IMIDAZOLE • **Glyoxaline, 1, 3-Diazole.** Derived from benzene *(see).* Consists of orange-colored needles. It is an antimetabolite and inhibitor of histamine, and is used to control pests. It is an inhibitor of growth rather than toxic.

IMIDAZOLIDINONE • **Ethylene Urea.** Prepared from ethylenediamine and carbon dioxide. Used in pressure-sensitive adhesives, lacquers, insecticides, and for coatings.

IMIDAZOLIDINYL UREA • The most commonly used cosmetic preservative after the parabens, it is the second most identified cosmetic preservative causing contact dermatitis, according to The American Academy of Dermatology's Standards on Vehicle and Preservative Patch Testing Tray results. It is colorless, odorless, and tasteless, and is employed in baby shampoos, lotions, oils, powders, eye shadows, permanent waves, rinses, fragrances, hair tonics, colognes, powders, creams, bath oils, blushers, rouges, moisturizers, and fragrances. No known toxicity. On the basis of the available animal and human data, the CIR Expert Panel *(see)* concludes that this ingredient is safe as used in cosmetics.

IMIDAZOLINE • A derivative of imidazole *(see)* also called glyoxalidine.

IMIDAZOLINE AMPHOTERIC • Surfactant used in "no tears" shampoos. An "anti-irritant" that neutralizes the effects of a cosmetic. See Imidazolidinyl Urea.

IMIDUREA • See Urea.

IMINO-BIS-PROPYLAMINE • See Propylamine.

IMITATION • With reference to a fragrance, containing all or some portion of nonnatural materials. For instance, unless a strawberry flavoring used in lipstick is made entirely from strawberries, it must be called imitation.

IMMORTELLE EXTRACT • A natural flavoring extract from a red-flowered tropical tree. The name derives from the French *immortel*—"immortal" or "everlasting." Used in raspberry, fruit, and liquor flavorings for beverages, ice cream, ices, baked goods, candy, gelatin desserts, and chewing gum. GRAS.

IMPATIENS • A large genus of widely distributed annual plants of the *Balsaminaceae* family. It has a watery juice and is used in "organic" cosmetics. The FDA issued a notice in 1992 that impatiens has not been shown to be safe and effective as claimed in OTC poison ivy, poison oak, and poison sumac products. It is used in cosmetics to reduce inflammation.

INDIAN CRESS EXTRACT • **Phytelene of Capucine.** The extract obtained from the flowers of *Tropaeolum majus.*

INDIAN HEMP • *Apocynum cannabinum.* **Dogbane.** A North American dogbane that yields a tough fiber formerly used in rope.

INDIGO • Probably the oldest known dye. Prepared from various *Indigofera* plants native to Bengal, Java, and Guatemala. Dark blue powder with a coppery luster. No known skin irritation, but continued use on hair can cause hair to become brittle.

INDIGOFERA • See Indigo.

INDOLE • A white, lustrous, flaky substance with an unpleasant odor, occurring naturally in jasmine oil and orange flowers, and used in perfumes. Also extracted from coal tar and feces; in highly diluted solutions, the odor is pleasant. Large doses have been lethal to dogs. No known toxicity on the skin.

INNER CELLULAR MEMBRANE COMPLEX • A vegetable-derived protein imitating cellular membrane complex *(see).* See also Hair.

INOSITOL • A dietary supplement of the Vitamin B family used in emollients. Found in plant and animal tissues. Isolated commercially from corn. A fine, white, crystalline powder, it is odorless with a sweet taste. Stable in air. No known toxicity.

INSOLUBLE METAPHOSPHATE • See Sodium Metaphosphate.

INTERMEDIATE • A chemical substance found as part of a necessary step between one organic compound and another, as in the production of dyes, pharmaceuticals, or other artificial products that develop properties only upon oxidation. For instance, it is used for hair-dye bases that have dyeing action only when exposed to oxygen.

INULIN • **Elecampane Extract.** A sugar from plants. Used by intravenous injection to determine kidney function; also used in bread for diabetics. Used in cosmetics as a humectant and as a skin conditioning ingredient.

IODIDE • The negative ion of iodine is made from iodine and water. See Iodine.

IODINE • Discovered in 1811 and classed among the rarer earth elements, it is found in the earth's crust as bluish black scales. Nearly 200 products contain this chemical. They are prescription and over-the-counter medications. Iodine compounds are used as expectorants and thinners, particularly in the treatment of asthma and in contrast media for X rays and fluoroscopy. They can produce a diffuse red pimply rash, hives, asthma, and sometimes anaphylactic shock. Iodine is also used as an antiseptic and germicide in cosmetics.

IODIZED • The addition of iodine often used in compounds as a stabilizer and preservative.

IODIZED CORN PROTEIN • See Corn and Iodine.

IODIZED GARLIC • Powdered garlic to which iodine has been added. See Iodine and Garlic.

IODIZED HYDROLYZED EXTENSIN • See Iodine and Extensin.

IODIZED ZEIN • See Iodine and Zein.

IODOFORM • Small, greenish yellow or lustrous crystals or powder with a penetrating odor. Derived from iodine *(see)*. Used as a preservative and antiseptic. Can be irritating to the skin.

IODOPHOR • Tamed Iodine. A complex of iodine with certain surface-active ingredients that have detergent properties.

IODOPROPYNL BUTYLCARBAMATE • A preservative widely used in cosmetics. Has been shown to adversely affect livers in rats in feeding studies. It also affected their behavior. It was also mildly irritating in human testing. On the basis of the available animal and human data, the CIR Expert Panel *(see)* concludes that this ingredient is safe as used in cosmetics at concentrations up to 0.1 percent but it should not be used in aerosolized products. See Carbamates.

IONONE • Used as a scent in perfumery and as a flavoring ingredient in foods, it occurs naturally in *Boronia,* an Australian shrub. Colorless to pale yellow, with an odor reminiscent of cedar wood or violets. It may cause allergic reactions.

IPBC • Abbreviation for Iodopropynl Butylcarbamate *(see).*

IPECAC • *Cephaelis ipecacuanha.* **Ipecacuanha.** From the dried rhizome and roots of a creeping South American plant with drooping flowers. Used by herbalists and sold in conventional pharmacies, ipecac is primarily used to induce vomiting when ingestion of noncaustic poisons has occurred. It may also be used in medicine to induce expulsion of mucus in lung congestion. Used as a denaturant in alcohol. Fatal dose in humans is as low as 20 milligrams per kilogram of body weight. Irritating when taken internally but no known toxicity on the skin.

IPOMOEA • A vinelike herb. Sweet potatoes and morning glories belong to this family.

IRIS FLORENTINA, GERMANICA AND PALLIDA • See Orris.

IRIS VERSICOLOR • See Blue Flag.

IRISH MOSS • See Carrageenan.

IRON OXIDES • Very widely used to color cosmetics. Any of several natural or synthetic oxides of iron (that is, iron combined with oxygen), varying in color from red to brown, black to orange or yellow, depending on the degree of water added and the purity. Ocher, sienna, and iron oxide red are among the colors used to tint face powders, liquid powders, and foundation creams. Black iron oxide is used for coloring eye shadow. See Colors for toxicity. Permanently listed in 1977.

IRON SALTS • Iron Sources: ferric, choline citrate; ferric orthophosphate; ferric phosphate; ferric sodium pyrophosphate; ferrous fumarate; ferrous gluconate; ferrous lactate; and ferrous sulfate. Widely used as enrichment for foods, they are used in cosmetics mainly for coloring and as astringents. Ingestion of large quantities can cause gastrointestinal disturbances, but there is no known toxicity in cosmetics.

IRONE • The fragrant principle of violets, usually isolated from the iris, and used in perfumery. A light yellow, viscous liquid, it gives off the delicate fragrance of violets when put in alcohol. It is also used to flavor dentifrices. See Orris for toxicity.

ISATIN • A hair coloring. See Indole.

ISATIS TINCTORIA • **Woad.** A biennial widely distributed in Europe, Asia, and North Africa, it is a member of the mustard family. The plant is used to treat St. Anthony's fire (gangrene and inflammation) and for plasters and ointments used to treat ulcers and inflammation.

ISO • Greek for "equal." In chemistry, it is a prefix added to the name of one compound to denote another composed of the same kinds and numbers of atoms but different from each other in structural arrangement.

ISOAMIDOPROPYL ETHYLDIMONIUM ETHOSULFATE • See Quaternary Ammonium Compounds.

ISOAMYL ACETATE • A synthetic flavoring ingredient that occurs naturally in bananas and pears. Colorless, with a pearlike odor and taste, it is used in perfumery. Exposure to 950 ppm for one hour has caused headache, fatigue, shoulder pain, and irritation of the mucous membranes. It has been found to stimulate acetylcholine release in the nerve endings and act as a competitive inhibitor of acetylcholine in isolated nerves. Acetylcholine is a nerve messenger and plays a big part in memory functioning. It is used up to 10 percent in fingernail formulations. The CIR Expert Panel *(see)* concludes this is a safe ingredient in cosmetics. See Amyl Acetate.

ISOAMYL ALCOHOL • A synthetic flavoring ingredient that occurs naturally in apples, cognac, lemons, peppermint, raspberry, strawberry, and tea. Used in chocolate, apple, banana, brandy, and rum flavorings for beverages, ice cream, ices, candy, baked goods, gelatin desserts, chewing gum, and brandy. A central nervous system depressant. Vapor exposures have caused marked irritation of the eyes, nose, and throat and headache. Amyl alcohols are highly toxic, and ingestion has caused human deaths from respiratory failure. Isoamyl alcohol may cause heart, lung, and kidney damage.

ISOAMYL LAURATE • The ester of isoamyl alcohol and lauric acid *(see both)* used as a synthetic fruit flavoring.

ISOAMYL p-METHOXYCINNAMATE • See Cinnamic Acid.

ISOBORNYL ACETATE • A synthetic pine odor in bath preparations. Also used as a synthetic fruit flavoring for beverages. No known toxicity.

ISOBUTANE • A constituent of natural gas and illuminating gas, colorless and insoluble in water, used in refrigeration plants. A propellant used for cosmetic sprays. On the basis of the available animal and human data, the CIR Expert Panel *(see)* concludes that this ingredient is safe as used in cosmetics. See Paraffin and Propellant.

ISOBUTOXYPROPANOL • See Isopropyl Alcohol.

ISOBUTYL ACETATE • The ester of isobutyl alcohol and acetic acid used as a synthetic flavoring ingredient. A clear, colorless liquid with a fruity odor, it may be mildly irritating to mucous membranes, and in high concentrations it is narcotic.

ISOBUTYL METHYL TETRAHYDROPYRANOL • A fragrance ingredient.

ISOBUTYL MYRISTATE • The ester of isobutyl alcohol and myristic acid *(see)*.

ISOBUTYL PALMITATE • See Palmitate.

ISOBUTYL PELARGONATE • The ester of isobutyl alcohol and pelargonic acid *(see)*.

ISOBUTYL QUINOLINE • See Quinoline.

ISOBUTYL SALICYLATE • See Salicylates.

ISOBUTYL STEARATE • The ester of isobutyl alcohol and stearic acid. Used in waterproof coatings, polishes, face creams, rouges, ointments, soaps, dyes, and lubricants. No known toxicity. Used as a skin conditioning ingredient. On the basis of the available animal and human data, the CIR Expert Panel *(see)* concludes that this ingredient is safe as used in cosmetics. See Fatty Alcohols.

ISOBUTYL TALLOWATE • The ester of isobutyl alcohol and tallow acid.

ISOBUTYLATED • A method to alkylate compounds to make them more soluble. See Butane.

ISOBUTYLATED BENZOATE • See Benzoic Acid and Isobutylated.

ISOBUTYLATED LANOLIN • The partial ester of lanolin oil *(see)*.

ISOBUTYLATED LANOLIN OIL • See Lanolin and Isobutylated.

ISOBUTYLENE/ISOPRENE COPOLYMER • A copolymer of isobutylene and isoprene monomers derived from petroleum and used as a resin.

ISOBUTYLENE/MALEIC ANHYDRIDE COPOLYMER • A copolymer of isobutylene and maleic anhydride monomers derived from petroleum and used as a resin. Strong irritant.

ISOBUTYLENE/SODIUM MALEATE COPOLYMER • A synthetic polymer used as a film-former.

ISOBUTYLPARABEN • Widely used in makeup, hair products, and skin conditioners as a preservative. On the basis of the available animal and human data, the CIR Expert Panel *(see)* concludes that this ingredient is safe as used in cosmetics See Parabens.

ISOBUTYRIC ACID • A pungent liquid that smells like butyric acid *(see)*. A mild irritant used chiefly in making fragrance materials.

ISOCETEARETH-8 STEARATE • See Ethylene Oxide and Stearic Acid.

ISOCETETH-10, -20, -30 • The polyethylene glycol ethers of isocetyl alcohol. See Cetyl Alcohol.

ISOCETETH-10 STEARATE • The ester of isoceteth-10 and stearic acid. See Stearic Acid.

ISOCETYL ALCOHOL • See Cetyl Alcohol.

ISOCETYL ISODECANOATE • See Cetyl Alcohol.

ISOCETYL ISOSTEARATE • A skin conditioning ingredient. See Isostearic Acid.

ISOCETYL LAURATE • A skin conditioning ingredient. See Lauric Acid.

ISOCETYL PALMITATE • See Cetyl Alcohol and Palmitate.

ISOCETYL STEARATE • See Cetyl Alcohol and Stearic Acid.

ISOCETYL STEAROYL STEARATE • The ester of isocetyl alcohol, stearic alcohol, and stearic acid. See Fatty Acids.

ISODECANE • A gel. See Decanoic Acid.

ISODECETH-4, -5, -6 • See Polyethylene Glycol and Decyl Alcohol.

ISODECYL HYDROXYSTEARATE • An emollient ingredient. See Decyl Alcohol and Stearic Acid.

ISODECYL ISONONANOATE • See Decyl Alcohol.

ISODECYL LAURATE • The ester of decyl alcohol and lauric acid *(see both)* used as a wetting ingredient *(see)*.

ISODECYL MYRISTATE • See Decyl Alcohol and Myristic Acid.

ISODECYL NEOPENTANOATE • See 1-Pentanol.

ISODECYL OCTANOATE • The ester of decyl alcohol and hexanoic acid.

ISODECYL OLEATE • An emollient. See Decyl Alcohol and Oleic Acid.

ISODECYL PALMITATE • See Decyl Alcohol and Palmitic Acid.

ISODECYL SALICYLATE • The ester of decyl alcohol and salicylic acid.

ISODECYLPARABEN • The ester of decyl alcohol and p-hydroxybenzoic acid. See Propylparaben.

ISODON JAPONICUS AND TRICHOCARPUS • Perennial herb growing in Japan, Korea, and Russia. Yields essential oil.

ISOEICOSANE • See Eicosane.

ISOEUGENOL • An aromatic, liquid, phenol oil obtained from eugenol *(see)* by mixing with an alkali. Used chiefly in perfumes but also employed in hand creams and in making the flavoring vanillin. Strong irritant. Not recommended for use.

ISOHEXADECANE • See Hexadecanoic Acid.

ISOHEXYL LAURATE • See Lauryl Alcohol.

ISOHEXYL PALMITATE • See Palmitic Acid.

ISOJASMONE • See Jasmone.

ISOLAURETH-3, -6, -10 • See Polyethylene Glycol and Lauric Acid.

ISOLEUCINE • An essential amino acid not synthesized within the human body. Isolated commercially from beet sugar, it is a building block of protein. GRAS.

ISOLONGIFOLENE KETON EXO • An ingredient in fragrances.

ISOMALT • A candidate for an artificial sweetener, it has 45 to 65 percent the sweetness of sugar. A component of bread obtained by the action of enzymes on starch. It contains calories and is physically similar to sugar. It is free flowing, white, and crystalline. It has a sweet taste reportedly without any aftertaste. While it is not as sweet as sugar, it may be enhanced with an intense sweetener such as acesulfame. It is used in 15 countries in candies, gums, ice cream, jams, and baked goods. Used in cosmetics as an anticaking ingredient, thickener, and flavoring ingredient.

ISOMERIZED JOJOBA OIL • Used in emollients. See Jojoba Oil.

ISONONAMIDOPROPYL ETHYLDIMONIUM ETHOSULFATE • See Quaternary Ammonium Compounds.

ISONONYL FERULATE • An ester *(see)* of Ferulic Acid used in emollients.

ISONONYL ISONONANOATE • The ester *(see)* produced by the reaction of nonyl alcohol with nonanoic acid. Used in fruit flavorings for lipsticks and mouthwashes. Occurs in cocoa and oil of lavender. No known toxicity.

ISOOCTYL THIOGLYCOLATE • The ester of thioglycolic acid *(see)*.

ISOPENTANE • Volatile, flammable, liquid hydrocarbon found in petroleum and used as a solvent in cosmetics. A skin irritant. Narcotic in high doses. On the basis of the available animal and human data, the CIR Expert Panel *(see)* concludes that this ingredient is safe as used in cosmetics.

ISOPENTYLDIOL • A solvent. See Butyl Alcohol.

ISOPROPANOL • Legal name for Isopropyl Alcohol *(see)*.

ISOPROPANOLAMINE • A water-soluble emulsifying ingredient with a light ammonia odor. It is used as a plasticizer and in insecticides, as well as in cosmetic creams as a solvent.

ISOPROPYL ACETATE • The ester of isopropyl alcohol and acetic acid, a colorless liquid with a strong odor, it is used as a solvent for resin, gums, and cellulose; for lacquers; and in perfumery. Flammable.

ISOPROPYL ALCOHOL • **Isopropanol.** An antibacterial, solvent, and denaturant *(see)*. Solvent for the spice oleoresins. Used in hair-color rinses, body rubs, hand lotions, after-shave lotions, and many other cosmetics. It is prepared from propylene, which is obtained in the cracking of petroleum. Also used in antifreeze compositions and as a solvent for gums, shellac, and essential oils. Ingestion or inhalation of large quantities of the vapor may cause flushing, headache, dizziness, mental depression, nausea, vomiting, narcosis, anesthesia, and coma. The fatal ingested dose is about 1 fluid ounce. No known toxicity to the skin.

ISOPROPYL CREOSOLS • See Creosols.

ISOPROPYL ESTER OF PVM/MA COPOLYMER • A synthetic resin. See Polyvinyl Alcohol.

ISOPROPYL ISOSTEARATE • An emollient. Used as a skin conditioning ingredient. Undiluted, it is a skin irritant. On the basis of the available animal and human data, the CIR Expert Panel *(see)* concludes that this ingredient is safe as used in cosmetics. See Stearic Acid and Propylene Glycol.

ISOPROPYL LANOLATE • A mixture of isopropyl esters of lanolin acids. After purification, the acids are esterified *(see ester)* with isopropyl alcohol *(see)*. One of the more versatile lanolin derivatives because of its surfactant *(see)* properties and pigment-dispersing ability, it is used in combination with mineral oil and isopropyl palmitate *(see)* for pigments such as Titanium Dioxide, Oxy Red, and Red No. 9. In lipsticks, creams, lotions, and aerosol emulsions it acts as a lubricant and gives high gloss. It has been used for more than 20 years. May cause skin sensitization. Its effects on lung tissue have not been studied, although it is used as an aerosol. Used as a skin-conditioning ingredient. On the basis of the available animal and human data, the CIR Expert Panel *(see)* concludes that this ingredient is safe as used in cosmetics. See Lanolin.

ISOPROPYL LAURATE • See Lauric Acid.

ISOPROPYL LINOLEATE • An emollient. Used as a skin-conditioning ingredient. On the basis of the available animal and human data, the CIR Expert Panel *(see)* concludes that there is insufficient data to support the safety of this ingredient in cosmetics. See Linoleic Acid.

ISOPROPYL MYRISTATE • A widely used fatty compound derived from isopropyl alcohol and myristic acid. It causes blackheads and is being removed from many of the newer formulations. However, a more serious potential danger exists, since when nitrate compounds such as n-nitrosodiethanolamine (NDELA), an impurity in many cosmetic preparations, was applied in isopropyl myristate, its absorption was increased 230 times. NDELA may be a reaction product of di- or triethanolamine, used in many cosmetic formulations. Scientists are concerned that when isopropyl myristate is applied over large areas of the skin for long periods of time, such as in suntanning lotion, there will be a significant absorption of NDELA if the contaminant is present. On the basis of the available data, the CIR Expert Panel *(see)* concludes that it is safe as a cosmetic ingredient. See Myristic Acid.

ISOPROPYL OLEATE • The ester of isopropyl alcohol and oleic acid *(see)*.

ISOPROPYL PALMITATE • Widely used binder, skin-conditioning ingredient and emollient. It is in makeup, moisturizers, hair products, baby lotions, colognes, and manicuring products. The CIR Expert Panel *(see)* concludes that this ingredient is safe for use in cosmetic products. See Palmitic Acid.

ISOPROPYL C12-15-PARETH-9 CARBOXYLATE • The ester of carboxylic acid *(see)*.

ISOPROPYL RICINOLEATE • See Isopropyl Alcohol and Ricinoleic Acid.

ISOPROPYL STEARATE • An emollient. Used as a skin conditioning ingredient. On the basis of the available animal and human data, the CIR Expert Panel *(see)* concludes that this ingredient is safe as used in cosmetics. See Stearic Acid.

ISOPROPYL TALLOWATE • See Fatty Acids.

ISOPROPYLAMINE DODECYLBENZENESULFONATE • See Quaternary Ammonium Compounds.

ISOPROPYLBENZYLSALICYLATE • See Salicylates.

ISOPROPYLPARABEN • On the basis of the available animal and human data, the CIR Expert Panel *(see)* concludes that this ingredient is safe as used in cosmetics See Parabens.

ISOSORBIDE • A skin conditioning ingredient. See Sorbic Acid.

ISOSTEARAMIDE DEA • A mixture of fatty acids from stearic acid. The CIR Expert Panel *(see)* concludes that this ingredient is safe at maximum concentration of 40 percent. There is however a potential problem of producing nitrosamines *(see)* and it should not be used in products in which these cancer-causing agents may be formed.

ISOSTEARAMIDE MIPA • A mixture of isopropanolamides of isostearic acid.

ISOSTEARAMIDOPROPALKONIUM CHLORIDE • See Surfactants.

ISOSTEARAMIDOPROPYL BETAINE • See Surfactants.

ISOSTEARAMIDOPROPYL DIMETHYLAMINE GLYCOLATE • An antistatic ingredient used in hair products. See Surfactants.

ISOSTEARAMIDOPROPYL DIMETHYLAMINE LACTATE • See Surfactants.

ISOSTEARAMIDOPROPYL EPOXYPROPYLMORPHOLINIUM CHLORIDE • Used in hair conditioners. See Quarternary Ammonium Compounds.

ISOSTEARAMIDOPROPYL ETHYLDIMONIUM ETHOSULFATE • See Quaternary Ammonium Compounds.

ISOSTEARAMIDOPROPYL LAURYLACETODIMONIUM CHLORIDE • A quarternary ammonium compound *(see)* used as an antistatic ingredient in hair preparations.

ISOSTEARAMIDOPROPYL MORPHOLINE LACTATE • A hair conditioner. The CIR Expert Panel *(see)* concludes that it is safe for "rinse-off" formulations but there is insufficient data available to support safety in "leave-on" formulations. See Surfactants.

ISOSTEARAMIDOPROPYLAMINE OXIDE • See Surfactants.

ISOSTEARETH-2 THROUGH -20 • See Fatty Alcohols.

ISOSTEARIC ACID • A complex mixture of fatty acids similar to stearic acid *(see)*. Used as a binder, solvent, surfactant, and emulsifier *(see all)*. On the basis of the available information, the CIR Expert Panel *(see)* concludes that it is safe as a cosmetic ingredient.

ISOSTEARIC HYDROLYZED COLLAGEN • The world "animal" was removed from the ingredient name. Used in creams. See Protein and Hydrolyzation.

ISOSTEARIC/MYRISTIC GLYCERIDES • Used in emollients. See Glycerides.

ISOSTEAROAMPHOGLYCINATE • See Surfactants.

ISOSTEAROAMPHOPROPIONATE • See Surfactants.

ISOSTEAROYL HYDROLYZED COLLAGEN • See Surfactants.

ISOSTEARYL ALCOHOL • See Stearyl Alcohol.

ISOSTEARYL AVOCADATE • A skin-conditioning ingredient. See Avocado.

ISOSTEARYL BENZOATE • A skin-conditioning ingredient. See Benzoic Acid.

ISOSTEARYL BENZYLIMIDONIUM CHLORIDE • See Surfactants.

ISOSTEARYL DIGLYCERYL SUCCINATE • See Surfactants.

ISOSTEARYL ERUCATE • See Surfactants.

ISOSTEARYL ETHYLIMIDAZOLINIUM ETHOSULFATE • Quarternary Ammonium Compound used as an antistatic ingredient in hair conditioners. See Quarternary Ammonium Compounds.

ISOSTEARYL GLYCERYL ETHER • A skin-conditioning ingredient. See Glycerin.

ISOSTEARYL GLYCERYL PENTAERYTHRITYL ETHER • A hair-conditioning ingredient. See Pentaerythritol.

ISOSTEARYL HYDROXYETHYL IMIDAZOLINE • See Surfactants.

ISOSTEARYL IMIDAZOLINE • See Surfactants.

ISOSTEARYL ISOSTEARATE • See Stearyl Alcohol.

ISOSTEARYL ISOSTEARYOL STEARATE • A skin-conditioning ingredient. See Stearic Acid.

ISOSTEARYL LACTATE • See Surfactants.

ISOSTEARYL MYRISTATE • The ester of isostearyl alcohol and myristic acid.

ISOSTEARYL NEOPENTANOATE • An emollient. On the basis of the available information, the CIR Expert Panel *(see)* concludes that it is safe as a cosmetic ingredient. See Surfactants.

ISOSTEARYL PALMITATE • See Surfactants.

ISOSTEAROYL PG-TRIMONIUM CHLORIDE • An antistatic ingredient in hair preparations. See Quarternary Ammonium Compounds.

ISOSTEARYL STEAROYL STEARATE • See Surfactants.

ISOTHIAZOLONONES • **5-Chloro-3-Methyl and 3-Methyl.** A preservative in European cosmetics. May cause allergies, but the incidence is low. Most of those who do show a reaction are also allergic to nickel. See Kathon CG.

ISOTRIDECYL ISONONANOATE • See Tridecyl Alcohol.

ISOVALERIC ACID • Occurs in valerian, hop oil, tobacco, and other plants. Colorless liquid with a disagreeable taste and odor, used in flavors and perfumes. See Valeric Acid.

IVY EXTRACT • Extract of climbing plant with evergreen leaves native to Europe and Asia. Widely used in body and hand products, bubble bath, bath soaps, mud packs, and moisturizers. Produces a color that ranges from dark grayish green to yellowish. No known toxicity.

J

JABORANDI • Pilocarpus. A tincture from the leaves of the pilocarpus plant, grown in South America. It supposedly stimulates the sebaceous glands and scalp, and was formerly used to induce sweating. Used in hair tonics. A source of pilo-carpine *(see)*. Poisonous when ingested. No known toxicity on the skin.

JAGUAR GUM • See Guar Gum.

JALAP RESIN • A resin *(see)* used in cosmetics. The dried purgative tuberous root of a Mexican plant. Was once used as a drastic cathartic. No known toxicity on the skin.

JAMBUL EXTRACT • **Jamboo. Java Plum.** An extract of the roots of *Syzyglum jambolanum*. The bark, resin, and oil contain volatile oils, fat, gallic acid *(see)*, and albumen. It is used medically as an antidiarrheal. Extracts of the bark are used in cosmetics to soothe the skin.

JAPAN WAX • *Rhus Succedanea.* **Vegetable Wax. Japan Tallow.** A fat squeezed from the fruit of a tree grown in Japan and China. Pale yellow, flat cakes, disks, or squares with a fatlike rancid odor and taste. Used as a substitute for beeswax in cosmetic ointments, also floor waxes and polishes. It is related to poison ivy and may cause allergic contact dermatitis. The CIR Expert Panel *(see)* concludes this is a safe ingredient.

JAPANESE ANGELICA • *Angelica acutiloba*. A shrub or small Japanese tree. Used in bath products. See Angelica.

JAPANESE QUINCE EXTRACT • Extract of the seeds of *Chaenomeles japonica*. See Quince Seed.

JASMINE • Used in perfumes. The essential oil extracted from the extremely fragrant white flowers of the tall, climbing, semi-evergreen jasmine shrub. May cause allergic reactions. Synthetic jasmine contains cinnamic aldehyde *(see)*.

JASMINE ABSOLUTE • Oil of jasmine obtained by extraction with volatile or nonvolatile solvents. Sometimes called the "natural perfume" because the oil is not subjected to heat and distilled oils. May cause allergic reactions. See Absolute.

JASOMONE • Derived from the oil of jasmine flowers, it is used in flavorings and perfumery.

JAVA JUTE EXTRACT • Extract of the flowers of *Hibiscus sabdariffa*. See Hibiscus.

JEWELWEED • See Impatiens.

JOB'S TEARS • *Coix lacryma-jobi*. **Tear Grass.** Asiatic grass now widely cultivated. A skin-conditioning ingredient.

JOJOBA ALCOHOL • Fatty alcohol from Jojoba. See Jojoba Oil.

JOJOBA BUTTER • Obtained from jojoba oil *(see)*.

JOJOBA OIL • *Buxux chinensis*. Widely used in cosmetics, it is the oil extracted from the beanlike seeds of the desert shrub *Simondsia chinensis*. A liquid wax used as a lubricant and as a substitute for sperm oil, carnauba wax, and beeswax. Mexicans and American Indians have long used the bean's oily wax as a hair conditioner and skin lubricant. U.S. companies are now promoting the ingredient in shampoos, moisturizers, sunscreens, and conditioners as a treatment for "crow's feet," wrinkles, stretch marks, and dry skin. May cause allergic reactions. On the basis of the available information, the CIR Expert Panel *(see)* concludes that it is safe as a cosmetic ingredient.

JOJOBA WAX • The semisolid fraction of jojoba oil *(see)*. On the basis of the available information, the CIR Expert Panel *(see)* concludes it is safe as a cosmetic ingredient.

JOJOBA WAX PEG 80, 120 ESTERS • Used as surfactants, cleansing ingredients, and solubilizing ingredients.

JONQUIL EXTRACT • Extract of *Narcissus jonquilla*.

JUJUBE EXTRACT • Da T'sao. Extract of the fruit of *Zizyphus jujube miller*. The Chinese jujube date is commonly used in a wide variety of herbal formulas. It is found dried in most oriental markets. It is used to enhance the taste and benefits of soups and stews and to energize the body. Chinese herbalists believe it relieves nervous exhaustion, insomnia, apprehension, forgetfulness, dizziness, and clamminess.

JUGLANS • See Walnut Extract.

JUGLONE • A coloring for hair dyes. Yellow needles, slightly soluble in hot water but soluble in alcohol. It is the active coloring principle in walnuts. When mixed in solution with an alkali, it gives a purplish red color. It has antihemorrhaging activity. The lethal oral dose in mice is only 2.5 milligrams per kilogram of body weight. No known skin toxicity.

JUNIPER BERRY • *Juniperus communis.* **Viscum. Mistletoe.** The berries are used by herbalists to treat urinary problems. According to herbalists, it acts directly on the kidneys, stimulating the flow of urine. Juniper berries and extracts are in several over-the-counter drugstore diuretic and laxative preparations. In fact, gin was created in the 1500s by a Dutch pharmacist using juniper berries to sell as an inexpensive diuretic. The berries have long been used by herbalists to treat gout caused by high uric acid in the blood. The berry is also recommended to aid digestion and eliminate gas and cramps. The berries are high in Vitamin C. It is used in "organic" cosmetics. Juniper is also used to lower cholesterol and to treat arthritis. Large amounts may irritate the kidneys. The FDA issued a notice in 1992 that juniper has not been shown to be safe and effective as claimed in OTC digestive aid products and oral menstrual drugs.

JUNIPER TAR • **Oil of Cade.** The volatile oil from the wood of a pine tree. Dark brown, viscous, with a smoky odor and acrid, slightly aromatic taste. Very slightly soluble in water. It is used as a skin peeler and anti-itching factor in hair preparations and as a scent in perfumes. Less corrosive than phenol *(see)*.

JUNIPERUS • See Juniper Berry.

JUNIPERUS OXYCEDRUS TAR • Obtained from the wood of the juniper bush. Used to scent hair products. See Juniper Berry.

K

KALANCHOE PINNATA • An African and Australian herb. See Cedar.

KALAYA OIL • See Emu Oil.

KANGAROO PAW FLOWER • An Australian sedgelike spring-flowering herb related to the *Amaryllis*. It has clustered flowers covered with greenish wool. Used in Australian-imported hairsprays. No known toxicity.

KAOLIN • **China Clay.** Aids in the covering ability of face powder and in absorbing oil secreted by the skin. Used in baby powders, bath powders, face masks, foundation cake makeups, liquid powders, face powders, dry rouges, and emollients. Originally obtained from Kaoling Hill in Kiangsi Province in Southeast China. Essentially a hydrated aluminum silicate *(see)*. It is a white or yellowish white mass or powder, insoluble in water and absorbent. Used medicinally to treat intestinal disorders, but in large doses it may cause obstructions, perforations, or granuloma (tumor) formation. It is also used in the manufacture of porcelain, pottery, bricks, and color lakes *(see)*. No known toxicity for the skin.

KARAYA GUM • See Gum Karaya.

KATHON CG • **Octhilinone.** A fungicide used in cosmetics and shampoos and for leather preservation. It has been extensively studied in cosmetics and toiletries. It is effective in low concentration and is very useful against bacteria, yeasts, and fungi. Although toxicity has not been a problem at usual use levels, sensitization, particularly among women, has been reported. The main source of sensitization has been kathon in cosmetics. Researchers in the United States and Europe are reporting an increasing number of patients becoming sensitized to the preservative.

KAVA KAVA • *Piper methysticum.* **Kawa. Ava.** The Polynesian herb's root is used by herbalists as a remedy for insomnia and nervousness. A compound in kava is marketed in Europe as a mild sedative for the elderly. Other ingredients in kava have been shown to have antiseptic properties in the laboratory, and it is used in "organic" cosmetics. It is also a reputedly potent analgesic and antiseptic that may be taken internally or applied directly to a painful wound.

KAWA EXTRACT • The extract of the roots, stems, and leaves of *Piper methysticum.* See Kava Kava.

KELP • Recovered from the giant Pacific marine plant *Macrocystis pyriferae,* it is used by herbalists to supply the thyroid gland with iodine, to help regulate the texture of the skin, and to help the body burn off excess fat. In Japan, where kelp is a large part of the diet, thyroid disease is almost unknown. Kelp was banned from over-the-counter diet pills by the FDA, February 10, 1992. Kelp does contain many minerals, and herbalists claim that it has anticancer, antirheumatic, antiinflammatory, and blood pressure–lowering properties. No known toxicity.

KERATIN • **Animal Keratin.** Protein *(see)* obtained from the horns, hoofs, feathers, quills, and hairs of various creatures. Yellowish brown powder. Insoluble in water, alcohol, or ether but soluble in ammonia. Used in permanent wave solutions and hair rinses. Nontoxic.

KERATIN AMINO ACIDS • **Animal Keratin Amino Acids.** The cosmetic manufacturers took out as many "animals" in the labels as possible. A mixture of amino acids from the hydrolysis of keratin *(see).* See also Hydrolyzed Keratin.

KERATOLYTICS • Products that appear to loosen skin flakes and allow them to be more easily washed away. Lotions containing salicylic acid *(see)* are used for this purpose.

KEROSENE • See Deodorized Kerosene.

KETOCONAZOLE • **Nizoral.** Introduced in 1981, it inhibits the growth of fungi, and is used to treat systemic candidiasis, chronic mucocandidiasis, oral thrush, candiduria, coccidioidomycosis, histoplasmosis, chromomycosis, and paracoccidioidomycosis—severe skin infections resistant to therapy with topical or oral griseofulvin. Adverse effects include headache, nervousness, dizziness, nausea, enlargement of the male breast, vomiting, stomach pain, diarrhea, constipation, elevated liver enzymes, and fatal liver toxicity. In skin preparations ketoconazole may cause severe irritation, itching, stinging, and localized allergic reactions. In topical applications, the potential adverse reactions include itching, stinging, or irritation. If athlete's foot is the problem, the patient should avoid wearing socks made from wool or synthetic materials and, instead, wear clean, cotton socks. May interact with many drugs, including antacids, anticholinergics, and some antihistamines. Rifampin and isoniazid may make the antifungal less effective. The medication is a powerful inhibitor of liver enzymes. Coadministration with triazolam *(see),* for example, inhibits the clearance of the sleep medication. Studies are now under way to detect other such interactions with ketoconazole. May be taken with food to reduce risk of stomach upset. A keto-conazole shampoo is a candidate for OTC status, as of this writing.

KETONES • Acetone, Methyl, or Ethyl. Aromatic substances obtained by the oxidation of secondary alcohols. Ethereal or aromatic odor, generally insoluble in water but soluble in alcohol or ether. Solvents used in nail polish and nail polish removers. When injected into the abdomens of rats, intermediate dosages are lethal. See Acetone for skin toxicity.

KIDNEY BEAN EXTRACT • Extract of *Phaseolus vulgaris,* the beans were used as a nutrient and a laxative by the American Indians. No known toxicity.

KIGELIA AFRICANA • Sausage Tree. Often cultivated in tropical countries for its brownish red, bell-shaped flowers and long sausage-shaped fruits. Used in skin care products.

KINETIN • Found in many yeast plants. Used as a plant growth regulator. In cosmetics, it is employed in skin care and "age-defying" products.

KINO • *Pterocarpus marsuipun. P. indicus. P. echinatus.* **Gummi. Narra. Bibla. Prickly Narra. Padauk.** The exudate from the trunk of this large tree is used as an astringent *(see)* for the treatment of wounds, scrapes, diarrhea, and skin ulcers. It contains a tanninlike substance. It was also used as an aphrodisiac in Africa.

KIWI EXTRACT • Extract of the fruit named for the kiwi bird, *Actinidia chinensise.* It is used in cosmetic flavorings and in emollients.

KNOTWEED EXTRACT • Extract of *Polygonum aviculare.* A common weed, the FDA issued a notice in 1992 that knotgrass, a member of the family, has not been shown to be safe and effective as claimed in OTC digestive aid products. As of this writing, no such caution has been made about its use in cosmetics.

KOHL • Kohol. Cohol. A preparation of antimony or soot mixed with other ingredients used especially in Arabia and Egypt to darken the edges of the eyelids. In Israel, it is used even on the eyes of some babies. The application to the eyes of babies or their mothers increases the blood lead levels in the infants. The incidence of adverse reactions is high, about 25 percent if applied daily and 18 percent if applied occasionally. Third World–manufactured kohls have been purchased in the United States and Britain, suggesting that this hazard is no longer confined to the Third World. The kohls that contain lead are being sold in violation of U.S. and British law.

KOJIC ACID • An antibiotic usually isolated from *Aspergillus (see) oryzae.* Used as an antioxidant.

KOLA NUT • *Cola acuminata.* **Cola. Guru Nut.** Collected from a tree that grows in tropical Africa and is cultivated in South America, the seeds contain caffeine, theobromine, tannin, and volatile oil *(see all).* It is used in "organic" cosmetic. It is used for stimulation to counteract fatigue and as a diuretic. Herbalists use it to treat some types of migraine headache and diarrhea caused by anxiety. It is also used to treat emotional depression.

KRAMERIA EXTRACT • Khatany Extract. A synthetic flavoring derived from the dried root of either of two American shrubs. Used in raspberry, bitters, fruit, and rum flavorings. Used in cosmetics as an astringent. Low oral toxicity. Large doses may produce gastric distress. Can cause tumors and death after injection, but not after ingestion.

KUKUI NUT OIL • *Aleurites moluccana*. **Candlenut Oil. Varnish Tree. Lumbang Oil.** The oily seed of a tropical tree widely distributed in the tropics and used locally to make candles and commercially as a source of oil for making soap. Has been used by native Hawaiians for thousands of years to treat dry skin, psoriasis, acne, and other common skin problems.

L

LABDANUM • **Synthetic Musk.** Used in perfumes, especially as a fixative, it is a volatile oil obtained by steam distillation from gum extracted from various rockrose shrubs. Golden yellow, viscous, with a strong balsamic odor and a bitter taste. Also used as a synthetic flavoring in foods.

LABRADOR TEA EXTRACT • **Hudson's Bay Tea. Marsh Tea.** The extract of the dried flowering plant or young shoots of *Ledum palustre* or *L. groelandicum,* a tall, resinous evergreen shrub found in bogs, swamps, and moist meadows. Brewed like tea, it has a pleasing antiscorbutic and stimulating quality. It was used by the American Indians and settlers as a tonic supposed to purify blood. It was also employed to treat wounds. *L. palustre* contains, among other things, tannin and valeric acid *(see both)*. No known toxicity.

LAC • A substance secreted by the lac insect and used chiefly in the form of shellac.

LACCAIC • A pigment found in sticky stuff produced by the insect *Coccus laccae* on certain trees in India.

LACQUER • A Japanese lacquer tree contains a lacquer related to poison ivy. See Shellac.

LACTAMIDE DEA • Skin conditioning ingredient and humectant.

LACTAMIDE MEA • A mixture of ethanolamines *(see)* of lactic acid *(see)*.

LACTATE ESTERS • Salt of lactic acid *(see)*. See also Ester.

LACTIC ACID • Used in skin fresheners. Odorless, colorless, usually a syrupy product normally present in blood and muscle tissue as a product of the metabolism of glucose and glycogen. Present in sour milk, beer, sauerkraut, pickles, and other food products made by bacterial fermentation. Also an acidulant. It is caustic in concentrated solutions when taken internally or applied to the skin. In cosmetic products it may cause stinging in sensitive people, particularly in fair-skinned women. The FDA issued a notice in 1992 that lactic acid has not been shown to be safe and effective as claimed in OTC digestive aid products. See Alpha-Hydroxy Acids.

LACTIC YEASTS • Obtained from milk. See Lactic Acid and Faex.

LACTIS LIPIDA • Milk Fat.

LACTIS PROTEINUM • Milk protein.

LACTITOL • Obtained from lactose *(see)* and used as a flavoring agent and humectant.

LACTOBACILLUS • Lactobacilli are any of the various rod-shaped bacteria of the genus *Lactobacillus*. These versatile bacteria ferment lactic acid *(see)*. Certain strains reside in the urogenital tract and intestinal tract of healthy people. Yogurt contains lactobacilli.

LACTOFERRIN • A substance found in the milk of mammals believed to be involved in the transport of iron to the red blood cells.

LACTOGLOBULIN • Protein isolated from milk. Used in hair and skin conditioning products.

LACTOPEROXIDASE • An enzyme obtained from milk.

LACTOSE • **Milk Sugar.** Used widely as a base in eye lotions. Present in the milk of mammals. Stable in air but readily absorbs odors. Used in preparing food for infants, in tablets, as a general base and diluent in pharmaceutical and cosmetic compounding, and in baked goods. In large doses it is a laxative and diuretic but generally nontoxic. However, it was found to cause tumors when injected under the skin of mice in 50-milligram doses per kilogram of body weight.

LACTOYL METHYLSILANOL ELASTINATE • The ester *(see)* of lactic acid and the salt of elastin *(see)*. Used in emollients.

LACTUCA SATIVA • See Lettuce Extract.

LADY'S MANTLE EXTRACT • From the dried leaves and flowering shoots of *Achemilla vulgaris*. A common European herb covered with spreading hairs, it has been used for centuries by herbalists to concoct love potions.

LADY'S SLIPPER • *Cypripedium calceoulus*. The root is used to treat anxiety, stress, insomnia, neurosis, restlessness, tremors, epilepsy, and palpitations. Herbalists claim it is also useful for depression. It is used in "organic" cosmetics. It contains volatile oils, resins, glucosides, and tannin *(see all)*.

LADY'S THISTLE EXTRACT • *Silybum marianum*. A recent class of substances, flavonlignans, produced by the plant are being studied for their liver-protecting capacity. See Thistle.

LAKES, COLOR • A lake is an organic pigment prepared by precipitating a soluble color with a form of aluminum, calcium, barium potassium, strontium, or zirconium, which then makes the colors insoluble. Not all colors are suitable for making lakes.

LAMINARIA • See Algae.

LAMIUM • **White Nettle.** A troublesome weed, with stingers, it has a long history and was used in folk medicine. Its flesh is rich in minerals and plant hormones, and it supposedly stimulates hair growth and shines and softens hair. Also used to make tomatoes resistant to spoilage, to encourage the growth of strawberries, and to stimulate the fermentation of humus. Hemp belongs to the nettle family.

LAMPBLACK • Used in eye makeup pencils. It is a bluish black, fine soot deposited on a surface by burning liquid hydrocarbons *(see)* such as oil. It is duller and less intense in color than other carbon blacks and has a blue undertone. It is also used in pigments for paints, enamels, and printing inks. See Carbon Black for toxicity.

LANETH-5 THROUGH -40 • Emulsifiers. See Lanolin Alcohols.

LANETH-9 AND -10 ACETATE • Emulsifiers. On the basis of the available information, the CIR Expert Panel *(see)* concludes that they are safe as a cosmetic ingredient. See Lanolin Alcohols.

LANOLIN • **Wool Fat. Wool Wax.** A product of the oil glands of sheep. Used in lipsticks, liquid powders, mascaras, nail polish removers, protective oils, rouges, eye shadows, foundation creams, foundation cake makeups, hair conditioners, eye creams, cold creams, brilliantine hairdressings, ointment bases, and emollients. A water-absorbing base material and a natural emulsifier, it absorbs and holds water to the skin. Chemically a wax instead of a fat. Contains about 25 to 30 percent water. Advertisers have found that the words "contains lanolin" help to sell a product and have promoted it as being able to "penetrate the skin better than other oils," although there is little scientific proof of this. Lanolin has been found to be a common skin sensitizer, causing allergic contact skin rashes. It will not prevent or cure wrinkles and will not stop hair loss. It is not used in pure form today because of its allergy-causing potential. Products derived from it are less likely to cause allergic reactions. The CIR Expert Panel *(see)* found it safe. The FDA issued a notice in 1992 that lanolin has not been shown to be safe and effective as claimed in OTC poison ivy, poison oak, and poison sumac products.

LANOLIN ACID • See Lanolin.

LANOLIN ALCOHOLS • **Sterols. Triterpene Alcohols. Aliphatic Alcohols.** Derived from lanolin *(see),* lanolin alcohols are available commercially as solid waxy materials that are yellow to amber in color or as pale to golden-yellow liquids. They are widely used as emulsifiers and emollients in hand creams and lotions, and while they are less likely to cause an allergic reaction than lanolin, they still may do so in the sensitive.

LANOLIN CERA • Lanolin Wax. See Lanolin.

LANOLIN LINOLEATE • See Lanolin.

LANOLIN OIL • Widely used in cosmetics including eyeliners, cold creams, suntan gels, bath soaps, hair conditioners, fragrance preparations, skin-care products, moisturizers, face powders, and baby oils, it consists of 15 to 17 percent cholesterol, with the remainder liquid lanolin. See Lanolin for toxicity.

LANOLIN RICINOLEATE • See Lanolin Alcohols.

LANOLIN WAX • An emollient. See Lanolin.

LANOLINAMIDE DEA • The ethanolamides of lanolin acid. See Lanolin.

LANOSTEROL • A widely used skin softener in hand creams and lotions, it is the fatty alcohol derived from the wool fat of sheep. See Lanolin.

LANTHANUM CHLORIDE • An inorganic salt. A rare earth mineral that occurs in cerite, monazerite, orthite, and certain fluorspars. Used as a reingredient *(see)* and catalyst *(see)* in cosmetic preparations. No known toxicity from topical use, but a small oral dose is lethal in rats.

LAPACHO EXTRACT • *Tabecuia heptaphylla* or *impetiginosa.* **Pau d'arco Lapacho.** The inner bark of a tree in the forests of Brazil, it was used by Brazilian Indians for the treatment of cancer. Contains quinones and lapachol. It also is used to treat fungal and parasitic infections, and to aid digestion. Also reportedly lowers blood sugar. Pau d'arco is now being studied in Brazil to treat cancers, including leukemia. Related structurally to vitamin K.

LAPIS LAZULI • No longer authorized for use in cosmetics. See Colors.

LAPPA EXTRACT • **Burdock Extract.** The extract of the roots of *Arctium lappa*, it contains tannic acid *(see)* and is used to soothe the skin. No known toxicity.

LAPYRIUM CHLORIDE • Germ killer and antistatic ingredient. See Quaternary Ammonium Compounds.

LARD • Easily absorbed by the skin, it is used as a lubricant, emollient, and base in shaving creams, soaps, and various cosmetic creams. It is the purified internal fat from the abdomen of the hog. It is a soft, white, unctuous mass, with a slight characteristic odor and a bland taste. Insoluble in water. No known toxicity.

LARD GLYCERIDE • See Lard.

LARKSPUR • *Consolida regalis.* The seeds are used to treat nits and lice on the skin and hair. It is a poison and should not be taken internally.

LARREA DIVARICATA • See Chaparral Extract.

LATEX • **Synthetic Rubber.** The milky, usually white juice or exudate of plants obtained by tapping. Used in beauty masks (see face masks and packs) for its coating ability. Any of various gums, resins, fats, or waxes in an emulsion of water and synthetic rubber or plastic are now considered latex. Ingredients of latex compounds can be poisonous, depending upon which plant products are used. Can cause skin rash.

LATHER • Produced by action of air bubbles in a soap solution. For satisfactory shaving, a lather must be dense. The air bubbles must be fine and stable for the duration of the shave. In bubble baths the air bubbles must be large and light.

LAURALKONIUM BROMIDE • See Quaternary Ammonium Compounds.

LAURALKONIUM CHLORIDE • May form nitrosamines *(see)*. Based on the available data, the CIR Expert Panel *(see)* concludes that this ingredient is safe as a cosmetic ingredient. However, it should not be used in cosmetic products containing nitrosating agents. See Quaternary Ammonium Compounds.

LAURAMIDE DEA • A widely used mixture of ethanolamides of lauric acid, the principal fatty acid of coconut oil, it is widely used in cosmetic soaps and detergents as a softener thickener, and foam booster. See Lauric Acid.

LAURAMIDE MEA • See Lauric Acid.

LAURAMIDE MIPA • A mixture of isopropanolamides of lauric acid widely used as a wetting ingredient in soaps and detergents. See Lauric Acid.

LAURAMIDOPROPYL ACETAMIDODIMONIUM CHLORIDE • See Quaternary Ammonium Compounds.

LAURAMIDOPROPYL BETAINE • See Quaternary Ammonium Compounds.

LAURAMIDOPROPYL DIMETHYLAMINE • See Lauric Acid and Dimethylamine.

LAURAMINE OXIDE • Widley used as an cleansing agent and conditioner in hair products such as shampoos and dressings. Can form nitrosamines *(see)*. In rats up to 40 percent was absorbed through the skin. On the basis of the available information, the CIR Expert Panel *(see)* concludes that it is safe as a cosmetic ingredient for "rinse-off" products but for "leave-on" products it should be limited to 5 percent. See Lauric Acid.

LAURAMINOPROPIONIC ACID • See Propionic Acid.

LAURDIMONIUM HYDROXYPROPYL HYDROLYZED SOY PROTEIN • An antistatic ingredient in hair conditioners. See Quaternary Ammonium Compounds.

LAURDIMONIUM HYDROXYPROPYL HYDROLYZED WHEAT PROTEIN • An antistatic ingredient in hair conditioners. See Quaternary Ammonium Compounds.

LAUREL • The fresh berries and leaf extract of the laurel tree *Laurus nobilis*. The berries are used as a flavoring for beverages, and the leaf extract is a spice flavoring for vegetables. See Laurel Leaf Oil. GRAS.

LAUREL GALLATE • An antioxidant, the laurel ester of gallic acid *(see)*.

LAUREL LEAF OIL • Derived from steam distillation of the leaves of *Laurus nobilis*, it is a yellow liquid with a spicy odor used as a flavoring ingredient. Moderately toxic by ingestion. A skin irritant. GRAS.

LAURETH-1, -23 • Surfactants. On the basis of the available information, the CIR Expert Panel *(see)* concludes that this ingredient is safe as a cosmetic. See Lauryl Alcohol.

LAURETH PHOSPHATE • A complex mixture of esters of phosphoric acid and ethoxylated lauryl alcohol. See Surfactants.

LAURIC ACID • **n-Dodecanoic Acid.** A common constituent of vegetable fats, especially coconut oil and laurel oil. Its derivatives are widely used as a base in the manufacture of soaps, detergents, and lauryl alcohol *(see)* because of their foaming properties. Has a slight odor of bay and makes copious large bubbles when in soap. A mild irritant but not a sensitizer. The CIR Expert Panel *(see)* concludes that this ingredient is safe for use in cosmetic products.

LAURIC ALDEHYDE • See Lauric Acid.

LAURIC DEA • Creates a good, long-lasting foam in shampoos. See Lauric acid.

LAURIC/PALMITIC/OLEIC TRIGLYCERIDE • **Turtle oil®.** A mixture of glycerin with lauric, palmitic, and oleic acids used as a skin moisturizer.

LAUROAMPHOACETATE • A preservative. See Imidazole.

LAUROAMPHODIACETATE • A preservative. See Imidazole.

LAUROAMPHODIPROPIONATE • See Propionic Acid and Lauric Acid.

LAUROAMPHODIPROPIONIC ACID • A preservative. See Lauric Acid and Propionic Acid.

LAUROAMPHODROXYPROPYLSULFONATE • See Imidazole.

LAUROAMPHOPROPINOATE • See Lauric Acid and Propionic Acid.

LAUROYL COLLAGEN AMINO ACIDS • A condensation product of lauric acid chloride and hydrolyzed (see) animal protein used in soaps. The word "animal" has been removed from this ingredient name.

LAUROYL ETHYL GLUCOSIDE • An emulsifier. See Laurel.

LAUROYL HYDROLYZED COLLAGEN • A condensation product of lauric acid chloride and hydrolyzed collagen *(see)*. The world "animal" has been removed from this ingredient name.

LAUROYL HYDROLYZED ELASTIN • Used in hair and skin conditioners. See Laurel and Elastin.

LAUROYL LYSINE • Widely used in makeup such as blushers and lipsticks. See Lauric Acid and Lysine.

LAUROYL SARCOSINE • See Sarcosines.

LAURTRIMONIUM CHLORIDE • See Quaternary Ammonium Compounds.

LAURUS NOBILIS • See Laurel.

LAURYL ALCOHOL • **1-Dodecanol.** A colorless, crystalline compound that is produced commercially from coconut oil. Used to make detergents because of its sudsing ability. Has a characteristic fatty odor. It is soluble in most oils but is insoluble in glycerin. Used in perfumery. See Lauric Acid for toxicity.

LAURYL AMINE • See Lauric Acid.

LAURYL AMINOPROPYLGLYCINE • See Lauryl Alcohol and Glyceric Acid.

LAURYL BEHENATE • Used as a skin conditioning ingredient and as a cover-up. The ester *(see)* of Lauric Acid and Behenic Acid *(see both)*.

LAURYL BETAINE • Widely used in bath products. See Lauric Acid.

LAURYL DIETHLENDIAMINEGLYCINE • See Lauryl Alcohol.

LAURYL DIMETHYLAMINE ACRYLINOLATE • See Lauric Acid and Dimethylamine.

LAURYL DIMETHYLAMINE ACRYLINOLEATE • See Acrylinic Acid.

LAURYL DIMONIUM HYDROXYPROPYL HYDROLYZED COLLAGEN • See Quaternary Ammonium Compounds.

LAURYL DIMONIUM HYDROXYPROPYL HYDROLYZED KERATIN • Protein derivative from skin. See Quarternary Ammonium Compounds.

LAURYL DIMONIUM HYDROXYPROPYL HYDROLYZED SOY PROTEIN • See Soy and Quaternary Ammonium Compounds.

LAURYL GLUCOSIDE • Widely used surfactant in hair dyes and shampoos. See Lauryl Alcohol and Glucose.

LAURYL GLYCOL • See Lauryl Alcohol and Glycol.

LAURYL HYDROSULTAINE • A salt of lauric acid *(see)* used as a softener.

LAURYL HYDROXYETHYL IMIDAZOLINE • A preservative. See Imidazoline.

LAURYL ISOQUINOLINIUM BROMIDE • A quaternary ammonium compound *(see)* active against a microorganism believed to cause a type of dandruff. Used in hair tonics and cuticle softeners. Slightly greater toxicity than benzalkonium chloride in rats. No skin irritation or sensitization in concentrations of 0.1 percent and lower. Used also as an agriculture fungicide.

LAURYL ISOSTEARATE • The ester of lauryl alcohol and isostearic acid *(see both)*.

LAURYL LACTATE • See Lauric Acid and Lactic Acid.

LAURYL METHACRYLATE • See Lauric Acid and Acrylates.

LAURYL PALMITATE • The ester *(see)* of lauryl alcohol and palmitic acid *(see both)*.

LAURYL PHOSPHATE • An emulsifier. See Phosphoric Acid and Lauric Acid.

LAURYL PYRIDINUM CHLORIDE • See Quaternary Ammonium Compounds.

LAURYL STEARATE • The ester of lauryl alcohol and stearic acid *(see both)*.

LAURYL SULFATE • Derived from lauryl alcohol *(see)*. Its potassium, zinc, magnesium, sodium, calcium, and ammonium salts are used in shampoos because of their foaming properties. See Sodium Lauryl Sulfate.

LAURYL SULTAINE • See Lauryl Alcohol and Betaine.

LAVANDIN OIL • Used in soaps and perfumes. It is the essential oil of a hybrid related to the lavender plant. Fragrant, yellowish, with a camphor-lavender scent. No known toxicity.

LAVANDULA • See Lavender Oil.

LAVENDER OIL • Widely used in skin fresheners, powders, shaving preparations, mouthwashes, dentifrices, and perfumes. The volatile oil from the fresh flowering tops of lavender. Also used in a variety of food flavorings. It can cause allergic reactions and has been found to cause adverse skin reactions when the skin is exposed to sunlight. Related to the lavender plant. Fragrant, yellowish, with a camphor-lavender scent. No known toxicity.

LAWSONE • Derived from the leaves of *Lawsonia inermis,* it is used as a sunscreen ingredient. See Henna.

LAWSONIA INERMIS • See Henna.

LEAD ACETATE • **Sugar of Lead.** Colorless, white crystals or grains with an acetic odor. Bubbles slowly. It has been used as a topical astringent but is absorbed through the skin, and therefore might lead to lead poisoning. Also used in hair dyeing and printing colors and in the manufacture of chrome yellow *(see* Colors). Still used to treat bruises and skin irritations in animals. Not recommended for use because of the possibility of lead buildup in the body. Permission was given in 1981 by the FDA to use this in progressive hair dyes, although it is a proven carcinogen. Permanently listed as a color component of hair dye in 1969 with a caution that it "should not be used on cut or abraded scalp." See Lead Compounds.

LEAD COMPOUNDS • Used in ointments and hair dye pigments. Lead may cause contact dermatitis. It is poisonous in all forms. It is one of the most hazardous of toxic metals because its poison is cumulative and its toxic effects are many and severe. Among them are leg cramps, muscle weakness, numbness, depression, brain damage, coma, and death. Ingestion and inhalation of lead cause the most severe symptoms.

LECITHIN • From the Greek, meaning "egg yolk." A natural antioxidant and emollient used in eye creams, lipsticks, liquid powders, hand creams and lotions, soaps, and many other cosmetics. Also a natural emulsifier and spreading ingredient. It is found in all living organisms, and is frequently obtained from common egg yolk and soybeans for commercial purposes. Egg yolk is 8 to 9 percent lecithin. Nontoxic.

LECITHIN AMIDE DEA • A reaction product of lecithin and diethanolamine with ammonia. See Quaternary Ammonium Compounds.

LEDUM GROENLANDICUM • **Labrador Tea.** See Labrador Tea Extract.

LEMON • The common fresh fruit and fruit extract is the most frequently used acid in cosmetics. It is 5 to 8 percent citric acid. Employed in cream rinses, hair color rinses, astringents, fresheners, skin bleaches, and for reducing alkalinity of many other products. Do-it-yourselfers can squeeze two lemons into a strainer, add the juice to 1 cup of water, and use it as a rinse after shampooing to remove scum and to leave a shine on the hair. Lemon can cause allergic reactions.

LEMON BALM • **Sweet Balm. Garden Balm.** Used in perfumes and as a soothing facial treatment. An Old World mint cultivated for its lemon-flavored, fragrant leaves. Often considered a weed, it has been used by herbalists as a medicine and to flavor foods and medicines. It reputedly imparts long life. Also used to treat earache and toothache. Nontoxic.

LEMON BIOFLAVONOIDS • See Lemon and Bioflavonoids.

LEMON EXTRACT • See Lemon Oil.

LEMON JUICE • See Lemon.

LEMON OIL • **Cedro Oil.** Used in perfumes and food flavorings, it is the volatile oil expressed from the fresh peel. A pale yellow to deep yellow, it has a characteristic odor and taste of the outer part of fresh lemon peel. It can cause an allergic reaction and has been suspected of being a co–cancer-causing ingredient.

LEMON PEEL • From the outer rind, the extract is used as a flavor in medicines and in beverages, confectionery, and cooking. See Lemon for toxicity.

LEMON VERBENA EXTRACT • Extract of *Lippia citriodoral.* See Lemongrass Oil.

LEMONGRASS OIL • **Indian Oil of Verbena.** Used in perfumes, especially those added to soap. It is the volatile oil distilled from the leaves of lemon grasses. A yellowish or reddish brown liquid, it has a strong odor of verbena. Also used in insect repellents and in fruit flavorings for foods and beverages. Death was reported when taken internally, and autopsy showed lining of the intestines was severely damaged. Skin toxicity unknown.

LENS ESCULENTA • See Lentil Extract.

LENTIL EXTRACT • The extract of the fruit of *Lens culinaris* or *esculenta.* A widely grown annual plant.

LEPTOSPERMUM SCOPARIUM • See Tea Tree Oil.

LESPEDEZA • An herb or shrub named for a Spanish governor of Florida. It is a member of the legume family.

LESQUERELLA OIL • The oil expressed from the seed of *Lesquerella fendleri.* A genus of low annual or perennial American herbs with yellow flowers and puffy pods.

LETTUCE EXTRACT • *Lactuca elongata.* An extract of various species of *Lactuca.* Used in commercial toning lotions and by herbalists to make soothing skin decoctions. During the Middle Ages, lettuce was used as a valuable narcotic, and its milky juice, *Lactuca,* was used with opium to induce sleep.

LEUCINE • An essential amino acid *(see)* for human nutrition not manufactured in the body. It is isolated commercially from gluten, casein, and keratin *(see all).* No known toxicity.

LEUKOCYTE EXTRACT • Extract of white blood cells used in "antiaging" products.

LEUKOTRIENES • Substances issued by cells that have physiologic activity, such as playing a part in inflammation and allergic reactions.

LEVULINIC ACID • Crystals used as an intermediate for plasticizers, solvents, resins, flavors, and pharmaceuticals.

LEVULOSE • See Fructose.

LIATRIS • See Deer's Tongue Leaves.

LICHEN EXTRACT • *Usnea barbata.* **Old Man's Beard. Usnea. Beard Lichen.** The plant, which is a lichen growing on branches of trees, is used internally and externally for fungus infections and for viral and bacterial infections. When combined with *Echinacea (see),* it is used as a general antibiotic and antifungal medication. Used externally for fungal infections.

LICORICE • **Liquorice. Glycyrrhizin.** A black substance derived from a plant, *Glycyrrhiza glabra,* "sweet root," belonging to the *Leguminosae* family and cultivated from southern Europe to Central Asia. It is used in fruit, licorice, anise, maple, and root beer flavorings for beverages, ice cream, ices, candy, baked goods, gelatin, chewing gum, and syrups. Licorice root is used in licorice and root beer flavorings for beverages, candy, baked goods, chewing gum, tobacco, and medicines. Some people known to have eaten licorice candy, regularly and generously, had raised blood pressure, headaches, and muscle weakness. It can cause asthma, intestinal upsets, and contact dermatitis. No known skin toxicity.

LIDOCAINE • Needles from benzene or alcohol, insoluble in water. A local anesthetic, it relieves itching, pain, soreness, and discomfort due to skin rashes, including eczema and minor burns, but can cause an allergic reaction.

LIGHT • Sensitivity to light may be caused by drugs, cosmetics, or foods or may be an allergy itself. When some people are exposed to sunlight, their skins erupt with eczema, hemorrhages, hives, and scales. In severe sunlight allergy, the person may break out all over in large hives, feel dizzy, and fall into shock. The allergy may appear suddenly, last for years, and then disappear, or it may remain for a lifetime. Some people allergic to sunlight are also sensitive to fluorescent light.

LIGNOCERIC ACID • Obtained from beechwood tar or by distillation of rotten oak wood. Occurs in most natural fats. Used in shampoos, soaps, and plastics. No known toxicity.

LIGNOL • See Lignoceric Acid.

LIGUSTRUM LUCIDIUM EXTRACT • A common plant used as a hedge in many yards, its fruits contain mannitol and glucose *(see both),* as well as oleanolic acid, and fatty oil. It is used to treat liver, kidney, and adrenal gland problems.

Herbalists also claim that it can prevent premature graying of the hair or loss of vision.

LILAC • Used in perfumes. Derived from the plant, especially the European shrub variety. It has fragrant bluish to purple-pink flowers. No known toxicity.

LILIUM • **Tiger Lily.** Grown in China and Japan, the plant flowers in July and August. The bloom is orange and spotted. A tincture is made from the fresh plant and is used by herbalists to treat uterine and nerve problems, congestion, and irritation. It is poisonous.

LILY OF THE VALLEY • **Convallaria Flowers.** A perfume ingredient extracted from the low perennial herb. It has oblong leaves and fragrant, nodding, bell-shaped, white flowers. Has been used as a heart stimulant. No known toxicity for the skin.

LIME • A perfume ingredient from the small, greenish yellow fruit of a spicy tropical tree. Its very acid pulp yields a juice used as a flavoring ingredient and as an antiseptic. A source of Vitamin C. Can cause an adverse reaction when skin is exposed to sunlight.

LIME OIL • A natural flavoring extracted from the fruit of a tropical tree. Colorless to greenish. Used in grapefruit, lemon, lemon-lime, lime, orange, cola, fruit, rum, nut, and ginger flavorings for beverages, ice cream, ices, candy, baked goods, gelatin desserts, chewing gum, and condiments. May cause a sensitivity to light.

LIME SULFUR • Topical antiseptic. A brown, clear liquid prepared by boiling sulfur and lime with water. Can cause skin irritation.

LIMEWATER • An alkaline water solution of calcium hydroxide that absorbs carbon dioxide from the air, forming a protective film of calcium carbonate *(see)* on the surface of the liquid. Used in medicines, as an antacid, and as an alkali in external washes, face masks, and hair-grooming products. No known toxicity.

LIMNANTHES ALBA • A family of North American herbs. Has succulent leaves.

LIMONENE • **D, L, and DL forms.** A synthetic flavoring ingredient that occurs naturally in star anise, buchu leaves, caraway, celery, oranges, coriander, cumin, cardamom, sweet fennel, common fennel, mace, marigold, oil of lavandin, oil of lemon, oil of mandarin, peppermint, petitgrain oil, pimento oil, orange leaf, orange peel (sweet oil), origanum oil, black pepper, peels of citrus, macrocarpa bunge, and hops oil. Used in lime, fruit, and spice flavorings for beverages, ice cream, ices, candy, baked goods, gelatin desserts, and chewing gum. A skin irritant and sensitizer.

LIMONIUM VULGARE • See Lavender.

LINALOE OIL • **Bois de Rose Oil.** An ingredient in perfumes that is the colorless to yellow, volatile, essential oil distilled from a Mexican tree. It has a pleasant flowery scent and is soluble in most fixed oils. May cause allergic reactions.

LINALOOL • **Linalol.** Used in perfumes and soaps instead of bergamot or French lavender. It is a fragrant, colorless liquid that occurs in many essential oils such as linaloe, Ceylon cinnamon, sassafras, orange flower, and bergamot. Also used in food flavorings such as blueberry, chocolate, and lemon. May cause allergic reactions.

LINALYL ACETATE • A colorless, fragrant liquid, slightly soluble in water, it is the most valuable constituent of bergamot and lavender oils, which are used in perfumery. It occurs naturally in basil, jasmine oil, lavandin oil, lavender oil, and lemon oil. It has a strong floral scent. Also used as a synthetic flavoring in food. No known toxicity.

LINALYL ESTERS • See Linalool and Ester.

LINDEN EXTRACT • *Tilia Cordata.* A natural flavoring ingredient from the flowers of the tree grown in Europe and the United States. Widely used in fragrances, skin fresheners, moisturizers, cold creams, shampoos, and many other products. It is also used in raspberry and vermouth flavorings.

LINLUM USITATISSIMUM • See Linseed Oil.

LINOLEAMIDE • See Linoleic Acid.

LINOLEAMIDE DEA • Alkyl amides produced by a diethanolamine *(see)* condensation of linoleic acid. Used as a foaming ingredient in soaps and shampoos. May form nitrosamines *(see)*. Based on the available data, the CIR Expert Panel *(see)* concludes that this ingredient is safe as a cosmetic ingredient. However, it should not be used in cosmetic products containing nitrosating agents. See Quaternary Ammonium Compounds and Coconut Acid.

LINOLEAMIDE MEA • A mixture of ethanolamides of linoleic acid *(see)*. Used as a surfactant *(see)*.

LINOLEAMIDE MIPA • A mixture of isopropanolamides of linoleic acid. Used as an emulsifier. See Linoleic Acid.

LINOLEAMIDOPROPALKONIUM CHLORIDE • See Quaternary Ammonium Compounds.

LINOLEAMIDOPROPYL ETHYDIMONIUM ETHOSULFATE • See Quaternary Ammonium Compounds.

LINOLEIC ACID • Used as an emulsifier. An essential fatty acid *(see)* prepared from edible fats and oils. Component of Vitamin F and a major constituent of many vegetable oils, for example, cottonseed and soybean. Used in emulsifiers and vitamins. Large doses can cause nausea and vomiting. No known skin toxicity and, in fact, may have emollient properties.

LINOLELEYL LACTATE • A skin-conditioning ingredient. See Linolenic Acid and Lactic Acid.

LINOLENIC ACID • Colorless, liquid glyceride found in most oils. Insoluble in water, soluble in organic solvents. Used to make nail polishes dry faster. Slightly irritating to mucous membranes.

LINSEED ACID • See Linseed Oil.

LINSEED OIL • Oil used in shaving creams, emollients, and medicinal soaps. Soothing to the skin. It is the yellowish oil expressed or extracted from flaxseed. Gradually thickens when exposed to air. It has a peculiar odor and a bland taste, and is also used in paint, varnish, and linoleum. Can cause an allergic reaction.

LIP BRUSH • A brush to trace a sharp outline of the lips with lipstick.

LIP CREAM • A mixture of oils that melt on contact with the skin to soften and soothe the lips. Almost identical to night creams or moisturizers. See Emollients.

LIP GLOSS • Usually comes in jars, sticks, sometimes in tubes. Contains different proportions of the same ingredient as lipstick but usually has less wax and more oil to make the lips shinier. Used alone or with lipstick and applied with the fingertip.

LIP PENCIL • A colored wax mixture in wood or metal casing for the same purpose as a lip brush *(see)*.

LIP PRIMER • A stick similar to lipstick but containing less wax, used to soften the lips and to serve as a base for lipstick. Makes the lips shinier.

LIPASE • An enzyme that breaks down fat, widely distributed in plants and animal tissues, especially in the pancreas. Isolated from castor beans. The FDA issued a notice in 1992 that lipase has not been shown to be safe and effective as claimed in OTC digestive aid products.

LIPO • Glyceryl, ethylene glycol, and propylene glycol esters used as emulsifiers and stabilizers. Widely used as emollients and thickeners in creams and lotions, and as opacifying and pearling ingredients in surfactants.

LIPO- • Fat.

LIPOCOL • Polyoxyethylene ethers used as nonionic surfactants in antiperspirants, depilatories, creams, lotions, and pigment dispersions. Also used as emulsifiers, defoamers, wetting ingredients, solubilizers, and conditioning ingredients in shampoos, detergents, bleaches, and dyes.

LIPOLAN • See Lanolin.

LIPONATE • Emollient used to give a velvety feel to creams, lotions, and bath preparations. Also used for thickening, viscosity control, and pigment.

LIPONIC • Humectant to control the moisture exchange between a product and the atmosphere, thus helping to retard drying of the product in the package.

LIPOPEG • Mild, fatty, polyoxyethylene glycol esters used in bath oils, creams, and lotions for solubilizing, spreading, emulsifying, dispersing, and lubricating.

LIPOSOMES • Microscopic sacs, or spheres, manufactured from a variety of fatty substances, including phospholipids. The material for cosmetics may be obtained either from natural or synthetic sources. When properly mixed with water, phospholipids form liposome spheres, which can "trap" any substance that will dissolve in water or oil. Manufacturers claim liposomes act like a delivery system. They say that, when present in a cream or lotion, liposomes can more easily penetrate the surface skin to underlying layers, "melt," and deposit other ingredients of the product. See also Phytosomes.

LIPOSORB • Sorbitan esters used as emulsifying, thickening, and lubricating ingredients. See Sorbitan Fatty Acid Esters.

LIPOVOL • Emollient oils for use as lubricants and conditioners in skin products, hair-care products, makeups, fine soaps, and bath oils.

LIPOWAX • Emulsifying waxes.

LIPSTICK • Regular, Frosted, Medicated, Sheer. Primarily a mixture of oil and wax in a stick form with a red-staining certified dye dispersed in oil, red pigments similarly dispersed, flavoring, and perfume. Bromo acid, D & C Red No. 21, and related dyes are most often used. Among other common lipstick dyes are D & C Red No. 27 and insoluble dyes known as lakes, such as D & C Red, No. 34 Calcium Lake, and D & C Orange No. 17 Lake. Pinks are made by mixing titanium dioxide with various reds. Among the oils and fats used are olive, mineral, sesame, castor, butyl stearate, polyethylene glycol, cocoa butter, lanolin, petrolatum, lecithin, hydrogenated vegetable oils, carnauba and candelilla waxes, beeswax, ozokerite, and paraffin. Colors of lipsticks on the market remain essentially the same, but the names, such as "strawberry rose," are frequently changed to induce customers to buy. A typical lipstick formula contains castor oil, about 65 percent; beeswax, 15 percent; carnauba wax, 10 percent; lanolin, 5 percent; certified dyes, soluble; color lakes, insoluble; and perfume. Frosted lipstick includes a pearling ingredient that adds luster to the color. Such an ingredient may be a bismuth compound or guanine. Medicated lipstick is used to treat or prevent chapped or sun-dried lips. It may or may not combine coloring with ingredients but usually contains petrolatum, mineral wax, and oils. It may or may not contain menthol or a sunscreen. Sheer lipsticks include transparent coloring and no indelible dyes so as to give a more natural look to the lips. The main difficulty with lipsticks results from allergy to the dyes or to specific ingredients. See Cheilitis.

LIPSTICK HOLDER • See Nickel.

LIQUEFYING CREAM • Cleansing cream designed to liquefy when rubbed into the skin. It usually contains paraffin, a wax, stearic acid, sodium borate, liquid petrolatum (54 percent), and water (26 percent).

LIQUID MAKEUP • See Foundation Makeup.

LIQUID POWDER • See Foundation Makeup.

LITCHI CHINENSIS • **Lychee Nut Extract.**

LITHIUM • A metal that has been used as a medicine since ancient Greece, when it was prescribed for gout, rheumatism, and kidney stone. Small amount of the salts are used as a nutraceutical to treat manic-depressive illness today. Lithium has a very narrow margin of safety and may have severe side effects.

LITHIUM CHLORIDE • A crystalline salt of the alkali metal, used as a scavenger in purifying metals, to remove oxygen, and in soap and lubricant bases. The crystals absorb water and then become neutral or slightly alkaline. It is also used in the manufacture of mineral waters, in soldering, and in refrigeration machines. Formerly used as a salt substitute. Prolonged absorption may cause disturbed electrolyte balance in humans and impair kidney function and cause central nervous system problems.

LITHIUM HYDROXIDE • Used in making cosmetic resins and esters *(see both)*. A granular, free-flowing powder, acrid, and strongly alkaline. It is the salt of the alkaline metal that absorbs water from the air and is soluble in water. Used in photo developers and in batteries. Very irritating to the skin, and flammable in contact with the air.

LITHIUM MAGNESIUM SILICATE • A synthetic clay used as a thickener. See Magnesium and Lithium.

LITHIUM STEARATE • White, fatty, solid, and soluble in water and alcohol. A metallic soap used as an emulsifier, lubricant, and plasticizer in various cosmetic creams and lotions. Also a coloring ingredient. On the basis of the available information, the CIR Expert Panel *(see)* concludes that it is safe as a cosmetic ingredient. See Aluminum Distearate.

LITHOSPERMUM EXTRACT • **Pucoon.** An extract of the roots of *Radix lithospermi,* an herb with polished, white, stony nutlets. The extract is supposed to be soothing to the mucous membranes.

LITSEA CUBEBA • A small plum tree with evergreen leaves. An essential oil used in fragrances.

LIVER EXTRACT • Extract of bovine livers used in antiwrinkle creams. No known toxicity.

LOCUST BEAN GUM • **St. John's Bread. Carob Bean Gum.** A thickener and stabilizer in cosmetics and foods. Also used in depilatories. A natural flavor extract from the seed of the carob tree cultivated in the Mediterranean area. The history of the carob tree dates back more than two thousand years, when the ancient Egyptians used locust bean gum as an adhesive in mummy binding. It is alleged that the "locust" (through confusion of the locusts with carob) and wild honey, which sustained John the Baptist in the wilderness, was from this plant; thus the name St. John's Bread. The carob pods are used as feed for stock today because of their high protein content. No known toxicity from cosmetic use. It is on the FDA list for study of side effects.

LOESS • An abrasive and absorbent. Believed to be deposited by the wind, it consists of shells, bones, and teeth of mammals as well as sand.

LOGWOOD • An active ingredient known as hematoxylin from the very hard brown, or brownish red, heartwood of a tree common to the West Indies and Central America. It was widely used as a liquid or as a solid extract obtained by evaporation in black hair colorings and for neutralizing red tones in dyed hair. It is also a mild astringent. May cause an allergic reaction in the hypersensitive. No longer authorized for use in cosmetics.

LONICERA CAPRIFOLIUM • See Honeysuckle.

LOOFAH • **Luffa. Dish Cloth Sponge.** A material obtained from the fruit of the sponge *Luffa cylindrica.* The fibrous skeleton of the loofah is used as a sponge and to exfoliate *(see)* the skin. When used, the sponges should be allowed to dry completely because they have been found to support the growth of numerous bacteria. When skin flakes are trapped in the fibers of the loofah, sponges can become a rich breeding ground for pathogens.

LOOSESTRIFE, PURPLE • *Lythrum salicaria.* A perennial herb grown in many parts of the world, in damp, marshy places. It is used as an astringent and tonic. It was also used in Europe to treat fevers and in Ireland for diarrhea and the healing of wounds. It was also used by herbalists in soothing eye drops and in salves for skin ulcers.

LOQUAT • *Eriobotrya japonica.* The leaves and fruit are used by herbalists to treat coughs and lung inflammations. It contains amygdalin *(see)*, which is also found in cherry bark and apricot kernel, both of which are used to treat coughs.

LOTION • Liquid applied to large areas of the skin.

LOTUS • The name of several water lilies. It grows in marshes from Egypt to China, and its leaves and pink flowers grow on stalks rising several feet from the water. The fruit, the sacred bean of Asia, is eaten, and the large rhizomes yield a starchy powder. Lotus is used in "organic" cosmetics.

LOVAGE • An ingredient in perfumery from an aromatic herb native to southern Europe and grown in monastery gardens centuries ago for medicine and food flavoring. It has a hot, sharp, biting taste. The yellow-brown oil is extracted from the root or other parts of the herb. It has a reputation for improving health and inciting love; Czechoslovakian girls reportedly wear it in a bag around their necks when dating boys. It supposedly has deodorant properties when added to bathwater. No known toxicity.

LUBRICATING CREAM • See Emollients.

LUFFA CYLINDRICA • **Sponge Gourd Powder.** See Loofah.

LUNGWORT • *Pulmonaria officinalis.* **Black Hellebore. Mullein. Wall Hawkweed. Virginia Cowslip.** Any of several plants thought to be helpful in combating lung diseases, coughs, and hoarseness. Lungworts are also used by herbalists to treat diarrhea. The leaves contain mucins, silicic acid, tannin, saponin, allantoin, quercetin, and Vitamin C *(see all)*. Externally, this plant is used to heal wounds. It is used in "organic cosmetics."

LUPIN EXTRACT • **Lupine.** Extract of *Lupinus albus.* The seed has been used as a food since earliest times. It produces a light blue dye. No known toxicity.

LUPINUS ALBUS • A member of the legume family, it has white, yellow, or blue flowers. See Lupin Extract.

LYCOPODIUM • **Ground Pine. Ground Fir.** A dusting powder derived from erect, or creeping, evergreen plants grown in North America, Europe, and Asia. The plant's spores create a fine yellow powder that sticks to the fingers when touched. It is odorless and absorbent. It may cause a form of inflammatory reaction in wounds or exposed tissues, and can cause allergic reactions such as a stuffy nose and hay fever.

LYCOPSIS ARVENSIS • **Bugloss Extract.** See Bugloss Extract.

LYSINE • An essential amino acid *(see)* isolated from casein, fibrin, or blood. It is used to improve the protein quality of a product. No known toxicity.

LYSOLECITHIN • The product obtained from treating lecithin with enzymes. Used as a base for creams.

LYTHRUM SALICARIA • See Loosestrife.

M

MA • Abbreviation for maleic anhydride *(see)*.

MACADAMIA NUT OIL • **Queensland Nut Oil.** Derived from the nut of a small evergreen tree, it is widely cultivated. Used in emollients. Contains magnesium and thiamine.

MACE • Oil and Oleoresin. Obtained by steam distillation from the ripe, dried seed of the nutmeg. Colorless to pale yellow, with the taste and odor of nutmeg. Used in bitters, meat, and spice flavorings for beverages, ice cream, ices, baked goods, condiments, and meats (2,000 ppm). The oil is used in chocolate, cocoa, coconut, cola, fruit, nut, spice, and ginger ale flavorings for beverages, ice cream, ices, candy, baked goods, chewing gum, condiments, and meats. The final report to the FDA of the Select Committee on GRAS Substances stated in 1980 that while no evidence in the available information on it demonstrates a hazard to the public at current use levels, uncertainties exist, requiring that additional studies be conducted. The FDA continued the GRAS status while tests were being completed and evaluated in 1980. Nothing new has been reported by the FDA since then.

MACERATION • The extraction of flower-oil production by immersion in warm fats.

MACROCYSTIS PYRIFERA • See Kelp.

MADDER • *Rubia tintorum*. **Dyers' Madder.** A shrub that is a member of the *Rubiaceae* family, it is widely distributed. In medicine it is a mild tonic and has astringent properties. It was once used for treating edema. The root was boiled in wine or water for palsy, jaundice, and sciatica, and for treating bruises. The leaves and roots were beaten and applied externally to remove freckles and other skin blemishes.

MAGNESIA • A skin freshener and dusting powder ingredient. Slightly alkaline, white powder taken from any one of several ores, such as periclase. Named after Magnesia, an ancient city in Asia Minor. An antacid. No known toxicity.

MAGNESIUM • A silver-white, light malleable metal that occurs abundantly in nature and is widely used in combination with various chemicals as a powder. It was reevaluated by the FDA in 1976 and found not harmful at presently used levels. The World Health Organization recommended further studies because of kidney damage found in dogs that ingested it.

MAGNESIUM ACETATE • A buffering agent. See Magnesium.

MAGNESIUM ACETYLMETHIONATE • The magnesium salt of *n*-acetylmethionine. See Magnesium and Methionine.

MAGNESIUM ALUMINUM SILICATE • A silver-white, light malleable metal that occurs abundantly in nature and is widely used in combination with various chemicals as a powder. It is used primarily as a thickener in cosmetics. It was reevaluated by the FDA in 1976 and found not harmful at presently used levels. The World Health Organization recommended further studies because of kidney damage found in dogs that ingested it.

MAGNESIUM ASCORBATE • An antioxidant and skin-conditioning ingredient. See Magnesium and Ascorbic Acid.

MAGNESIUM ASCORBYL PHOSPHATE • An antioxidant used in suntan products. See Magnesium and Ascorbic Acid.

MAGNESIUM ASPARTATE • Used widely as a skin conditioning ingredient. See Magnesium and Aspartic Acid.

MAGNESIUM BENZOATE • A preservative. See Benzoic Acid.

MAGNESIUM BROMIDE • The inorganic salt of magnesium *(see)*.

MAGNESIUM CARBONATE • Perfume carrier, anticaking ingredient, and coloring ingredient. Used in baby powder, bath powder, tooth powders, face masks, liquid powders, face powders, and dry rouges. It is a silver-white, very crystalline salt that occurs in nature as magnetite or dolomite. Can be prepared artificially and is also used in paint, printing ink, table salt, and as an antacid. Nontoxic to the intact skin but may cause irritation when applied to abraded skin.

MAGNESIUM CHLORIDE • The inorganic salt of magnesium *(see)*.

MAGNESIUM CITRATE • Used in hair sets or hair-bodying ingredients. The magnesium salt of citric acid. Soluble in water. It leaves a glossy film after drying. No known toxicity.

MAGNESIUM COCOATE • The magnesium salt of coconut acid *(see)*.

MAGNESIUM FLUORIDE • Used in toothpastes. See Fluoride and Magnesium.

MAGNESIUM FLUOROSILICATE • Used in toothpastes. See Fluoride and Silicates.

MAGNESIUM GLUCONATE • The inorganic salt of gluconic acid *(see)*.

MAGNESIUM GLYCEROPHOSPHATE • Used in toothpaste. See Magnesium and Glycerol.

MAGNESIUM HYDROXIDE • Used as an alkali in dentrifices and skin creams, in canned peas, and as a drying ingredient and color retention ingredient for improved gelling in the manufacture of cheese. Slightly alkaline, crystalline compound obtained by hydration of magnesia *(see)* or precipitation of seawater by lime. Toxic when inhaled. Harmless to skin and in fact soothes it.

MAGNESIUM LANOLATE • Magnesium salt of lanolin. See Magnesium and Lanolin.

MAGNESIUM LAURETH SULFATE • Widely used as a surfactant because of its low irritation potential in shampoos. See Anionic Surfactants.

MAGNESIUM LAURYL SULFATE • A detergent. See Sodium Lauryl Sulfate.

MAGNESIUM METHYL COCOYL • Used as a surfactant and a cleansing ingredient. See Coconut Oil.

MAGNESIUM MONTMORILLONITE • See Montmorillonite.

MAGNESIUM MYRETH SULFATE • The inorganic salt of myristyl alcohol *(see)*.

MAGNESIUM MYRISTATE • The magnesium salt of myristic acid *(see)*.

MAGNESIUM NITRATE • Used in shampoos. See Nitrates.

MAGNESIUM OLEATE • Salt of magnesium used in liquid powders as a texturizer. It is a yellowish powder of mass that is insoluble in water. No known toxicity.

MAGNESIUM OLETH SULFATE • See Oleyl Alcohol.

MAGNESIUM OXIDE • **White Charcoal.** The inorganic salt of magnesium *(see)*.

MAGNESIUM PALMITATE • The inorganic salt of magnesium and palmitic acid *(see both)*.

MAGNESIUM PCA • Used as a skin-conditioning ingredient and a humectant.

MAGNESIUM PEG-3 COCAMIDE SULFATE • A magnesium salt of coconut oil used as an emulsifier.

MAGNESIUM PROPIONATE • A preservative. See Propionic Acid.

MAGNESIUM SALICYLATE • A drug related to aspirin that is used to treat rheumatoid arthritis. Produces analgesia by an ill-defined effect on the hypothalamus and by blocking generation of pain impulses. The peripheral action may involve inhibition of prostaglandin synthesis. Relieves fever by acting on the hypothalamic heat-regulating center to produce blood vessel dilation. This increases peripheral blood flow and promotes sweating, which leads to loss of heat and cooling by evaporation. Potential adverse effects include ringing in the ears and hearing loss, nausea, vomiting, GI distress, abnormal liver function, rash, bruising, and hypersensitivity manifested by asthma or anaphylaxis. Ammonium chloride and other urine acidifiers increase blood levels of salicylates. See Magnesium.

MAGNESIUM SILICATE • An insoluble, effervescent, white powder that is slowly decomposed by acids to form a soluble salt and an insoluble silica, which has strong absorptive properties. Used to opacify shampoos; also medicinally to reduce stomach acidity, with slow neutralizing action. Toxic by inhalation.

MAGNESIUM STEARATE • Coloring ingredient used in face powder, protective creams, and baby dusting powders. It is a white soapy powder, insoluble in water. Also used for tablet making. No known toxicity. On the basis of the available information, the CIR Expert Panel *(see)* concludes that it is safe as a cosmetic ingredient. See Aluminum Distearate.

MAGNESIUM SULFATE • **Epsom Salts.** A magnesium salt used to treat deficiency during stress, to decrease the release of certain nerve impulses in the brain to prevent or control seizures in pregnancy (preeclampsia or eclampsia), and to stop hypomagnesemic seizures. Also used as a laxative and a bath additive. Potential adverse reactions include sweating, drowsiness, depressed reflexes, paralysis, low temperature, low blood pressure, flushing, circulatory collapse, depressed heart function, heart block, respiratory paralysis, and low blood calcium. In 1992, the FDA proposed a ban on magnesium sulfate in oral menstrual drug products because it has not been shown to be safe and effective for its stated claims. No known toxicity when used in the bath. See Magnesium.

MAGNESIUM SULFIDE • A depilatory ingredient. See Sulfides.

MAGNESIUM TALLOWATE • The magnesium salt of tallow *(see)*.

MAGNESIUM THIOGLYCOLATE • Used in depilatories. See Thioglycolic Acid.

MAGNESIUM TRISILICATE • Coloring ingredient. See Magnesium Aluminum Silicate.

MAGNESIUM/TEA-COCO-SULFATE • A cleansing ingredient. See Coconut Oil.

MAGNOLIA • **Sweet Bay.** Used in perfumery. A genus of North American and Asian shrubs and trees named after the French botanist Pierre Magnol. The plants have evergreen or deciduous leaves and usually snowy white, yellow, rose or purple flowers appearing in early spring. The dried bark is used in folk medicine to induce sweating and as a bitter tonic. No known toxicity.

MAIDEN HAIR FERN EXTRACT • **Venus Hair.** Extract of the leaves of the fern *Adiantum capillus veneris.* Used in herbal creams to soothe irritated skin.

MAKEUP BASE, FOUNDATION • See Foundation Makeup.

MALEATED SOYBEAN OIL • Modified soybean oil in which some of the unsaturation has been converted to carboxylic acid. See Maleic Acid and Soybean Oil.

MALEIC ACID • Colorless crystals with a bad taste. Toxic by ingestion. Used as a preservative for oils and fats.

MALEIC ANHYDRIDE • Colorless needles derived from oxidation of benzene. Used in the manufacture of polyester resins, pesticides, as a preservative for oils and fats, and in permanent-press resins. Irritating to tissue.

MALIC ACID • A colorless, crystalline compound with a strong acid taste that occurs naturally in a wide variety of fruits, including apples and cherries. An alkali in cosmetics, foods, and wines. Also used as an antioxidant for cosmetics and as an ingredient in hair lacquer. Irritating to the skin and can cause an allergic reaction when used in hair lacquers. See Alpha-Hydroxy Acids.

MALLOW EXTRACT • From the herb family. A moderate purplish red that is paler than magenta rose. Used in coloring and also as a source of pectin *(see)*. No known toxicity.

MALONIC ACID • An antioxidant prepared synthetically. Occurs naturally in many plants. The colorless crystals obtained from the oxidation of malic acid are used in the manufacture of barbiturates. It is a strong irritant. Large doses injected into mice are lethal.

MALPIGHIA GLABRA • See Acerola.

MALT EXTRACT • Extracted from barley that has been allowed to germinate, then heated to destroy vitality and dried. It contains sugars, proteins, and salts from barley. The extract is mixed with water and allowed to solidify. It is used as a nutrient and in cosmetics as a texturizer. No known toxicity.

MALTITOL • Obtained from maltose *(see)*.

MALTODEXTRIN • The sugar obtained by hydrolysis of starch.

MALTOL • A white, crystalline powder with a butterscotch odor, found in the bark of young larch trees, pine needles, chicory, wood tars, and roasted malt. It imparts a "freshly baked" odor and flavor to bread and cakes. Used as a synthetic chocolate, coffee, fruit, maple, nut, and vanilla flavoring ingredient for beverages, ice cream, ices, candy, baked goods, gelatin desserts, chewing gum, and jelly. No known toxicity.

MALTOSE • **Malt Sugar.** Colorless crystals derived from malt extract and used as a nutrient, sweetener, culture medium, and stabilizer. No known toxicity.

MALVA MOSCHATA • *Malvacae.* An erect European perennial herb with rosy purple flowers. Contains mucilage, essential oil, and a trace of tannin. The herb is used to soothe inflammation in the mouth and throat, and to treat earache. Also used in bathwater or in a compress to heal boils, abscesses, and minor burns.

MAMMARIAN HYDROLYSATE • The hydrolysate *(see)* of animal mammarian tissue derived by acid, enzyme, or other method of hydrolysis. See Mammary Extract.

MAMMARY EXTRACT • The extract of cow's mammary tissue.

MANDARIN ORANGE OIL • Obtained by expression of the peel of a ripe mandarin orange. Clear, dark orange to reddish yellow, with a pleasant orangelike odor. It is an orange, tangerine, cherry, and grape flavoring for beverages, ice cream, ices, candy, baked goods, chewing gum, and gelatin desserts. GRAS.

MANDELIC ACID • **Amygdalic Acid.** Large white crystals or powder with a faint odor. Toxic by ingestion. Used in manufacturing of chemical compounds and as a urinary antiseptic.

MANGANESE ACETYLMETHIONATE • See Manganese Sources and Methionine.

MANGANESE ASPARTATE • See Aspartic Acid and Manganese Sources.

MANGANESE CARBONATE • Rose-colored crystals derived from manganese. Used as a pigment.

MANGANESE GLUCONATE • Used in skin fresheners and cold creams. See Gluconic Acid and Salts and Manganese Sources.

MANGANESE GLYCEROPHOSPHATE • Used in oral care products. See Glycerol and Phosphate.

MANGANESE PCA • Used in skin conditioners. See Manganese Pyrrolidone, and Carboxylic Acid.

MANGANESE SOURCES • **Manganese Acetate, Manganese Carbonate, Manganese Chloride, Manganese Citrate, Manganese Sulfate, Manganese Glycerophosphate, Manganese Hypophosphite,** and **Manganese Oxide.** A mineral supplement first isolated in 1774, it occurs in minerals and in minute quantities in animals, plants, and water. Many forms are used in dyeing. Manganous salts are activators of enzymes, and are necessary to the development of strong bones. They are used as nutrients and as dairy substitutes. Toxicity occurs by inhalation. Symptoms include languor, sleepiness, wakefulness, emotional disturbances, and Parkinsonlike symptoms. **Manganese chloride, citrate, glycerophosphate,** and **hypophosphite** are all considered GRAS according to the final report of the Select Committee on GRAS Substances and should continue their GRAS status as nutrients with no limitations other than good manufacturing practices. However, **manganese oxide,** according to the Select Committee, does not have enough known about it upon which to base an evaluation when it is used as a food ingredient.

MANGANESE STEARATE • See Stearic Acid and Manganese Sources.

MANGANESE SULFATE • Usually prepared by dissolving dolomite *(see)* or magnetite in acid. It is the salt of the element manganese, a metal ore. Its pale red crystals are used in red hair dye and to make red glazes on porcelain. Also used medicinally as a purgative and as a dressing for cotton goods. No known toxicity to the hair or scalp, but very small doses injected into mice are lethal.

MANGANESE VIOLET • **Burgundy Violet. Permanent Violet. Ammonium Manganese Pyrophosphate.** A moderate purple that is redder and duller than heliotrope and bluer than amethyst. Toxic when inhaled. Permanently listed in 1976 for cosmetic coloring, including around the eyes.

MANGIFERRERA INDICA • See Mango.

MANGO • A tropical evergreen tree from India and Malaysia. It produces a rich, juicy fruit with a hard pit. Mangoes are eaten in many parts of the world. They are used in "organic" cosmetics.

MANIHOT UTILISSIMA • A tropical herb. Contains glycosides *(see)* and Vitamin E. It is used as a thickener.

MANNITAN LAURATE • The monoester of lauric acid and mannitol *(see both)*.

MANNITOL • A humectant in hand creams and lotions, and used in hair-grooming products as an emulsifier and antioxidant. It is widespread in plants but mostly prepared from seaweed. White, crystalline solid, odorless, and sweet tasting. Its use as a food additive is under study by the FDA because it can cause gastrointestinal disturbances. However, there is no known toxicity from its use as a cosmetic. In cosmetics it is used as a flavoring ingredient, humectant, and skin conditioner.

MARE MILK • Milk from female horses.

MARIS AQUA • Seawater.

MARIS LIMUS • Sea silt.

MARIS SAL • Sea salt.

MARITIME PINE EXTRACT • Extract of the bark and pine buds of *Pinus maritima. Pinus pinaster.* See Pine Tar.

MARJORAM OIL • Used in hair preparations, perfumes, and soaps, it is the yellowish essential oil from sweet marjoram. Insoluble in water, soluble in alcohol and chloroform. Can irritate the skin. The redness, itching, and warmth experienced when applied to the skin are carried by local dilation of the blood vessels or by local reflex. May produce allergic reactions. Essential oils such as marjoram are believed to penetrate the skin easily and produce systemic effects.

MARMOT OIL • Oil from a short-legged rodent. Related to the woodchuck or prairie dog. Used in hair and skin conditioning products. It is occulsive.

MARROW EXTRACT • Extract from bovine bone marrow.

MARRUBIUM VULAGRE • See Horehound.

MARSDENIA CONDURANGO • See Condurango Extract.

MARSHMALLOW ROOT • *Althea officinalis.* A demulcent containing up to 35 percent mucilage, it is an old-time remedy for digestive disorders. It soothes mucous membranes and has been used externally for hundreds of years as a wound healer. Marshmallow ointments and creams are used on chapped hands and lips. It is used internally to treat inflammation of the genitourinary tract, including painful urination. It is also used to treat diarrhea and cholera. It is used to soothe a respiratory tract irritated by bronchitis, asthma, or coughs. It is used as a mouthwash and gargle and to soothe teething infants. Herbalists claim it has a general calming effect on the body.

MASCARA • A cosmetic for coloring the eyelashes and eyebrows. Contains insoluble pigments, carnauba wax, triethanolamine stearate, paraffin, and lanolin. Pigments in eye makeup must be inert and are usually carbon black, iron oxides, chromium oxide, ultramarine, or carmine. Coal tar dyes are not permitted. The excipients may contain beeswax, cetyl alcohol, glyceryl monostearate, gums such as tragacanth, mineral oil, perfume, preservatives such as *p*-hydroxybenzoic acid, propylene glycol, spermaceti, and synthetics such as isopropyl myristate, as well as vegetable oils. The newer lash extenders may carry certain tiny fibers of rayon or nylon. Almost any one of the ingredients may cause an allergic reaction in the susceptible.

MASKING FRAGRANCE • A small amount of fragrance used literally to mask the unpleasant odors in a product such as soaps.

MATÉ EXTRACT • **Paraguay Tea Extract. St. Bartholomew's Tea. Jesuit's Tea.** A natural flavoring extract from small gourds grown in South America, where maté is a stimulant beverage. Among its constituents are caffeine, purines, and tannins. See Caffeine and Tannic Acid for toxicity. GRAS.

MATILJA POPPY • **Romneya Coulteri.** See Poppy Oil.

MATRICARIA EXTRACT • **Wild Chamomile Extract.** Extract of the flower heads of *Matricaria chamomilla.* Used internally as a tonic and externally as a soothing medication for contusions and other inflammation. Widely used in cold creams, cleansing lotions, shampoos, suntan gels, hair care products, skin fresheners, and eye makeup. See Tannic Acid.

MATRICARIA OIL • **Camomile Oil.** The volatile oil distilled from the dried flower heads of *Matricaria chamomilla.* See Matricaria Extract.

MATTE FINISH MAKEUP • Designed to be an all-in-one makeup combining foundation and powder. It is a more concentrated version of standard makeup and contains more powder, pigment, and emollient than standard makeup. Effective in covering blemishes. Skin toxicity depends upon ingredients used.

MAYAPPLE • *Podophyllum peltatum.* **Duck's Foot. Hogapple. Mandrake.** A perennial plant of the barberry family, it is native to North America. It was used by early American settlers as a laxative, and to treat diarrhea, arthritis, and kidney problems. American Indians reportedly used it as a poison to commit suicide.

MAYBLOSSOM • See Hawthorn.

MAYONNAISE • The common salad dressing. Semisolid, made with eggs, vegetable oil, and vinegar or lemon juice. Used by natural cosmeticians as a dry hair conditioner. The hair is rubbed liberally with mayonnaise, a hot towel is wrapped around the hair and kept on for 15 minutes, and then it is removed. Two soapings and plenty of rinsing follow. As effective as any of the more expensive commercial products.

MDM • Abbreviation for monomethyl dimethyl.

MDM HYDANTOIN • **Monomethylol Dimethyl Hydantoin.** Used as a preservative in cosmetic preparations, the compound liberates an allergen steadily at a slow rate in the presence of water. The resin is used in hair lacquers.

MEA • The abbreviation for monoethanolamine.

MEA-BORATE • The ester of ethanolamine borate. See Ethanolamines and Boric Acid.

MEA-BENZOATE • A preservative. See Benzoic Acid.

MEA-DICETEARYL PHOSPHATE • An emulsifier. See Cetrearyl Alcohol.

MEADOW SAFFRON • *Colchicum autumnale.* The perennial plant, the leaves of which appear in the spring and the flowers in the autumn, is a native of the temperate parts of Europe where it grows wild in meadows. All parts of the meadow saffron plant contain colchicine *(see)* which is used to treat the pain and inflammation of gout. Meadow saffron can be toxic and may even be fatal if ingested.

MEADOWFOAM SEED OIL • The oil expressed from the seeds of the meadowfoam plant, *Limnanthes alba.* A skin conditioning ingredient used in lipstick, body and hand preparations.

MEADOWSWEET • *Spiraea ulmaria.* A perennial common to Europe, eastern United States, and Canada, it grows in meadows. It was used to treat diarrhea and stomach upsets. It was also given for gout, arthritis, and flu. It is rich in Vitamin C and contains salicylic acid and citric acid *(see both).* Widely used in "organic" cosmetics as a skin-conditioning ingredient.

MEA-HYDROLYZED COLLAGEN • The monoethanolamine salt of hydrolyzed animal protein. The word "animal" has been removed from this ingredient's name.

MEA-IODINE • See Iodine.

MEA-LAURETH-6 CARBOXYLATE • See Polyethylene Glycol.

MEA-LAURETH SULFATE • The monoethanolamine salt of ethylated lauryl sulfate. See Quaternary Ammonium Compounds.

MEA-LAURYL SULFATE • The monoethanolamine salt of sulfated lauryl alcohol. See Quaternary Ammonium Compounds.

MEA-PPGP6P-LAURETH-7-CARBOXYLATE • See Quaternary Ammonium Compounds.

MEA-SALICYLATE • A preservative. See Salicyclic Acid.

MEA-THIOLACTATE • Used in hair straightening and hair curling products. See Thiolactic Acid.

MEDICAGO SATIVA • See Alfalfa Extract.

MEDICATED MAKEUP • Cosmetic manufacturers advertise medicated makeup that both "covers" and treats the skin simultaneously. Such cosmetics contain antibacterials such as bithionol and tribromsalan. The American Medical Association frowns on such preparations because such anti-infective ingredients are useful in medical preparations for the treatment of minor cuts and abrasions, but in cosmetics and toilet preparations they serve merely to limit the bacterial contamination of the product during use. Furthermore, their potential harm often outweighs their benefit because such ingredients may cause allergic reactions and sensitivity to sunlight or bright lights; when the skin is exposed, it breaks out or reddens.

MEK • Methyl Ethyl Ketone. A flammable, colorless liquid compound resembling acetone and most often made by taking the hydrogen out of butyl alcohol. Used chiefly as a solvent. Similar to, but more irritating than, acetone; its vapor is irritating to mucous membranes and eyes. Central nervous system depression in experimental animals has been reported, but the irritating odor usually discourages further inhalation in humans. No serious poisonings reported in humans, except for skin irritation when nail polish was applied with MEK as a solvent. Large doses inhaled by rats are lethal.

MEL • See Honey.

MELALEUCA • See Tea Tree Oil and Cajeput Oil.

MELAMINE • White, free-flowing, powdered resin. Used in nail enamel. First introduced into industry in 1939, it is now used in a wide variety of products, including boilproof adhesives and scratch-resistant enamel finishes. Combined with urea resins, it forms the heat-resistant amino plastics. It may cause skin rashes, but that is believed to be caused by the formaldehyde component rather than the melamine. See Urea-Formaldehyde Resin.

MELAMINE/FORMALDEHYDE RESIN • A film-former. Respiratory distress, bleeding in the lungs, significant weight loss, and other lung problems were observed during inhalation studies in rats. Feeding studies in animals did not show toxicity. Human sensitization to this has been reported in medical literature. The safety of this ingredient has not been documented and substantiated according to the CIR Expert Panel *(see)*. See Melamine.

MELANIN • The pigment is responsible for the color of skin, hair, feathers, and fur. Use of this ingredient is prohibited in the United States and may be restricted in other countries.

MELASYN • A synthetic melanin *(see)* protects against ultraviolet light.

MELIA AZADIRACHTA • See Neem Tree.

MELILOT OIL • **Esberiven. Sweet Clover.** Dried leaves and flowering tops of *Melilotus officinalis.* Contains coumarin, resins, and volatile oils *(see all).*

MELILOTUS OFFICINALIS • See Clover.

MELISSA OIL • *Melissa officinalis.* **Lemon Balm. Sweet Balm.** A sweet-tasting herb introduced into Britain by the Romans, it has been used from early times in England for nervousness, menstrual irregularity, and surgical dressings. The Greeks used it for fevers and to treat scorpion stings and the bites of mad dogs. A hot tea made from it causes perspiration and is said to stop the early symptoms of a cold. See Balm.

MELISSIC ACID • See Bayberry.

MELON EXTRACT AND JUICE • *Cucumis Melo.* **Honey Dew.** Used in products for dry hair and as a skin conditioner.

MENADIONE • **Vitamin K₃.** Used as a preservative in emollients. A synthetic with properties of Vitamin K. Bright yellow crystals that are insoluble in water. They are used medically to prevent blood clotting and in food to prevent souring of milk products. Can be irritating to mucous membranes, respiratory tract, and the skin.

MENHADEN OIL • **Pogy Oil. Mossbunker Oil.** Obtained along the coast of Africa from the menhaden fish, which are a little larger than herrings. The fish glycerides of menhaden are reddish and have a strong fishy odor. Used in soaps and creams. No known toxicity.

MENTHA AQUATICA • Water mint. See Mint.

MENTHA ARVENSIS • See Wild Mint Extract.

MENTHA PIPERITA • See Mint.

MENTHA PULEGIUM • See Pennyroyal Extract.

MENTHA VIRIDIS • See Spearmint Oil.

P-MENTHAN-7-OL • A fragrance ingredient. See Mint.

MENTHOL • Used in perfumes, emollient creams, hair tonics, mouthwashes, shaving creams, preshave lotions, after-shave lotions, body rubs, liniments, and skin fresheners. It gives that "cool" feeling to the skin after use. It can be obtained naturally from peppermint or other mint oils and can be made synthetically by hydrogenation *(see)* of thymol *(see)*. It is a local anesthetic. It is nontoxic in low doses, but in concentrations of three percent or more it exerts an irritant action that can, if long continued, induce changes in all layers of the mucous membranes. The Food and Drug Administration issued a notice in 1992 that menthol has not been shown to be safe and effective for stated claims in OTC products, including those for the treatment of fever blisters and cold sores, poison ivy, poison oak, poison sumac, and insect bites and stings, as well as in astringents. Also used in grooming aids, skin fresheners, mouthwashes, fragrances, creams, cleansing lotions, bathsoaps and many other cosmetic products.

MENTHOXYPROPANEDIOL • A cooling ingredient. See Menthol and Propylene Glycol.

MENTHYL ACETATE • The ester *(see)* of menthol and acetic acid *(see both)*.

MENTHYL ANTHRANILATE • The ester *(see)* of menthol *(see)*.

MENTHYL LACTATE • See Menthol and Lactic Acid.

MENTHYL SALICYLATE • The ester of menthol and salicylic acid used in medicines and sunscreen preparations. See Salicylic Acid.

MENYANTHES TRIFOLIATA • See Buckbean Extract.

MERCAPTANS • **Quicksilver.** Used in depilatories. A class of compounds that contain sulfur and have a disagreeable odor. Depilatories containing mercaptans can cause irritation and allergic reactions, as well as infections of hair follicles.

MERCAPTOPROPIONIC ACID • See Mercaptans.

MERCURIALIS EXTRACT • **Dog Mercury.** An extract of the herb *Mercurialis perennis,* a small slender species. Formerly dried and used as a diuretic and to treat syphilis.

MERCURIC OXIDE • **Red Mercuric Oxide. Yellow Mercuric Oxide.** Derived by heating mercurous nitrate, it is used in perfumery as a topical disinfectant and as a fungicide. Highly toxic.

MERCURY COMPOUNDS • **Quicksilver.** Until July 5, 1973, mercury was widely used in cosmetics, including wax face masks, hair tonics, medicated soaps, and bleach and freckle creams. Mercury compounds are heavy, silver liquids from the metal that occurs in the earth's crust. Mercury is potentially dangerous by all portals of entry, including the skin. It may cause a variety of symptoms, ranging from chronic inflammation of the mouth and gums to personality changes, nervousness, fever, and rash. If ingested in small amounts, it may be fatal. The ban on mercury was brought about because it was found that its use in bleaching creams and other products over a long period of time caused mercury buildup in the body. Mercury is still used in eye preparations as a preservative to inhibit growth of germs. It is now the only use permitted. Because the prevention of eye infection warrants the use of mercury, eye makeup contains up to 0.0065 percent. See also Calomel.

MEROXAPOL-105, -108, -171, -172, -174, -178, -251, -252, -254, -255, -258, -311, -312, -314 • **Pluronic.** The polyoxypropylene block polymer that is derived from petroleum, it is a liquid nonionic—resists freezing and shrinkage—surfactant used in hand creams. The numbers after the name identify the liquidity of the compound: the higher the number, the more solid.

METABROMSALAN • See Bromates.

METALLIC HAIR DYES • Metals such as copper are used to change the color of hair. They are not used very often because they tend to dull the hair. However, they are used in products that are designed for daily application over a week or so to effect color changes gradually. Combs impregnated with dye or hair lotions may contain metals for this purpose. See Hair Coloring for further information, including toxicity.

METHACRYLOYL ETHYL BETAINE/METHACRYLATES COPOLYMER • See Methacrylic Acid.

METHANOL • **Methyl Alcohol. Wood Alcohol.** A solvent and denaturant obtained by the destructive distillation of wood. Flammable, poisonous liquid with a nauseating odor. Better solvent than ethyl alcohol. See Ethanol for skin toxicity.

METHENAMINE • An odorless, white, crystalline powder made from formaldehyde and ammonia. Used as an antiseptic and bacteria killer in deodorant creams and powders, mouthwashes, and medicines. It is one of the most frequent causes of skin rashes in the rubber industry, and is omitted from hypoallergenic cosmetics. Skin irritations are believed to be caused by formic acid, which occurs by the action of perspiration on the skin. On the basis of the available information, the CIR Expert Panel *(see)* concludes that it is safe as a cosmetic ingredient.

METHENAMMONIUM CHLORIDE • **Busan 1500®.** A water-soluble bactericide active over a wide pH range. See Ammonia.

METHICONE • Widely used as a skin conditioning ingredient in foundations, eye shadows, face powders, lipsticks, blushers, eyeliners, moisutrizers, masacara, makeup bases, and powders. Also after-shave lotions. See Silicones.

METHIONINE • An essential amino acid *(see)* that occurs in protein. Used as a texturizer in cosmetic creams. Also used as a dietary substance and is attracted to fat. Nontoxic.

METHOCARBAMOL • A skeletal muscle relaxant prepared from phenol.

o-METHOXY CINNAMIC ALDEHYDE • See Cinnamic Aldehyde.

METHOXY PEG 10-40 • Humectants. See Polyethylene Glycol.

METHOXY PEG-22/DODECYL GLYCOL • See Polymers.

METHOXY PROPANOL • See Propylene Glycol.

p-METHOXYACETOPHENONE • *p*-**Acetanisole.** Crystalline solid with a pleasant odor. Soluble in alcohol and fixed oils, and derived from the interaction of anisole and acetyl chloride with aluminum chloride and carbon disulfide. Used in perfumery as a synthetic floral odor and in flavoring.

3-METHOXYBUTANOL • A solvent. See Butanoic Acid.

METHOXYDIGLYCOL • See Polyethylene Glycol.

METHOXYETHANOL • **2-Methoxy Ethanol. Ethylene Glycol Monomethyl Ether.** A widely used solvent in industrial products such as surface coatings, inks, dyes, cleaning fluids, degreasing ingredients, metalworking, and hydraulic brake fluids. The permissible human exposure levels of this ethylene glycol ether is 25 ppm to 5 ppm, and a further reduction has been proposed. It is both a reproductive and developmental toxicant. May cause birth defects. See Ethylene Glycol.

METHOXYINDANE • **Phoralid.** A synthetic fragrance.

METHOXYISOPROPANOL • A solvent. See Propylene Glycol.

2-METHOXYMETHYL-p-AMINOPHENOL • See Phenol.

2- AND 4-METHOXY-m-PHENYLENEDIAMINE • See *p*-Phenylenediamine.

4-METHOXY-m-PHENYLENEDIAMINE • Hair dye ingredient. On the basis of the available information, the CIR Expert Panel *(see)* concludes that it is unsafe as a cosmetic ingredient. See Phenylenediamine.

4-METHOXY-m-PHENYLENEDIAMINE SULFATE • A hair dye ingredient. On the basis of the available information. The CIR Expert Panel *(see)* concludes that it is unsafe as a cosmetic ingredient. See Phenylenediamine.

2-METHOXY-p-PHENYLENEDIAMINE SULFATE • See Phenylenediamine.

4-METHOXY-m-PHENYLENEDIAMINE-HCL • A hair dye ingredient. On the basis of the available information, the CIR Expert Panel *(see)* concludes that it is unsafe as a cosmetic ingredient.

6-METHOXY-2-3-PYRIDINEDIAMINE • See Pyridine.

METHOXYSALEN • **8-Methoxypsoralen.** White to cream-colored, odorless crystalline solid; slightly soluble in alcohol and almost insoluble in water. Used as a suntan accelerator and a sunburn protectant.

4-METHOXYTOLUENE-2, 5-DIAMINE HCL • A colorless liquid used in perfumery and flavorings. See Toluene.

METHYACRYLIC ACID • **2-Methylpropenoic Acid.** Occurs in Roman chamomile oil. It has a bad odor and is corrosive. It is used to make clear plastic.

METHYL ACETAMIDE • See Methyl Acetate.

METHYL ACETATE • **Acetic Acid.** Colorless liquid that occurs naturally in coffee, with a pleasant apple odor. Used in perfume to emphasize floral notes *(see)*, especially that of rose, and in toilet waters having a lavender odor. Also occurs naturally in peppermint oil. Used as a solvent for many resins and oils. May be irritating to the respiratory tract, and in high concentrations may be narcotic. Since it has an effective fat solvent drying effect on skin, it may cause skin problems such as chafing and cracking.

METHYL ACETOACETATE • **3-Oxobutanoic Acid. Methyl Ester.** See Butanoic Acid.

METHYL ACETYL RICINOLEATE • See Ricinoleic Acid.

METHYL ACRYLATE • **2-Propanoic Acid. Methyl Ester.** Derived from ethylene chlorohydrin, it is transparent and elastic. Used to coat paper and plastic film. Can be highly irritating to the eyes, skin, and mucous membranes. Convulsions occur if vapors are inhaled in high concentrations. See Acrylates.

METHYL ALCOHOL • See Methanol.

METHYL ANTHRANILATE • Used as an "orange" scent for ointments, in the manufacture of synthetic perfumes, and in suntan lotions. Occurs naturally in neroli, ylang-ylang, bergamot, jasmine, and other essential oils. Colorless to pale yellow liquid with a bluish fluorescence and a grapelike odor. It is made synthetically from coal tar *(see)*. Can irritate the skin.

METHYL ASPARTIC ACID • See Aspartic Acid.

METHYL BEHENATE • A skin-conditioning ingredient. See Behenic Acid and Alcohol.

METHYL BENZOATE • **Essence of Oil of Niobe.** Made from methanol and benzoic acid *(see both)*. Used in perfumes. Colorless, transparent liquid with a pleasant fruity odor. Also used as a flavoring in foods and beverages. No known toxicity.

METHYL BUTENES • Solvent.

METHYL CAPROATE • **Methyl Hexanoate.** The ester produced by the reaction of methyl alcohol and caproic acid. Used as a stabilizer and plasticizer for hand and face creams. No known toxicity.

METHYL CAPRYLATE • See Methyl Caproate.

METHYL CHLORIDE • **Chloromethane.** Colorless gas or colorless liquid with a sweet taste, it is used as a spray for pesticides in food storage and processing areas. It is not supposed to contact fatty foods. Poisonous, it can cause severe injury to liver and kidney.

METHYL CINNAMATE • White crystals, strawberrylike odor, and soluble in alcohol. Derived by heating methanol, cinnamic acid, and sulfuric acid. Used in perfumes and flavoring. See Cinnamic Acid.

METHYL COCOATE • **Methyl Alcohol and Fatty Acids.** See Methanol and Coconut Oil.

6-METHYL COUMARIN • A synthetic compound once used in suntan products. A potent photosensitizer. Not recommended for use in fragrance ingredients.

METHYL CYCLODEXTRIN • See Dextrin.

METHYL DEHYDROABIETATE • See Abietic Acid.

METHYL DICOCOAMINE • An anti-static ingredient for hair preparations. See Coconut Oil.

METHYL DIISOPROPYL PROPIONAMIDE • A fragrance ingredient. See Propionic Acid.

METHYL ETHYL KETONE • See MEK.

METHYL EUGENOL • **Eugenol. Methyl Ether.** See Eugenol and Ether.

METHYL GLUCETH-10 or -20 • The polyethylene glycol ether of methyl glucose. See Glucose Glutamate.

METHYL GLUCETH-20 SESQUISTEARATE • **Glucamate.** Used in moisturizers. See Glucose Glutamate.

METHYL GLUCOSE SESQUIOLEATE • A mixture of diesters of methyl glucoside and oleic acid. See Glutamic Acid.

METHYL GLUCOSE SESQUISTEARATE • A mixture of diesters of methyl glucoside and stearic acid. See Glutamic Acid.

METHYL HYDROGENATED ROSINATE • The ester of methyl alcohol and hydrogenated acids derived from rosin *(see)*.

METHYL p-HYDROXYBENZOATE • See Methylparaben.

METHYL HYDROXYETHYLCELLULOSE • See Methylcellulose.

METHYL HYDROXYMETHYL OLEYL OXAZOLINE • A synthetic wax. See Oxazoline.

METHYL HYDROXYSTEARATE • The ester of methyl alcohol and hydroxystearic acid used in cosmetic creams. See Methanol and Stearic Acid.

METHYL LACTATE • The ester of menthol and lactic acid (see both).

METHYL LAURATE • The ester of methyl alcohol and lauric acid. Derived from coconut oil, it is used in detergents, emulsifiers, wetting ingredients, stabilizers, resins, lubricants, plasticizers, and flavorings. No known toxicity.

METHYL LINOLEATE • The ester of methyl alcohol and linoleic acid, it is a colorless oil derived from safflower oil and used in detergents, emulsifiers, wetting ingredients, stabilizers, resins, lubricants, and plasticizers. It is used in skin conditioners. No known toxicity.

METHYL METHACRYLATE CROSSPOLYMER • See Methacrylic Acid and Polymer.

METHYL METHACRYLATE MONOMER • Banned in nail products because of adverse effects.

METHYL 3-METHYLRESORCYLATE • See Resorcinol.

METHYL MYRISTATE • A skin conditioning ingredient. See Myristic Acid.

METHYL NICOTINATE • Derived from nicotinic acid (see) and used as a rubefacient (see). No known toxicity.

METHYL OLEATE • An emollient ingredient. See Oleic Acid.

METHYL PALMITATE • The ester of methyl alcohol and palmitic acid. Colorless liquid derived from palm oil. Used in detergents, emulsifiers, wetting ingredients, stabilizers, resins, lubricants, and plasticizers. Low toxicity.

METHYL PARABEN • **Methyl p-Hydroxybenzoate.** One of the most widely used preservatives in cosmetics, it has a broad spectrum of antimicrobial activity and is relatively nonirritating, nonsensitizing, and nonpoisonous. It is stable over the acid-alkalinity range of most cosmetics and is sufficiently soluble in water to produce the effective concentration in the water phase. Can cause allergic reactions.

METHYL PELARGONATE • **Nonanoic Acid. Methyl Ester.** The ester of ethyl alcohol and pelargonic acid (see) used as an emollient in perfume and flavorings. No known toxicity.

METHYL PHENYLACETATE • Colorless liquid with a honeylike odor used in perfumery and as a flavoring. See Phenylacetic Acid.

METHYL PHTHALYL ETHYL GLYCOLATE • See Phthalic Acid and Polyethylene Glycol.

METHYL RICINOLEATE • The ester of methyl alcohol and ricinoleic acid. A colorless liquid used as a plasticizer, lubricant, cutting oil, and wetting ingredient. See Castor Oil, Methol Alcohol, and Ricinoleic Acid.

METHYL ROSINATE • **Rosin Acid. Methyl Ester.** The ester of acids recovered from rosin (see). See Methyl Alcohol.

METHYL SALICYLATE • **Oil of Wintergreen.** A counterirritant, local anesthetic, and disinfectant used in perfumes, toothpaste, tooth powder, and mouthwash. The volatile oil obtained by maceration and subsequent steam distillation in a species of leaves, including those of sweet birch, cassie, and wintergreen. A strong irritant to the skin and mucous membranes, and may be absorbed readily through the skin. Used as a flavor in foods, beverages, and pharmaceuticals, and used as an odorant in perfumery and as an ultraviolet absorber in sunburn lotions. Toxic by ingestion. Use in foods restricted by the FDA. Lethal dose 30 cc in adults, 10 cc in children. See Salicylates.

METHYL SILICONE • Prepared by hydrolyzing *(see)* dimethyldichlorosilane or its esters, it is used to help compounds resist oxidation. No known toxicity. See Silicones.

METHYL STEARATE • See Stearic Acid and Methyl Alcohol.

METHYL THIOGLYCOLATE • Hair straightening and hair waving ingredient. See Thioglycolic Acid.

METHYLAMINES • Occur in herring brine, in the urine of dogs, in certain plants such as mints, and in methanol. Used in tanning and in organic processing. Irritating to the eyes, skin, and respiratory tract.

3-METHYLAMINO-4-NITROPHENOXYETHANOL • See *p*-Methylamino-phenol Sulfate.

p-METHYLAMINOPHENOL SULFATE • Crystals that discolor in air and are soluble in water. They are used in photographic developers, for dyeing furs, and for hair dyes. May cause skin irritation, allergic reactions, and a shortage of oxygen in the blood. In solution applied to the skin, restlessness and convulsions have been produced in humans.

METHYLATED SPIRITS • **Toilet Quality.** Alcohol denatured with methanol *(see)*. Used in fragrances and other cosmetic products in amounts of over 85 percent ethyl alcohol, 5 percent methyl alcohol, and 5 percent water. See Ethanol for toxicity.

METHYLBENZETHONIUM CHLORIDE • **Diaparene Chloride.** A quaternary ammonium compound used as a germicide in cosmetics and baby products such as baby oils. Also used as a topical disinfectant. See Quaternary Ammonium Compounds for toxicity.

4-METHYLBENZYLIDENE CAMPHOR • See Camphor.

METHYLCELLULOSE • **Cellulose Methyl Ether. Citrucel. Cologel.** A binder, thickener, and emulsifying ingredient used in wave-setting lotions, bath oils, and other cosmetic products. Introduced in 1947, this compound is prepared from wood pulp or chemical cotton by treatment with alcohol. It swells in water and increases bulk. It is not absorbed systemically and is nontoxic. On the basis of the available animal and human data, the CIR Expert Panel *(see)* concludes that this ingredient is safe as used in cosmetics.

METHYLCHLOROISOTHIAZOLINONE • A preservative used in shampoos, hair, skin and after-shave and bath products that was taken from industry to replace formaldehyde. While it has been shown to be a sensitizer in animals, it has not been shown to be a sensitizer in humans. See Imidazole.

METHYLDIBROMO GLUTARONITRILE • A preservative used in bubble baths, indoor tanning preparations, and hair conditioners. Application to the skin of rats for 21 days at a level of 4.0 g/kg produced severe irritation, whereas skin studies in rabbits showed only slight to moderate irritation. It is readily absorbed through the skin. Based on available data, the CIR Expert Panel *(see)* concludes it is safe as used in "rinse-off" products and safe up to 0.025 percent in "leave-on" products. See Bromates and Glutaric Acid.

METHYLDIHYDROJASMONATE • See Jasmone.

METHYLENE CHLORIDE • A solvent for nail enamels and for cleansing creams. A colorless gas that compresses into a colorless liquid of pleasant odor and sweet taste. Used as an anesthetic in medicine. High concentrations are narcotic. Damage to the liver, kidneys, and central nervous system can occur, and persistent postrecovery symptoms after inhalation include headache, nervousness, insomnia, and tremor. Can be absorbed through the skin and converted to carbon monoxide, which can cause stress on the cardiovascular system. It is also a skin irritant. No longer permitted in cosmetics. In 1988, the CIR Expert Panel *(see)* determined it was safe in cosmetics designed for brief use.

METHYLENEDIOXYPHENOL • See Phenol.

METHYLETHANOLAMINE • See Ethanolamine and Methyl.

2-METHYL-5-HYDROXYETHYLYAMINOPHENOL • A hair dye ingredient. Only slight absorption was observed in mice skin studies. On the basis of the available data, the CIR Expert Panel *(see)* concludes that it is safe as a cosmetic ingredient. See Phenols.

2-METHYL-4-HYDROXYPYRROLINE • A plasticizer derived from acetylene and formaldehyde. See latter for toxicity.

METHYLISOTHIAZOLINONE • Widely used with methylchloroisothiazolinone as a preservative in shampoos to replace formaldehyde. While it is a sensitizer in animals, it has not been shown to be a sensitizer in shampoos. Also used in baby products, moisturizers, body and hand preprations, and cleansing creams as well as makeup removers and suntan preparations. See Kathon CG.

METHYLISOTHIAZOLINONE/METHYLCHLOROISOTHIAZOLINONE • Used in cosmetics as a broad spectrum preservative. It is highly toxic in rats and rabbits orally but only moderately toxic when applied to the skin. Can be a skin sensitizer in humans. On the basis of the available data, the CIR Expert Panel *(see)* concludes that it can be safely used in "rinse-off" products at a concentration not to exceed 15 ppm and in "leave-on" products at concentrations not to exceed 7.5 ppm. The stated safe use concentration refers to a mixture containing 23.3 percent methylisothiazolinone and 76.7 percent methylchloroisothiazolinone.

N-METHYL-3-NITRO-p-PHENYLENEDIAMINE • Coal tar *(see)* hair coloring.

METHYLPHENYLPOLYSILOXANE • Cresol *(see)* with a blend of silicone *(see)* oils. An oily, fluid resin, stable over a wide temperature range, used in lubricating creams. No known toxicity.

2-METHYLRESORCINOL • Orcin. An aromatic compound with white crystalline prisms derived from lichen and used in medicine and as a reingredient for sugars and starches. A mild skin irritant. On the basis of the available data, the CIR Expert Panel *(see)* concludes that it is safe as a cosmetic ingredient. See Resorcinol.

METHYLSILANOL • See Silicon.

METHYLSILANOL ELASTINATE • A product of methylsilanol and elastin *(see all)*.

METHYLSTYRENE/VINYLTOLUENE COPOLYMER • The polymer of methylstyrene and vinyltoluene monomers. Used as a wax. See Styrenes.

MIBK • **Methyl Isobutyl Ketone.** Colorless liquid with a pleasant odor that is used as a solvent for paints, varnishes, and nitrocellulose lacquers, and as a denaturant for alcohol. Hazardous by either ingestion or inhalation.

MICA • **Pearls.** Any of a group of minerals that are found in crystallized, thin, elastic sheets that can be separated easily. They vary in color from pale green, brown, or black to colorless. Ground and widely used as a lubricant, coloring in cosmetics, and to create a glow in makeup. Irritant by inhalation; may be damaging to the lungs. Nontoxic to the skin. Coloring permanently listed for cosmetic use in 1977.

MICROCOCCUS LYSATE • A catalase is an enzyme in plant and animal tissues. It exerts a chemical reaction that converts hydrogen peroxide into water and oxygen. Derived from bacteria by a pure culture fermentation process, bacterial catalase may be used safely, according to the FDA, in destroying and removing the hydrogen peroxide that has been used in the manufacture of cheese—providing "the organism *Micrococcus lysodeikticus* from which the bacterial catalase is to be derived, is demonstrated to be nontoxic and non-pathogenic." The organism is removed from the bacterial catalase prior to the use of the catalase, the catalase to be used in an amount not in excess of the minimum required to produce its intended effect.

MICROCRYSTALLINE CELLULOSE • Abrasive, anticaking and bulking ingredient in emulsions. It is the colloid crystalline portion of cellulose fibers. See Cellulose Gums.

MICROCRYSTALLINE WAX • Any of various plastic materials that are obtained from petroleum. They are different from paraffin *(see)* waxes in that they have a higher melting point, higher viscosity, and much finer crystals that can be seen only under a microscope. Widely used in nail polishes and in cake cosmetics. No known toxicity. See Ceresin.

MICROFINE ZINC OXIDE • Zinc oxide is one of the best sunblockers but it is not "esthetic" to wear. Microfine is a zinc oxide that has been synthesized at a specific particle size to make it more acceptable and it is expected to replace other sunblockers that are not as effective or that have more unwanted side effects.

MILFOIL • See Yarrow.

MILK • Used in bath preparations and face masks as a soothing skin cleanser. Also used by natural cosmeticians as a face wash: for dry skin, cream is used; for oily skin, skim milk. It is as effective as many more expensive products. Nontoxic, but if not rinsed thoroughly from the skin with water, rancidity sets in and becomes a focus of bacteria. Consequently, the skin may break out in pimples.

MILK LIPIDS • Fats from milk used in skin-conditioning ingredients for emollients.

MILK PROTEIN • Obtained from cows' milk and used in skin and hair-conditioning products.

MILKAMIDOPROPYL AMINE OXIDE • A fatty acid derived from milk used in hair-conditioning products and as a foam booster.

MILKAMIDOPROPYL BETAINE • A fatty acid derived from milk used as an antistatic agent in hair products. See Betaines.

MILLET • A cereal and forage grass used in "natural cosmetics."

MIMOSA • Reddish yellow solid with a long-lasting, pleasant odor resembling ylang-ylang, used in perfumes. Derived from trees, shrubs, and herbs native to tropical and warm regions. Mimosa droops and closes its leaves when touched. Also used in tanning. May produce allergic skin reactions. It is used in skin care products.

MINERAL OIL • **White Oil.** Used in baby creams, baby lotions, bay oil, brilliantine hairdressings, cleansing creams, cold creams, emollients, moisturizing creams, eye creams, foundation creams and makeup, hair conditioners, hand lotions, lipsticks, mascaras, rouge, shaving creams, compact powders, makeup removers, suntan creams, oils, and ointments. Also a cosmetic lubricant, protective ingredient, and binder. It is a mixture of refined liquid hydrocarbons *(see)* derived from petroleum. Colorless, transparent, odorless, and tasteless. When heated, it smells like petroleum. It stays on top of the skin and leaves a shiny protective surface. Nontoxic.

MINERAL SALTS • Used as a skin conditioner.

MINERAL SPIRITS • **Ligroin.** A refined solvent of naphtha. Contains naphthenes and paraffin *(see)*. Used as a solvent in cosmetic oils, fats, and waxes. See Kerosene for toxicity.

MINERAL WAX • See Ceresin.

MINK OIL • Used in emollients, it supposedly softens the skin. It became popular as a cosmetic ingredient when a mink farmer noticed his hands were softer after handling minks. According to the American Medical Association, mink oil is no more effective than other oils in minimizing the evaporation of moisture from the skin and smoothing the surface scales of excessively dry skin. No known toxicity. However, on the basis of the available data, the CIR Expert Panel *(see)* concludes there is not enough data to conclude that it is safe as a cosmetic ingredient.

MINK WAX • The solid fraction derived from mink oil *(see)*.

MINKAMIDO • Fatty acids derived from mink oil *(see)*. Used as a thickener and foam booster.

MINKAMIDOPROPYL DIETHYLAMINE • Fatty acids derived from mink oil. See MIPA.

MINT • *Mentha.* Peppermint and spearmint are alike in their actions but peppermint is the stronger of the two. They are both used as flavorings, and in herbal teas to aid digestion. Peppermint also is used for headaches, vomiting, and insomnia, as a bath additive for general aches and pains, and as a salve for massage. Spearmint is used in folk medicine for "women's complaints." See Spearmint Oil, Peppermint Oil, Wintergreen Oil, and Sassafras Oil.

MIPA • Abbreviation for monoisopropanolamine.

MIPA-BORATE • Boric acid *(see)* mixed with propanol isopropanolamine.

MIPA-HYDROGENATED COCOATE • See Coconut Oil.

MIPA-DODECYLBENZENESULFONATE • See Quaternary Ammonium Compounds.

MIPA-LANOLATE • See Lanolin.

MIPA-LAURYL SULFATE • The monoisopropanolamine salt of lauryl sulfate. See Quaternary Ammonium Compounds.

MISTLETOE • *Viscum album* (**European Mistletoe**); *Phoradendron flavescens* (**American Mistletoe**). A parasitical plant with a root firmly attached to the wood of the tree on which it grows, it was sacred to the Druids and reputedly used by them to cure sterility and epilepsy; and as an antidote for poisons. Hippocrates and Galen used it as an external remedy and internally to treat sleep disorders. It is also used in "organic" cosmetics. See also Juniper Berry.

MITRACARPUS SCABER • A South American vine.

MIXED CRESOLS • A preservative. See Cresols.

MIXED IONONES • Fragrance ingredients.

MIXED ISOPROPANOLAMINES MYRISTATE • A mixture of amine salts formed by neutralizing myristic acid with mixed isopropanolamines. See Myristic Acid and Isopropyl Alcohol.

MIXED TERPENES • Terpenes are a class of organic compounds widely distributed in nature. They are components of volatile or essential oils and are found in substantial amounts in cedar wood oil, camphor, thymol, eucalyptol, menthol, turpentine, and pure oil. They are used in cosmetics as wetting ingredients and surfactants. Can cause local irritation.

MODERN BLENDS • One of the basic perfume types, it has indefinable top-notes *(see)* that cannot be linked to either the floral or the oriental. These blends contain aldehydes *(see),* meaning that whether they are basically floral or woody, they have a sparkle in their more insistent notes that enhances all the others.

MODIFIED SEA SALT • Salt derived from seawater with a reduced sodium chloride content.

MODIFIED STARCH • Ordinary starch that has been altered chemically to modify such properties as thickening or jelling. Among chemicals used to modify starch are succinic anhydride, aluminum sulfate, and sodium hydroxide *(see all).* On the FDA top priority list for reevaluation since 1980. Nothing new reported by the FDA since.

MODIFIER • A term in cosmetics to describe a substance that induces or stabilizes certain shades in hair coloring.

MOISTURIZERS • **Emollients. Skin Softeners. Creams. Lotions.** The selection of a night cream, hand cream, eye cream, skin softener, moisturizer, etc., is really the selection of an emollient. They all perform the same function—to make the skin feel softer and smoother and to reduce the roughness, cracking, and irritation of the skin. Most are a mixture of oils. The most common ingredients are: mineral oil, stearic acid, lanolin, beeswax, sorbitol, and polysorbates. Among the other ingredients added may be natural fatty oils such as olive, coconut, corn, peach and sesame; natural fats such as stearate and diglycol laurate; hydrocarbon solids such as paraffin; alcohols such as cetyl, stearyl, and oleyl; emulsifiers, preservatives, and antioxidants, including Vitamin E and paraben; antibacterials and perfumes, especially menthol and camphor. As you can see from the list above, many of the ingredients are common allergens described in this book.

MOLYBDENUM ASPARTATE • Skin-conditioning agent. The molybendum salt of aspartic acid *(see)*.

MOLYBDIC ACID • White or slightly yellow powder, used in ceramic glazes and as a clarifying ingredient. No known toxicity.

MONASCUS/RICE FERMENT • The fermentation of rice by the organism *Monascus purpureus.*

MONO AMMONIUM GLYCYRRHIZINATE • See Ammonia and Glycyrrhizic Acid.

MONOAZO COLOR • A dye made from diazonium and phenol, both coal tar derivatives. See Coal Tar.

MONOBENZONE • **Hydroquinone Monobenzyl Ether.** Prepared synthetically and used as an antioxidant and to retard melanin production. Used also in bleach and freckle creams. It may cause blotchiness and allergic skin reactions.

MONOGLYCERIDES • Produced synthetically by treating fats with glycerol and alcohol. Used as emulsifiers, cosmetics, and lubricants. See Glycerol.

MONOMER • A molecule that by repetition in a long chain builds up a large structure, or polymer *(see)*. The gas ethylene, for instance, is the monomer of polyethylene *(see)*.

MONOPOTASSIUM GLUTAMATE • Flavor enhancer and salt substitute used on meat. Mildly toxic by ingestion. May cause headaches. See Glutamate.

MONOSACCHARIDE LACTATE CONDENSATE • The condensation product of sodium lactate and the sugars glucose, fructose, ribose, glucosamine, and deoxyribose.

MONOSODIUM CITRATE • Used to adjust pH.

MONTAN WAX • **Lignite Wax.** White, hard, earth wax derived of extraction of lignite, which is coal made from wood. Its physical properties vary with the source of lignite. It is used as a substitute for carnauba and beeswax *(see both)*.

MONTMORILLONITE • A type of clay that is the main ingredient of bentonite and fuller's earth. Widely used in the petroleum industry. It is used in the manufacture of many chemical compounds. Inhalation of the dust can cause respiratory irritation. See Fuller's Earth.

MORANTEL • **Paratect. Suiminth.** A worm medicine used to treat cattle that leaves residues in beef and milk. FDA limits residues to from 1.2 ppm to 4.8 ppm in cattle and to 0.4 ppm in milk.

MORDANTS • Chemicals that are insoluble compounds that serve to fix a dye, usually a weak dye, to hasten the development of the desired shade or to modify it in hair colorings. Toxicity depends upon specific ingredients.

MORINGA OIL • **Ben Oil.** Oil from the seeds of the tropical tree *Moringa oleafera.* See Horseradish Extract.

MORPHOLINE • A salty fatty acid used as a surface-active ingredient *(see)* and an emulsifier in cosmetics. Prepared by taking the water out of diethanolamine *(see)*. A mobile, water-absorbing liquid that mixes with water. It has a strong ammonia odor. A cheap solvent for resins, waxes, and dyes. Also used as a corrosion inhibitor, antioxidant, plasticizer, viscosity improver, insecticide, fungicide, local anesthetic, and antiseptic. Irritating to the eyes, skin, and mucous membranes. It may cause kidney and liver injury, and can produce sloughing of the skin. The safety of this ingredient has not been documented and substantiated. The CIR Expert Panel *(see)* "cannot conclude that it is safe for use in cosmetic products until such time that the appropriate safety data has been obtained and evaluated."

MORPHOLINE STEARATE • A coating and preservative. See Morpholine.

MORTIERELLA OIL • Oil from the seeds of *Mortierella isabellina*. Used in emollients. No known toxicity.

MORUS ALBA • See Mulberry.

MOSCHUS MOSCHIFERUS • A musk from an Asian deer. See Musk.

MOUNTAIN ASH EXTRACT • The extract from the berries of the European tree or shrub *Sorbus aucuparia*. High in Vitamin C, it has been used by herbalists to cure and prevent scurvy and to treat nausea. Used in cosmetics as an antioxidant. No known toxicity.

MOUNTAIN MAPLE EXTRACT • Extract from a tall shrub or bushy tree found in the eastern United States. Used in chocolate, malt, and maple flavoring for beverages, ice cream, ices, candy, and baked goods. No known toxicity.

MOUTHWASH • Promoted as a method to cleanse the mouth and overcome objectionable odors. Claims for such abilities have not been proven. Among ingredients used in mouthwashes are sodium bicarbonate, alcohol, mixed flavoring oils, cinnamon, methyl salicylate, menthol, anethole, thyme, certified colors, resorcinol, sorbitol, urea, methyl salicylate, boric acid, benzalkonium chloride, benzoic acid, propylene glycol, cetylpyridinium chloride, and chlorophyllin. Several of the above, particularly the colorings and the flavorings, are common allergens. Resorcinol is a resin *(see)*, and methyl salicylate is related to aspirin and other salicylates.

MUCILAGE • A solution in water of the sticky principles of vegetable substances. Used as a soothing application to the mucous membranes.

MUCINS • Any of a group of proteins found in various secretions and tissues of humans and lower animals such as saliva, lining of the stomach, and skin. They are white or yellowish powders when dry and thick when moist.

MUCOPOLYSACCHARIDES • A complex of proteins *(see)*. Used in moisturizers.

MUCOUS MEMBRANES • The thin layers of tissue that line the respiratory and intestinal tracts and are kept moist by a sticky substance called mucus. These membranes line the nose and other parts of the respiratory tract, and are found in other parts of the body that have communication with air.

MUD PACKS • Long in use as a facial treatment. Today, they consist of a paste for the face composed chiefly of fuller's earth and astringents *(see both)*. There is no evidence that mud packs are effective. No known toxicity.

MUGWORT • The extract of the flowering herb *Artemisia absinthium*. See Wormwood and Sesquiterpene Lactones.

MUIRA PUAMA EXTRACT • A wood extract used as an aromatic resin and fat. No known toxicity.

MULBERRY EXTRACT • An extract of the dried leaves of various species of *Morus,* which produces a purplish black dye.

MULLEIN EXTRACT • The extract of common mullein, *Verbascum thapsis,* used in henna dyes.

MULLEIN FLOWERS • The flowers from common mullein, *Verbascum thapsis.* Used as a flavoring in alcoholic beverages only and in henna hair coloring.

MUSA SAPIENTUM • Banana *(see).*

MUSCLE EXTRACT • The oil extracted from cow muscle.

MUSHROOM EXTRACT • The extract of various species of mushrooms used as an oil and plasticizer.

MUSK • Used in perfumes. It is the dried secretion from preputial follicles of the northern Asian small hornless deer, which has musk in its glands. Musk is a brown, unctuous, smelly substance associated with attracting the opposite sex and which is promoted by stores for such purposes. Also used in food flavorings and at one time as a stimulant and nerve sedative in medicine. Can cause allergic reactions.

MUSK AMBRETTE • A synthetic fixative, it is widely used as a fragrance ingredient in perfumes, soaps, detergents, creams, lotions, and dentifrices in the United States at an estimated 100,000 pounds per year. It reportedly damages the myelin, the covering of nerve fibers. It can cause photosensitivity *(see)* and contact dermatitis. The problem is mostly with after-shave lotions. Musk tetralin, in use for twenty years as a fragrance ingredient, was identified as a neurotoxin and removed from the market in 1978. Musk ambrette has been generally recognized as safe as a food additive by the FDA, but see Introduction.

MUSK MOSKENE • A soft, sweet fragrance resembling musk ambrette. It is a creamy powder and is used in fragrances. It costs less than other musks and is not as sensitive to sunlight. It is therefore being increasingly used. Rouges and perfumes containing musk moskene have been reported to cause hyperpigmentation of the skin of some patients. The hyperpigmentation slowly disappeared after discontinuation of the products.

MUSK ROSE OIL • **Delta Rose.** The oil obtained from *Rosa rubiginosa*. Used in fragrances.

MUSKMELLON EXTRACT • Extract of the common mullein, *Verbascum thapsis.*

MUSSEL EXTRACT • The extract from sea mussels.

MUSTARD OIL • **Allyl isothiocyanate.** The greenish yellow, bland fatty oil expressed from the seeds of the mustard plant. Used in soaps, liniments, and lubricants. It has an intensely pungent odor that can be irritating. It is a strong skin blisterer and is used diluted as a counterirritant *(see)* and rubefacient *(see)*. Can cause allergic reactions.

MUSTARD SEED • See Mustard Oil.

MUSTELA • See Mink Oil.

MYOSOTIS SYLVATICA • **Forget-Me-Not Extract.** A perennial herb that has blue and white flowers.

MYRCIA • **Bay Rum.** See Bay Rum.

MYRETH-3 • The polyethylene glycol ether of myristyl alcohol *(see)*.

MYRETH-3 CAPRATE • **Myristic Ethoxy Caprate.** See Capric Acid.

MYRETH-3 LAURATE • The ester of lauric acid and myreth-3 *(see both)*.

MYRETH-4 • The polyethylene glycol ether of myristyl alcohol *(see)*.

MYRICA CERIFERA • See Bayberry.

MYRICYL ALCOHOL • **Triacontanol.** A waxy alcohol used as a substitute for bayberry wax.

MYRISTALKONIUM CHLORIDE • See Quaternary Ammonium Compounds.

MYRISTAMIDE DEA • **Myristic Diethanolamide.** See Myristic Acid and Diethanolamide.

MYRISTAMIDE MIPA • A mixture of isopropanolamides of lauric acid *(see)*.

MYRISTAMIDOPROPYL BETAINE • See Surfactants.

MYRISTAMIDOPROPYL DIETHYLAMINE • See Quaternary Ammonium Compounds.

MYRISTAMIDOPROPYLAMINE OXIDE • See Quaternary Ammonium Compounds.

MYRISTAMINE OXIDE • See Myristic Acid.

MYRISTAMINOPROPIONIC ACID • See Propionic Acid and Myristic Acid.

MYRISTATE • The ester of myreth-3 and myristic acid *(see both)*.

MYRISTIC ACID • Used in shampoos, shaving soaps, and creams. A solid, organic acid that occurs naturally in butter acids (such as nutmeg butter to the extent of 80 percent), oil of lovage, coconut oil, mace oil, *cire d'abeille* in palm seed fats, and in most animal and vegetable fats. Also used in food flavorings. When combined with potassium, myristic acid soap gives a very good copious lather. No known toxicity. The CIR Expert Panel *(see)* concludes that this ingredient is safe for use in cosmetic products. See Lauric Acid.

MYRISTICA FRAGRANS • See Nutmeg.

MYRISTIMIDE MEA • A mixture of ethanolamide of myristic acid *(see)*.

MYRISTOAMPHOACETATE • See Surfactants.

MYRISTOL GLUTAMIC ACID • A hair-conditioning ingredient. See Myristic Acid.

MYRISTOYL HYDROLYZED PROTEIN • The condensation product of myristic acid and hydrolyzed animal protein *(see both)*. Used as a setting ingredient and film-former, it allows the incorporation of protein into nonwater-based cosmetics. The "animal" was taken out of the ingredient name but not out of the ingredient.

MYRISTOYL GLUTAMIC ACID • An emulsifying agent. See Myristic Acid and Lactic Acid.

MYRISTOYL SARCOSINE • See Sarcosines.

MYRISTYL ALCOHOL • Used as an emollient in hand creams, cold creams, and lotions to give them a smooth velvety feel. It is made up of white crystals prepared from fatty acids *(see)*. Practically insoluble in water. Nontoxic. See Behenyl Alcohol.

MYRISTYL BETAINE • See Myristyl Alcohol.

MYRISTYL STEARATE • An emollient. Used as a skin-conditioning ingredient. On the basis of the available animal and human data, the CIR Expert Panel *(see)* concludes that this ingredient is safe as used in cosmetics. See Myristic Acid.

MYROXYLON BALSAMUM • See Balsam Tolu.

MYRRH EXTRACT • *Commiphora Abyssinica Extract.* Used in perfumes, dentifrices, and skin topics. One of the gifts of the Magi, it is a yellowish to reddish brown, aromatic, bitter-gum resin that is obtained from various trees, especially from east Africa and Arabia. Used by the ancients as an ingredient of incense and perfumes and as a remedy for localized skin problems. The gum is used in fruit, liquor, tobacco, and smoke flavorings for beverages, baked goods, ice cream, ices, candy, chewing gum, and soups. The oil is used in honey and liquor flavorings for beverages, ice cream, ices, candy, and baked goods. The gum resin has been used to break up intestinal gas and as a topical stimulant.

MYRTIMONIUM BROMIDE • A Quaternary Ammonium Compound *(see)*.

MYRTUS COMMINUS • The extract of the leaves of myrtle, a European shrub. It is used in alcoholic beverages.

N

NAIL A'PEEL • A peel-off polish that eliminates a major source of exposure to many hazardous substances for people that wear nail polish. Most high-quality nail polishes contain hazardous and flammable solvents, which must be removed with acetone solvent removers. In contrast, Nail a'Peel is water-based, fume-free nail polish that reportedly can be worn by most people who suffer from allergic reactions to current solvent-based polishes and nail polish removers.

NAIL, ARTIFICIAL • See Artificial Nails.

NAIL BLEACHES • Compounds designed to remove ink, nicotine, vegetable, and other stains from fingernails. They consist mainly of an oxidizing ingredient and chlorinated compounds. A typical formula includes titanium dioxide, 20 percent; talc, 20 percent; zinc peroxide, 7.5 percent; petrolatum, 26 percent; mineral oil, 26.5 percent; and perfume *(see all)*. Toxicity depends upon ingredients used.

NAIL ENAMEL • See Nail Polish.

NAIL FINISHES • **Top Coat.** Usually a colorless nail polish *(see)* or it can be slightly pink. Contains Celluloid®, amyl acetate, and acetone *(see all)*. Protects the nail by strengthening it physically, helps to keep the nail polish from chipping, and produces a shiny surface.

NAIL HARDENERS • Keep the nails from breaking or chipping. Most nail hardeners formerly contained formaldehyde but now contain polyesters, acrylics, and polyamides. Sensitization rarely occurs.

NAIL MENDING KITS • Tissue paper, high solids, and enamel. May have acrylic adhesives, which are sensitizers. Can be an eye irritation.

NAIL POLISH • Used to paint the nails with colors, usually some shade of red. Polishes contain cellulose nitrate (nitrocellulose), butyl acetate, ethyl acetate, toluene, dibutyl phthalate, alkyl esters (amyl, acetate, ethyl acetate), dyes, glycol derivatives, gums, hydrocarbons (aromatic and aliphatic), ketones (acetone, methyl, ethyl), lakes, and phosphoric acid. Common colors used are D & C Red No. 19 or 31 *(see)*. Skin rashes of the eyelids and neck are common in those allergic to nail polish. Among recent complaints to the FDA about nail polishes were irritation of the nail area, discolored nails, nails permanently stained black, splitting of nails, and nausea.

NAIL POLISH REMOVER • Usually a liquid, it is used to remove nail polish. It contains acetone, toluene, alcohol, amyl acetate, butyl acetate, benzene, and ethyl acetate. It also contains castor oil, lanolin, cetyl alcohol, olive oil, perfume, spermaceti, synthetic oil (ethyl oleate, butyl stearate) *(see all)*. Many components are very toxic and can cause central nervous system depression, especially the toluene and aliphatic acetates. A report to the FDA described a "tight smothering feeling in the chest" after use of a nail polish remover.

NAIL (FAKE) REMOVER • See Artificial Nail Remover.

NAIL STRENGTHENERS • See Nail Hardeners.

NAIL WHITENERS • The cream nail whiteners may contain titanium dioxide, beeswax, cetyl alcohol, petrolatum, cocoa butter, sodium borate, tincture of benzoin *(see all)*, and water. The liquid nail whites may contain titanium dioxide, glyceryl monostearate, beeswax, almond oil, petrolatum *(see all)*, and water. Toxicity is dependent upon ingredients.

NAILS, PRESS-ON • Fake nails made of resins and acrylic glues. The acrylic glues may sensitize.

NAPHTHALENE • A coal tar *(see)* derivative, it is used to manufacture dyes, solvents, and lubricants; as a moth repellent; and as a topical and internal antiseptic. It has been used as a dusting powder to combat insects on animals. Can cause allergic contact dermatitis.

1, 3-NAPHTHALENEDIOL • A hair coloring. See Naphthas.

2, 7-NAPHTHALENEDIOL • See Naphthas.

NAPHTHAS • Obtained from the distillation of petroleum, coal tar, and shale oil. It is a common diluent *(see)* found in nail lacquer. Among the common naphthas that are used as solvents are coal tar/naphtha and petroleum/naphtha. See Kerosene for toxicity.

NAPHTHAZOLINE HYDROCHLORIDE • **Privine Hydrochloride.** Prepared from acids, it is composed of bitter-tasting crystals, which are soluble in water. Used as a nasal and eye decongestant. It may cause sedation in infants, and high blood pressure and central nervous system excitement followed by depression in adults.

NAPHTHOL • A coal tar *(see)* derivative, it is used as an antiseptic, in hair dyes, and to treat eczema, ringworm, and psoriasis. May cause allergic contact dermatitis.

1-NAPHTHOL • **a-Naphthol.** Used in hair dyes and treatment of skin diseases, as an antiseptic, and as an antioxidant for fats and oils. Also used in perfumery. White crystals with phenolic odor and disagreeable burning taste. Slightly soluble in water. Toxic by ingestion and skin absorption. Hair dyes containing this ingredient when applied to the skin were neither teratogenic or carcinogenic. On the basis of the available data, the CIR Expert Panel *(see)* concludes that it is safe as a cosmetic ingredient.

2-NAPHTHOL • **b-Naphthol.** Used as an antiseptic and modifier in hair preparations, with tendency to darken gray hair. Sometimes used in treatment of eczema, ringworm, and psoriasis. See 1-Naphthol for toxicity.

B-NAPHTHYL ETHYL ETHER • White crystals with an orange-blossom odor. It is used in perfumes, soaps, and flavorings. See Nerol.

B-NAPHTHYL METHYL ETHER • White crystals with a menthol odor. Used to perfume soaps. See Naphthol.

NARCISSUS OIL • *Anarylidiaceae.* A genus of Old World bulbous herbs. Can numb skin.

NASTURTIUM EXTRACT • The extract of the leaves and stems of *Tropaeolum majus.* A member of the mustard family, it has pungent and tasty leaves. It is very rich in Vitamins A and C, as well as containing Vitamins B and B_2. It is soothing to the skin and supposedly has blood-thinning factors and increases the flow of urine. No known toxicity.

NATIONAL TOXICOLOGY PROGRAM (NTP) • Tests chemicals for all federal agencies.

NATTO GUM • The fermentation product of soy protein by *Bacillus nato.* Used as a thickener.

NATURAL • Ingredients extracted directly from plants or animal products as opposed to being produced synthetically. See Organic Cosmetics.

NATURAL RED 26 • **Carthamic Acid.** A red, crystalline, glucoside coloring constituting the coloring matter of the safflower *(see).* No known toxicity.

NEAT'S-FOOT OIL • Lubricant used in creams and lotions. A pale yellow fatty oil made by boiling the feet and shinbones of cattle. Used chiefly as a leather dressing and waterproofing. In cosmetics it is used as a cover-up in skin care products. Can cause allergic reactions in the hypersensitive.

NECTARINE • *Prunius persica nectarina.* The leaves or bark from young trees native to China, but widely cultivated, are used by herbalists to make sedatives, diuretics, expectorants, and soothing compounds.

NEEM TREE • *Azadriachta indica.* **Nim. Margosa.** The bark, leaves, and seeds are used in India as a treatment for many skin diseases. The extract of the leaves has been shown to have antibacterial and antiviral activity. Neem is also taken internally to eliminate worms. The branches of the tree are chewed and used to clean the teeth and to prevent gum inflammation.

NELUMBIUM SPECIOSUM • See Lotus.

NENOLONE HEMISUCCINATE • See Succinic Acid.

NEODECANOIC ACID • Colorless liquid used in plasticizers and lubricants. See Decanoic Acid.

NEOFOLINONE • Occurs naturally in oil of lavender, orange leaf (absolute), palmarosa oil, rose, neroli, and oil of petitgrain. Used in citrus, honey, and neroli flavorings for beverages, ice cream, ices, candy, baked goods, chewing gum, gelatin desserts, and puddings. No known toxicity.

NEOHESPERIDINE DIHYDROCHALCONE • See Dihydrochalcones.

NEOMYCIN • Used in underarm deodorants, it is a product of the growth of microorganisms inhabiting the soil. It inhibits the growth of bacteria and, therefore, the odor from sweat. It can cause the skin to swell, redden, or break out when exposed to light. It produces allergic reactions in many people. Highly toxic to the eighth nerve, which involves hearing, and to the kidneys. The FDA does not believe the use of neomycin in deodorants is justified because it caused resistant strains of staphylococci to develop. Such staph infections are extremely difficult to treat and could be lethal.

NEOMYCIN SULFATE • Introduced in 1951, it is one of the most widely used antibiotics for humans. In a cream or ointment, it is used to treat skin infections, minor burns, wounds, skin grafts, itching, inflammation of the outer ear, and skin ulcers. Potential adverse skin reactions include rashes, contact dermatitis, hives, and possible kidney, ear, and nerve toxicity when absorbed systemically. The skin product should not be used on more than 20 percent of the body surface and should not be used to treat deep wounds, puncture wounds, or serious burns without medical advice.

NEOPENTYL GLYCOL • White, crystalline solid from propanediol that is used in polyester foams, insect repellents, plasticizers and lubricants.

NEOPENTYL GLYCOL DICAPRATE • The diester of glycol dicaprate is the diester of neopentyl glycol and decanoic acid *(see)*.

NEOPENTYL GLYCOL DICAPRYLATE/DIPELARGONATE/DICARPRATE • The esters of neopentyl glycol and caprylic, pelargonic, and capric acids. Used in creams and lotions.

NEOPENTYL GLYCOL DIOCTANOATE • The ester of neopentyl glycol and octanoic acid *(see)*.

NEOPENTYL GLYCOL DISTEARATE • The ester of neopentyl glycol and stearic acid *(see)*.

NEPETA • See Catnip.

NERIUM OLEANDER • See Oleander.

NEROL • A primary alcohol used in perfumes, especially in rose and orange blossom scents. Occurs naturally in oil of lavender, orange leaf, palmarosa oil, rose, neroli, and oil of petitgrain. It is colorless, with the odor of rose. Also used in food flavorings. Similar to geraniol *(see)* in toxicity.

NEROLI BIGARADE OIL • Used chiefly in cologne and in perfumes. Named for the putative discoverer, Anna Mariade la Tremoille, princess of Nerole (1670). A fragrant, pale yellow essential oil obtained from the flowers of the sour orange tree. It darkens upon standing. Also used in food flavorings. No known toxicity.

NEROLIDOL • A sesquiterpene alcohol. A straw-colored liquid with an odor similar to rose and apple. Occurs naturally in Balsam Peru and oils of orange flower, neroli, sweet orange, and ylang-ylang. Also made synthetically. Used in perfumery and flavoring. See Nerol.

NEROSOL • See Nerol.

NERYL ACETATE • A synthetic citrus, fruit, and neroli flavoring for beverages, ice cream, ices, candy, and baked goods. No known toxicity.

NERYL BUTYRATE • A synthetic berry, chocolate, cocoa, citrus, and fruit-flavoring ingredient for beverages, ice cream, ices, candy, and baked goods. No known toxicity.

NERYL FORMATE • **Formic Acid.** A synthetic berry, citrus, apple, peach, and pineapple flavoring ingredient for beverages, ice cream, ices, candy, and baked goods. See Formic Acid for toxicity.

NERYL ISOBUTYRATE • A synthetic citrus and fruit-flavoring ingredient for beverages, ice cream, ices, candy, and baked goods. No known toxicity.

NERYL ISOVALERATE • A synthetic berry, rose, and nut-flavoring ingredient for beverages, ice cream, ices, candy, and baked goods. No known toxicity.

NERYL PROPIONATE • A synthetic berry and fruit-flavoring ingredient for beverages, ice cream, ices, candy, and baked goods. No known toxicity.

NETTLES • Used in hair tonics and shampoos. It is obtained from the troublesome weed, with stingers. It has a long history and was used in folk medicine. Its flesh is rich is minerals and plant hormones, and it supposedly stimulates hair growth and shines and softens hair. Also used to make tomatoes resistant to spoilage, to encourage the growth of strawberries, and to stimulate the fermentation of humus. No known toxicity.

NEURAL EXTRACT • The extract of animal nerve tissue.

NGDA • See Nordehydroguaiaretic Acid.

NIACIN • **Nicotinic Acid.** White or yellow, crystalline powder, it is an essential nutrient that participates in many energy-yielding reactions. It is a component of the B Vitamin complex.

NIACINAMIDE • **Nicotinamide. Vitamin B.** Used as a skin stimulant. A white or yellow, crystalline, odorless powder used to treat pellagra, a vitamin-deficiency disease, and in the assay of enzymes for substrates. No known skin toxicity.

NICKEL • Metal that occurs in the earth. See Nickel Sulfate.

NICKEL SULFATE • Used in hair dyes and astringents. Occurs in the earth's crust as a salt of nickel. Obtained as green or blue crystals and is used chiefly in nickel plating. It has a sweet astringent taste and acts as an irritant and causes vomiting when swallowed. Its systemic effects include blood vessel, brain, and kidney damage and nervous depression. Frequently causes skin rash when used in cosmetics. It is used in eye pencils and some containers.

NICOTIANA TABCUM • **Tobacco Extract.** See Nicotinyl Alcohol.

NICOTINE REMOVERS • See Nail Bleaches.

NICOTINIC ACID • See Niacin.

NICOTINYL ALCOHOL • Used as a skin-conditioning ingredient reportedly for its ability to dilate blood vessels. It is also a solvent.

NISIN • Crystals from *Streptococcus lactis* used as a preservative and antimicrobial agent in cosmetics and cheese spreads. FDA limits residue to 250 ppm nisin in the finished cheese product. It is also used in canned vegetables and fruit. GRAS.

NITRATE • **Potassium and Sodium.** Potassium nitrate, also known as saltpeter and niter, is used as a color fixative in cured meats. Sodium nitrate, also called Chile saltpeter, is used as a color fixative in cured meats. Both nitrates combine with amines found in the stomach, saliva, food and other substances to create nitrosamines, powerful cancer-causing agents. Nitrates are natural constituents of plants.

NITRILOTRIACETIC ACID • **NTA.** Chelating and sequestering ingredient. Used in detergents. Can be irritating.

NITRITE • **Potassium and Sodium.** Used as color fixatives and preservatives. The question about nitrites concerns their combining with substances in organic substances in cosmetics called amines. This combination known as nitrosamines *(see)* has been found to be a potential cancer-causing agent.

NITRO- • A prefix denoting one atom of nitrogen and two of oxygen. Nitro also denotes a class of dyes derived from coal tars. Nitro dyes can be absorbed through the skin. When absorbed or ingested they can cause a lack of oxygen in the blood. Chronic exposure may cause liver damage. See Colors.

3-NITRO-4-AMINOPHENOXYETHANOL • An aromatic ether alcohol used as a fungicide. See *o*-Phenylphenol.

NITROBENZENE • **Essence of Mirabane.** A colorless to pale yellow, oily, poisonous liquid (nitric acid and benzene). It is used to scent cheap soaps, and in the manufacture of aniline. It is also a solvent for cellulose, an ingredient of metal polishes, shoe polishes, and many other products. It is rapidly absorbed through the skin. Workers are warned not to get it in their eyes, or on their skin, and not to breathe the vapor. Exposure to essence of mirabane may cause headaches, drowsiness, nausea, vomiting, lack of oxygen in the blood (methemoglobinemia), and cyanosis.

NITROCELLULOSE • Any of several esters *(see)* obtained as white fibrous flammable solids by adding nitrate to cellulose, the cell walls of plants. Used in skin protective creams, nail enamels, and lacquers. No known toxicity.

3-NITRO-p-CRESOL • A hair coloring. See Coal Tar Colors.

NITROGEN • A gas that is 78 percent of the atmosphere by volume and essential to all living things. Odorless. Used as a preservative for cosmetics, in which it is nontoxic. In high concentrations, it can asphyxiate. Toxic concentration in humans is 90 ppm; in mice, 250 ppm.

2-NITRO-5-GLYCERYL METHYLANILINE • See Aniline Dyes.

3-NITRO-p-HYDROXYETHYLAMINOPHENOL • See *o*-Phenylphenol.

2-NITRO-n-HYDROXYETHYL-p-ANISIDINE • See Azo Dyes.

NITROPHENOL • A hair coloring. See Coal Tar Colors.

4-NITRO-m-PHENYLENEDIAMINE • A hair coloring. The safety has not been documented and substantiated. The CIR Expert Panel *(see)* "cannot conclude that this ingredient is safe for use in cosmetic products until the appropriate safety data have been obtained and evaluated." See *p*-Phenylenediamine.

4-NITRO-o-PHENYLENEDIAMINE • A hair coloring. The safety has not been documented and substantiated. The CIR Expert Panel *(see)* "cannot conclude that this ingredient is safe for use in cosmetic products until the appropriate safety data have been obtained and evaluated." See *p*-Phenylenediamine.

2-NITRO-p-PHENYLENEDIAMINE • See Phenylenediamine.

4-NITROPHENYL AMINOETHYLUREA • See Phenol and Urea.

6-NITRO-2, 5-PYRIDINEDAMINE • See Coal Tar Dyes.

6-NITRO-o-TOLUIDINE • See Coal Tar Dyes.

NITROSAMINES • Compounds formed when chemicals containing nitrites react with amine, natural chemicals found in foods and in the body. Many nitrosamines are among the most potent cancer-causing agents found. Because there are numerous chemicals capable of reacting with nitrite, nitrosamines have been found in air, water, tobacco smoke, cured meats, cosmetics, pesticides, and alcoholic beverages. It is also believed that they may be formed in our bodies. Some epidemiological studies have associated increased incidence of human cancer with the presence of nitrosamines.

NITROSATING • The introduction of a nitrogen and oxygen (nitroso) of molecules into a compound that may cause the compound to form cancer-linked nitrosamines *(see)*.

NITROUS OXIDE • **Laughing Gas.** A whipping ingredient for whipped cosmetic creams and a propellant in pressurized cosmetic containers. Slightly sweetish odor and taste. Colorless. Used in rocket fuel. Less irritating than other nitrogen oxides but narcotic in high concentrations, and it can asphyxiate.

g-NONALACTONE • See Coconut Oil.

NONANAL • Colorless liquid with an orange-rose odor. Used in perfumery and flavoring. See Aldehyde.

NONANE-1, 3-DIOL MONOACETATE • Colorless to slightly yellow mixture of isomers used in perfumery and flavoring. See Nonanoic Acid and Acetic Acid.

NONANOIC ACID • A colorless, oily liquid that is insoluble in water, it occurs in the oil of pelargonium plants such as the geranium. It is practically insoluble in water and is used in producing salts and in the manufacture of lacquers. Can be very irritating to the skin.

NONCOMEDOGENIC • Does not cause pimples and blackheads by blocking pores.

NONETH-8 • The polyethylene glycol ether of nonyl alcohol *(see)*.

NONFAT DRY COLOSTRUM • The residue produced by the dehydration of defatted colostrum, the first milk secreted after the birth of a baby.

NONFAT DRY MILK • The solid residue produced by removing the water from defatted cow's milk. See Milk.

NONIONIC • A group of emulsifiers used in hand creams. They resist freezing and shrinkage. Toxicity depends upon specific ingredients.

NONOXYNOL-2 • Polyoxyethylene (2) Nonyl Phenyl Ether. Used as a non-ionic *(see)* surface-active ingredient and as a dispersing ingredient in cosmetics. The numbers signify the viscosity of the compound. No known toxicity. See Polyethylene Glycol.

NONOXYNOL-4, -8 THROUGH -100 • Surfactants and emulsifying ingredients. The CIR Expert Panel *(see)* concludes that these ingredients are safe for use in "rinse-off" products and safe at concentrations of less than 5 percent in "leave-on" products. See Nonoxynol-2.

NONOXYNOL-9 IODINE • See Nonoxynol-2 and Iodine.

NONOXYNOL-12 IODINE • See Nonoxynol-2 and Iodine.

NONYL ACETATE • Used in perfumery. An ester produced by the reaction of nonyl alcohol and acetic acid *(see)*. Pungent odor, suggestive of mushrooms, but when diluted it resembles the odor of gardenias. Insoluble in water. No known toxicity.

NONYL ALCOHOL • Nonalol. A synthetic flavoring, colorless to yellow with a citronella-oil odor. Occurs in oil of orange. Used in butter, citrus, peach, and pineapple flavorings for beverages, ice cream, ices, candy, and chewing gum. Also used in the manufacture of artificial lemon oil. In experimental animals it has caused central nervous system and liver damage.

y-NONYL LACTONE • Yellowish to almost colorless liquid with a coconutlike odor. Used in perfumery and flavors. See Nonyl Alcohol.

NONYL NONANOATE • Nonyl Pelargonate. Liquid with a floral odor used in flavors, perfumes, and organic synthesis. See Nonyl Alcohol.

NONYL NONOXYNOL-5 THROUGH -100 • The ethoxylated *(see)* phenol alcohol. See Phenol.

NOOTKA • See Cedar Wood Oil.

NOPYL ACETATE • A fragrance ingredient.

NORDIHYDROGUAIARETIC ACID • NGDA. An antioxidant used in brilliantines and other fat-based cosmetics. Occurs in resinous exudates of many plants. White or grayish white crystals. Lard containing .01 percent NGDA stored at room temperature for 19 months in diffuse daylight showed no appreciable rancidity or color change. Canada banned the additive in food in 1967, after it was shown to cause cysts and kidney damage in a large percentage of rats tested. The FDA removed it from the Generally Recognized As Safe list of food additives in 1968. No known toxicity for use in cosmetics.

NORVALINE • A protein amino acid *(see)*, soluble in hot water and insoluble in alcohol. See Valeric Acid.

NORWAY SPRUCE EXTRACT • The extract of the buds of *Picea abies.* A widely cultivated pine tree. See Pine Oil.

NOTE • A distinct odor or flavor. "Top" note is the first note normally perceived when a flavor is smelled or tasted; usually volatile and gives "identity." "Middle" or "main" note is the substance of the flavor, the main characteristic. "Bottom" note is what is left when top and middle notes disappear. It is the residue when the aroma or flavoring evaporates.

NSAIDS • Abbreviation for nonsteroidal anti-inflammatory drugs. Aspirin, diclofenac, etodolac, ibuprofen, indomethacin, and naproxen are among the popular NSAIDs in use.

NTA • Abbreviation for Nitrilo Triacetic Acid *(see)*.

NTP • Abbreviation for National Toxicology Program *(see)*.

NURTURE® • A new oat-based material produced from oat grain. The microparticles are porous and supposedly able to entrap most water- or oil-based liquids, thereafter releasing them gradually to the skin.

NUTMEG • A natural flavoring extracted from the dried ripe seed of *Myristica fragrans*. Used in cola, vermouth, sausage, eggnog, and nutmeg flavorings for beverages, ice cream, ices, baked goods, condiments, meats, and pickles. The oil is used in loganberry, chocolate, lemon, cola, apple, grape, muscatel, rum, sausage, eggnog, pistachio, root beer, cinnamon, dill, ginger, mace, nutmeg, and vanilla flavorings for beverages, ice cream, ices, candy, baked goods, chewing gum, condiments, meats, syrups, and icings. Can cause flushing of the skin, irregular heart rhythm, and contact dermatitis.

NYLON • The commonly known synthetic material used as a fiber in eyelash lengtheners and mascaras and as a molding compound to shape cosmetics. Comes in clear or white opaque plastic for use in making resins. Can cause allergic reactions. Resistant to organic chemicals but is dissolved by phenol, cresol *(see both)*, and strong acids. No known toxicity.

NYLON-6 THROUGH -66 • Thickeners and opacifiers.

NYMPHAEACEAE ALBA • **Water Lily. Water Rose. Nenuphar. Candock.** Cultivated in pools, this beautiful and romantic flower was used in folk medicine to depress sexual function. Externally, white and yellow water lilies were used to treat various skin disorders such as boils, inflammations, tumors, and ulcers.

NYMPHAEACEAE ODORATA • Extract of the root of *Nymphaea alba*. Used in fragrances.

NYSTATIN • **Mycostatin. Nilstat.** Yellow to light-tan powder with a cereallike odor. Antifungal medication introduced in 1954. It is used in human medicine to treat oral, vaginal, and intestinal infections caused by *Candida albicans* (Monilia) and other *Candida* species. In cream or ointment it is used to treat infant eczema, itching around the anus or vagina, and localized forms of candidiasis. Skin applications may cause occasional contact dermatitis from preservatives in some formulations. Nystatin is in the Environmental Protection Agency's Genetic Toxicology Program to determine its effects on DNA. Causes birth defects in experimental animals. Moderately toxic by ingestion.

O

OAK BARK EXTRACT • **Oak Chip Extract.** The extract from the white oak used in bitters and whiskey flavorings for beverages, ice cream, and baked goods. Contains tannic acid *(see)* and is exceedingly astringent. The American Indians used it in a wash for sore eyes and as a tonic. Used in astringents in herbal cosmetics. No known toxicity.

OAT BRAN • The broken coat of oats, *Avena sativa*. See Oat Flour.

OAT EXTRACT • The extract of the seeds of oats, *Avena sativa*. See Oat Flour.

OAT FLOUR • Flour from the cereal grain that is an important crop grown in the temperate regions. Light yellowish or brown to weak greenish or yellow powder. Slight odor; starchy taste. Makes a bland ointment for cosmetic treatments, including soothing baths. No known toxicity.

OAT GUM • A plant extract used as a thickener and stabilizer in foods and cosmetics. Also an antioxidant in butter, creams, and candy. It is used as a thickener and stabilizer in pasteurized cheese spread and cream cheese. In foods, it can cause an allergic reaction, including diarrhea and intestinal gas. No known toxicity.

OAT ROOT EXTRACT • The extract of the roots of the oak tree species *Quercus,* grown in the eastern United States and Canada. The bark contains tannic acid, oak-red resin, pectin, levulin, and quercitol. The extract is used as an astringent.

OATMEAL • *Avena sativa*. Meal obtained by the grinding of oats from which the husks have been removed. Used through the ages by women as a face mask. Here is a modern version: In a blender put 4 tablespoons quick-cooking or regular oatmeal and 1 teaspoon dried mint leaves and turn to high until the mix is finely ground; add enough hot water to make a spreadable paste; smooth and pat on the face gently. When the paste is dry, remove with lukewarm water, then rinse well with cool water. Apply chilled witch hazel. Soothing. Nontoxic.

OAKMOSS • Any one of several lichens that grow on oak trees and yield a resin for use as a fixative *(see)* in perfumery. Stable green liquid with a long-lasting characteristic odor. Soluble in alcohol. No known toxicity but a common allergen in after-shave lotions.

OCHRONOSIS • A disturbance of metabolism in which the skin of the face, the whites of the eyes, and other tissues such as muscle and cartilage become discolored brown. The urine is also dark brown. Exogenous ochronosis is a condition characterized by hyperpigmentation of the face secondary to the long-term use of hydroquinone-containing bleaching creams. It is characterized by yellowish brown bumps, coarsening of the skin, and eventually scars. It is epidemic in South African blacks. See also Hydroquinone.

OCIMENE • A terpene obtained from sweet basil oil. Used in flavors and perfumes.

OCIMUM • See Basil.

OCTACOSANOL • A constituent of vegetable wax. Isolated from the green blades of wheat and from carnauba wax.

OCTACOSANYL • An emulsifier and stabilizer. See Octanoic Acid.

OCTADECANE • A solvent for emollients. See Octanoic Acid.

OCTADECENE/MA COPOLYMER • An emulsion stablizer and film-former. See Octanoic Acid.

OCTANOIC ACID • Colorless, oily liquid with a bad odor, derived from coconut, it is used as an antimicrobial ingredient in other food additives and as a defoaming ingredient, flavoring ingredient, and lubricant. It is used in baked goods, soft candies, cheese, fats, frozen dairy desserts, gelatins, meat products, oils, packaging materials, puddings, and snack foods. Mildly toxic by ingestion and a skin irritant, it has caused mutations in experimental animals.

1-OCTANOL • **Caprylic Alcohol.** Used in the manufacture of perfumes. Colorless, viscous liquid, soluble in water, insoluble in oil. Occurs naturally in oil of lavender, oil of lemon, oil of lime, oil of lovage, orange peel, and coconut oil. It has a penetrating, aromatic scent. May cause skin rash.

2-OCTANOL • **Caprylic Alcohol.** An oily aromatic liquid with a somewhat unpleasant odor. For use in the manufacture of perfumes and disinfectant soaps. See 1-Octanol.

OCTOCRYLENE • An absorbent. See Phenol.

OCTODODECANOL • **2-Octyl Dodecanol.** See Stearyl Alcohol.

OCTODODECETH-16, -20, -25 • Polyethylene ethers of octyldodecanol and stearic acid *(see both)*.

OCTODODECYL MYRISTATE • See Myristic Acid.

OCTODODECYL NEODECANOATE • The ester of octyldodecanol and neodecanoic acid *(see both)*.

OCTOXYGLYCERYL BEHENATE • An ester of glycerin and behenic acid *(see both)*. Used in lipsticks.

OCTOXYGLYCERYL PALMITATE • See Glycerin and Palmitic Acid.

OCTOXYNOL-1, -3, -10, -13, -40, -70 • Waxlike emulsifiers, dispersing ingredients, and detergents used in hand creams, lotions, and lipsticks. Derived from phenol *(see)* and used as a surfactant. The number signifies the viscosity.

OCTOXYNOL-9 or -20 CARBOXLYLIC ACID • See Octoxynols and Carboxylic Acid.

OCTRIZOLE • An absorbent derived from phenol *(see)*.

OCTYL ACETOXYSTEARATE • See Stearic Acid.

OCTYL COCOATE • See Coconut Acid.

OCTYL DIMETHYL PABA • Used in sunscreens and makeup. See Para-aminobenzoic Acid and Sunscreens.

OCTYL DODECANOL • Widely used emulsifier, opacifying ingredient, hair conditioner, emollient, and surfactant. See Stearyl Alcohol.

OCTYL HYDROXYSTEARATE • See Ester and Stearic Acid.

OCTYL ISONONANOATE • See Ester and Nonanoic Acid.

OCTYL ISOPALMITATE • An ester of palmitic acid *(see)*, it is used as a skin-conditioning ingredient in body and hand products, eye shadows, skin care products, blushers and frangrances.

OCTYL METHOXYCINNAMATE • Widely used as an ultraviolet light absorber in makeup bases, foundations, suntan lotions, and hair preparations. See Ester and Methyl Cinnamate.

OCTYL MYRISTATE • See Ester and Myristic Acid.

OCTYL OCTANOATE • See Ester and Octanoic Acid.

OCTYL PALMITATE • Widely used as an emollient in makeup, cold creams, lipsticks, and shaving creams. The CIR Expert Panel *(see)* concludes that this ingredient is safe for use in cosmetic products. See Ester and Palmitate.

OCTYL PELARGONATE • See Ester and Pelargonic Acid.

OCTYL SALICYLATE • A sunscreen widely used in makeup, lipsticks, hairsprays, and hand creams. See Salicylates.

OCTYL STEARATE • Widely used as an emollient in makeup bases, skin care products, eye shadows, cold cream, and indoor tanning preparations. Used as a skin-conditioning ingredient. On the basis of the available animal and human data, the CIR Expert Panel *(see)* concludes that this ingredient is safe as used in cosmetics. See Stearic Acid.

OCTYL TRIAZONE • The use of this ingredient as a colorant in cosmetics is prohibited in the United States and may be restricted in other countries.

OCTYLACRYLAMIDE/ACRYLATES/BUTYLAMINOETHYL METHACRYLATE COPOLYMERS • Used in hair products as a fixative. See Acrylates.

OCTYLACRYLAMIDE/ACRYLATES COPOLYMER • See Acrylates and Polymers.

OCTYLDECANOL • Widely used as a skin-conditioning ingredient in hair products, body and hand products, moisutrizing preparations, cold creams, cleansing lotions, eyebrow pencils, blushers, suntan gels, makeup, deodorants, and preshave lotions. See Decanol.

OCTYLDODECETH-16, -20, -25 • Emulsifiers and surfactants. Polyethylene ethers of octyldodecanol *(see)*.

OCTYLDODECYL BEHENATE • The ester *(see)* of octyldodecanol and behenic acid *(see)*. Used in skin creams.

OCTYLDODECYL BENZOATE • The ester *(see)* of octyldodecanol and benzoic acid (see).

OCTYLDODECYL MYRISTATE • Widely used as a skin-conditioning ingredient in moisturizers and body and hand cosmetics. See Ester and Myristic Acid.

OCTYLDODECYL NEODECANOATE • See Ester and Neodecanoic Acid.

OCTYLDODECYL NEOPENTANOATE • See Ester and Neopentanoic Acid.

OCTYLDODECYL OLEATE • See Ester and Oleic Acid.

OCTYLDODECYL OLIVATE • The ester *(see)* of olive oil used as a skin-conditioning ingredient.

OCTYLDODECYL STEARATE • The ester of octyldodecanol and stearic acid *(see both)*.

OCTYLDODECYL STEAROYL STEARATE • A skin-conditioning ingredient widely used in face powders, eye shadows, foundations, blushers, eye makeup, makeup bases, and moisturizers. See Stearic Acid.

OENOTHERA BIENNIS • See Evening Primrose.

OLAFLUR • A dentifrice. See Fluoride.

OLAX • An evergreen tree that yeilds an essential oil used in fragrances. It grows in Asia, Africa and Australia.

OLEA EUROPAEA • See Olive Oil.

OLEALKONIUM CHLORIDE • See Quaternary Ammonium Compounds.

OLEAMIDE • **Oleylamide.** See Oleic Acid.

OLEAMIDE DEA • **Oleic Diethanolamide.** Widely used as a foam booster and thickener in hair products and bubble baths. May form nitrosamines (see). Based on the available data, the CIR Expert Panel (see) concludes that this ingredient is safe as a cosmetic ingredient. However, it should not be used in cosmetic products containing nitrosating agents. See Quaternary Ammonium Compounds, Oleic Acid, and Diethanolamide.

OLEAMIDE MIPA • See Oleic Acid and MIPA.

OLEAMIDOPROPYL BETAINE • See Quaternary Ammonium Compounds.

OLEAMIDOPROPYL DIMETHYLAMINE • See Quaternary Ammonium Compounds.

OLEAMIDOPROPYL DIMETHYLAMINE GLYCOLATE • Antistatic ingredient in hair products. See Quaternary Ammonium Compounds.

OLEAMIDOPROPYL DIMETHYLAMINE HYDROLYZED COLLAGEN • Antistatic ingredient in hair products. Hydrolyzed animal protein (see).

OLEAMIDOPROPYL DIMETHYLAMINE LACTATE • See Lactic Acid and Quaternary Ammonium Compounds.

OLEAMIDOPROPYL DIMETHYLAMINE PROPIONATE • See Quaternary Ammonium Compounds.

OLEAMIDOPROPYL HYDROXYSULTANE • See Quaternary Ammonium Compounds.

OLEAMIDOPROPYL PG-DIMONIUM CHLORIDE • See Quaternary Ammonium Compounds.

OLEAMIDOPROPYLAMINE OXIDE • See Quaternary Ammonium Compounds.

OLEAMIDOPROPYLDIMONIUM HYDROXYPROPYL HYDROLYZED COLLAGEN • Hair and skin conditioning ingredient. See Quaternary Ammonium Compounds.

OLEAMIDOPROPYLETHYLDIMONIUM ETHOSULFATE • See Quaternary Ammonium Compounds.

OLEAMINE • **Oleyl Amine.** A fatty amine derived from oleic acid (see) and used as a stabilizer and plasticizer in creams, lotions, lipsticks, and perfumes. Not as greasy as oil-type stabilizers and plasticizers. No known toxicity.

OLEAMINE BISHYDROXYPROPYLTRIMONIUM CHLORIDE • See Quaternary Ammonium Compounds.

OLEAMINE OXIDE • Hair conditioning and cleansing ingredient. See Oleamine.

OLEANDER • **Oleandrin.** The extract of *Nerium oleander*. The extract is used medically as a diuretic. It is used in cosmetic fragrances.

OLEIC ACID • Obtained from various animal and vegetable fats and oils. Colorless. On exposure to air, it turns a yellow to brown color and develops a rancid odor. Used in preparations of Turkey-red oil *(see)*, soft soap, permanent wave solutions, vanishing creams, brushless shave creams, cold creams, brilliantines, nail polish, toilet soaps, and lipsticks. Possesses better skin-penetrating properties than vegetable oils. Also employed in liquid makeup, liquid lip rouge, shampoos, and preshave lotions. Low oral toxicity but is mildly irritating to the skin. The CIR Expert Panel *(see)* concludes that this ingredient is safe for use in cosmetic products.

OLEIC/PALMITIC/LAURIC/MYRISTIC/LINOLEIC TRIGLYCERIDE • The mixed esters *(see)* of fatty acids used in skin creams.

OLEOAMPHODIPROPIONATE • See Surfactants.

OLEOAMPHOHYDROXYPROPYLSULFONATE • See Surfactants.

OLEORESIN • A natural plant product consisting of essential oil and resin extracted from a substance, such as ginger, by means of alcohol, ether, or acetone. The solvent—alcohol, for example—is percolated through the ginger. Although the oleoresin is very similar to the spice from which it is derived, it is not identical because not all the substances in the spice are extracted. Oleoresins are usually more uniform and more potent than the original product. The normal use range of an oleoresin is from one-fifth to one-twentieth the corresponding amount for the crude spice. Certain spices are extracted as oleoresins for color rather than for flavor. Examples of color-intensifying oleoresins are those from paprika and turmeric.

OLEOSTEARINE • See Tallow and Fatty Acids.

OLEOYL HYDROLYZED COLLAGEN • Used as a hair-conditioning and skin-conditioning ingredient as well as a cleanser. The condensation product after oleic acid chloride and hydrolyzed animal protein have been processed. The word "animal" was taken out of the ingredient name but not out of the ingredient. See Hydrolyzed Protein.

OLEOYL HYDROXYETHYL IMIDAZOLINE • See Imidazoline.

OLEOYL PG-TRIMONIUM CHLORIDE • See Quaternary Ammonium Compounds.

OLEOYL SARCOSINE • The condensation product of oleic acid with *n*-methyl glycine, widely used in polishing compounds, soaps, and lubricating oils. Can be mildly irritating to the skin.

OLETH-2 AND -3 • Emulsifiers. The polyethylene glycol *(see)* esters of oleyl alcohol. They are surfactants and emulsifiers, and cleansing agents. Limited data is available. The CIR Expert Panel *(see)* concludes that this ingredient is safe for use in cosmetic products. See Oleyl Alcohol.

OLETH-5 and -10 • See Oleyl Alcohol.

OLETH-20 • An oily liquid derived from fatty alcohols. Used as a surface-active ingredient *(see)*. No known toxicity.

OLETH-25 AND -50 • See Oleyl Alcohol.

OLETH-3, -6, -10 CARBOXYLIC ACID • See Oleic Acid and Carboxylic Acid.

OLETH-2, -3, -4, -10, -20 PHOSPHATE • See Phosphoric Acid and Oleic Acid.

OLEYL ACETATE • The acetyl ester of oleyl alcohol *(see)*. See also acetylated.

OLEYL ALCOHOL • Ocenol®. Widely used cosmetic ingredient found in fish oils. Oily and usually pale yellow. Gives off an offensive burning odor when heated. Chiefly used in the manufacture of detergents and wetting ingredients and as an antifoam ingredient; also a plasticizer for softening and lubricating fabrics and as a carrier for medications. No known toxicity.

OLEYL ARACHIDATE • The ester of oleyl alcohol and arachidic acid *(see both)* used as a wax.

OLEYL BETAINE • See Oleamine.

OLEYL ERUCATE • A skin-conditioning ingredient. The ester of erucic acid and oleyl alcohol *(see both)*.

OLEYL HYDROXYETHYL IMIDAZOLINE • See Oleyl Alcohol and Imidazoline.

OLEYL IMIDAZOLINE • See Oleyl Alcohol and Imidazoline.

OLEYL LACTATE • The ester of lactic acid and oleyl alcohol *(see both)*.

OLEYL LANOLATE • See Lanolin.

OLEYL MYRISTATE • See Myristic Acid.

OLEYL OLEATE • See Oleic Acid.

OLEYL PALMITAMIDE • See Quaternary Ammonium Compounds.

OLEYL STEARATE • See Oleic Acid and Stearic Acid.

OLIBANUM EXTRACT • **Frankincense Extract.** The extract of *Boswellia carterri* of various species. The volatile, distilled oil from the gum resin of a plant found in Ethiopia, Egypt, and Arabia. It was one of the Gifts of the Magi. It is used in flavorings and fragrances. No known toxicity.

OLIVAMIDOPROPYL BETAINE • The salt of olive oil used as a quaternary ammonium compound *(see)*.

8-OLIVAMIDOPROPYL DIMETHYLAMINE • See Quaternary Ammonium Compounds.

OLIVAMIDOPROPYLAMINE OXIDE • Fatty acids derived from olive oil *(see)*.

OLIVE HUSK OIL • The solvent extraction of olive oil *(see)*.

OLIVE LEAF EXTRACT • The extract of the leaves of *Olea europaea*. See Olive Oil.

OLIVE OIL • *Olea europaea*. Superior to mineral oils in penetrating power. Used in brilliantine hair dressings, emollients, eyelash oils, lipstick, nail polish removers, shampoos, soaps, face powders, and hair colorings. Antiwrinkle and massage oils. It is a pale yellow or greenish fixed oil obtained from ripe olives grown around the Mediterranean Sea. May cause allergic reactions.

OLIVE OIL PEG-6 ESTERS • A complex mixture of the esterification *(see* ester) of olive oil and polyethylene glycol *(see both)*.

OLIVE OIL UNSAPONIFIABLES • See Olive Oil and Saponification.

OLUS • **Black Lovage.** Similar to Angelica *(see)*, it is a perennial herb with globular fruit. When ripe it is almost black. It is used in skin care products. See Lovage.

OMENTAL LIPIDS • Fats obtained from bovine omentum, a fold of tissue that connects a cow's stomach to the intestines. Used in skin conditioners.

ONION EXTRACT • Extract of the bulbs of the onion, *Allium cepa*. Used in flavorings and as a skin-conditioning ingredient. No known toxicity.

ONONIS • See Restharrow Extract.

OPACIFIERS • Substances such as the fatty alcohols stearyl and cetyl *(see both)* that make shampoos and other liquid cosmetics impervious to light.

OPHIOGON JAPONICUS • **Allheal.** An herb related to celery. A fragrance ingredient.

OPOPNAX OIL • An odorous gum resin formerly used in medicine and believed to be obtained from Hercules Allheal. A fragrance ingredient.

OPUTNIA TUNA • **Prickly Pear.**

ORANGE-FLOWER OIL • See Nerol.

ORANGE-FLOWER WATER • The watery solution of the sweet-smelling principles of the flowers of *Citrus sinensis.*

ORANGE OIL • *Citrus sinensis.* **Sweet Orange Oil.** Yellow to deep orange, highly volatile, unstable liquid with a characteristic orange taste and odor expressed from the fresh peel of the ripe fruit of the sweet orange plant species. Once used as an expectorant, it is now employed in perfumery, soaps, and flavorings. Inhalation or frequent contact with oil of orange may cause severe symptoms such as headache, dizziness, and shortness of breath. Perfumes, colognes, and toilet water containing oil of orange may cause allergic reaction in the hypersensitive. Omitted from hypoallergenic cosmetics.

ORANGE PEEL WAX • The wax obtained from the peel of the orange and used as a skin-conditioning ingredient.

ORANGE ROUGHY OIL • The oil obtained from the fat under the skin of the deep sea fish *Hoplostethus atlanticus.* Used as a skin-conditioning ingredient.

ORBIGNYA OLEIFERA • See Babassu Oil.

ORCHID • *Orchis morio.* A very large family of plants that produce colorful and elaborate flowers. Orchids produce minute seeds that are devoid of stored food and thus require the aid of fungi to supply the nourishment needed for germination. They are used in "organic" cosmetics.

ORCHIS • See Orchid.

OREGON GRAPE ROOT • *Berberis aquifolium.* **Wild Oregon Grape. Rocky Mountain Grape. Trailing Mahonia. Berberis.** Employed by early American physicians to treat skin diseases or other illnesses that dried out the skin or produced sores, including syphilis and chronic hepatitis. Oregon grape root contains hydrastine, used to stop uterine bleeding, and berberine *(see both),* used today as an antiseptic and decongestant in eye lotions. Modern studies have found that Oregon grape also contains oxyacanthine chloride and columbine chloride, which show antibacterial properties. Herbalists have also used the root to treat hepatitis, arthritis, cancer, and heart problems.

ORGANIC COSMETICS • Cosmetics made from only animal or vegetable products. Used as a gimmick to sell some cosmetics to those who believe "natural" is better, although most cosmetic ingredients are derived from natural sources.

ORIENTAL BLENDS • One of the basic perfume types, this group gives an impression of subtlety and warmth, with an intense note of spices and incense. They usually include amber, musk, and civet. They vary between heavily floral and richly resinous. They are more insistent in their predominating notes than any other type, and usually are worn at night.

ORIGANUM OIL • The volatile oil is obtained by steam distillation from a flowering herb. Yellowish red to dark brown, with a pungent odor. Used in flavorings. A teaspoonful can cause illness, and less than an ounce has killed adults. GRAS.

ORIZANOL • See Oryzanol.

ORNITHINE • An amino acid *(see)* used as a skin-conditioning ingredient.

ORNITHOGALUM UMBELLATUM • **Star of Bethlehem.** A lily with white, green, or yellow flowers. Used in fragrances.

OROBANCHE RAPUM • **Bitter Vetch. Broomrape. Chick Pea.** Plant native to western America.

OROTIC ACID • **Pyrimidecarboxylic Acid.** Found in milk and certain molds, it is a growth factor for certain microorganisms.

ORRIS • **Orrisroot Oil. White Flag. Love Root.** Distilled for use in dusting powders, perfumes, dry shampoos, toothpastes, and sachets. Made from the roots of the plant. Yellowish, semisolid, and fragrant oil. Discontinued in the United States because of frequent allergic reactions to orris, including infantile eczema, hay fever, stuffy nose, red eyes, and asthma. It is, however, used in raspberry, blackberry, strawberry, violet, cherry, nut, and spice flavorings for beverages, ice cream, ices, candy, baked goods, gelatin desserts, chewing gum, and icings.

ORRIS ABSOLUTE • One of the most widely used perfume ingredients, it is the oldest and most expensive of all natural perfume materials. It is twice the price of Rose Bulgaria *(see)* and three times that of French Jasmine (*see* Jasmine). The so-called oil is produced by steam distillation from the underground stems of the iris. The rhizomes are washed, dried, and then stored for three years to acquire their fragrance. Prior to distillation, they are pulverized, and the absolute is distinctly violetlike with a fruity undertone—sweet, floral, warm, and lasting. The bulk of the material is produced in Italy, distillation taking place mostly in France and sometimes in England and Italy. Can cause allergic reactions. See Orris.

ORRISROOT EXTRACT • Obtained from dried orrisroot. Has an intense odor and is used in perfumery. Used in chocolate, fruit, nut, vanilla, and cream soda flavorings for beverages, ice cream, ices, candy, baked goods, gelatin desserts, and chewing gum. Causes frequent allergic reactions.

ORTHOSIPHON STAMINEUS • A perennial herb with thick wood. There are about 45 species. There are three in China and others in Africa, Asia, Australia. It contains essential oils and resins that are used in fragrances.

ORYZA SATIVA • See Rice Bran Oil. Contains fatty acids used in emollients.

ORYZANOL • **Orizanol.** The ester of ferulic acid and terpene alcohol widely found in plants used in flavorings and perfumes. See Cinnamate.

OSTREA • **Oyster Shell Extract.** Used as an abrasive.

OSTRICH OIL • Used in hair conditioners and skin emollients.

OURICURY WAX • The wax exuded from the leaves of the Brazilian palm tree. The hard, brown wax has the same properties and uses as carnauba wax *(see)*.

OVARIAN EXTRACT • The extract of cow ovaries.

OVUM • See Egg Yolk.

OX BILE • **Oxgall.** Emulsifier from the fresh bile of male castrated bovines. Brownish green or dark green; viscous. Characteristic odor. Bitter, disagreeable taste. Used in dried egg whites up to .1 percent. No known toxicity. The final report to the FDA of the Select Committee on GRAS Substances stated in 1980 that it should continue its GRAS status with no limitations other than good manufacturing practices.

OXALIC ACID • Occurs naturally in many plants and vegetables, particularly in the *Oxalis* family; also in many molds. Used in freckle and bleaching cosmetic preparations. Caustic and corrosive to the skin and mucous membranes; may cause severe intestinal upsets and kidney damage if ingested. Used industrially to remove paint, varnish, rust, and ink stains. Used in dentistry to harden plastic models. Fingernails exposed to it have turned blue, become brittle, and fallen off.

OXAZOLINE • A series of synthetic waxes that are versatile and miscible with most natural waxes and can be applied to the same uses.

OXGALL • See Ox Bile.

OXIDIZED POLYETHYLENE • Polyethylene *(see)* and oxygen combined.

OXIDIZER • A substance that causes oxygen to combine with another substance. Oxygen and hydrogen peroxide are examples of oxidizers.

OXYBENZONE • **Aquaderm Combination Treatment. Chap Stick Petroleum Jelly Plus with Sunblock. PreSun for Kids. Vaseline Intensive Care Moisturizing Sunblock Lotion.** Derived from isopropanol *(see)*, it is used as a sunscreening ingredient. Sunscreens may irritate the skin and in some people cause an allergic rash. According to studies at Columbia Presbyterian Medical Center in New York City, photosensitivity *(see)* to this ingredient is increasing. Similar results were reported from French university researchers in Tours.

OXYQUINOLINE • **8-Hydroxyquinoline.** White, crystalline powder, almost insoluble in water. Used as a fungistat and for reddish orange colors when combined with bismuth. Used internally as a disinfectant. Has caused cancer in animals both orally and when injected. The CIR Expert Panel *(see)* concludes that the available data are insufficient to support the safety of this ingredient in cosmetic products. See Oxyquinoline Sulfate.

OXYQUINOLINE BENZOATE • **8-Quinolinol Benzoate.** The salt of benzoic acid *(see)* and oxyquinoline *(see)*.

OXYQUINOLINE SULFATE • Made from phenols; composed of either white crystals or powder, almost insoluble in water and ether but soluble in alcohol, acetone, and benzene. Used as a preservative in cosmetics for its ability to prevent fungus growth and to disinfect. The CIR Expert Panel *(see)* concludes that the available data are insufficient to support the safety of this ingredient in cosmetic products. See Phenol for toxicity.

OYSTER SHELL EXTRACT • Shells of *Ostrea viriginca* taken from the Gulf of Mexico coast in Texas and Louisiana and from the Chesapeake Bay. Used as a source of lime and in cattle feed. Used as a thickener and skin conditioner.

OZOKERITE • **Ceresin.** A naturally occurring, waxlike mineral; a mixture of hydrocarbons. Colorless or white when pure; horrid odor. Upon refining, it yields a hard, white, microcrystalline wax known as ceresin *(see)*. Widely used as an emulsifier and thickening ingredient used in lipstick and cream rouge. No known toxicity.

OZONE • A colorless gas or dark blue liquid used as an antimicrobial agent in bottled water. Under the EPA Genetic Toxicology Program. Toxic effects are from inhalation.

OZONIZED JOJOBA OIL • Jojoba oil *(see)* treated with ozone. It is used in skin-conditioning creams.

P

PABA • **4-Aminobenzoic Acid. p-Aminobenzoic Acid.** See Para-Aminobenzoic Acid.

PAEONIA • **Peony. Shao-yao.** The root is used by herbalists as a liver tonic. Also used to treat all female "complaints," especially menstrual irregularity and abdominal pains associated with the menstrual cycle. It is also used to treat gallstones and liver complaints. Externally, it has been used to treat wounds and skin growths. Peony is toxic when used internally in excessive doses. Potential adverse effects from herbal use include colic, nausea, and diarrhea. It may also produce uterine contractions. Contraindicated in pregnancy.

PALM KERNEL ACID • A mixture of fatty acids from palm-kernel oil *(see)*. Used as an opacifier, surfactant, and emulsifier.

PALM KERNEL ALCOHOL • The mixture of fatty alcohols derived from palm-kernel oil *(see)*. Used as an emulsifier and stabilizer.

PALM KERNEL GLYCERIDES • A mixture of glycerides *(see)* derived from palm-kernel oil *(see)*.

PALM-KERNEL OIL • *Elaeis guineensis.* **Palm Nut.** The oil from palms, particularly the African palm oil tree. White to yellowish edible fat, it resembles coconut oil more than palm oil. It is used chiefly in making soaps and ointments. On the basis of the animal and clinical data, the CIR Expert Panel *(see)* concludes that it is safe as used in cosmetic formulations.

PALM KERNELAMIDE DEA • A mixture of ethanolamide of the fatty acids derived from palm-kernel oil *(see)*. See Quaternary Ammonium Compounds.

PALM KERNELAMIDE MEA • See Palm-Kernel Oil and Quaternary Ammonium Compounds.

PALM KERNELAMIDE MIPA • See Quaternary Ammonium Compounds.

PALM KERNELAMIDOPROPYL BETAINE • See Quaternary Ammonium Compounds.

PALM OIL • *Elaesis guineensis.* **Palm Butter. Palm Tallow.** Oil used in baby soaps, ordinary soaps, liniments, and ointments. Obtained from the fruit or seed of the palm tree. A reddish yellow to dark, dirty red. A fatty mass with a faint violet odor. Also used to make candles and lubricants. Was teratogenic in albino rats given 3 ml. daily. On the basis of the animal and clinical data, the CIR Expert Panel *(see)* concludes that it is safe as used in cosmetic formulations. No known toxicity.

PALM OIL GLYCERIDE • See Palm Oil.

PALMAMIDE DEA • A mixture of ethanolamides of the fatty acids derived from palm oil. See Palm Oil.

PALMAMIDE MEA • A mixture of ethanolamides of the fatty acids derived from palm oil *(see)*.

PALMAMIDE MIPA • A mixture of isopropanol amides of the fatty acids derived from palm oil *(see)*.

PALMAMIDOPROPYL BETAINE • See Palm Oil and Betaine.

PALMARIA PALMATA EXTRACT • **Dulse.** A natural flavoring extract from red seaweed. Used as a food condiment. No known toxicity. GRAS.

PALMAROSA OIL • **Geranium Oil.** The volatile oil obtained by steam distillation from a variety of partially dried grasses grown in East India and Java. Used in rose, fruit, and spice flavorings for beverages, ice cream, ices, candy, and baked goods. Believed as toxic as other essential oils, causing illness after ingestion of a teaspoonful and death after ingestion of an ounce. A skin irritant. GRAS.

PALMITAMIDE DEA, MEA • See Palmitic Acid.

PALMITAMIDOPROPYL BETAINE • Widely used as an antistatic ingredient in hair conditioners. Also used as a cleansing ingredient and foam booster. See Palmitic Acid and Surfactants.

PALMITAMIDOPROPYL DIMETHYLAMINE LACTATE • See Quaternary Ammonium Compounds and Lactic Acid.

PALMITAMIDOPROPYL DIMETHYLAMINE PROPIONATE • See Quaternary Ammonium Compounds and Propionic Acid.

PALMITAMIDOPROPYLDIETHYLAMINE • See Palmitic Acid and Surfactants.

PALMITAMINE • The CIR Expert Panel *(see)* concludes that this ingredient is safe for use in cosmetic products.

PALMITAMINE OXIDE • **Palmityl Dimethylamine Oxide.** See Palmitic Acid and Dimethylamine.

PALMITATE • A salt of palmitic acid *(see)* used as an oil in baby oils, bath oils, eye creams, hair conditioners, and cream rouges. Occurs in palm oil, butterfat, and most other fatty oils and fats. See Palmitic Acid for toxicity.

PALMITIC ACID • A mixture of solid organic acids obtained from fats consisting chiefly of palmitic acid with varying amounts of stearic acid *(see)*. Used as a texturizer in shampoos, shaving creams, and soaps. It is white or faintly yellow and has a fatty odor and taste. Palmitic acid occurs naturally in allspice, anise, calamus oil, cascarilla bark, celery seed, butter acids, coffee, tea, and many animal fats and plant oils. It forms 40 percent of cow's milk. Obtained from palm oil,

Japan wax, or Chinese vegetable tallow. No known toxicity to skin and hair, provided no salts of oleic or lauric acids *(see both)* are present. The CIR Expert Panel *(see)* concludes that this ingredient is safe for use in cosmetic products.

PALMITOYL COLLAGEN AMINO ACIDS • The condensation product of animal collagen amino acid and palmitic acid *(see both)*.

PALMITOYL HYDROLYZED COLLAGEN • The condensation product of palmitic acid and hydrolyzed animal protein. The word "animal" was removed from this ingredient's name. See Hydrolyzed Protein.

PALMITOYL HYDROLYZED MILK PROTEIN • The condensation product of palmitic acid chloride and hydrolyzed milk protein. See Hydrolyzed and Milk.

PALMITOYL KERATIN AMINO ACIDS • The condensation product of palmitic acid chloride and amino acids from animal skin. See Keratin Amino Acids.

PALMITOYL PG-TRIMONIUM CHLORIDE • See Quaternary Ammonium Compounds.

PANAX GINSENG • See Ginseng.

PANCREASE • See Pancrelipase.

PANCREATIN • **Hi-Vegi-Lip. Pancreatin Enseals.** A preparation of pancreatic hormones used to aid digestion of starches, fats, and proteins. Potential adverse reactions include nausea and diarrhea. Antacids may negate pancreatin's beneficial effects. Should be used cautiously in people who are allergic to pork. Used in processing cosmetics.

PANCRELIPASE • **Pancrease. Viokase. Zymase.** A preparation of pancreatic hormones used in disorders of the pancreas to aid digestion of starches, fats, and proteins. Used to treat cystic fibrosis. Should be used cautiously in patients who are allergic to pork. Used in processing cosmetics.

PANSY, WILD (H) • *Viola tricolor.* **Johnny Jump-Up. Heart's Ease. Violet.** A European herb, it is grown for its large, attractive flowers. Used for colorings. The herb contains mucilaginous material that is used as a soothing lotion for boils, swellings, and skin diseases. It also contains salicylates, saponins, alkaloid, flavonoids, and tannin *(see all)*. It is also used as a gentle laxative and to treat kidney diseases. The root is both emetic and cathartic.

PANTETHINE • A growth factor for *Lactobacillus bulgaricus.* Glassy, lightly yellow substance. Used in hair products such as hairsprays and moisturizing preparations.

PANTHENOL • **Dexpanthenol. Vitamin B Complex Factor.** Widely used in hair products and emollients, and as a supplement in foods. Employed medically to aid digestion. It is good for human tissues. No known toxicity.

PANTHENYL ETHYL ETHER • The ethyl ether of the B vitamin panthenol *(see)*.

PANTHENYL ETHYL ETHER ACETATE • The ester of acetic acid and the ethyl ether of the B vitamin panthenol *(see)*.

PANTOTHENIC ACID • **Vitamin B$_5$.** A necessity in the human diet. It is involved in the metabolism of fats and proteins. Nontoxic.

PANTOTHENYL TRIACETATE • See Panthenol.

PAPAIN • See Papaya.

PAPAVER • See Poppy Oil.

PAPAYA • A base of organic makeup. It is a fruit grown in tropical countries. It contains an enzyme, papain, used as a meat tenderizer and medicinally to prevent adhesions. It is deactivated by cooking. Because of its protein-digesting ability, it can dissolve necrotic (dead) material. It may cause allergic reactions. It is used in cosmetics as a hair conditioner.

PAPRIKA • The finely ground pods of dried, ripe, sweet pepper. The strong, reddish orange powder is used in sausage and spice flavorings. The oleoresin *(see)* is used in fruit, meat, and spice flavorings for beverages, ice cream, ices, candy, baked goods, condiments, and meats. Both paprika and paprika oleoresins are used as red coloring. No known toxicity. Permanently listed since 1966 for use in foods consistent with good manufacturing practices.

PARA-AMINOBENZOIC ACID • The colorless or yellowish acid found in Vitamin B complex. In an alcohol and water solution plus a little light perfume, it is sold under a wide variety of names as a sunscreen lotion to prevent skin damage. It is also used as a local anesthetic in sunburn products. It is used medicinally to treat arthritis. However, it can cause allergic eczema and a sensitivity to light in susceptible people whose skin may react to sunlight by erupting with a rash, sloughing, and/or swelling.

PARA-AMINOSALICYLIC ACIDS • See Salicylic Acid.

PARABENS • The parabens, methyl-, propyl-, and parahydroxybenzoate, are the most commonly used preservatives in the United States. In 1977, about 30 percent of the cosmetic products registered with the Food and Drug Administration contained parabens. Water is the only ingredient used more frequently in cosmetics. The parabens have a broad spectrum of antimicrobial activity, are safe to use—relatively nonirritating, nonsensitizing, and nonpoisonous—are stable over the pH *(see)* range in cosmetics, and are sufficiently soluble in water to be effective in liquids. The typical paraben preservative system contains 0.2 percent methyl- and 0.1 percent propylparaben. See Methylparaben and Butylparaben.

PARA-DICHLOROBENZENE • **p-Dichlorobenzene. Paracide. PDB.** Crystals made from chlorine and benzene have a penetrating odor, are almost insoluble in water, and are noncorrosive and nonstaining. A solvent for many organic materials, it is employed in degreasing hides and wool, metal polishes, moth repellents, general insecticides, germicides, spray deodorants, and fumigants. PDB is commonly found in room deodorizers and moth-killing products. Vapors may cause irritation to the skin, throat, and eyes, and prolonged exposure to high concentrations may cause weakness, dizziness, loss of weight, and liver damage. A well-known animal cancer-causing ingredient, the chemical can linger in the home for months or even years after use. Toxic by ingestion and inhalation, and is irritating to mucous membranes. You can lessen your exposure to it by reading product labels and avoiding preparations that contain it (not all labels list it).

PARAFFIN • Used in solid brilliantines, cold creams, wax depilatories, eyelash creams, and oils, eyebrow pencils, lipsticks, liquefying creams, protective creams, and mascaras; also used for extracting perfumes from flowers. Obtained from the distillate of wood, coal, petroleum, or shale oil. Colorless or white, odorless, greasy, and not digestible or absorbable in the intestines. Easily melts over boiling water and is used to cover food products. Pure paraffin is harmless to the skin, but the presence of impurities may give rise to irritations and eczema.

PARAFORMALDEHYDE • A white solid with the odor of formaldehyde, it is derived from it. It is used as a fungicide, to kill bacteria, and in disinfectants. It is also used in adhesives and as a waterproofing ingredient. Toxic by ingestion. See Formaldehyde.

PARAGUAY TEA • See Maté Extract.

PARA-HYDROXYBENZOIC ACID • See *p*-Hydroxybenzoic Acid.

PARA-PHENYLENE DIAMINE • PPDA. See Phenylenediamine.

PARETH-15-3 • See C11-15 Pareth 9.

PARETH-25-12 • A detergent. See C12-15 Pareth 12.

PARFUM • European name for "fragrance." The term is not permitted on United States labels.

PARIETARIA OFFICINALIS • See Pellitory Extract and Spanish Pellitory Extract.

PARSLEY EXTRACT • *Petroselinum cripsum. P. sativum.* A perennial of the carrot family, it is native to Europe, especially to Sardinia, where it is believed it may have originated. It was given in a tea to colicky infants and to settle the stomachs of adults after a meal. The oil is used to induce menstruation. The crushed seeds were made into an eyewash. A tea was used for urinary infections and for insect bites and swollen glands. It is rich in Vitamin C. Ancient herbalists maintained that it would help hair grow if it were rubbed into the scalp. It is a source of chlorophyll, nature's breath freshener. It also contains Vitamin B, potassium, protein, apiol—an anti-inflammatory in parsley oil—and myristicin, another oil. In 1992, the FDA proposed a ban on parsley in oral menstrual drug products because it has not been shown to be safe and effective for its stated claims. See Parsley Oil.

PARSLEY OIL • Used as a preservative in perfume and flavoring in cosmetics, it is obtained by steam distillation of the ripe seeds of the herb. Yellow to light brown, with a harsh odor. Parsley may cause skin to break out with a rash, redden, and swell when exposed to light. It may also cause an allergic reaction in the sensitive.

PARSLEY SEED OIL • See Parsley Oil.

PASQUE FLOWER • *Anemone pulsatilla.* A low, perennial herb with white or purple flowers, it is used by herbalists to treat insomnia and other tension-induced conditions; it is also used to treat painful periods and painful conditions of the testes. The antibacterial effects are used by herbalists to treat skin infections and asthma.

PASSIFLORA • See Passionflower Extract.

PASSIONFLOWER EXTRACT • Extract of the various species of *Passiflora camata.* Indians used passionflower for swellings and sore eyes, and to induce vomiting. It has been shown that an extract of the plant depresses the motor nerves of the spinal cord.

PATCHOULI OIL • Used in perfume formulations to impart a long-lasting oriental aroma in soaps and cosmetics. It is the essential oil obtained from the leaves of an East Indian shrubby mint. Yellowish to greenish brown liquid, with the pleasant fragrance of summer flowers. May produce allergic reactions.

PAULLINA CUPANA • See Guarana Extract.

PAWPAW EXTRACT • **Custard Apple.** The extract of the fruit *Caraya papaya*. The dried and pulverized large brown seeds have been rubbed into the scalp to eradicate head lice. The fruit is rich in vitamins and minerals. No known toxicity for the skin, but if taken internally, it can cause vomiting.

PCA • **Pyrrolidone Carboxylic Acid.** Employed in the manufacture of polyvinylpyrrolidone *(see)*, which goes into hairsprays. Also a high boiling solvent in petroleum processing, and a plasticizer and coalescing ingredient for floor polishes. On the basis of the animal and clinical data, the CIR Expert Panel *(see)* concludes that it is safe as used in cosmetic formulations but should not be used in products containing nitrosating *(see)* agents.

PEA EXTRACT • The extract of *Pisum sativum*.

PEA PALMITATE • The compound obtained by crushing peas with palmitic acid chloride. Used as a skin conditioner.

PEACH EXTRACT • *Prunus persica*. See Peach Juice Extract.

PEACH JUICE EXTRACT • The liquid obtained from the pulp of the peach, *Prunus persica*. It is used as a natural flavoring and as an emollient. Nontoxic.

PEACH KERNEL OIL • **Persic Oil.** Used as an oil base in emollients, eyelash creams, and brilliantines. It is a light yellow liquid expressed from a seed. Smells like almonds. Also a flavoring in foods. No known toxicity.

PEACH PIT POWDER • The powder obtained by grinding the pits of *Prunus persica*. It is used as an exfoliant *(see)*.

PEANUT • *Arachis hypogaea*. Widely used in cosmetics as an abrasive, thickener, and skin conditioner in body and hand products, cleansing lotions, hair conditioners, and lipsticks.

PEANUT ACID • Used as a surfactant and cleansing ingredient.

PEANUT GLYCERIDES • A mixture of glycerides *(see)* derived from Peanut Oil *(see)*.

PEANUT OIL • **Arachis Oil.** Used in the manufacture of soaps, baby preparations, hair-grooming aids, nail dryers, shampoos, and as a solvent for ointments and liniments; also in night creams and emollients. A solvent in salad oil, shortening, mayonnaise, and confections. Also used in conjunction with natural flavorings. Peanut butter is about 50 percent peanut oil suspended in peanut fibers. Greenish yellow, with a pleasant odor. Prepared by pressing shelled and skinned seeds of the peanut. It is used as a substitute for almond and olive oils in cosmetic creams, brilliantines, antiwrinkle oils, and sunburn preparations. Has been reported to be a mild irritant in soap, but is considered harmless to the skin.

PEANUTAMIDE • A mixture of the ethanolamines *(see)* of the fatty acids derived from peanuts. Used as a thickener and foam booster.

PEANUTAMIDE MEA • Loramine Wax. See Peanut Oil.

PEANUTAMIDE MIPA • A mixture of isopropanol amides of the fatty acids derived from peanut oil *(see)*.

PEAR EXTRACT • The extract of the fruit of *Pyrus communis*.

PEARL ESSENCE • Guanine. A suspension of crystalline guanine *(see)* in nitrocellulose *(see)* and solvents. Guanine is obtained from fish scales. Used in nail polish to give it a shine. Implants of small amounts of guanine hydrochloride were lethal in mice. No known toxicity to the skin or nails.

PEARL POWDER • The dried powder obtained from freshwater pearls. Used to add shine to lipsticks and powders.

PEARLS • See Mica.

PEARLY EVERLASTING • *Anaphalis margarotacea*. An American everlasting having floccose-woolly herbage and small corymbose heads with pearly white whorls. Used in "organic" cosmetics.

PECAN SHELL POWDER • From *Carya illinoinensis* shells. A coloring ingredient used in cosmetics. Employed medicinally by the American Indians. It is the nut from a hickory of the southern central United States with a rough bark and hard but brittle wood. Edible. No known toxicity.

PECTIN • Emulsifying ingredient used in place of various gums in toothpastes, hair-setting lotions, and protective creams. The pectins are found in roots, stems, and fruits of plants and form an integral part of such structures. They are used in cosmetics as a gelling and thickening ingredient. They are soothing and mildly acidic. Also used in foods as a "cementing ingredient" and as an antidiarrheal medication. No known toxicity to the skin.

PEG • Abbreviation for polyethylene glycol/polyethylene, used in making nonionic surfactants. The low molecular polyethylene glycols from 200 to 400 may cause hives and eczema. The higher polyethylenes are not sensitizers. See Surfactants and Nonionic.

PEG-4, -6, -8, -9, -10, -12, -14, -16, -18, -32, -40, -150, -200, -350 • Polymers *(see)* of ethylene oxide. Usually, a waxy compound. The number refers to the liquidity; the higher the number, the harder the composition.

PEG-8-C 12-18 ALKYL ESTER • See C12-18 PEG-8-Ester.

PEG-8 CAPRATE • The polyethylene glycol ester of capric acid. See Capric Acid and Polyethylene Glycol.

PEG-9 CAPRYLATE • The polyethylene glycol ester of caprylic acid *(see)*.

PEG-8 CAPRYLATE/CAPRATE • The polyethylene glycol ester of a mixture of caprylic and capric acids *(see all)*.

PEG-6 CAPRYLIC/CAPRIC GLYCERIDES • The ethoxylated glycerides of caprylic and capric acid derivatives. See Caprylic and Capric Acids and Glycerides.

PEG-3 TO -200 CASTOR OIL • The polyethylene glycol derivative of castor oil *(see)*. The higher the number after the listing, the more solid the compound. See Polyethylene Glycol.

PEG-3 TO -11 COCAMIDE • The polyethylene glycol amides of coconut acid. The higher the number, the more solid the compound. Used as emulsifiers. See Polyethylene Glycol and Coconut Oil.

PEG-2 TO -15 COCAMINE • The polyethylene glycol amines of coconut acid. The higher the number, the harder the compound.

PEG-5, -8 OR -15 COCOATE • The polyethylene glycol esters of coconut acid. The lower the number, the more liquid the compound. See Polyethylene Glycols and Coconut Oil.

PEG-2 OR -15 COCOMONIUM CHLORIDE • See Quaternary Ammonium Compounds.

PEG-15 COCOPOLYAMINE • The polyethylene glycol polyamine and coconut acid. See Polyethylene Glycol and Coconut Oil.

PEG-4 THROUGH -150 DILAURATE • The polyethylene glycol diesters of lauric acid *(see)*. The higher the number, the more solid the compound. See also Polyethylene Glycol.

PEG-6 TO -150 DIOLEATE • The polyethylene glycol diesters of oleic acid *(see)*. The lower the number, the more liquid the compound. See Polyethylene Glycol.

PEG-3 DIPALMITATE • The polyethylene glycol diester of palmitic acid *(see)*.

PEG-2 THROUGH -175 DISTEARATE • The polyethylene glycol diesters of stearic acid. The higher the number, the more solid the compound. See Stearic Acid and Polyethylene Glycol.

PEG-8 OR -12 DITALLATE • The polyethylene glycol diesters of tall oil *(see)*.

PEG-8 DITRIRICINOLEATE • See Ricinoleic Acid and Polyethylene Glycol.

PEG-22 OR -45 DODECYL GLYCOL COPOLYMERS • See Polyethylene Glycol.

PEG-7 OR -30 GLYCERYL COCOATE • The polyethylene glycol ethers of glyceryl cocoate. See Coconut Oil.

PEG-15 OR -20 GLYCERYL RICINOLEATE • The polyethylene glycol ether of glyceryl ricinoleate. The number signifies the liquidity of the compound. See Polyethylene Glycol and Castor Oil.

PEG-5 THROUGH -120 GLYCERYL STEARATE • See Polyethylene Glycol and Stearic Acid.

PEG-28 GLYCERYL TALLOWATE • See Tallow Glycerides and Polyethylene Glycol.

PEG-25 GLYCERYL TRIOLEATE • See Oleic Acid and Polyethylene Glycol.

PEG-5 THROUGH -200 HYDROGENATED CASTOR OIL • See Polyethylene Glycol and Castor Oil.

PEG-5 HYDROGENATED CORN GLYCERIDES • The polyethylene glycol derivative of mixed glycerides derived from hydrogenated corn oil. See Hydrogenation and Corn Oil.

PEG-8 HYDROGENATED FISH GLYCERIDES • The polyethylene glycol derivative of hydrogenated fish glycerides. See Hydrogenation and Fish Oil.

PEG-5 THROUGH -70 HYDROGENATED LANOLIN • The polyethylene glycol derivative of hydrogenated lanolin. The higher the number, the more solid the compound. See Polyethylene Glycol and Lanolin.

PEG-13 HYDROGENATED TALLOW AMIDE • See Polyethylene Glycol and Tallow.

PEG-6 THROUGH -10 ISOLAURYL THIOETHER • The polyethylene glycol ether of dodecyl mercaptan. The number signifies liquidity. See Polyethylene Glycol and Lauryl Alcohol.

PEG-6 OR -12 ISOSTEARATE • The polyethylene glycol ester of isostearic acid. See Polyethylene Glycol and Stearic Acid.

PEG-5 TO -20 LANOLATE • See Lanolin.

PEG-5 THROUGH -100 LANOLIN • The polyethylene glycol derivative of lanolin. The number signifies liquidity. Widely used in cosmetics. See Lanolin.

PEG-75 LANOLIN OIL AND WAX • See Lanolin.

PEG-3 TO -6 LAURAMIDE • The polyethylene glycol amide of lauric acid *(see)*.

PEG-3 LAURAMINE OXIDE • See Lauric Acid.

PEG-LAURATE (2 THROUGH 150) • The polyethylene glycol esters of lauric acid. The number signifies liquidity. Yellow, oily liquid insoluble in water. Widely used in soaps and detergents. Emulsifier in cosmetic creams and lotions. Gives an oil-in-water emulsion. No known toxicity other than allergic reactions in some persons sensitive to laurates. See Lauric Acid.

PEG-6 METHYL ETHER • See Methanol.

PEG-20 METHYL GLUCOSE SESQUISTEARATE • A mixture of polyethylene glycol mono- and diesters of methyl glucose and stearic acid *(see all)*.

PEG-2 MILK SOLIDS • See Milk and Polyethylene Glycol.

PEG-4 OCTANOATE • The polyethylene glycol ester of caprylic acid *(see)*.

PEG-2 THROUGH -9 OLEAMIDE • The polyethylene glycol amide of oleic acid *(see)*. Widely used as a stabilizer and plasticizer.

PEG-2 THROUGH -30 OLEAMINE • The polyethylene glycol amine of oleic acid *(see)*. Widely used in vanishing creams, soft soaps, cold creams, and many other cosmetics.

PEG-2 OLEAMONIUM CHLORIDE • See Quaternary Ammonium Compounds.

PEG-12, -20, or -30 OLEATE • The polyethylene glycol ether of glyceryl oleate. See Polyethylene Glycol and Glycerin.

PEG-3 THROUGH -150 OLEATE • The polyethylene glycol esters of oleic acid *(see)*. Widely used in cosmetic bases and shampoos. Emulsifying ingredient in creams and lotions. A dark red oil that can be dispersed in water; soluble in alcohol and miscible with cottonseed oil. No known toxicity.

PEG-6 THROUGH -20 PALMITATE • The polyethylene glycol esters of palmitic acid *(see)*.

PEG-8 PALMITOYL METHYL DIETHONIUM METHOSULFATE • See Quaternary Ammonium Compounds.

PEG-5 PENTAERYTHRITOL ETHER • The polyethylene glycol ether of pentaerythritol that is used as a plasticizer and synthetic lubricant. See Formaldehyde and Acetaldehyde.

PEG/PPG-17/6 OR 18/4 OR 23/50 OR 35/9 OR 125/30 COPOLYMERS • The copolymers produced by the interaction of ethylene oxide with propylene oxide. Used as plasticizers and bases for cosmetics. See Ethylene Oxide and Propylene Glycol.

PEG-8 PROPYLENE GLYCOL COCOATE • The polyethylene glycol ether of polyethylene glycol cocoate derived from coconut acid *(see)* and used as an emulsifier.

PEG-25 THROUGH -125 PROPYLENE GLYCOL STEARATE • See Stearic Acid.

PEG-2 OR -7 RICINOLEATE • The polyethylene glycol esters of ricinoleic acid *(see)*.

PEG-8 SESQUILAURATE • The mixture of polyethylene glycol mono- and diesters of lauric acid with ethylene oxide. See Lauric Acid.

PEG-8 SESQUIOLEATE • The mixture of polyethylene glycol mono- and diesters of oleic acid with ethylene oxide. See Oleic Acid.

PEG-6, -8, -20 SORBITAN BEESWAX • The ethoxylated sorbitol derivative of beeswax with ethylene oxide. See Sorbitol and Beeswax.

PEG-5 OR -20 SORBITAN ISOSTEARATE • The ethoxylated sorbitol monoester of isostearic acid and ethylene oxide. See Sorbitol and Stearic Acid.

PEG-40 OR -75 OR -80 SORBITAN LANOLATE • The ethoxylated sorbitol derivative of lanolin and ethylene oxide of 40, 75, or 80 molecules. See Lanolin and Sorbitol.

PEG-3 or -6 SORBITAN OLEATE • The ethoxylated sorbitan ester of oleic acid. See Oleic Acid and Sorbitan.

PEG-80 SORBITAN PALMITATE • The ethoxylated sorbitol monoester of palmitic acid *(see)*.

PEG-40 SORBITAN PEROLEATE • The mixture of oleic acid esters of sorbitol. See Sorbitol and Oleic Acid.

PEG-3 OR -40 SORBITAN STEARATE • See Sorbitol and Stearic Acid.

PEG-30, -40, OR -60 SORBITAN TETRAOLEATE • See Oleic Acid and Sorbitol.

PEG-60 SORBITAN TETRASTEARATE • See Stearic Acid and Sorbitol.

PEG-2 TO -15 SOYAMINE • See Polyethylene Glycol and Soy Acid.

PEG-SOYA STEROLS • See Soybean Oil and Polyethylene Glycol.

PEG-2 THROUGH -150 STEARATE • Widely used emulsifying ingredients. See Polyethylene Glycol and Stearic Acid.

PEG-2 OR -15 STEARMONIUM CHLORIDE • See Quaternary Ammonium Compounds.

PEG-5 STEARYL AMMONIUM CHLORIDE • See Quaternary Ammonium Compounds.

PEG-12 OR -20 TALLATE • See Polyethylene Glycol and Tall Oil.

PEG-2 THROUGH -50 TALLOW AMINE • See Tallow and Polyglycerol.

PEG-3, -10, OR -15 TALLOW AMINOPROPYLAMINE • See Polyethylene Glycol and Tallow.

PEG-15 TALLOW POLYAMINE • See Tallow.

PEG-20 TALLOWATE • See Polyethylene Glycol and Tallow.

PEG-66 OR -200 TRIHYDROXYSTEARIN • See Surfactants.

PEI • Abbreviation for polyethylenimine.

PEI-7 • **Polyethylenimine 7.** Highly viscous liquid used as an adhesive or anchoring ingredient for cellophane and as a disinfectant for the skin. Also used in water purification.

PEI-15 THROUGH -2500 • See PEI-7.

PELARGONIC ACID • **Nonanoic Acid.** A synthetic flavoring ingredient that occurs naturally in cocoa and oil of lavender. Used in berry, fruit, nut, and spice flavorings. A strong irritant.

PELARGONIUM CAPITATUM • See Rose Geranium.

PELLIS LIPIDA • Skin fats.

PELLITORY EXTRACT • **Extract of Pellitory. Parietary Extract.** The extract obtained from the leaves and stem of *Parietaria officinalis.* Used as an emollient, particularly in baby creams and lotions. No known toxicity.

PELVETIA CANALICULATA • A family of rockweed. See Bladder Wrack Extract.

PENGAWAR DJAMBI OIL • Oil obtained from a variety of ferns of the family *Cyatheaceae.* Used in emollients.

PENICILLINS • A group of beta-lactam antibiotics produced by several species of mold and/or semisynthetically. There are many kinds, and they offer a broad clinical spectrum of activity. They act by inhibiting bacterial enzymes involved in the making of cell walls. Used topically, they may cause skin rash.

PENNYROYAL EXTRACT • An extract of the flowering herb *Mentha pulegium.* Used since ancient days as a medicine, scent, flavoring, and food. Obtained from the dried flower tops and leaves, it contains tannin, which is soothing to the skin.

PENTA- • A prefix meaning containing five atoms or groups.

PENTADECALACTONE • **Angelica Lactone.** Used as a cosmetic fragrance and in berry, fruit, and liquor flavorings. It is obtained from the fruit and root of a plant grown in Europe and Asia. No known toxicity.

PENTADESMA BUTTER • **Kanya Butter.** The vegetable fat extracted from the nut of the *Pentadesma butyracea.* See Shea Butter.

PENTAERYTHRITOL • Prepared from acetaldehyde and formaldehyde *(see both).* It is used in synthetic resins.

PENTAERYTHRITOL HYDROGENATED ROSINATE • The ester of acids derived from hydrogenated rosin *(see)* mixed with pentaerythritol *(see).*

PENTAERYTHRITYL ROSINATE • The ester of acids derived from rosin *(see)* mixed with pentaerythritol *(see).* It is used as a skin-conditioning agent and a thickener. The CIR Expert Panel *(see)* concludes that the data available are insufficient to support the safety of this ingredient as used in cosmetic products.

PENTAERYTHRITYL STEARATE/CAPRATE/CAPRYLATE ADIPATE • The mixed ester *(see)* of pentaerythritol and stearic, capric, caprylic, and adipic acids. Used as emulsifiers.

PENTAERYTHRITYL TETRAABIETATE • See Pentaerythritol and Abietic Acid.

PENTAERYTHRITYL TETRABEHENATE • The ester of pentaerythritol and behenic acid *(see both)*.

PENTAERYTHRITYL TETRAOCTANOATE • See Caprylic Acid.

PENTAERYTHRITYL TETRAOLEATE • The ester of pentaerythritol and oleic acid *(see both)*.

PENTAERYTHRITYL TETRASTEARATE AND CALCIUM STEARATE • See Stearic Acid.

PENTAERYTHRITYL TRIOLEATE • The ester of pentaerythritol and oleic acid *(see both)*.

PENTAHYDROSQUALENE • The end product of hydrogenation *(see)* of squalene *(see)*.

PENTANE • The aliphatic hydrocarbon derived from petroleum. Used as a solvent. Narcotic in high doses.

1-PENTANOL • **Pentyl Alcohol. n-Amyl Alcohol.** Liquid with a mild odor, slightly soluble in water. Used as a solvent. Irritating to the eyes and respiratory passages, and absorption may cause a lack of oxygen in the blood.

PENTAPOTASSIUM TRIPHOSPHATE • See Pentasodium Pentetate.

PENTASODIUM AMINOTRIMETHYLENE PHOSPHONATE • An emulsifier. See Phosphoric Acid and Pentasodium Pentetate.

PENTASODIUM PENTETATE • **Pentasodium Diethylenetriaminepentaacetate. Sodium Tripolyphosphate.** Prepared from dehydration of mono- and disodium phosphates. An inorganic salt used as a water softener, sequestering ingredient *(see)*, emulsifier, and dispersing ingredient in cosmetic cleansing creams and lotions. Moderately irritating to the skin and mucous membranes. Ingestion can cause violent purging.

PENTETIC ACID • **Penthanil. Diethylenetriaminepentaacetic Acid.** A chelating ingredient *(see)* to remove iron particles floating in cosmetic solutions. No known toxicity.

PENTYL DIMETHYL PABA • The ester of pentyl alcohol and dimethyl *p*-aminobenzoic acid. Used as a preservative. See Parabens.

PEONY • *Paeonia lactiflora.* **Shao-yao.** The root is used by herbalists as a liver tonic. It is also used to treat all female complaints, especially menstrual irregularity and abdominal pains associated with the menstrual cycle. It is used in "organic" cosmetics.

PEPPER OIL, BLACK • A pungent oil obtained from the dried, unripe berries of the East Indian pepper plant, *Piper nigrum.* Used in flavorings. Pepper was formerly used as a carminative to break up intestinal gas and cause sweating, and as a gastric ingredient to promote gastric secretion. No known toxicity.

PEPPERMINT EXTRACT • See Peppermint Oil.

PEPPERMINT LEAVES • See Peppermint Oil.

PEPPERMINT OIL • Used in toothpaste and tooth powders, eye lotions, shaving lotions, and toilet waters. It is the oil made from the dried leaves and tops of a plant common to Asian, European, and American gardens. Widely used as a food and beverage flavoring. It can cause allergic reactions such as hay fever and skin rash.

PEPSIN • A digestive enzyme found in gastric juice that helps break down protein. Used in hair conditioners. The pepsin product used to aid digestion is obtained from the glandular layer of the fresh stomach of a hog. Slightly acid taste and a mild odor. No known toxicity. In 1992, the FDA proposed a ban on pepsin in oral menstrual drug products because it has not been shown to be safe and effective for its stated claims. Used in processing cosmetics.

PEPTONES • Secondary protein derivatives formed during the process of digestion—the result of the action of the gastric and pancreatic juices upon protein. Peptones are used as a foam stabilizer for beer and as a processing aid in baked goods, confections, and frostings. No known toxicity. Determined to be GRAS in 1982.

PERCUTANEOUS • Movement through or into the skin.

PERFLUORODIMETHYLCYCLOHEXANE • A solvent. See Hexanoic Acid.

PERFLUOROPOLYMETHYLISOPROPYL ETHER • A skin conditioner. See Fluorine Compounds and Polymer.

PERFUMES • Literally means "through smoke" because the first perfumes were incense. Thereafter, powdered flowers, leaves, wood spices, and aromatic resins were used for fragrances during religious festivals, for the home, and for the body. Some perfumes have as many as 200 ingredients. The essential oils used for today's scents come from leaves, needles, roots, and peels of plants. Floral oils come from petals, whole flowers, gums, and resins. Animal exudates such as musk and ambergris are all used in perfumes. Isolates used in perfumes are made of individual factors in natural oils, which may also be treated chemically. Synthetic chemicals imitate natural aromas and are being used in increasing quantities today. There are three basic scents today: florals, fruits, and modern blends such as woodsy-mossy-leafy-spicy and oriental. Woodsy-mossy-leafy types have a warm aromatic scent with sandalwood, cedar-wood, and balsam predominating. Orientals have subtly heavier odors. Fruity perfumes have a clean fresh fragrance. A typical basic flower perfume (rose) would include phenylethyl alcohol, 35 percent; geraniol, 48 percent; amyl cinnamaldehyde, 2 percent; benzyl acetate, 4 percent; ionone, 4 percent; eugenol, 2 percent; and terpineol, 5 percent. Perfumes are among the most frequent allergens and are left out of many hypoallergenic products. Complaints to the FDA concerning perfumes include headaches, dizziness, rash, hyperpigmentation (*see* Berloque Dermatitis), violent coughing and vomiting, skin irritation, and the explosion of the perfume container.

PERHYDROSQUALENE • See Squalene.

PERILLA • An Asiatic mint. Yields a dark purple coloring.

PERIWINKLE EXTRACT • The extract of *Vinca minor*. See Myrtle.

PERMANENT WAVE NEUTRALIZER • Used to neutralize the acids that curl the hair (*see* Permanent Waves). May contain sodium perborate, bromates, or sodium hexametaphosphate *(see all)*. Before 1940, bromate poisoning was rare, but when bromate was put into permanent wave neutralizers for home use, incidents became more common. Many manufacturers then substituted sodium perborate and sodium hexametaphosphate, a product used as a laundry detergent and in water softeners.

PERMANENT WAVES • **Cold Waves.** Chemicals designed to "permanently" bend or curl the hair. Once done only in beauty parlors, kits have been developed for home use. The process in both the beauty parlor and at home consists of applying a waving lotion containing thioglycolic acid, ammonia, and 93 percent water, as well as borax, ethanolamine, or sodium lauryl sulfate *(see all)*. Then, after a period of time, depending upon the lotion used and the tightness of the curl desired, a neutralizer is applied. Chemicals in the neutralizer may be sodium or potassium bromate, sodium perborate, or hydrogen peroxide (*see* Permanent Wave Neutralizer). The thioglycolates are toxic and may cause skin irritation and low blood sugar. Among the injuries reported to the FDA were hair damage; swelling of legs and feet; eye irritations; rash in the area of the ears, neck, scalp, and forehead; and swelling of the eyelids.

PEROXIDE • Used in hair bleaches. It is a strong oxidant and can injure the skin and eyes. Chemists are cautioned to wear rubber gloves and goggles when handling it. May cause hair breakage and is an irritant. See Hydrogen Peroxide.

PERSIC OIL • See Apricot and Peach Kernel Oil.

PERSIMMON • A medium-sized tree that grows in the southern and eastern United States. Has a hard wood and greenish yellow or greenish white bell-shaped flowers followed by an orange to red berry that is edible. Used as a wax in cosmetics.

PERSULFATES • A salt derived from persulfuric acid, a strong oxidizer. Persulfates are excellent catalysts that speed hair color changes in hair dye. See Hydrogen Peroxide for toxicity.

PERUVIAN BALSAM • See Balsam Peru.

PETASITES HYBRIDUS • **Butterbur.** An herb that is native to temperate climates. Has a thick root and leaves that reputedly possess medicinal powers similar to coltsfoot *(see)*.

PETITGRAIN OIL • Used extensively in perfumes. It is the volatile oil obtained from the leaves, twigs, and unripe fruit of the bitter orange tree. Brownish to yellow with a bittersweet odor. Used in food flavorings. Supposedly dissolves in sweat, and under the influence of sunlight becomes an irritant. May cause allergic skin reactions.

PETROLATUM • **Vaseline. Petroleum Jelly. Paraffin Jelly.** Used in cold creams, emollient creams, conditioning creams, wax depilatories, eyebrow pencils, eye shadows, liquefying creams, liquid powders, nail whites, lipsticks, protective creams, baby creams, and rouge. It is a purified mixture of semisolid hydrocarbons from petroleum. Yellowish to light amber or white, semisolid unctuous mass, practically odorless and tasteless, almost insoluble in water. As a lubricant in lipsticks, it gives them a shine, and it makes creams smoother. Helps to soften and smooth the skin in the same way as any other emollient and is less expensive. The oily film helps prevent evaporation of moisture from the skin and protects the skin from irritation. However, petrolatum does cause allergic skin reactions in the hypersensitive. It is generally nontoxic.

PETROLATUM DISTILLATE • Clear, colorless, highly flammable distillate used as a solvent for fats, oils, and detergents. See Kerosene for toxicity.

PETROLEUM DISTILLATES • **Hydrocarbons, Naphtha, Waxes.** Condensations of a highly complex mixture of paraffinic, naphthalenic, and aromatic hydrocarbons containing some sulfur and trace amounts of nitrogen and oxygen compounds. Believed to have originated from both plant and animal sources millions of years ago. When petroleum is cracked into fractions, the gases butane, ethane, and propane, as well as naphtha, gasoline, kerosene, fuel oils, gas oil, lubricating oils, paraffin wax, and asphalt are obtained. A defoaming ingredient in cosmetics and yeast and a coating on cheese, raw fruits, and vegetables. Used as a coating on eggshells; in froth-flotation cleaning of vegetables; as a float on fermentation fluids; in the manufacture of vinegar, wine, and pickle brine; as a component of pesticide formulations; as a defoamer in processing beet sugar and yeast; in modified hop extract of beer; and in many other formulations. Formerly used for bronchitis and tapeworm, and externally for arthritis and skin problems. Many petroleum products are reported to be cancer-causing ingredients. Others, presumably those used on food, are inert. The CIR Expert Panel *(see)* concludes that these are safe as a cosmetic ingredients as currently used.

PEUCEDANUM GRAVEOLENS • See Dill.

pH • The scale used to measure acidity and alkalinity. pH is the hydrogen (H) ion concentration of a solution; "p" stands for the power factor of the hydrogen ion. The pH of a solution is measured on a scale of 14. A truly neutral solution, neither acidic nor alkaline, such as water, is 7. Acid is less than 7; alkaline is more than 7. The pH of blood is 7.3; vinegar is 3.1; lemon juice is 2.3; and lye is 13. Skin and hair are naturally acidic. Soap and detergents are alkaline.

PHASEOLUS • See Green Bean Extract and Kidney Bean Extract.

PHELLODENDRON • **Oubaku.** A family of aromatic trees of Eastern Asia that have greenish yellow flowers. Used in Eastern medicine to treat boils, carbuncles, and eczema. It is usually pounded with talc.

PHENACETIN • **Acetophenetidin.** Obtained from phenol and salicylic acid *(see both)*. Slightly bitter, crystalline powder, used in sunscreen lotions and soothing creams. Used medicinally as an analgesic and antifever ingredient. Less toxic than acetanilid *(see),* but may cause kidney damage in prolonged and excessive internal doses. No known toxicity on the skin.

PHENETHYL ALCOHOL • **2-Phenylethyanol.** Used as a floral scent in rose perfumes and as a preservative in cosmetics. It occurs naturally in oranges, raspberries, and tea. Used in synthetic fruit flavorings. In some studies it was found to cause birth defects in rats. It was not shown to be an irritant or sensitizer in humans. The CIR Expert Panel *(see)* concludes that is safe as a cosmetic ingredient as currently used.

PHENOL • Carbolic Acid. Used in shaving creams and hand lotions. Obtained from coal tar. Occurs in urine and has the characteristic odor present in coal tar and wood. It is a general disinfectant and anesthetic for the skin. Ingestion of even small amounts may cause nausea, vomiting, and circulatory collapse, paralysis, convulsions, coma, and greenish urine as well as necrosis of the mouth and gastrointestinal tract. Death results from respiratory failure. Fatalities have been reported from ingestion of as little as 1.5 grams (30 grams to the ounce). Fatal poisoning can occur through skin absorption. Although there have been many poisonings from phenolic solutions, it continues to be used in commercial products. A concentration of 1 percent used to prevent itching from insect bites and sunburn, applied for several hours, caused gangrene resulting from spasm of small blood vessels under the skin. Swelling, pimples, hives, and other skin rashes following application to the skin have been widely reported. A concentration of 2 percent causes gangrene, burning, and numbness.

PHENOXYETHANOL • 2-Phenoxyethanol. Oily liquid with a faint aromatic odor and a burning taste derived from treating phenol with ethylene oxide in an alkaline medium. Widely used as a fixative for perfumes, bactericide, insect repellent, and topical antiseptic. Also used as a fragrance. It is in many cosmetics including hairsprays, bubble baths, eye lotions, skin and body preparations, makeup, makeup removers, and shampoos. Undiluted, it is a strong eye irritant but is not irritating when diluted at 2.2 percent. It has not been found to be a skin irritant or sensitizer. The CIR Expert Panel *(see)* concludes that it is safe as a cosmetic ingredient as currently used. See Phenol.

PHENOXYISOPROPANOL • 1-Phenoxy-2-Propanol. See Phenol.

PHENYL ACETALDEHYDE • Used in perfumes. An oily, colorless liquid with a harsh odor. Upon dilution, emits the fragrance of lilacs and hyacinths. Derived from phenethyl alcohol. Less irritating than formaldehyde *(see),* but a stronger central nervous system depressant. In addition, it sometimes produces fluid in the lungs upon ingestion. Because it is considered an irritant, it is not used in cosmetic preparations for babies.

PHENYL ANTHRANILATES • See Coal Tar.

PHENYL BENZOATE • Used in fragrances. See Benzoic Acid.

PHENYL GLYCINE • See Glycine.

PHENYL METHYL PYRAZOLONE • A white powder made from phenylhydrazine with ethyl acetoacetate used as an intermediate in hair dyes and plastics. See Pyrazole.

o-PHENYLPHENOL • White, flaky crystals with a mild characteristic odor. Prepared from phenyl ether. Practically insoluble in water. An intermediate in the manufacture of cosmetic resins. Also a germicide and fungicide in cosmetics. See Phenol for toxicity.

N-PHENYL-p-PHENYLENEDIAMINE • 4-Amino Diphenylamine. White crystals, very soluble in alcohol. Used in hair dyes. Intense skin irritation and blisters reported. Similar to other compounds of the group.

N-PHENYL-p-PHENYLENEDIAMINE HCL • White crystals, slightly soluble in water. A constituent of hair dyes. Derived from diphenolic acid *(see)*. Probably of moderate toxicity, but reports of several skin rashes from its use have been described in the literature. It is thought to be less irritating than its parent compound.

PHENYL SALICYLATE • See Salicylates.

PHENYL THIOGLYCOLIC ACID • See Thioglycolic Acid Compounds.

PHENYL TRIMETHICONE • Methyl Phenyl Polysiloxane. Silicone oil used as a skin protectant and to give it gloss. It is treated to make it water-repellent. The CIR Expert Panel *(see)* concludes that it is safe as a cosmetic ingredient as currently used. See Silicones.

PHENYLACETIC ACID • Used as a starting material in the manufacture of perfumes and soaps. Occurs naturally in Japanese mint, oil of neroli, and black pepper. It has a honeylike odor. Also used as a synthetic flavoring for foods and in the manufacture of penicillin. No known toxicity.

PHENYLALANINE • An amino acid *(see)* considered essential for growth in normal human beings and not synthesized by the body. It is associated with phenylketonuria (PKU), an affliction that, if not detected soon after birth, leads to mental deterioration in children. Restricting phenylalanine in diets results in improvement. Whole egg contains 5.4 percent and skim milk 5.1 percent. Used to improve penetration of emollients. The FDA has asked for further study of this amino acid as a food additive. In cosmetics it is used in hair conditioners.

PHENYLDIMETHICONE • A mixture of silica gels used in tanning creams. See Dimethicone.

m-PHENYLENE DIAMINE SULFATE • See Phenylenediamine.

p-PHENYLENE DIAMINE SULFATE • See Phenylenediamine.

PHENYLENEDIAMINE, m-,o-,p- • Most permanent home and beauty parlor dyes contain this chemical or a related one such as 4-nitro-*o*-phenylenediamine. Also called oxidation dyes, amino dyes, para dyes, or peroxide dyes. PPD was first introduced in 1890 for dyeing furs and feathers. It comes in about 30 shades and is used as an intermediate in coal tar dyes. May produce eczema, bronchial asthma, gastritis, skin rash, and death. Can cross-react with many other chemicals, including azo dyes used for temporary hair colorings. Can also produce photosensitization. It has reportedly caused cancer in some animal experiments and not in others. In 1979, the National Cancer Institute reported tests showing coal tar ingredients in some permanent hair dyes caused cancer when fed to laboratory rats. The Food and Drug Administration then announced it was powerless to ban the suspect hair dyes since they were exempted from such action by the 1938 Food, Drug and Cosmetic Act. The FDA tried to make manufacturers put a warning label on the hair dye containers, but the cosmetic manufacturers successfully defeated that. The manufacturers, after the publicity, voluntarily removed a commonly used permanent hair coloring, 4-MMPD—4-methoxy-*m*-phenylenediamine—one of six hair dyes found to cause cancer in animals. The others were 2,4-toluene diamine (used in a few permanent hair colors), 4-amino-2-nitrophenol, and 2-nitrophenylenediamine (used in many gold and reddish shade highlighters), Direct Black 38; and Direct Blue 6 (both voluntarily removed from hair dyes). Bruce Ames reported in 1978 that 150 semipermanent hair dyes he tested (*see* Ames Test) were mutagenic. An estimated 70 to 75 percent of the carcinogens showed up as mutagens in his test. In January 1978, NIOSH reported that a new study of beauticians and cosmetologists showed they have a higher-than-expected incidence of six kinds of cancer. That study, along with NCI's findings, led NIOSH to recommend that 2,4-diaminoanisole be treated as a human carcinogen. On April 6, 1978, the FDA issued an order that manufacturers place warnings on the labels of some permanent hair dyes that read "Warning: contains an ingredient that can penetrate your skin and has been determined to cause cancer in laboratory animals." The FDA also proposed that beauty parlors post notices urging customers to check the labels on products used in salons. The industry representatives successfully fought these suggestions and, as of this writing, no signs are posted and the labels do not carry warnings. The FDA still has no power to ban the ingredients in hair dyes or even require manufacturers to demonstrate safety. Not everyone agrees hair dyes are dangerous. Dr. E. Cuyler Hammond of the American Cancer Society conducted a 13-year test of 5,000 hairdressers and a matched group of nonhairdressers and did not find any difference in the groups. However, the ACS on February 22, 1978, did issue a statement that said: "The results of studies among beauticians and women who use hair dyes have been mixed. But the regulatory agencies feel that in the absence of hard data, they must be cautious. They feel that because of the wide use by the public, even a small potential risk of cancer caused by little exposure could be associated with significant additional cancer cases. While available information does not prove or disprove that hair dyes cause cancer in humans, the ACS advises caution in the use of the substances under question until more definitive evidence is developed."

A study by New York University researchers suggests that women who have used hair dye for 10 years or more face an increased risk of developing breast cancer. In this study, published in the February 1979 issue of the *Journal of the National Cancer Institute,* the use of hair dye by 129 women with breast cancer was compared to 193 matched controls. In 1981, F. N. Marzulli and his colleagues at the FDA's Division of Toxicology reported skin penetration by five substances present in cosmetics. The greatest skin penetration was recorded with 2,4-toluenediamine and the least with 2,4-diaminoanisole when applied to the skin of monkeys and humans. They found 2-nitro-*p*-phenylenediamine and *N*-nitrosodiethanolamine showed intermediate degrees of skin penetration. Other researchers reported that hair dye containing *p*-toluenediamine sulfate (2,5-diaminotoluene) resulted in human absorption of about 0.2 percent of the material if the dye was left on for 40 minutes and then rinsed off. The CIR Expert Panel *(see)* concludes that these ingredients are safe as currently used. Dr. John Bailey of the FDA agrees that they are safe as currently used but, check his quotations and the results of scientific studies concerning the dyes in the Introduction. The final proof about whether hair dyes based on coal tar are carcinogenic or not is not available. The CIR *(see)* and many other regulatory and scientific groups are studying the phenylenediamine family of chemicals. See also Hair Coloring.

p-PHENYLEPHRINE HCL • **Hydrochloride.** Same as nasal decongestant Neo-Synephrine HCL®. Used topically to contract blood vessels and as a nasal decongestant; also in eye lotions to "take the red out." Prepared from *m*-hydroxy-*w*-chloroacetophenone and methylamine in water-alcohol solution. Some hypersensitive individuals may experience a mild stinging sensation. Prolonged exposure to air, metal, or strong light will cause oxidation and some loss of potency. Therefore, deeply discolored solutions, although harmless, should be discarded.

PHENYLETHYL PHENYL ACETATE • A synthetic fruit and honey–flavoring ingredient for beverages, ice cream, ices, candy, maraschino cherries, and baked goods. See Coal Tar.

PHENYLMERCURIC ACETATE • White, creamy prisms derived from benzene and mercuric acetate. Used as a preservative, fungicide, herbicide, mildewicide for paints, and to keep swimming pool water free of slime. Slightly soluble in water. Very toxic internally, and blisters have been reported when it is applied to the skin. Also toxic by inhalation. See Mercury.

PHENYLMERCURIC BENZOATE • See Benzoic Acid and Mercury Compounds.

PHENYLMERCURIC BORATE • Crystalline powder. Soluble in water and alcohol. Local external antiseptic. Much less toxic than most mercury compounds.

PHILODENDRON • The extract of powdered bark of *Philodendron,* a genus of a tropical, American, climbing plant.

PHLOROGLUCINOL • An antioxidant prepared from various acids for use in hair dyes. Consists of white crystals with a sweet taste. Discolors in the light. The aqueous solution gives a blue-violet color. The CIR Expert Panel *(see)* concludes that it cannot conclude it is safe for use in cosmetic products until the appropriate safety data have been obtained and evaluated. See Pyrogallol for toxicity.

PHOSPHATE • A salt of ester of phosphoric acid *(see).* Used as an emulsifier, texturizer, and sequestrant in cosmetics and foods. No known toxicity.

PHOSPHATE ESTERS, ORGANIC • See Phosphate and Esters.

PHOSPHOLIPIDS • **Phosphatides.** Complex fat substances found in all living cells. Lecithin is an example. Widely used in hand creams and lotions. Phospholipids contain phosphoric acid and nitrogen, and are soluble in the usual fat solvents, with the exception of acetone *(see).* They are used in moisturizers because they bind water and hold it in place. No known toxicity.

PHOSPHORIC ACID • An acid, sequestrant, and antioxidant used in hair tonics, nail polishes, and skin fresheners. A colorless, odorless solution made from phosphate rock. Mixes with water and alcohol. No known toxicity in cosmetic use. Concentrated solutions are irritating to the skin.

PHOSPHORIC ANHYDRIDE • Soft, white powder absorbs moisture from the air. Derived by burning phosphorus in dry air. Used in surfactants *(see).*

PHOTOSENSITIVITY • A condition in which the application or ingestion of certain chemicals, such as propylparaben *(see)*, causes skin problems—including rash, hyperpigmentation, and swelling—when the skin is exposed to sunlight. In a five-year study at Columbia Presbyterian Medical Center in New York, photosensitivity responses were most often due to fragrance ingredients (musk ambrette and 6-methyl coumarin) and sunscreen ingredients (*p*-aminobenzoic acid and esters and oxybenzone). The Columbia researchers concluded that photoallergy due to fragrances is declining, whereas reactions to sunscreen ingredients, in particular oxybenzone, are increasing.

PHOTOTOXICITY • Reaction to sunlight or ultraviolet light resulting in inflammation.

PHTHALATES • A large group of chemical compounds used in the production of plastics, household articles, packages, cosmetics, and plant pesticides. World production of phthalates is estimated to be several million tons a year. Recent observations indicate some may be mutagenic, cancer-causing, and adversely affect human male sperm. The Instituto de Medicina Forense Framboyanes in Veracruz, Mexico, is now studying the effect of phthalates on sperm. See Phthalic Acid.

PHTHALIC ACID • Obtained by the oxidation of various benzene derivatives, it can be isolated from the fungus *Gibberella fujikuroi*. When rapidly heated, it forms phthalic anhydride *(see)* and water. It is used chiefly in the manufacture of cosmetic esters, dyes, and nail polishes. Moderately irritating to the skin and mucous membranes.

PHTHALIC ANHYDRIDE • Prepared from naphthalene by oxidation, it consists of lustrous white needles. It is used in the manufacture of cosmetic dyes and artificial resins. It is moderately irritating to the skin and mucous membranes.

PHTHALIC/TRIMELLITIC/GLYCOLS COPOLYMER • See Phthalic Anhydride and Polymer.

PHYSALIS ALKEKENGI • See Cherry Pit Oil.

PHYSOSTIGMINE • Eserine. Antilirium. Obtained from the dried ripe seed (Calabar bean) of *Physostigma venenosum*. It is used topically to produce a contraction of the pupil and decrease pressure inside the eye in glaucoma. It is used to inhibit the destruction of acetylcholine *(see)*. It is also used to treat central nervous system toxicity associated with tricyclic antidepressant and anticholinergic poisonings and experimentally to treat Alzheimer's disease.

PHYTIC ACID • Occurs in nature in the seeds of cereal grains and is derived commercially from corn. It is used to chelate heavy metals, as a rust inhibitor, in metal cleaning, and in the treatment of hard water. Nontoxic, although those allergic to corn may have a reaction.

PHYTOL • An alcohol obtained by the decomposition of chlorophyll.

PHYTOLACCA DECANDRA • A tropical herb.

PHYTONADIONE • Vitamin K.

PHYTOSOMES • A new term cosmetologists are using for the combination of liposomes *(see)* and plant extracts. They claim that the desirable substances then pass more easily through the skin. In the works are phytosomes to carry catechin, quercitron, escin, and glycyrrhetinic acid *(see all)*.

PHYTOSPHINGOSINE • A fatty alcohol used as a skin and hair conditioning ingredient.

PHYTOSTEROLS • Plant fatty alcohols.

PICEA EXCELSA • See Norway Spruce Extract.

PICES MARINE COLLAGEN • A source of collagen from cod and pollack skin. It has a high collagen content and is almost odorless. It is claimed to be pathogen-free, unlike bovine collagen, which is not always free of contaminants.

PICHI • *Fabiana imbricata.* A Peruvian shrub whose herbage yields a tonic and diuretic. It is used in "organic" cosmetics.

PICRAMIC ACID • **4, 6-Dinitro-2-Aminophenol.** A red, crystalline acid obtained from phenol *(see)* and used chiefly in making azo dyes *(see)*. Highly toxic material. Readily absorbed through intact skin. Vapors absorbed through respiratory tract. Produces marked increase in metabolism and temperature, profuse sweating, collapse, and death. May cause skin rash, cataracts, and weight loss.

PIGMENT BLUE 15 • Classed chemically as a phthalocyanine (copper complex) color. See Chlorophyllin and Colors.

PIGMENT BLUE 15:2 • The solvent stable form of pigment blue prepared by the introduction of chlorine.

PIGMENT GREEN 7 • Classed chemically as a phthalocyanine (copper complex) color. See Chlorophyllin and Colors.

PIGMENT ORANGE 5 • A monoazo color whose name can be used only when applied to batches of uncertified colors. The CTFA name for certified batches is D & C Orange No. 17 *(see)*.

PIGMENT RED 4 • A monoazo color whose name can be used only when applied to batches of uncertified color. The CTFA adopted name for certified batches is D & C Red No. 36 *(see)*.

PIGMENT RED 5 • A monoazo color *(see)*.

PIGMENT RED 48:4 • A monoazo color *(see)*.

PIGMENT RED 53 • A monoazo color whose name can be used only when applied to batches of uncertified color. The CTFA adopted name for certified batches is D & C Red No. 8.

PIGMENT RED 53:1 • The barium salt of Pigment Red 53, whose name can be applied only to uncertified batches of color. The CTFA adopted name for certified color batches is D & C Red No. 9.

PIGMENT RED 57 • A monoazo color whose name can be applied only to uncertified batches of color. The CTFA adopted name for certified batches is D & C Red No. 6.

PIGMENT RED 57:1 • A monoazo color, it is the calcium salt of Pigment Red No. 57. The name can be applied only to batches of uncertified color. The CTFA adopted name for certified batches is D & C Red. No. 7.

PIGMENT RED 57:2 BARIUM LAKE • An insoluble color composed of the barium salt of Pigment Red 57. The CTFA name for the uncertified batch of this color is D & C Red No. 6 Barium Lake.

PIGMENT RED 63:1 • A monoazo color whose name can be used only for batches of uncertified color. The CTFA adopted name for certified batches is D & C Red No. 34.

PIGMENT RED 64:1 • A monoazo color whose name can be applied only to uncertified batches. The CTFA adopted name for certified batches is D & C Red. No. 31.

PIGMENT RED 68 • A monoazo color *(see)*.

PIGMENT RED 90:1 ALUMINUM LAKE • An insoluble pigment composed of the aluminum salt of Solvent Red 43. The CTFA name for the certified batches of this color is D & C Red No. 21 Aluminum Lake.

PIGMENT RED 112 • A monoazo color. See Azo Dyes.

PIGMENT RED 172 ALUMINUM LAKE • The insoluble pigment composed of the aluminum salt of Acid Red 51. The CTFA certified name of this color is FD & C Red No. 3 Aluminum Lake. It has been prohibited in cosmetic products in the United States. Its use as a cosmetic colorant may also be restricted in other countries.

PIGMENT RED 173 ALUMINUM LAKE • An insoluble pigment composed of the aluminum salt of Basic Violet 10. The CTFA name for certified batches of this color is D & C Red No. 19 Aluminum Lake. This color has been prohibited in cosmetic products in the United States. Its use as a cosmetic colorant may also be restricted in other countries.

PIGMENT VIOLET 19 • A quinacridone color. A light fast pigment derived from coal tar *(see)*. It provides a wide range of shades, and cosmetic manufacturers are increasing its use.

PIGMENT YELLOW 1 • A monoazo color. See Azo Dyes.

PIGMENT YELLOW 3 • A monoazo color. See Azo Dyes.

PIGMENT YELLOW 12 • A diazo color. See Azo Dyes.

PIGMENT YELLOW 13 • A diazo color. See Azo Dyes.

PIGMENT YELLOW 73 • A monoazo color. See Azo Dyes.

PIGSKIN EXTRACT • An extract of the skin of young pigs. Used in hand and hair conditioners.

PILEWORT EXTRACT • An extract of *Ranunculus ficuria,* the coarse, hairy, perennial figwort of the eastern and central United States. It was once used to treat tuberculosis. No known toxicity.

PILOCARPINE • Used in hair tonic to stimulate the sweat glands. Derived from a tree grown in Brazil and Paraguay. Soluble in water, alcohol, and chloroform. White, water-absorbing crystals with a bitter taste. Also an antidote for atropine poisoning. Readily absorbed through the skin from the concentrations employed in hair tonics. High concentrations are known to be irritating and toxic, but no available information on toxicity in cosmetics is reported.

PIMENTA LEAF OIL • Jamaica Pepper. Allspice. Derived from the dried ripe fruit of the evergreen shrub grown in the West Indies and Central and South

America. Used in raspberry, fruit, nut, and spice flavorings for beverages, ice cream, ices, candy, baked goods, gelatin desserts, chewing gum, condiments, and meat products. Moderately toxic by ingestion. A severe skin irritant. GRAS.

PIMPINELLA ANISUM • See Anise.

PINECONE EXTRACT • An extract from the cones of *Pinus sylvestris*. See Pine Oil.

PINE NEEDLE EXTRACT • An extract of various species of *Pinus* used to scent bath products and as a natural flavoring in pineapple, citrus, and spice flavorings. Ingestion of large amounts can cause intestinal hemorrhage.

PINE OIL • The extract from a variety of pine trees. As a pine tar it is used in hair tonics; also a solvent, disinfectant, and deodorant. As an oil from twigs and needles, it is used in pine bath-oil emulsions, bath salts, and perfumery. Irritating to the skin and mucous membranes. Bornyl acetate, a substance obtained from various pine needles, has a strong pine odor and is used in bath oils. It can cause nausea, vomiting, convulsions, and dizziness if ingested. In general, pine oil in concentrated form is an irritant to human skin and may cause allergic reactions. In small amounts it is nontoxic.

PINE TAR • A product obtained by the distillation of pinewood. A blackish brown, viscous liquid, slightly soluble in water. Used as an antiseptic in skin diseases. May be irritating to the skin.

PINE TAR OIL • A synthetic flavoring obtained from pinewood and used in licorice flavorings for ice cream and candy. Used as a solvent, disinfectant, and deodorant in cosmetics. May be irritating to the skin and mucous membranes, and large ingested doses cause central nervous system depression.

PINEAPPLE EXTRACT • See Pineapple Juice.

PINEAPPLE JUICE • The common juice from the tropical plant. Contains a protein-digesting and milk-clotting enzyme, bromelin *(see)*. An anti-inflammatory enzyme, it is used in cosmetic treatment creams. It is also used as a texturizer. No known toxicity.

PINUS PUMILIO OIL • **Oil of Dwarf Pine Needles. Oil of Mountain Pine.** *Pinus montana.* Colorless or faintly yellow liquid with a pleasant odor. Used in flavoring and perfume. Used medically as an expectorant.

PINUS SYLVESTRIS OIL • See Pinus Pumilio Oil.

PIPER • See Pepper Oil, Black.

PIPERAZINE • **Adipate and Citrate. Entacyl. Antepar. Bryrel. Pin-Tega Tabs. Pipril. Ta-Verm. Vermirex. Vermizine.** An anthelmintic ingredient that paralyzes worms, causing their expulsion by normal movement of the human intestines. Adverse reactions include incoordination, numbness, seizures, memory problems, headache, dizziness, eye problems, nausea, vomiting, diarrhea, abdominal cramps, hives, skin rashes, joint pain, fever, bronchospasm, and anemia.

PIPERIDINE • A synthetic flavoring that occurs naturally in black pepper. Used in beverages, candy, baked goods, meats, soups, and condiments. Soapy texture. Has been proposed for use as a tranquilizer and muscle relaxant. No known toxicity.

PIPERITONE • A synthetic flavoring ingredient that occurs naturally in Japanese mint. Used to give dentifrices a minty flavor and to give perfumes their peppermint scent. No known toxicity.

PIPERONAL • **Heliotropin.** A synthetic flavoring and perfume ingredient that occurs naturally in vanilla and black pepper. White crystalline powder with a sweet floral odor. Used chiefly in perfumery. Ingestion of large amounts may cause central nervous system depression. Has been reported to cause skin rash. In lipsticks, said to produce marking of the skin. Not recommended by some cosmetic chemists because of its ability to produce skin irritation.

PIPERONYL BUTOXIDE • **A-200 Pediculicide Shampoo. Lice. Enz Foam. Pronto Lice Killing Shampoo. R & C Shampoo. Rid Lice Killing Shampoo.** A compound derived from petroleum used in combination with pyrethrins to treat skin parasites. For external use only. Should not be inhaled or used on irritated, infected, or broken skin. Should not be used by a person sensitive to ragweed. Harmful if swallowed.

PISCUM LECUR • **Fish Liver Oil.**

PISUM SATIVUM • **Pea Extract.**

PISTACHIA VERA • See Pistachio Nut Oil.

PISTACHIO NUT OIL • The oil from the nut of a small tree, *Pistaclum,* grown in Europe, Asia Minor, and recently in the United States.

PITUITARY HORMONES • **Pituitrin.** Used to stimulate smooth muscle contractions.

PLACENTAL ENZYMES, LIPIDS, AND PROTEINS • Derived from animal placenta, the vascular membrane that nourishes the fetus.

PLACENTAL EXTRACT • Prepared from the placenta, the nourishing lining of the human womb that is expelled after birth. Promoted by cosmetic manufacturers as capable of removing wrinkles. The American Medical Association maintains no such evidence has been presented, nor is it likely. (Even newborn babies emerge from the womb with wrinkled skin.) Nontoxic.

PLACENTAL PROTEIN • See Placental Extract.

PLANKTON EXTRACT • An extract of the marine organisms *Thalasso plankton,* a green micro-algae or seaweed.

PLANTAGO • See Plantain Extract.

PLANTAIN EXTRACT • The extract of various species of plantain. The starchy fruit is a staple item of diet throughout the tropics, and is used for bladder infections by herbalists. It is a natural astringent and antiseptic with soothing and cooling effects on blemishes and burns.

PLASTICIZERS • Chemicals added to natural and synthetic resins and rubbers to impart flexibility, workability, or distensibility without changing the chemical nature of the material. Dibutyl phthalate *(see)* is a plasticizer for nitrocellulose used in nail lacquers.

PLUM EXTRACT • The extract of the fruit of the plum tree, *Prunus domestica;* the American Indians boiled the wild plum and gargled with it to cure mouth sores.

PLUMERIA • See Frangipani.

PODOPHYLLUM PELTATUM EXTRACT • An ingredient in topical medications to treat warts. A few hours after podophyllin is applied to a wart, the growth becomes whitened and, in one to three days, begins to disintegrate. Podophyllin can cause severe irritation of normal skin. Therefore, petrolatum is usually applied on the perimeter of the wart to keep podophyllin from touching healthy tissue. It can be toxic if too much is absorbed into the body, causing confusion, diarrhea, abdominal pain, and convulsions. See Mayapple.

POGOSTEMON CABLIN • See Patchouli Oil.

POKEWEED • *Phytolacca americana.* **Pokeroot. Coakum.** Native to the southern United States and the Mediterranean area, the dried roots reduces inflammation and arthritic pains. It has antibiotic, antiviral, and anti-inflammatory properties. Among its constituents are tannin, formic acid, saponins, and alkaloids *(see all).* It is prescribed by herbalists for a variety of ailments, from swollen glands to weight loss. It is used in "organic" cosmetics. A member of the bloodberry family, it is an emetic and laxative with narcotic properties. Both berries and roots contain a dangerous drug. Some people are more sensitive to pokeweed's adverse effects than others, and fatalities have occurred.

POLIANTHES TUBEROSA • See Tuberose Oil.

POLISH REMOVER • See Nail Polish Remover.

POLISHING INGREDIENTS • Used in dentrifices to shine teeth. Even after removing debris and stains, teeth may still be dull. Polishing whitens and brightens teeth, and teeth that are polished are less receptive to dental plaque. Substances used to polish teeth are hydrated alumina, sodium metaphosphate, calcium phosphate, and calcium carbonate *(see all).*

POLLEN EXTRACT • An extract of flower pollen.

POLOXAMER 101 THROUGH 407 • See Poloxamer 188.

POLOXAMER 188 • **Poloxalene.** A liquid, nonionic, surfactant polymer. If chain lengths of polyoxyethylene and polyoxypropylene are increased, the product changes from liquid to paste to solid. No known toxicity. See Polymer.

POLOXAMINE 304 TO 1508 • The polyethylene, polyoxypropylene block of polymer of ethylenediamine. The numbers signify the various properties of the chemicals and whether one is to be used in food, drugs, or cosmetics. In cosmetics, it is used primarily as a surfactant *(see).*

POLY- • A prefix meaning many.

POLYACRYLAMIDE • The polymer of acrylamide monomers, it is white, solid, water-soluble, and used as a thickening ingredient, suspending ingredient, and an additive to adhesives. Used in tanning creams. Used in the manufacture of plastics and in nail polishes. Highly toxic and irritating to the skin. Causes central nervous system paralysis. Can be absorbed through unbroken skin. The CIR Expert Panel *(see)* concludes that it is safe as a cosmetic ingredient if used at less than 0.01 percent.

POLYACRYLIC ACID • See Acrylic Resins.

POLYAMINO SUGAR CONDENSATE • A skin conditioner and humectant. The condensation product of the sugars fructose, galactose, glucose, lactose, maltose, mannose, rhamnose, ribose, or xylose, with a minute amount of amino acids such as alanine, arginine, aspartic acid, glutamic acid, glycine, histidine, hydroxyproline, isoleucine, leucine, lysine, methionine, phenylalanine, proline, pyroglutamic acid, serine, threonine, tyrosine, or valine. The CIR Expert Panel *(see)* concludes that it is safe as a cosmetic ingredient as currently used. See Amino Acids.

POLYBETA-ALANINE • See Alanine.

POLYBUTENE • **Indopol. Polybutylene.** A plasticizer. A polymer *(see)* of one or more butylenes obtained from petroleum oils. Used in lubricating oil, adhesives, sealing tape, cable insulation, films, and coatings. May asphyxiate. The CIR Expert Panel *(see)* concludes that it is safe as a cosmetic ingredient as currently used.

POLYCHLOROTRIFLUOROETHYLENE • Colorless, impervious to corrosive chemicals, it resists most organic solvents and heat. Nonflammable. Used as a transparent film.

POLYDECENE • A polymerization of decylene. A colorless liquid used in flavors and fragrances.

POLYETHYLENE • A polymer *(see)* of ethylene; a product of petroleum gas or dehydration of alcohol. One of a group of lightweight thermoplastics that have a good resistance to chemicals, low moisture absorption, and good insulating properties. Widely used in hand lotions. No known skin toxicity, but implants of large amounts in rats caused cancer. Ingestion of large oral doses has produced kidney and liver damage.

POLYETHYLENE 6000 OR MORE • Excellent barrier to water vapor and moisture, it resists solvents and corrosive solutions. It is combustible but nontoxic.

POLYETHYLENE GLYCOL • **PEG.** Used in hair straighteners, antiperspirants, baby products, fragrances, polish removers, hair tonics, lipsticks, and protective creams. It is a binder, plasticizing ingredient, solvent, and softener widely used for cosmetic cream bases and pharmaceutical ointments. Improves resistance to moisture and oxidation.

POLYGALA SENEGA • See Senega Extract.

POLYGLYCEROL • Prepared from edible fats, oils, and esters of fatty acids. Derived from corn, cottonseed, palm, peanuts, safflower, sesame, and soybean oils, lard, and tallow. Used as an emulsifier in cosmetics. No known toxicity. See Glycerol.

POLYGLYCEROL ESTER • One of several partial or complete esters of saturated and unsaturated fatty acids with a variety of derivatives of polyglycerols ranging from diglycerol to triglycerol. Used as lubricants, plasticizers, gelling ingredients, humectants, surface-active ingredients, dispersants, and emulsifiers in foods and cosmetic preparations.

POLYGLYCERYL-4 COCOATE • See Coconut Acid and Polyglycerol.

POLYGLYCERYL-10 DECALINOLEATE • See Glycerin and Linoleic Acid.

POLYGLYCERYL-10 DECAOLEATE • See Oleic Acid and Polyglycerol.

POLYGLYCERYL-2 DIISOSTEARATE • See Isostearic Acid and Polyglycerol.

POLYGLYCERYL-6 DIOLEATE • See Oleic Acid and Glycerin.

POLYGLYCERYL-6 DISTEARATE • See Stearic Acid and Glycerin.

POLYGLYCERYL-3 HYDROXYLAURYL ETHER • See Lauryl Alcohol and Glycerin.

POLYGLYCERYL-4 ISOSTEARATE • See Isostearic Acid and Glycerin.

POLYGLYCERYL-2 LANOLIN ALCOHOL ETHER • See Lanolin Alcohol and Glycerin.

POLYGLYCERYL-LAURYL ETHER • See Lauryl Alcohol and Glycerin.

POLYGLYCERYL-3 OR -4 OLEATE • Oily liquid prepared by adding alcohol to coconut oil or other triglycerides with a polyglyceryl. Used in foods, drugs, and cosmetics as fat emulsifiers in conjunction with other emulsifiers to prepare creams, lotions, and other emulsion products. In addition, they may also be used as lubricants, plasticizers, gelling ingredients, and dispersants. No known toxicity.

POLYGLYCERYL-2 OR -4 OLEYL ETHER • The ether of oleyl alcohol and glycerin *(see both)* polymer.

POLYGLYCERYL-3-PEG-2 COCOAMIDE • See Coconut Oil and Glycerin.

POLYGLYCERYL-2-PEG-4 STEARATE • An ether of PEG-4 stearate *(see)* and glycerin *(see)*.

POLYGLYCERYL-2-SESQUIISOSTEARATE • A mixture of esters of isostearic acid and glycerin *(see both)*.

POLYGLYCERYL-2-SESQUIOLEATE • A mixture of ester of oleic acid and glycerin *(see both)*.

POLYGLYCERYL SORBITOL • A condensation product of glycerin and sorbitol *(see both)*.

POLYGLYCERYL-3, -4, OR -8 STEARATE • An ester of stearic acid and glycerin *(see both)*.

POLYGLYCERYL-10 TETRAOLEATE • An ester of oleic acid and glycerin *(see both)*.

POLYGLYCERYL-2 TETRASTEARATE • See Stearic Acid and Glycerin.

POLYGONATUM OFFICINALE • **Solomon's Seal.** See Buckwheat Extract.

POLYGONUM • A large family of herbs. See Knotweed Extract.

POLYHYDROXYSTEARIC ACID • A widely used suspending ingredient in cosmetics.

POLYISOBUTENE • See Polybutene.

POLYISOPRENE • The major component of natural rubber but also made synthetically. Nontoxic.

POLYMER • A substance or product formed by combining many small molecules (monomers). The result is, essentially, recurring long-chain structural units that have tensile strength, elasticity, and hardness. Examples of polymers (literally, having many parts) are plastics, fibers, rubber, and human tissue.

POLYMETHYL METHACRYLATE • A widely-used film-former in many creams, makeup, powders and skin care products. See Acrylates.

POLYMYXIN B • Aerosporin. Aquaphor Antibiotic Ointment. Bactine First Aid Antibiotic. Campho Penique Triple Antibiotic Ointment. Mycitracin. Neosporin Cream and Ointment. Polysporin Ointment. An antibacterial drug mainly used topically to treat infections of the skin, eyes, and ears. May cause hives, fever, and possibly fatal allergic reactions.

POLYNAPHTHALENE SULFONATE • Used as a solvent in wrinkle creams. See Naphthalene.

POLYOLS • Alcohol compounds that absorb moisture. They have a low molecular weight: polyols with a weight above 1,000 are solids and less toxic than those that weigh 600 or below. The latter are liquid and, although higher in toxicity, very large doses are required to kill animals. Such deaths in animals have been found to be due to kidney damage. See Propylene Glycol and Polyethylene Glycol as examples.

POLYOXYETHYLENE COMPOUNDS • The nonionic emulsifiers used in hand creams and lotions. Usually oily or waxy liquids. No known toxicity.

POLYOXYMETHYLENE UREA • A bulking ingredient. The CIR Expert Panel *(see)* concludes that it is safe as a cosmetic ingredient but should not be used in aerosols. See Urea.

POLYOXYPROPYLENE GLYCOL • A mixture of polymers of ethylene oxide and propylene glycol *(see)* used as emollients, antistatic agents, and surfactants.

POLYPOROUS UMBELLATUS • See Mushroom Extract.

POLYPROPYLENE GLYCOL • 1,2-Propanediol. A clear, colorless, viscous liquid, slightly bitter-tasting, derived from propylene oxide. In cosmetics it is the most common moisture-carrying vehicle other than water itself. It has better permeation through the skin than glycerin and is less expensive, although it has been linked to more sensitivity reactions. Absorbs moisture, acts as a solvent and a wetting ingredient. Used in liquid makeup, as a solvent for fats and oils, waxes, and resins; in cellophane, antifreeze solution, brake fluids, humectants, and preservatives. It is being reduced and replaced by safer glycols, such as butylene and polyethylene glycol.

POLYQUARTERNIUM 1 THROUGH 14 • Antistatic ingredients and filmformers. See Quaternary Ammonium Compounds.

POLYSACCHARIDES • Carbohydrates that are organic compounds consisting of carbon, hydrogen, and oxygen. The polysaccharides include starch, dextrin, glycogen, and cellulose.

POLYSILICONES • Used in lipsticks and hair products as a fixative. See Silicones.

POLYSORBATE 40 • Widely used as an emulsifier in cosmetic creams and lotions and as a stabilizer of essential oils in water. All the polysorbates are nontoxic. The CIR Expert Panel *(see)* concludes that it is safe as a cosmetic ingredient as currently used.

POLYSORBATE 60 AND POLYSORBATE 80 • Both are emulsifiers that have been associated with the contaminant 1, 4 dioxane, known to cause cancer in animals. The 60 is a condensate of sorbitol with stearic acid, and the 80 is a condensate of sorbitol and oleic acid *(see all)*. The 60 is waxy and soluble in solvents. The 80 is a viscous liquid with a faint caramel odor and is widely used in baby lotions, cold creams, cream deodorants, antiperspirants, suntan lotions, and bath oil products. The CIR Expert Panel *(see)* concludes that these are safe as cosmetic ingredients as currently used.

POLYSORBATES 1 THROUGH 85 • These are widely used emulsifiers and stabilizers. For example, Polysorbate 20 is a viscous, oily liquid derived from lauric acid. It is an emulsifier used in cosmetic creams and lotions, and a stabilizer of essential oils in water. It is used as a nonionic surfactant *(see)*. Polysorbate 85 is used in tanning lotions. The CIR Expert Panel *(see)* concludes that these are safe as cosmetic ingredients as currently used.

POLYSTYRENE • Used in the manufacture of cosmetic resins. Colorless to yellowish oily liquid with a penetrating odor. Obtained from ethylbenzene by removing the hydrogen or by chlorination. Sparingly soluble in water; soluble in alcohol. Used in the manufacture of cosmetic resins. Used to make foam coffee cups, plates, and fast-food carry-out containers. May be irritating to the eyes and mucous membranes; in high concentrations, may be narcotic.

POLYSTYRENE LATEX • A white, plastic solid derived from petroleum and used in preparing opaque hair-waving lotions. It has outstanding moisture resistance. No known toxicity.

POLYURETHANE • A heat-tolerating plastic produced by condensation of polyisocyanate and a hydroxyl-containing material. Used in spandex fibers, for bristles, and for coatings. Urethane has been found to be carcinogenic in animals.

POLYVINYL ACETATE • A binder, emulsion stabilizer, film-former, and hair fixative. The CIR Expert Panel *(see)* concludes that it is safe as a cosmetic ingredient as currently used. See Polyvinylpyrrolidone.

POLYVINYL ALCOHOL • Synthetic resins used in lipstick, setting lotions, and various creams. A polymer prepared from polyvinyl acetates by replacement of the acetate groups with the hydroxyl groups. Dry, unplasticized polyvinyl alcohol powders are white to cream-colored and have different viscosity. Solvent in hot and cold water, but certain ones require alcohol-water mixtures. The CIR Expert Panel *(see)* concludes that it is safe as a cosmetic ingredient as currently used.

POLYVINYL BUTYRAL • The condensation of polyvinyl alcohol and butyraldehyde *(see both)*, it is a synthetic flavoring found in coffee and strawberry, and is used in the manufacture of rubber and synthetic resins and plasticizers. May be an irritant and narcotic.

POLYVINYL CHLORIDE • PVC. Chloroethylene Polymer. Derived from vinyl chloride *(see)*, it consists of a white powder or colorless granules that are resistant to weather, moisture, acids, fats, petroleum products, and fungus. It is widely used for everything from plumbing to raincoats. It is used in cosmetics and toiletries in containers, nail enamels, and creams. PVC has caused tumors when injected under the skin of rats in doses of 100 milligrams per kilogram of body weight.

POLYVINYL IMIDAZOLINIUM ACETATE • The polymer of vinyl imidazolinium acetate. See Polyvinylpyrrolidone.

POLYVINYL METHYL ETHER • See Polyvinyl Alcohol.

POLYVINYLPYRROLIDONE • PVP. A faintly yellow, solid, plastic resin resembling albumen. Used to give a softer set in shampoos, hairsprays, and lacquers; also a carrier in emollient creams, liquid lip rouge, and face rouge; also a clarifier in vinegar and a plasma expander in medicine. Ingestion may produce gas and fecal impaction or damage to lungs and kidneys. It may last in the system for months to a year. Strong circumstantial evidence indicates thesaurosis—foreign bodies in the lung—may be produced in susceptible individuals from concentrated exposure to PVP in hairsprays. Modest intravenous doses in rats caused them to develop tumors. The CIR Expert Panel says based on available data, it is safe as a cosmetic ingredient.

POMADES • Almost synonymous with solid brilliantines *(see)* but of older origin. Pomades were originally made with the residual fatty material left from the enfleurage process *(see)* of extracting floral odors. Poma (apples) were used, hence giving the hairdressing its name.

POMEGRANATE • *Punica granatum.* An extract of the fruit pomegranate.

PONCEAU SX • A monoazo color. The name can be applied only to uncertified batches of color. The CTFA adopted name for certified batches is FD & C Red. No. 4 *(see).*

PONGAMOL • A fragrance ingredient.

POPLAR EXTRACT • **Balm of Gilead.** Extract of the leaves and twigs of *Populus nigra.* In ancient times, the buds were mashed to make a soothing salve that was spread on sunburned areas, scalds, scratches, inflamed skin, and wounds. They were also simmered in lard for use as an ointment and for antiseptic purposes. The leaves and bark were steeped by American colonists to make a soothing tea. It supposedly helped allergies and soothed reddened eyes. No known toxicity.

POPPY OIL • A yellow to reddish oil obtained from the seeds of the poppy for use in emulsions and soaps and as a lubricant for fine machinery. Nontoxic.

POPULUS • See Poplar Extract.

PORIA COCOS • A fungi.

PORPHYRA UMBILICALIS • See Algae.

POTASSIUM • The healthy human body contains about nine grams of potassium. Most of it is found inside body cells. Potassium plays an important role in maintaining water balance and acid-base balance. It participates in the transmission of nerve impulses and in the transfer of messages from nerves to muscles. It also acts as a catalyst in carbohydrate and protein metabolism. Potassium is important for the maintenance of normal kidney function. It has a major effect on the heart and all the muscles of the body.

POTASSIUM ACETATE • White, crystalline, water-absorbing powder with a salt taste. Used in synthetic flavors and as a dehydrating ingredient.

POTASSIUM ACRYLINOLEATE • See Acrylinoleic Acid.

POTASSIUM ALGINATE • See Alginates.

POTASSIUM ALUM • See Alum.

POTASSIUM ALUMINUM POLYACRYLATE • A mixture of potassium and aluminum salts of polyacrylic acid used as an absorbant. See Acrylates.

POTASSIUM ASPARTATE • The potassium salt of aspartic acid *(see)*.

POTASSIUM BICARBONATE • **Carbonic Acid. Monopotassium Salt.** Colorless, odorless, transparent crystals or powder, slightly alkaline, with a salty taste. Used in baking, soft drinks, and low pH liquid detergents.

POTASSIUM BINOXALATE • **Potassium Acid Oxalate. Salt of Sorrel.** White odorless crystals, which are poisonous, used in nail bleaches and as a stain remover.

POTASSIUM BIPHTHALATE • **Phthalic Acid Potassium Acid Salt.** A buffer used to affect alkalinity/acidity ratios. See Phthalic Acid.

POTASSIUM BORATE • A crystalline salt used as an oxidizing ingredient and as a preservative in cosmetics and in flour. See Borates for toxicity.

POTASSIUM BROMATE • Antiseptic and astringent in toothpastes, mouthwashes, and gargles as a 3 to 5 percent solution. Colorless or white crystals. Very toxic when taken internally. Burns and skin irritation have been reported from its industrial uses. In toothpaste it has been reported to have caused inflammation and bleeding of gums. It is a weak carcinogen in rats in oral feedings. Applied to the animal skin, it was not carcinogenic. The CIR Expert Panel says based on available data, it is safe as a cosmetic ingredient not to exceed 10.17 percent.

POTASSIUM BUTYLPARABEN • See Parabens.

POTASSIUM CARBONATE • **Salt of Tartar. Pearl Ash.** Inorganic salt of potassium. Odorless, white powder soluble in water but practically insoluble in alcohol. Used in freckle lotions, liquid shampoos, vanishing creams, setting lotions, and permanent wave lotions; also in the manufacture of soap, glass, pottery, and to finish leather. Irritating and caustic to human skin, and may cause dermatitis of the scalp, forehead, and hands.

POTASSIUM CARRAGEENAN • The potassium salt of carrageenan *(see)*.

POTASSIUM CASEINATE • The potassium of milk proteins. See Casein.

POTASSIUM CASTORATE • The potassium salt of fatty acids derived from castor oil *(see)*.

POTASSIUM CETYL PHOSPHATE • A mixture of esters of phosophoric acid and cetyl alcohol *(see both)*.

POTASSIUM CHLORATE • Antiseptic, astringent in mouthwashes, toothpastes, and gargles as 2 to 5 percent solution. Used in bleach and freckle lotions and in permanent-wave solutions. A colorless or white powder that dissolves slowly in water. Also used in explosives, fireworks, matches, dyeing, and in printing. May be absorbed through the skin. Irritating to the intestines and kidneys. Can cause dermatitis of the scalp, forehead, and hands. In toothpastes, reported to have caused inflammation of the gums. The salts are toxic to humans. The safety of this ingredient has not been documented and substantiated, the CIR Expert Panel says that it cannot conclude whether potassium chlorate is safe for cosmetic products until such time that the appropriate safety data have been obtained and evaluated.

POTASSIUM CHLORIDE • Colorless or white crystals with a strong salty taste. It occurs naturally as sylvite deposits. Used in pharmaceutical and food additives as well as cosmetic ingredients. Ingestion of large doses can cause gastrointestinal irritation, purging, weakness, and circulatory collapse.

POTASSIUM COCOATE • See Coconut Oil.

POTASSIUM COCO-HYDROLYZED PROTEIN • Hair conditioner and cleansing ingredient. The CIR Expert Panel *(see)* concludes that it is safe as a cosmetic ingredient as currently used. See Hydrolyzed Protein.

POTASSIUM COCOYL HYDROLYZED COLLAGEN • The potassium salt of the condensation product of coconut acid and hydrolyzed collagen. See Collagen.

POTASSIUM CORNATE • The potassium salt of fatty acids derived from corn oil. See Corn Oil.

POTASSIUM CYCLOCARBOXYPROPYLOLEATE • The potassium salt of cyclocarboxypropyloleate.

POTASSIUM DIHYDROXYETHYL COCAMINE OXIDE PHOSPHATE • See Coconut Oil and Surfactants.

POTASSIUM DNA • The potassium salt of DNA *(see)*, used in "youth creams" and other creams in which protein is included.

POTASSIUM DODECYLBENZENE SULFONATE • See Quaternary Ammonium Compounds.

POTASSIUM ETHYLPARABEN • See Parabens.

POTASSIUM GLYCOL SULFATE • See Polyethylene Glycol.

POTASSIUM GUAIACOL SULFONATE • See Quaternary Ammonium Compounds.

POTASSIUM HYALURONATE • See Hyaluronic Acid.

POTASSIUM HYDROXIDE • **Caustic Potash.** Used as an emulsifier in hand lotions, as a cuticle softener, and as an alkali in liquid soaps, protective creams, shaving preparations, and cream rouges. Prepared industrially by electrolysis of potassium chloride *(see)*. White or slightly yellow lumps. It may cause irritation of the skin in cuticle removers. Extremely corrosive, and ingestion may cause violent pain, bleeding, collapse, and death. When applied to the skin of mice, moderate dosages cause tumors. May cause skin rash and burning. Concentrations above 5 percent can destroy fingernails as well. Good quality toilet soaps do not contain more than 0.25 percent free alkali.

POTASSIUM IODIDE • **Potassium Salt.** A dye remover and an antiseptic. Used in table salt as a source of dietary iodine. It is also in some drinking water. May cause allergic reactions.

POTASSIUM LAURATE • The potassium salt of lauric acid *(see)*.

POTASSIUM LAUROYL HYDROLYZED COLLAGEN • The potassium salt of the condensation product of lauric acid chloride and hydrolyzed collagen. See Hydrolyzed Collagen.

POTASSIUM LAURYL SULFATE • A water softener used in shampoos. See Sodium Lauryl Sulfate.

POTASSIUM METABISULFITE • Potassium Pyrosulfite. White granules or powder with a sharp odor, used as an antiseptic, preservative, antioxidant, and as a developing ingredient in dyes. Low toxicity.

POTASSIUM METHYLPARABEN • See Parabens.

POTASSIUM MYRISTATE • The potassium salt of myristic acid *(see)*.

POTASSIUM MYRISTOYL HYDROLYZED COLLAGEN • Potassium salt of the condensation product of myristic acid chloride and hydrolyzed collagen. See Hydrolyzed Collagen and Myristic Acid.

POTASSIUM OCTOXYNOL-12 PHOSPHATE • The potassium salt of a mixture of esters of phosphoric acid and octoxynol *(see both)*.

POTASSIUM OLEATE • Oleic Acid Potassium Salt. Used as a detergent. Yellowish or brownish soft mass. Soluble in water or alcohol. No known toxicity.

POTASSIUM OLEOYL HYDROLYZED COLLAGEN • The potassium salt of the condensation product of oleic acid chloride and hydrolyzed collagen *(see)*.

POTASSIUM PALMITATE • The potassium salt of palmitic acid *(see)*.

POTASSIUM PCA • See Proline.

POTASSIUM PERSULFATE • Colorless, or white, odorless crystals. A powerful oxidant. Soluble in water. The solution is acid and is used in the manufacture of soaps and as a germicidal preparation for the bathroom. Aqueous solutions of 2.5 to 3 percent are not irritating to humans. Twenty-five percent is irritating to animals.

POTASSIUM PHOSPHATE • Monobasic, Dibasic, and Tribasic. Used as a buffering ingredient in shampoos and in cuticle removers. Colorless to white powder, also used as a yeast food in brewing industries in the production of champagne and other sparkling wines. Has been used medicinally as a urinary acidifier. No known toxicity.

POTASSIUM POLYACRYLATE • See Acrylates.

POTASSIUM RICINOLEATE • The potassium salt of ricinoleic acid *(see)*.

POTASSIUM SALTS OF FATTY ACIDS • The reaction of potassium salts on fatty acids *(see)* creates liquid soap.

POTASSIUM SILICATE • Soluble Potash Glass. Colorless or yellowish translucent to transparent glasslike particles. Used as a binder in cosmetics and in soap manufacturing. Also used as a detergent and in the glass and ceramics industries. Usually very slowly soluble in cold water. No known toxicity.

POTASSIUM SODIUM COPPER CHLOROPHYLLIN • Chlorophyllin. Copper Complex. Does not require certification. It has been permanently listed to color dentifrices that are cosmetics and is not to be used in excess of 0.1 percent in combination. See Chlorophyllin for toxicity.

POTASSIUM SODIUM TARTRATE • Rochelle Salt. Used in the manufacture of baking powder and in the silvering of mirrors. Translucent crystals or white, crystalline powder with cooling saline taste. Slight efflorescence in warm air. Probably used in mouthwashes, but use not identified in cosmetics. No known toxicity.

POTASSIUM SORBATE • Sorbic Acid Potassium Salt. Used as a mold and yeast inhibitor. May cause mild irritation of the skin. On the basis of available information, the CIR Expert Panel *(see)* concludes that it is safe as presently used in cosmetic formulations.

POTASSIUM STEARATE • Stearic Acid Potassium Salt. White powder with a fatty odor. Strongly alkaline. Used in the manufacture of soap, hand creams, emulsified fragrances, hair conditioners, lotions, and shaving creams. Acts as a defoaming ingredient. No known toxicity. On the basis of the available information, the CIR Expert Panel *(see)* concludes that it is safe as a cosmetic ingredient.

POTASSIUM STEAROYL HYDROLYZED COLLAGEN • The potassium salt of the condensation product of stearic acid chloride and hydrolyzed collagen *(see)*.

POTASSIUM SULFATE • Does not occur free in nature but is combined with sodium sulfate. Colorless, or white, crystalline powder with a bitter taste. Used as a reingredient *(see)* in cosmetics and as a salt substitute; also a water corrective in brewing, a fertilizer, and a cathartic. Large doses can cause severe gastrointestinal bleeding. No known toxicity to the skin.

POTASSIUM SULFITE • See Sulfites.

POTASSIUM TALLATE • See Tall Oil.

POTASSIUM TALLOWATE • The potassium salt of tallow acid *(see)*.

POTASSIUM THIOCYANATE • An inorganic salt used in moisturizers. See Thiocyanate.

POTASSIUM THIOGLYCOLATE • See Thioglycolic Acid Compounds.

POTASSIUM TOLUENESULFONATE • A water-soluble powder that may be used in cosmetics as a solubilizing (see solubilization) ingredient in conjunction with other detergent materials. This is primarily used in household chemical products and for various industrial purposes. See Toluene for toxicity.

POTASSIUM TROCLOSENE • Troclosene. Potassium. Used in solid bleaches and detergents, and as a local anti-infective ingredient. No known toxicity.

POTASSIUM UNDECYLENATE • Fine white powder used as a bacteriostat and fungistat in cosmetics and pharmaceuticals. Toxic in high concentrations.

POTASSIUM UNDECYLENOYL HYDROLYZED COLLAGEN • See Hydrolyzed Protein.

POTASSIUM XYLENE SULFONATE • See Xylene.

POTATO EXTRACT • The extract of *Solanum tuberosum*.

POTATO STARCH • A flour prepared from potatoes, ground to a pulp, and washed of fibers. Swells in hot water to form a gel on cooling. A demulcent used in dusting powder, an emollient in dry shampoos and baby powders. With glycerin forms soothing, protective applications for eczema, skin rash, and chapped skin. May cause allergic skin reactions and stuffy nose in the hypersensitive.

POTENTILLA • See Great Burnet and Tormentil.

POTERIUM OFFICINALE • See Great Burnet.

POULTICE • A warm mass of powdered herbs applied directly to the skin to reduce swelling.

POWDER • Face, Compact, and Dusting. Applied to the face with a puff. Usually done at the end of the makeup process. Its objective is to remove the "shine" from the face and to give a healthy subtle glow. Face powders are either loose or compacted. Talc is the principal ingredient (about 50 percent), but face powders also include about 15 percent of a clay, kaolin, and about 10 percent precipitated calcium carbonate, 10 percent zinc oxide, 10 percent zinc stearate, 5 percent magnesium carbonate *(see all)*, perfume, and pigments. Also included are fractions of barium sulfate, boric acid, cetyl alcohol, titanium dioxide, rice, or corn starch *(see all)*. The absorbing, covering, and adherent properties of the face powder may be changed by varying the amounts of the ingredients or by elimination of some of them. For instance, eliminating titanium dioxide makes the powder more transparent. Various pigments are used for shades of face powder, including yellow ocher, red ocher, umber, ultramarine blue, and violet, all inorganic pigments. Organic pigments used may include D & C Red No. 7 Calcium Lake or D & C Orange No. 4 *(see both)*. Problems with face powders are rare. The FDA recorded a concern with rash. Compact powder is similar to face powder but includes binders such as gums *(see);* cake makeup employs a binder such as lecithin. Also used in compact powder to make it keep its shape are glyceryl monostearate glycols or mineral oil *(see all)* and other oils. Dusting powder, usually used after a bath or shower, generally contains talc, perfumes, and zinc stearate *(see)*. Toxicity concerns mechanical blocking of pores and subsequent irritation by the powders. See Talc and Starch for toxicity.

PG • Abbreviation for propylene glycol *(see)*.

PPDA • Abbreviation for Para-Phenylenediamine. See Phenylenediamine.

PPG • Abbreviation for polypropylene glycol and polyoxypropylene glycol *(see both)*.

PPG BUTETH-260 THROUGH -5100 • Emulsifiers. See Propylene Glycol.

PPG BUTETH ETHER-200 • Emulsifiers. Polymer *(see)* prepared from butyl alcohol with propylene glycol *(see both)*.

PPG BUTYL ETHER-300 TO -1715 • Emulsifiers. See PPG Butyl Ether-200.

PPG-4-CETEARETH-12 • Emulsifier. See Cetearyl Alcohol.

PPG-10-CETEARETH-20 • See Cetearyl Alcohol.

PPG-4-CETETH-1 OR -5 OR -10 • See Cetyl Alcohol.

PPG-10-CETYL ETHER • See Cetyl Alcohol.

PPG-28 CETYL ETHER • See Cetyl Alcohol and Propylene.

PPG-30 CETYL ETHER • A liquid, nonionic, surface-active ingredient *(see)*. No known toxicity. See Cetyl Alcohol.

PPG-5-CETETH-10-PHOSPHATE • Used in tanning creams. See Cetyl Alcohol and Phosphates.

PPG-20-DECYLTETRADECETH-10 • See Decanoic Acid.

PPG-2 DIBENZOATE • See Dipropylene Glycol Dibenzoate.

PPG-24 OR -66 GLYCERETH-24 OR -12 • See Glycerin.

PPG-27, AND -55 GLYCERYL ETHER • See Glycerin and Propylene Glycol.

PPG-ISOCETYL ETHER • See Cetyl Alcohol.

PPG-3-ISOSTEARETH-9 • See Stearyl Alcohol and Propylene Glycol.

PPG-2, -5, -10, -20, -30 LANOLIN ALCOHOL ETHERS • See Lanolin Alcohol.

PPG-30 LANOLIN ETHER • Derived from lanolin alcohols *(see)*.

PPG-5 LANOLIN WAX • An emollient. Based on the available data, the CIR Expert Panel concludes that it is safe as used in cosmetics. See Lanolin and Propylene Glycol.

PPG-9 LAURATE • See Lauric Acid.

PPG-2 METHYL ETHER • See Methylene Glycol.

PPG-20-METHYL GLUCOSE ETHER • See Propylene Glycol and Glucose.

PPG-20-METHYL GLUCOSE ETHER DISTEARATE • See Propylene Glycol, Glucose, and Stearic Acid.

PPG-3-MYRETH-11 • See Polyethylene Glycol and Myristic Acid.

PPG-4 MYRISTYL ETHER • See Myristyl Alcohol.

PPG-26 OLEATE • **Polyoxypropylene 2000 Monooleate. Carbowax.** A solid polyethylene glycol *(see)*. Each PPG is a mixture of several polymers *(see)* with various consistencies. Used as a base or carrier in hand lotions, hair dressings, and various other cosmetic lotions. No known toxicity.

PPG-36 OLEATE • **Polyoxypropylene (36) Monooleate.** See PPG-26 Oleate.

PPG-10 OLEYL ETHER • See PPG-26 Oleate.

PPG-30, -50 OLEYL ETHER • See PPG-26 Oleate.

PPG-6-C12-18 PARETH • A mixture of synthetic alcohols. See Fatty Alcohols.

PPG-12-PEG-50 LANOLIN • See Polypropylene and Lanolin.

PPG-2 SALICYLATE • See Dipropylene Glycol Salicylate.

PPG-9-STEARETH-3 • See Stearyl Alcohol.

PPG-11 OR -15 STEARYL ETHER • See Polypropylene Glycol and Stearyl Alcohol.

PPM • Parts per million.

PRECIPITATE • To separate out from solution or suspension. A deposit of solid separated out from a solution or suspension as a result of a chemical or physical change, as by the action of a reingredient *(see)*.

PREDNISOLONE • Introduced in 1955, prednisolone is related chemically to hydrocortisone *(see)* and is used in tablet, syrup, liquid, salve, suppository, enema, and injection form. It is used to treat severe inflammation, as an immunosuppressant, and in the treatment of ulcerative colitis and proctitis. Most adverse reactions are the result of dose or length of time of administration. Contraindicated in systemic fungal infections. Prednisolone is also used in eyedrops to treat inflammation of the eyes. Potential adverse reactions for that use include increased eye pressure, thinning of the cornea, and increased susceptibility to viral and fungal eye infections.

PREDNISONE • Introduced in 1955 and related chemically to corticosteroids *(see)*, prednisone is widely used to treat severe inflammation, as an immunosuppressant, and to treat acute attacks of multiple sclerosis, arthritis, and irritable bowel syndrome. Most adverse reactions are the result of dose or length of time of administration.

PREGNENOLONE ACETATE • Derived from the urine of pregnant women. Used topically as an anti-inflammatory, anti-itch ingredient. Very slightly soluble in water. A corticosteroid. No known toxicity.

PRESERVATIVES • Because the presence of viable microorganisms in cosmetic products can lead to separation of emulsions, discoloration, the formation of gas and odors, and changes in the general properties, as well as possible infection for the users, a preservative must be effective against a wide range of microorganisms. It must not be toxic internally or externally. It must not alter the character of the product, and it is required to be long-lasting and inexpensive. Many kinds of yeasts, fungi, and bacteria have been identified in cosmetics, including pseudomonas, staphylococcus, and streptococcus. In many instances a product might show no visible evidence of microbial contamination and yet contain actively growing, potentially harmful germs. Esters of *p*-hydroxybenzoic acid *(see)* are the most widely used preservatives.

PRESHAVING LOTIONS • See Shaving Lotions.

PRICKLY ASH EXTRACT • *Zanthoxylum americanum.* **Toothache Tree.** A native American herb, the bark and berries have been used for more than 200 years to treat cholera, syphilis, rheumatism, gonorrhea, fevers, dysentery, neuritis, and ulcers. It has been found to contain coumarins, alkaloids *(see both),* and lignins. One of the lignins, asarinin, has been found by modern pharmaceutical researchers to have antitubercular action. The plant is a stimulant and was also used to produce perspiration. It was a popular remedy for chronic rheumatism, and was used extensively in the United States for this purpose. The bark was chewed raw, or inserted into cavities, as a toothache remedy. Prickly ash bark was also used in the treatment of flatulence and diarrhea.

PRIMROSE • *Primula vulgaris.* **Easter Rose.** A perennial native to Britain and Europe, it flourishes in meadows, hedges, and ditches. The name comes from the Latin word for first, *primu,* because it was the first rose of spring. Herbalists used it in a tea to treat arthritis, gout, and migraine, and as a general blood cleanser. A decoction of the root is given for catarrh, coughs, and bronchitis. It is also used to cure insomnia. It is used in "organic" cosmetics.

PRIMULA EXTRACT • The extract of various species of *Primula* taken from the rhizome and roots of the primrose or cowslip. It has been used as an expectorant, diuretic, and worm medicine. In some sensitive persons, it may cause a rash.

PRISTANE • A liquid hydrocarbon obtained from the liver oil of sharks and from ambergris *(see both).* Used as a lubricant and anticorrosive ingredient in cosmetics.

PROANTHOCYANIDINS • See Anthocyanins.

PROCAINE • **Novocain.** A local anesthetic used for spinal anesthesia during childbirth or in operative vaginal procedures. Onset is two to five minutes, and duration is 60 minutes. Potential adverse reactions include skin reactions, swelling, continuous asthma attacks, severe allergic reactions, anxiety, nervousness, and respiratory arrest.

PROCOLLAGEN • The precursor of collagen *(see)*. Used in hair conditioners.

PROGESTERONE • A female sex hormone used in face cream for its supposed antiwrinkle properties. There is no proven benefit to the skin, and it may be absorbed through the skin and have adverse systemic effects. See Hormone Creams.

PROLINE • An amino acid *(see)* used as a food supplement but classified as nonessential. Usually isolated from wheat or gelatin. L-Proline is the naturally occurring form, and DL Proline is the synthetic. GRAS.

PROPANE • A gas heavier than air; odorless when pure. It is used as a fuel and refrigerant. Cleared for use in a spray propellant and as an aerating ingredient for cosmetics in aerosols. May be narcotic in high doses. On the basis of the available animal and human data, the CIR Expert Panel *(see)* concludes that this ingredient is safe as used in cosmetics

PROPANOL • Another name for propyl alcohol. It is derived from propane, a flammable, gaseous paraffin hydrocarbon that occurs naturally in crude petroleum and natural gas. It is used in the manufacture of cosmetics.

PROPELLANT • A compressed gas used to expel the contents of containers in the form of aerosols. Chlorofluorocarbons were widely used because of their non-flammability. The strong possibility that they contribute to depletion of the ozone layer of the upper atmosphere has resulted in prohibition of their use for this purpose. Other propellants used are hydrocarbon gases, such as butane and propane, carbon dioxide, and nitrous oxide. The materials dispersed include shaving cream, whipping cream, and cosmetic preparations.

PROPENYL GUAETHOL • Free-flowing white powder with an odor and taste similar to vanilla but much more powerful. Used as artificial vanilla flavoring and flavor enhancer.

PROPIONIC ACID • Occurs naturally in apples, strawberries, tea, and violet leaves. An oily liquid with a slightly pungent, rancid odor. Can be obtained from wood pulp and waste liquor, and by fermentation. Used in perfume bases and as a mold inhibitor, antioxidant, and preservative in cosmetics. Its salts have been used as antifungal ingredients to treat skin mold. Large oral dose in rats is lethal. The Food and Drug Administration issued a notice in 1992 that propionic acid has not been shown to be safe and effective for stated claims in OTC products.

PROPIONIC ANHYDRIDE • Used in perfume oils. It has a more pungent odor than that of propionic acid *(see)*. No known toxicity to the skin.

PROPIONYL COLLAGEN AMINO ACIDS • See Collagen.

PROPOLIS WAX • Extracted from propolis, a resin found in beehives.

PROPYL ACETATE • Colorless liquid, soluble in water, derived from propane and acetate *(see both)*. It has the odor of pears. Used in the manufacture of perfumes and as a solvent for resins. It may be irritating to the skin and mucous membranes.

PROPYL ALCOHOL • Obtained from crude fuel oil. Alcoholic and slightly overpowering odor. Occurs naturally in cognac green oil, cognac white oil, and onion oil. A synthetic fruit flavoring. Used instead of ethyl alcohol as a solvent for shellac, gums, resins, and oils; as a denaturant *(see)* for alcohol in perfumery.

Not a primary irritant but, because it dissolves fat, it has a drying effect on the skin and may lead to cracking, fissuring, and infections. No adverse effects have been reported from local application as a lotion, liniment, mouthwash, gargle, or sponge bath.

PROPYL GALLATE • A fine, white, odorless powder with a bitter taste used as an antioxidant in creams and lotions. The CIR Expert Panel says based on available data, it is safe as a cosmetic ingredient.

PROPYL OLEATE • See Oleic Acid.

PROPYL THIOURACIL • White powder derived from thiourea and used as a thyroid inhibitor.

PROPYLAMINE • **1-Aminopropane.** An alkaline base for cosmetics, it is a colorless liquid with strong ammonia odor. Miscible in water, alcohol, and ether. Strong skin irritant. May cause allergic reactions.

PROPYLENE CARBONATE • Colorless liquid used as a solvent and plasticizer. The CIR Expert Panel says based on available data, it is safe as a cosmetic ingredient.

PROPYLENE GLYCOL • **1, 2-Propanediol.** One of the most widely used cosmetic ingredients, it is a clear, colorless, viscous liquid, slightly bitter-tasting. It is the most common moisture-carrying vehicle other than water itself in cosmetics. It has better permeation through the skin than glycerin and is less expensive, although it has been linked to more sensitivity reactions. Absorbs moisture, acts as a solvent and a wetting ingredient. Used in liquid makeup, foundation makeup, foundation creams, mascaras, spray deodorants, hair straighteners, liquid powders, preshave lotions, after-shave lotions, baby lotions, cold creams, emollients, antiperspirants, lipsticks, mouthwashes, stick perfumes, and suntan lotions. Its use is being reduced, and it is being replaced by safer glycols such as butylene and polyethylene glycol. In 1992, the FDA proposed a ban on propylene glycol in louse-killing products because it has not been shown to be safe and effective for its stated claims. The CIR Expert Panel says based on available data, it is safe as a cosmetic ingredient in concentrations up to 50 percent.

PROPYLENE GLYCOL ALGINATE • **Kelcoloid®.** The propylene glycol ester of alginic acid *(see)*, derived from seaweed, the most common moisture-carrying vehicle in cosmetics other than water. Used as a stabilizer and defoaming ingredient in cosmetics and food. No known toxicity.

PROPYLENE GLYCOL CAPRYLATE • See Polyethylene Glycol and Capric Acid.

PROPYLENE GLYCOL DICAPRYLATE/DICAPRIATE • A gel used in emollients. The CIR Expert Panel says based on available data, it is safe as a cosmetic ingredient. See Propylene Glycol and Capric Acid.

PROPYLENE GLYCOL DICOCONATE • Mixture of propylene glycol esters of coconut fatty acids. The CIR Expert Panel says based on available data, it is safe as a cosmetic ingredient. See Propylene Glycol.

PROPYLENE GLYCOL DIPELARGONATE • The CIR Expert Panel says based on available data, it is safe as a cosmetic ingredient. See Propylene Glycol.

PROPYLENE GLYCOL LAURATE • An ester of propylene glycol and lauric acid. An emulsifying ingredient for solvents, cosmetic creams, and lotions; also a stabilizer of essential oils in water. Light orange oil, dispersible in water, soluble in alcohol and oils. Nontoxic but can cause allergic reactions in the hypersensitive. The CIR Expert Panel says based on available data, it is safe as a cosmetic ingredient.

PROPYLENE GLYCOL MYRISTATE • The CIR Expert Panel says based on available data, it is safe as a cosmetic ingredient. See Propylene Glycol and Myristic Acid.

PROPYLENE GLYCOL RICINOLEATE • Ester of propylene glycol and ricinoleic acid *(see both)*.

PROPYLENE GLYCOL STEARATE • Cream-colored wax. Dispenses in water, soluble in hot alcohol. Lubricating ingredient and emulsifier in cosmetic creams and lotions. Stabilizer of essential oils. No known toxicity.

PROPYLENE GLYCOL STEARATE SE • A widely used emulsifier. See Propylene Glycol.

PROPYLPARABEN • **Propyl p-Hydroxybenzoate.** Developed in Europe, the esters of *p*-hydroxybenzoic acid are widely used in the cosmetic industry as preservatives and bacteria- and fungus-killers. They are active against a variety of organisms, are neutral, low in toxicity, slightly soluble, and active in all solutions, alkaline, neutral, or acid. Used in shampoos, baby preparations, foundation creams, beauty masks, dentifrices, eye lotions, hair-grooming aids, nail creams, and wave sets. Used medicinally to treat fungus infections. Can cause contact dermatitis. Less toxic than benzoic or salicylic acid *(see both)*.

PROPYLTRIMONIUM HYDROLYZED COLLAGEN • See Hydrolyzed Collagen.

PROSTAGLANDINS • **PGA. PGB. PGC. PGD.** A group of extremely potent hormonelike substances present in many tissues. There are more than 16 known with effects such as dilating or constricting blood vessels, stimulation of intestinal or bronchial smooth muscle, uterine stimulation, and antagonism to hormones and influencing fat metabolism. Various prostaglandins in the body can cause fever, inflammation, and headaches. Prostaglandins or drugs that affect prostaglandins are used medically to induce labor, prevent and treat peptic ulcers, control high blood pressure, in the treatment of bronchial asthma, and to induce delayed menstruation. Aspirin tends to inhibit prostaglandin production.

PROTEASE • An enzyme that breaks down protein. In 1992, the FDA issued a notice that protease had not been shown to be safe and effective as claimed in OTC digestive aid products. Used in cosmetics as a skin conditioning ingredient.

PROTECTIVE CREAMS • Water-repellent or oil-repellent creams designed to act as barrier ingredients against irritating chemicals, including water. Some products, such as the widely used silicones, are both water- and oil-repellent. Among the chemicals used in protective creams are stearic acid, beeswax, glycerin, casein, ammonium hydroxide, zinc stearate, titanium dioxide, butyl stearate, petrolatum, polyethylene glycol, paraffin, potassium hydroxide, magnesium stearate, aluminum compounds, benzoic acid, borates, calamine, ceresin, lanolin, salicylates, sodium silicate, talc, and triethanolamine *(see all)*.

PROTEIN FATTY ACID CONDENSATES • See Amides.

PROTEIN PAC • New name for hair moisturizers.

PROTEINS • The chief nitrogen-containing constituents of plants and animals—the essential constituents of every living cell. They are complex but by weight contain about 50 percent carbon, about 20 percent oxygen, about 15 percent nitrogen, about 7 percent hydrogen, and some sulfur. Some also contain iron and phosphorus. Proteins are colorless, odorless, and generally tasteless. They vary in solubility. They readily undergo putrefaction, hydrolysis, and dilution with acids or alkalies. They are regarded as combinations of amino acids *(see)*. Cosmetic manufacturers, particularly makers of hair products, claim that "protein enrichment" is beneficial to the hair and skin. Hair, of course, is already dead. It does consist of a type of protein, keratin *(see),* but the surface of the hair is cornified tissue that cannot be revitalized. Such products will add body to thin hair and add gloss or luster, but so will other hair conditioners *(see)*. As for face creams with protein, the lubricant is more beneficial than the protein. No known toxicity.

PRUNELLA VULGARIS • A family of herbs that yields popular fruits.

PRUNES • A source of fiber. A plum that is dried. Fruit from a shrub related to almond, apricot, cherry, and peach.

PRUNIS AVIUM • See Sweet Cherry Extract and Oil.

PRUNUS AMYGDALUS AMARA • See Almond Oil.

PRUNUS ARMENIACA • See Apricot.

PRUNUS DOMESTICA • See Prunes.

PRUNUS PERSICA • See Peach Juice Extract.

PRUNUS SEROTINA • See Wild Cherry Bark.

PSALLIOTA CAMPESTRIS • See Mushroom Extract.

PSEUDOTSUGA • See Balsam.

PSIDIUM GUAJAVA • See Guava.

PSORALEA EXTRACT • An extract of the fruit and seeds of *Psoralea.*

PSORALEN® • Named for the Latin *psora,* meaning itch, and derived from a plant. Used in the treatment of vitiligo (lack of skin pigment), in sunscreen to increase tanning, and in perfumes. It can cause photosensitivity *(see)*.

PSYLLIUM • Plantago psyllium. Metamucil. Naturacil. Perdiem. Serutan Toasted Granules. Siblin. Syllact. Laxative in use since the early 1930s that absorbs water and expands to increase bulk and moisture content. Allergic reactions may occur.

PTEROCARPUS SANTALINUS • See Sandalwood Oil.

PTFE • **Teflon.** Used as a bulking agent.

PTYCHOPETALUM OLACOIDES • See Muira Puama Extract.

PUERARIA LOBATA • **Kudzu.** A woody herb that is causing a problem in the southern United States. Has many seeded pods.

PULMONARIA OFFICINALIS • See Lungwort.

PUMICE • Used in hand-cleansing pastes, skin-cleansing grains, toothpastes, powders, and some soaps for acne treatment. A tooth whitener in Elizabethan times. Used to rub hair from legs and as a nicotine remover paste. Light, hard, rough, porous mass of gritty, gray-colored powder of volcanic origin. Used in cosmetics for removing tough or rough skin. Pumice consists mainly of silicates *(see)* found chiefly in the Lipari Islands and in the Greek archipelagos. Because of its abrasive action, daily use in dentifrices is not recommended. If used continuously on dry sensitive skin, it may cause irritation. Reported to be an irritant when used with soapless detergents, but is generally considered harmless.

PUMPKIN • **Cucurbita Pepo.** Native Americans used this seed to treat problems with enlarged prostate. It has a reputation among herbalists as being a nonirritating diuretic. Among its ingredients are fatty oil, albumin, lecithin, and phytosterol, an alcohol. Used by herbalists today to get rid of worms.

PUNICA GRANATUM • See Pomegranate.

PURCELLINE OIL SYN • A synthetic mixture of fatty esters simulating the natural oil obtained from the preen glands of waterfowl. Used as a fixative in perfumes. No known toxicity.

PURPLE HEATH EXTRACT • Extract of the flowers of *Erica cinerea.*

PVM/MA • Abbreviation for polyvinyl methyl ether/maleic anhydride.

PVM/MA COPOLYMER • A copolymer of methyl vinyl ether and maleic anhydride. See Polyvinyl Alcohols.

PVP • **1-Vinyl-2-Pyrrolidone.** Abbreviation for Polyvinylpyrrolidone.

PVP/DIMETHYLAMINOETHYL-METHYLACRYLATE COPOLYMER • A polymer prepared from vinylpryrrolidone and dimethylaminoethylmethacrylate. See Polyvinylpyrrolidone and Acrylates.

PVP/EICOSENE COPOLYMER • A polymer of vinylpyrrolidone and eicosine. See Polyvinylpyrrolidone.

PVP/ETHYL METHACRYLATE/METHACRYLIC ACID COPOLYMER • See Polyvinylpyrrolidone and Acrylate.

PVP-IODINE • Complex of polyvinylpyrrolidone and iodine *(see both).*

PVP/VA COPOLYMER • A film former used in hair sprays. The CIR Expert Panel says based on available data, it is safe as a cosmetic ingredient. See Polyvinyls and Polyvinylpyrrolidone.

PVP/VINYL ACETATE/ITACONIC ACID COPOLYMER • See Polyvinylpyrrolidone and Vinyl Polymers.

PYCNOGENOL • An ingredient from the French maritime pine tree, this substance is purported to be a powerful antioxidant and a blood-vessel and colagen strengthener. Used in "antiaging" products.

PYRAZOLE • A crystalline compound used to overcome acidity of aluminum chloride in antiperspirants. Soluble in water, alcohol, ether, and benzene. No known toxicity when used externally. A modest injection into the abdomens of mice is lethal.

PYRETHRINS • Thick esters that are the most potent insecticidal ingredients of chrysanthemum. Used in household insecticidal sprays and powders, and deodorant sprays. Also used in paper bags for shipping cereals. Insecticides labeled nontoxic to humans and pets usually contain pyrethrins.

PYRETHRUM • *Tanacetum cinerariifolium.* The natural insecticide obtained by extraction of chrysanthemum flowers. Can cause severe allergic dermatitis and systemic allergic reactions. Very toxic if ingested.

PYRIDINE • Occurs naturally in coffee and coal tar. Disagreeable odor, sharp taste. Used in chocolate flavorings for beverages, ice cream, ices, candy, and baked goods. Also used as a solvent for organic liquids and compounds. Once used to treat asthma, but may cause central nervous system depression and irritation of the skin and respiratory tract.

PYRIDIUM COMPOUNDS • A toxic, water-soluble, flammable liquid with a disagreeable odor that is obtained by distillation of bone oil or as a by-product of coal tar. Used as a modifier and preservative in shaving creams, soaps, hand creams, and lotions; also as a solvent, a denaturant in alcohol, and an industrial waterproofing ingredient. No known toxicity when used externally. The lethal dose injected into the abdomens of rats is only 3.2 milligrams per kilogram of body weight.

PYRIDOXINE • See Pyridoxine HCL.

PYRIDOXINE DICAPRYLATE • See Pyridoxine Dioctenoate.

PYRIDOXINE DILAURATE • See Vitamin B_6.

PYRIDOXINE DIOCTENOATE • **Vitamin B_6 Hydrochloride.** Texturizer. A colorless, or white, crystalline powder present in many foodstuffs. A coenzyme that helps in the metabolism of amino acids *(see)* and fats. Also soothing to skin. Nontoxic.

PYRIDOXINE DIPALMITATE • See Vitamin B_6.

PYRIDOXINE HCL • See Vitamin B_6.

PYRIDOXINE TRIPALMITATE • **Vitamin B_6 Tripalmitate.** See Pyridoxine HCL.

PYRITHIONE ZINC • **Head and Shoulders Antidandruff Shampoo. X-Seb Shampoo. Zincon Dandruff Shampoo.** A zinc derivative that acts as an antibacterial and antifungal ingredient for the skin. Relieves the itching and scalp flaking associated with dandruff and with seborrheic dermatitis of the scalp.

PYROCATECHOL • Used as an antiseptic. Colorless leaflets, soluble in water; prepared by treating salicylaldehyde with hydrogen peroxide. Used in blond-type dyes as an oxidizing ingredient and for dyeing furs; also in photography. It can cause eczema and systemic effects similar to phenol *(see)*. The CIR Expert Panel says based on available data, it is unsafe for use in "leave-on" products and that the available data are insufficient to support the safety of pyrocatechol as used in hair dyes.

PYROGALLOL • Antiseptic hair dye for hair restorers. The first synthetic organic dye used in human hair. Discovered in 1786 and suggested for use in hair in 1845. Solution grows darker as it is exposed to air. Consists of white, odorless crystals. An aromatic alcohol of pyrogallic acid. Used medicinally as an external antimicrobial and to soothe irritated skin. Ingestion may cause severe gastrointestinal irritation, kidney and liver damage, circulatory collapse, and death. Application to extensive areas of the skin is extremely dangerous. Even with careful use, it can cause a skin rash. Its adverse effects supposedly can be reduced by adding sulfide. The CIR Expert Panel says based on available data, it is safe as a cosmetic ingredient.

PYROPHOSPHATE • **Salt of Pyrophosphoric Acid.** It increases the effectiveness of antioxidants in creams and ointments. In concentrated solutions it can be irritating to the skin and mucous membranes.

PYROPHYLLITE • **Pencil Stone Agalmatolite.** White to yellowish gray mineral consisting predominantly of anhydrous aluminum silicate *(see)* mixed with silica *(see)*. Used as a coloring and opacifying ingredient. Permanently listed in 1966 for externally applied cosmetics. No known toxicity.

PYRROLIDONE • Derived from acetylene and formaldehyde, it is used as a plasticizer, solvent, insecticide, and in special inks.

PYRUS COMMUNIS • See Pear Extract.

PYRUS CYDONIA • See Quince Seed.

PYRUS SORBUS • See Sorbus Extract.

Q

QUASSIN • Bitter alkaloid obtained from the wood of *Quassia amara.* Chiefly used as a denaturant for ethyl alcohol. Shavings from a plant found in Jamaica and the Caribbean islands. Yellowish white to bright yellow chips. Used to poison flies. Toxic to humans.

QUATERNARIUM-1 THROUGH -6 • A germicide derived from lauric acid, a common constituent of vegetable fats, especially coconut oil. Positively charged with a low irritation potential, it is effective against a wide range of organisms. It is a preservative present in skin preparations. See Quarternarium-7.

QUATERNARIUM-7 • A surfactant and germicide derived from lauric acid *(see)*. Positively charged with a low irritation potential, it is effective against a wide range of organisms.

QUATERNARIUM-8 THROUGH -14 • See Quarternarium-15.

QUATERNARIUM-15 • A water-soluble antimicrobial ingredient that is active against bacteria but not very active against yeast. It is a formaldehyde *(see)* releaser, and is the number-one cause of dermatitis from preservatives, according to the American Academy of Dermatology's Testing Tray results. It is a teratogen *(see)* in rats when administered orally but not on the skin. Conditions which favor rapid absorption from the skin, therefore, might be expected to increase the risk of birth defects. Although it is a potential sensitizer, the CIR Expert Panel says based on available data, it is safe as a cosmetic ingredient.

QUATERNARIUM-16 THROUGH -29 • Antistatics and surfactants. See Quaternarium-18.

QUATERNARIUM -18, -19, -20, -23 • Derived from cellulose *(see)*, it is a film-former and binding ingredient used in products to give hair a sheen.

QUATERNARIUM-28 DODECYLBENZYL TRIMETHYLAMMONIUM CHLO-RIDE • See Quaternary Ammonium Compounds.

QUATERNARIUM-29 DODECYLXYLYL BIS • **Trimethyl Ammonium Chloride.** See Quaternary Ammonium Compounds.

QUATERNARIUM-18 HECTORITE • See Quaternary Ammonium Compounds.

QUATERNARY AMMONIUM COMPOUNDS • A wide variety of preservatives, surfactants, germicides, sanitizers, antiseptics, and deodorants used in cosmetics. Benzalkonium chloride *(see)* is one of the most popular. Quaternary ammonium compounds are synthetic derivatives of ammonium chloride *(see)* and are used in aerosol deodorants, after-shave lotions, antidandruff shampoos, antiperspirants, cuticle softeners, hair colorings, hair-grooming aids, hand creams, hair-waving preparations, mouthwashes, hand creams, and regular shampoos. Diluted solutions are used in medicine to sterilize the skin and mucous membranes. All the quaternary ammonium compounds can be toxic, depending upon the dose and concentration. Concentrated solutions irritate the skin and can cause necrosis of the mucous membranes. Concentrations as low as 0.1 percent are irritating to the eye and mucous membranes except benzalkonium chloride, which is well tolerated at such low concentrations. Ingestion can be fatal.

QUEEN OF THE PRAIRIE • See *Filipendula rubra.*

QUEEN'S DELIGHT • *Stillingia sylvatica.* The root of this North American herb contains volatile oil, tannin, and resin. It is used for the treatment of chronic skin conditions such as eczema and psoriasis. It is also used by herbalists to treat bronchitis and laryngitis, especially when they are accompanied by loss of the voice. The astringent *(see)* qualities have led herbalists to use it for hemorrhoid problems.

QUERCETIN • The inner bark of a species of oak tree common in North America. Its active ingredient, isoquercitin, is used in dark brown hair-dye shades but employed mainly for dyeing artificial hairpieces. Allergic reactions have been reported.

QUERCITOL • A sweet crystalline alcohol found in acorns and oak bark and in viburnums and other plants. It is used in astringents.

QUERCITRIN • *Aesculus hippocastanus.* Yellow crystals used as a dye. Found in elder flowers and in quercitron bark.

QUERCUS ALBA • The European Union's name for White Oak Bark *(see).*

QUILLAJA EXTRACT • **Soap Bark. Quillay Bark. Panama Bark. China Bark.** The extract of the bark of *Quillaja saponaria.* The inner dried bark of a tree grown in South America. Used in fruit, root beer, and spice flavorings for beverages, ice cream, and candy. Formerly used to treat bronchitis and externally as a detergent and local irritant. No known toxicity.

QUINCE SEED • The seed of a plant grown in southern Asia and Europe for its fatty oil. Thick jelly is produced by soaking seeds in water. Used in setting lotions, as a suspension in skin creams and lotions, as a thickening ingredient in depilatories, and as an emulsifier in fragrances, hand creams, lotions, rouges, and wave sets; medicinally as a demulcent. Has been largely replaced by cheaper substitutes. It may cause allergic reactions.

QUINIC ACID • A pH *(see)* adjuster.

QUINIDINE • An antiarrhythmic drug introduced in 1920, it is used to treat heart flutter or fibrillation. Used as a cooling and analgesic ingredient.

QUININE • The most important alkaloid of cinchona bark, which grows wild in South America. White crystalline powder, almost insoluble in water. Used as a local anesthetic in hair tonics and sunscreen preparations. Used in bitters as flavoring for beverages in limited amounts. When taken internally, it reduces fever. It is also used as a flavoring ingredient in numerous over-the-counter cold and headache remedies as well as in "bitter lemon" and tonic water, which may contain as much as 5 milligrams per 100 milliliters. Cinchonism, which may consist of nausea, vomiting, disturbances of vision, ringing in the ears, and nerve deafness, may occur from an overdose of quinine. If there is a sensitivity to quinine, such symptoms can result after ingesting tonic water. Quinine more commonly causes a rash.

QUINOA EXTRACT • The extract of the leaves and flowers of *Chenopodium quinoa.*

QUINOLINE • A coal-tar derivative used in the manufacture of cosmetic dyes. Also a solvent for resins. Made either by the distillation of coal tar, bones, and alkaloids or by the interaction of aniline *(see)* with acetaldehyde and formaldehyde *(see both)*. Absorbs water, has a weak base. Soluble in hot water. Also used as a preservative for anatomical specimens. See Coal Tar for toxicity. See also Colors.

QUINOLINE SALTS • A colorless, oily, very hygroscopic liquid with a disagreeable odor. Occurs in coal tar. Used in suntan preparations and perfumes as a preservative and solvent. Also a preservative for anatomical specimens. No known toxicity when used externally.

QUINONES • Derived from benzene *(see)*, used in yellow and orange to red colorings. Potent sensitizers.

R

RADISH EXTRACT • Extract of *Raphanus sativus*. The small seeds of the radish remain viable for years. Has been used as a food since ancient times. Used as a counterirritant *(see)* in herbal cosmetics.

RAFFINOSE MYRISTATE • A skin-conditioning ingredient. See Myristic Acid and Radish Extract.

RAISIN-SEED OIL • Oil from dried grapes or berries used in lubricating creams. See Grape-seed Oil.

RANUNCULUS FICARIA • See Pilewort Extract.

RAPESEED ACID • A mixture of fatty acids from rapeseed. Used as a cleansing ingredient. See Rapeseed Oil.

RAPESEED AMIDOPROPYL BENZYLDIMONIUM CHLORIDE • See Rapeseed Oil and Quaternary Ammonium Compounds.

RAPESEED AMIDOPROPYL ETHYLDIMONIUM ETHOSULFATE • See Rapeseed Oil and Quaternary Ammonium Compounds.

RAPESEED OIL • Brownish yellow oil from a turniplike annual herb of European origin. Widely grown as a forage crop for sheep in the United States. A distinctly unpleasant odor. Used chiefly as a lubricant, an illuminant, and in rubber substitutes; also used in soft soaps and margarine. Can cause acnelike skin eruptions.

RAPESEED OIL UNSAPONIFIABLES • The fraction of rapeseed oil *(see)* that is not changed into a fatty alcohol when it is saponified (heated with an alkali and an acid).

RAPHANUS SATIVUS • See Radish Extract.

RASPBERRY JUICE • Juice from the fresh ripe fruit grown in Europe, Asia, the United States, and Canada. used as a flavoring for lipsticks, food, and medicines. It has astringent properties. No known toxicity.

RAUWOLFIA EXTRACT • Raudixin. Rauzide. Rauverid. Wolfina. Deserpidine. Reserpine. A small shrub native to the Orient from India to Sumatra, where it has been used for medicinal purposes for hundreds of years. The active ingredients are usually in the root. Rauwolfia contains the basics for many widely used modern drugs, including reserpine, serpasil, and yohimbine. Rauwolfia extracts work by blocking nerve signals that trigger constriction of blood vessels.

RAYON • Regenerated cellulose. Rayon is composed of man-made textile fibers of cellulose and yarn; produced from wood pulp. Its appearance is similar to silk. Used to give shine and body to face powders and in eyelash extenders in mascaras. No known toxicity.

RED OIL • A commercial grade of oleic, linoleic, and stearic acids *(see all)*.

RED PEPPER • Cayenne Pepper. A condiment made from the pungent fruit of the plant. Used in sausage and pepper flavorings. Also used as a stimulant in hair tonics, but may be an irritant and also cause allergic reactions.

RED PETROLATUM • A minimally refined variety of petrolatum *(see)*, used as a sunscreen ingredient.

RED RASPBERRY EXTRACT • See Raspberry Juice.

RED RASPBERRY LEAF EXTRACT • An extract of the leaves of the red raspberry.

RED SANDALWOOD EXTRACT • The extract of the wood of *Pterocarpus santalinus*. The use of this ingredient as a colorant in cosmetics is prohibited in the United States, and may be restricted in other countries. See Sandalwood.

REDUCING INGREDIENT • A substance that decreases, deoxidizes, or concentrates the volume of another substance. For instance, a reducing ingredient is used to convert a metal oxide to the metal itself. It also means a substance that adds hydrogen ingredients to another, for example, when acetaldehyde is converted to alcohol in the final step of alcoholic fermentation.

REDUCTION • The process of reducing by chemical or electrochemical means. The gain of one or more electrons by an ion or compound. It is the reverse of oxidation.

REHMANNIA • *Radix Rehmanniae.* **Shennong Bencao Jing.** A Chinese herb used to clear heat and cool blood. The roots are dug in spring or autumn and dried in the sun.

REINGREDIENT • A chemical that reacts or participates in a reaction; a substance that is used for the detection or determination of another substance by chemical or microscopical means. The various categories of reingredients are colorimetric—to produce color-soluble compounds; fluxes—used to lower the melting point; oxidizers—used in oxidation; precipitants—to produce insoluble compounds; reducers—used in reduction *(see);* and solvents—used to dissolve water-insoluble compounds.

RESEDA LUTEOLA • **Dyer's rocket.** An essential oil from the dyer's rocket. European plant cultivated for its yellow dye.

RESINS • The brittle substance, usually translucent or transparent, formed from the hardened secretions of plants. Among the natural resins are dammar, elemi, and sandarac. Synthetic resins include polyvinyl acetate, various polyester resins, and sulfonamide resins. Resins have many uses in cosmetics. They contribute depth, gloss, flow adhesion, and water resistance. Toxicity depends upon ingredients used.

RESORCINOL • A preservative, antiseptic, antifungal, astringent, and anti-itching ingredient, particularly in dandruff shampoos. Also used in hair dyes, lipsticks, and hair tonics. Also used in tanning, explosives, printing textiles, and the manufacture of resins. Obtained from various resins. Resorcinol's white crystals become pink on exposure to air. A sweetish taste. Irritating to the skin and mucous membranes. May cause allergic reactions, particularly of the skin. While using resorcinol, you should avoid abrasive soaps or cleansers, medicated cosmetics, preparations containing alcohol, or any other acne preparations. The FDA issued a notice in 1992 that resorcinol has not been shown to be safe and effective for stated claims in OTC products. On the basis of the available data, the CIR Expert Panel *(see)* concludes that it is safe as a cosmetic ingredient.

RESORCINOL ACETATE • See Resorcinol.

RESTHARROW EXTRACT • A European woody herb, *Onones spinosa,* with pink flowers and long, tough roots used for medicinal purposes and in emollients. No known toxicity.

RETIN-A • A prescription drug for the treatment of acne, it is a Vitamin A derivative. The medication is available in five strengths and in cream, gel, and liquid form. It has a faint medicinal odor, is greaseless and easily absorbed. It reportedly plumps the skin, smoothes fine wrinkles, and begins to reverse other, less visible signs of sun damage. The drug is believed to increase cell turnover, so dull surface cells are shed more quickly. It thickens the epidermis and improves texture, elasticity, and blood circulation. And it helps normalize uneven cell growth. It is not said to reduce deep wrinkles. It is expected, as of this writing, to eventually be an ingredient in over-the-counter cosmetics. The FDA began a nationwide crackdown on unlicensed manufacturers who have begun to advertise and distribute bogus Retin-A drugs and cosmetics. Some manufacturers are also promoting Vitamin A in products as producing effects similar to Retin-A.

RETINOIC ACID • A derivative of Vitamin A. See Tretinoin and Retinoids.

RETINOIDS • Derived from Retinoic Acid, Vitamin A, it is used to treat acne and other skin disorders. See Vitamin A.

RETINOL • Vitamin A *(see)*.

RETINYL ACETATE • See Vitamin A.

RETINYL PALMITATE • The ester of Vitamin A and palmitic acid, sometimes mixed with Vitamin D_2 *(see all)*. It was nonmutagenic in several animal species. The CIR Expert Panel says based on available data, it is safe as a cosmetic ingredient.

RETINYL PROPIONATE • See Vitamin A.

RHATANY • *Krameria triandra.* The root of a shrub native to Peru that contains up to 9 percent tannin *(see)*. It is a powerful astringent long used in conventional pharmacy. It is used by herbalists to treat diarrhea, hemorrhoids, and hemorrhages, or as a styptic. Rhatany is often found in herbal toothpastes and powders to treat bleeding gums.

RHEUM PALMATUM • See Rhubarb.

RHODINOL • Used in perfumes, especially those of the rose type. Isolated from geranium or rose oils. It has the strong odor of rose and consists essentially of geraniol and citronellol *(see both)*. Also used in food and beverage flavorings. No known toxicity.

RHODODENDRON EXTRACT • Extract of various species of *Rhododendron.*

RHUBARB • The common plant with large edible leaves. It is combined with henna, black tea, and chamomile for hair dye. Its active principle is chrysophanol, which produces a desirable blond shade. No known skin toxicity.

RIBES • See Currant Extract.

RIBOFLAVIN • **Vitamin B₂. Lactoflavin.** Formerly called Vitamin G. Riboflavin is a factor in the Vitamin B complex and is used in emollients. Every plant and animal cell contains a minute amount. Good sources are milk, eggs, and organ meats. It is necessary for healthy skin and respiration, protects the eyes from sensitivity to light, and is used for building and maintaining human body tissues. A deficiency leads to lesions at the corner of the mouth and to changes in the cornea.

RIBONUCLEIC ACID • RNA. A material found in both the nucleus and cytoplasm of the cell, it contains directions for the genetic code of the cell, DNA.

RICE BRAN OIL • Oil expressed from the broken coat of rice grain.

RICE BRAN WAX • The wax obtained from the broken coat of rice grain.

RICE POWDER • Used in cosmetics and as a drying ingredient. May cause contact dermatitis. However, rice as a food is hypoallergenic.

RICE STARCH • The finely pulverized grains of the rice plant, used in baby powders, face powders, and dusting powders. It is a demulcent and emollient, and forms a soothing, protective film when applied. May cause mechanical irritation by blocking the pores and putrefying. May also cause an allergic reaction.

RICINOLEAMIDE • See Ricinoleic Acid.

RICINOLEAMIDE DEA • See Ricinoleic Acid.

RICINOLEATE • Salt of ricinoleic acid found in castor oil. Used in the manufacture of soaps. No known toxicity.

RICINOLEIC ACID • A mixture of fatty oils found in the seeds of castor beans. Castor oil contains 80 to 85 percent ricinoleic acid. The oily liquid is used in soaps, added to Turkey-red oil *(see),* and used in contraceptive jellies. It is believed to be the active laxative in castor oil. Also used externally as an emollient. No known toxicity.

RICINOLEOAMPHOGLYCINATE • See Castor Oil.

RICINOLETH-40 • See Castor Oil.

RNA • The abbreviation for Ribonucleic Acid. RNA is one of the molecules involved in carrying out a cell's DNA (deoxyribonucleic acid) instructions for reproduction, growth, and maturation. DNA provides the blueprint for any living organism.

ROCHELLE SALT • Potassium Sodium Tartrate. Used in the manufacture of baking powder and in the silvering of mirrors. Translucent crystals or white crystalline powder with cooling saline taste. Slight efflorescence in warm air. Probably used in mouthwashes, but use not identified in cosmetics. No known toxicity.

ROCK SALT CRYSTALS • See Sodium Chloride.

ROCKET EXTRACT • Extract of the leaves of *Eruca sativa.* Used in hair shampoos and in skin preparations to cut grease.

ROMAN CHAMOMILE • See Chamomile.

ROSA CENTIFOLIA • See Cabbage Rose Extract.

ROSA EGLANTERIA • Sweet Briar Rose.

ROSA MOSCHATA • Musk Rose.

ROSA MULITFLORA • See Rose Extract.

ROSA ROXBURGHI • Chestnut Rose.

ROSA SPINOSISSIMA EXTRACT • Burnet Rose.

ROSA SPP • Rose Extract.

ROSE BENGAL • A bluish red fragrant liquid taken from the rose of the Bengal region of the Asian subcontinent. Used to scent perfumes and as an edible color product to make lipstick dyes. Nontoxic.

ROSE BULGARIAN • True Otto Oil. Attar of Roses. Rose Otto Bulgaria. One of the most widely used perfume ingredients, it is the essential oil steam-distilled from the flowers of *Rosa damascena*. The rose flowers are picked early in the morning, when they contain the maximum amount of perfume, and are distilled quickly after harvesting. Bulgaria is the main source of supply, but Russia, Turkey, Syria, and Indo-China also grow it. The liquid is pale yellow and has a warm, deep floral, slightly spicy, and extremely fragrant, red rose smell. It is used as a flavoring ingredient in loganberry, raspberry, strawberry, orange, rose, violet, cherry, grape, peach, honey, muscatel, maple, almond, pecan, and ginger ale flavorings for beverages, ice cream, ices, candy, baked goods, gelatin desserts, chewing gum, and jellies. Also used in mucilage, coloring matter, and as a flavoring in pills. May cause allergic reactions.

ROSE EXTRACT • An extract of the various species of rose, it is used in raspberry and cola beverages and in fragrances. No known toxicity except for allergic reactions. GRAS.

ROSE GERANIUM • Distilled from any of several South African herbs grown for their fragrant leaves. Used in perfumes and to scent toothpaste and dusting powders. May cause allergic reactions.

ROSE HIPS EXTRACT • Extract of the fruit of various species of wild roses, it is rich in Vitamin C and is used as a natural flavoring. No known toxicity.

ROSE LEAVES EXTRACT • Derived from the leaves of a species of *Rosa*. Used in raspberry and cola beverages.

ROSE OIL • Attar of Roses. The fragrant, volatile, essential oil distilled from fresh flowers. Colorless or yellow, with a strong fragrant odor and taste of roses. Used in perfumes, toilet waters, and ointments. Nontoxic but may cause allergic reactions.

ROSE OTTO BULGARIA • See Rose Bulgarian.

ROSE SEED EXTRACT • Extract from the seed of *Rosa canina*. See Dog Rose Extract.

ROSE WATER • The watery solution of the odoriferous constituents of roses, made by distilling the fresh flowers with water or steam. Used as a perfume in emollients, eye lotions, and freckle lotions. No known toxicity, but may cause allergic reactions.

ROSE WATER OINTMENT • See Cold Cream.

ROSEMARINIC ACID • See Rosemary Extract.

ROSEMARY • Used in perfumery. The flowers and leaves of the plant are a symbol of love and loyalty. Rosemary oil is the volatile oil from the fresh flowering tops of rosemary and is used in liniments and hair tonics. Colorless to yellow, with the characteristic odor of rosemary and a warm camphorlike taste. Rosemary has the folk reputation of stimulating the growth of hair and is used in rinse water. It supposedly is also beneficial to the skin. It is used internally as a tonic and astringent, and by herbalists as a stimulant for the nerves. No known toxicity when used externally. A teaspoonful may cause illness in an adult, and an ounce may cause death.

ROSEMARY EXTRACT • Garden Rosemary. A flavoring and perfume from the fresh aromatic flowering tops of the evergreen shrub grown in the Mediterranean. Light blue flowers and gray-green leaves. Used for beverages, condiments, and meat. It is also used in citrus, peach, and ginger flavorings as well as in perfumes. Widely used in hair products, bubble baths, body and hand preparations, lipsticks, suntan products, and bath soaps. A teaspoonful of the oil may cause illness in an adult, and an ounce may cause death.

ROSEMARY OIL • The oil obtained from the flowering tops of *Rosemarinus officinalis.* See Rosemary.

ROSEWOOD OIL • From *Aniba Rosaeodora.* Used in fragrances.

ROSIN • Colophony. Used in soaps, hair lacquers, wax depilatories, and ointments. It is also used in masacaras. It is the pale yellow residue left after distilling the volatile oil from the oleoresin obtained from various species of pine trees produced chiefly in the United States. Also used in the manufacture of varnishes and fireworks. It can cause contact dermatitis.

ROSIN HYDROLYZED COLLAGEN • A protein used in hair and skin conditioners. See Rosin and Hydrolyzed.

ROSMARINIC ACID • An antioxidant. See Rosemary.

ROSMARINUS OFFICINALIS • See Rosemary.

ROUGE • One of the oldest types of makeup. Rouge is applied to the cheeks to give a rosy, healthy look. It is usually a finely divided form of ferric oxide, generally prepared by heating ferrous sulfate. Cake or compact rouge usually contains talc, kaolin, brilliant red lake (certified), zinc oxide, zinc stearate, liquid petrolatum, tragacanth, mucilage *(see all),* and perfume. Liquid rouge usually contains carmine coloring, ammonium hydroxide, glycerin *(see all),* and red coloring pigment. It may also contain polyvinylpyrrolidone or sodium carboxymethyl cellulose, glycerin, color, propylene glycol *(see all),* alcohol, perfume, and water. Rouge paste may contain carmine coloring, ammonium hydroxide, beeswax, cetyl alcohol, stearic acid, cocoa butter, and petrolatum *(see all).* Cream rouge may contain erythrosine as a coloring, stearic acid, cetyl alcohol, potassium hydroxide, glycerin, and water; or sorbitol, lanolin, mineral oil, petrolatum, a color pigment, perfume, and water; or anhydrous or emulsified carnauba wax, ozokerite, isopropyl palmitate, titanium dioxide, talc, certified colors, pigments, and perfume *(see all).* Dry rouge may contain kaolin, talc, precipitated calcium carbonate, magnesium carbonate, titanium dioxide, zinc stearate, certified colors and lakes, inorganic oxides, and perfume *(see all).* A typical formula for an emulsified rouge includes white beeswax, 12 percent; petrolatum, 24 percent; spermaceti, 8 percent; mineral oil, 22 percent; borax, 0.8 percent; water, about 30 percent; pigment, 3.1 percent; *p*-hydroxybenzoic acid, 0.1 percent; and perfume *(see all).* Rouge does not figure often in FDA complaints. In recent years there have been complaints of eye irritation and fungus.

ROYAL JELLY • Highly touted as a magic ingredient in cosmetics to restore one's skin to youthfulness. Royal jelly is the very nutritious secretion of the throat glands of the honeybee workers that is fed to the larvae in a colony, to all queen larvae, and possibly to the adult queen. It is a mixture of proteins plus about 31 percent fats, 15 percent carbohydrates, 15 percent minor growth factors, and 24 percent water and trace elements. If stored, royal jelly loses its capacity to develop queen bees. Even when fresh, it has no proven value in a cosmetic preparation. No known toxicity.

RUBBER • Rubber, as well as rubber-based adhesives, is a common cause of contact dermatitis. The natural gum obtained from the rubber tree is not allergenic; the offenders are the chemicals added to natural rubber gum to make it a useful product. Such chemicals are accelerators, antioxidants, stabilizers, and vulcanizers, many of which can cause allergies. Two are the most frequent but certainly not the only sensitizers in rubber. They are mercaptobenzothiazole and tetramethylthiuram. Don't forget that the edge of eyelash curlers may have rubber, as well as the false eyelashes themselves.

RUBBING ALCOHOLS • Isopropyl alcohol *(see),* probably the most common rubbing alcohol, is used in astringents, skin fresheners, colognes, and perfumes. It can be irritating to the skin. Ethanol *(see)* is used in perfumes and as a solvent for oils. It also can be irritating. Rubbing alcohols are denatured with chemicals to make them poisonous so they will not be ingested as an alcoholic beverage.

RUBEFACIENTS • Help stimulate blood circulation to the scalp and the activity of the oil-secreting glands. Pilocarpine *(see)* is an example.

RUBIA TINCTORIUM • See Madder.

RUBUS DELICIOSUS • See Boysenberry.

RUBUS IDAEUS • See Raspberry Juice.

RUBUS VILLOSUS • See Blackberry Extract.

RUE OIL • *Ruta graveolens.* A spice ingredient obtained from the fresh, aromatic, blossoming plants grown in southern Europe and the Orient. It has a fatty odor and is used in baked goods. The oil is obtained by steam distillation and is used in fragrances and in blueberry, raspberry, and other fruit flavorings. Formerly used in medicine to treat disorders and hysteria. It is on the FDA list for study of mutagenic, teratogenic, subacute, and reproductive effects. It may cause photosensitivity.

RUMEX CRISPUS • See Curled Dock.

RUMEX ACETOSELLA • See Sorrel Extract.

RUSCOGENIN • A sterol *(see)* used as a skin conditioning ingredient.

RUSCUS ACULEATUS • See Butcher's-Broom.

RUTA GRAVEOLENS • See Rue Oil.

RUTIN • Found in many plants, especially buckwheat, tobacco, and myrtle. Used to protect blood vessels in medicines. In cosmetics, it used as a skin- and hair-conditioning ingredient and as an anxitoxidant.

RYE FLOUR • Used in powders. Flour made from hardy annual cereal grass. Seeds are used for feed and in the manufacture of whiskey and bread. May cause allergic reactions.

S

SABBATIA • See American Centaury.

SACCHARATED LIME • Produced by the action of lime upon sugar. Used as a buffer *(see)* in cosmetics and as a preservative. No known toxicity.

SACCHARIDE HYDROLYSATE • A mixture of sugars derived from using an alkali and water on a mixture of glucose and lactose *(see)*.

SACCHARIDE ISOMERATE • See Saccharide Hydrolysate.

SACCHARIN • An artificial sweetener in use since 1879. It is 300 times as sweet as natural sugar. Used as a sweetener for mouthwashes, dentifrices, and lipsticks. It sweetens dentifrices and mouthwashes in 0.05 to 1 percent concentration. On the FDA's top priority list to retest for mutagenic, subacute, and reproductive effects. White crystals or crystalline powder. Odorless or with a faint aromatic odor. It was used with cyclamates in the experiments that led to the ban on cyclamates. The FDA has proposed restricting saccharin to 15 milligrams per day for each kilogram of body weight or 1 gram per day for a 150-pound person. Now being studied by NTP *(see)* for possible de-listing as a carcinogen.

SACCHAROMYCES • Yeast extracts.

SACCHARUM OFFICINARIUM • Black Strap Molasses Extract or Sugar Cane Extract.

SAFFLOWER GLYCERIDE • See Safflower Oil.

SAFFLOWER OIL • *Carthamus tinctorius Oil.* Used in creams and lotions to soften the skin and in hair conditioners. Oil is expressed from the seed of an Old World herb that has large bright red or orange flowers and resembles a thistle. Widely cultivated for its oil, which thickens and becomes rancid on exposure to air. The CIR Expert Panel says based on available data, it is safe as a cosmetic ingredient.

SAFFLOWERAMIDOPROPYL ETHYLDIMONIUM ETHOSULFATE • Fatty acid derived from safflower oil *(see)*. Antistatic hair conditioner.

SAFFRON CROCUS EXTRACT • An extract of the flowers of *Crocus sativus.* Used in perfumery and coloring in cosmetics. It is the dried stigma of the crocus cultivated in Spain, Greece, France, and Iran. Used also in bitters, liquors, and spice flavorings. Formerly used to treat skin diseases. No known toxicity.

SAFROLE • Found in certain natural oils such as star anise, nutmeg, and ylang-ylang, it is a stable, colorless to brown liquid with an odor of sassafras and root beer. Used in the manufacture of heliotropin *(see)* and in inexpensive soaps and perfumes. Also used as a beverage flavoring. The toxicity of this fragrance ingredient is being questioned by the FDA. It is an animal carcinogen.

SAGE EXTRACT • Used by herbalists to treat sore gums and mouth ulcers and to remove warts. The oil was used as a meat preservative. No known toxicity.

SAGE OIL • Obtained by steam distillation from the flowering tops of the plant believed by the Arabs to prevent dying. A pale yellow liquid that smells and tastes like camphor. Used to cover gray hair in some rinses and as an astringent in skin fresheners and steam baths. Supposedly has healing power. No known toxicity.

SAGEBRUSH • See Sesquiterpene Lactones.

SAINT JOHN'S BREAD • See Locust Bean Gum.

SAINT JOHN'S WORT • *Hypericum perforatum.* **Amber. Blessed. Devil's Scourge. God's Wonder Herb. Grace of God. Goatweed. Hypericum. Klamath Weed.** A perennial native to Britain, Europe, and Asia, it is now found throughout North America. The plant contains glycosides, volatile oil, tannin, resin, and pectin *(see all)*. It is used in "organic" cosmetics. It was believed to have infinite healing powers derived from the saint, the red juice representing his blood. It was used as an antivenereal. It is used to treat pains and diseases of the nervous system, arthritic pains, and injuries. An infusion made from its leaves is used for stomach disorders, diarrhea, depression, and bladder problems and to remove threadworms in children. A salve made from the flowers is used by herbalists to treat scratches, swellings, and small wounds. The oil is used for burns. A spray has been used for colds. It reputedly also eases fibrositis, sciatica, and varicose veins. It is now being studied by researchers from the National Cancer Institute and universities as a potential treatment for cancer and AIDS. The FDA listed Saint John's Wort as an "unsafe herb" in 1977. The FDA issued a notice in 1992 that St. John's Wort has not been shown to be safe and effective as claimed in OTC digestive aid products. That does not mean, however, that it cannot be used for other purposes.

SALAD OIL • Any edible vegetable oil. Dermatologists advise rubbing salad oils or fats on the skin, particularly on babies and older persons. Vegetable oils are used in commercial baby preparations, cleansers, emollient creams, face powders, hair-grooming preparations, hypoallergenic cosmetics, lipsticks, nail creams, shampoos, shaving creams, and wave sets. Nontoxic.

SALICARIA EXTRACT • **Spiked Loosestrife.** Extract of the flowering herb *Lythrum salicaria,* which has purple or pink flowers. Used since ancient Greek times as an herb that calms nerves and soothes the skin.

SALICYLAMIDE • An analgesic, fungicide, and anti-inflammatory ingredient used to soothe the skin. White to slightly pink crystalline bitter powder. Gives a sensation of warmth on the tongue. Soluble in hot water. In 1992, the FDA proposed a ban on the use of salicylamide to treat fever blisters and cold sores, poison ivy, poison oak, and poison sumac because it has not been shown to be safe and effective for stated claims in OTC products.

SALICYLANILIDE • Usually made from salicylic acid with aniline. Odorless leaflets, slightly soluble in water, freely soluble in alcohol. Used as a topical antifungal ingredient and in antibacterial soaps and topical preparations. In concentrated form may cause irritation of the skin and mucous membranes. When exposed to sunlight, it can cause swelling, reddening, and/or rash of the skin. Halogenated salicylanilides (those with chlorine added) are no longer permitted in cosmetics.

SALICYLATES • **Amyl. Phenyl. Benzyl. Menthyl. Glyceryl. Dipropylene Glycol Esters.** Salts of salicylic acid. Those who are sensitive to aspirin may also be hypersensitive to FD & C Yellow No. 5, a salicylate, and to a number of foods that naturally contain salicylate, such as almonds, apples, apple cider, apricots, blackberries, boysenberries, cherries, cloves, cucumbers, currants, gooseberries, grapes, nectarines, oil of wintergreen, oranges, peaches, pickles, plums, prunes, raisins, raspberries, strawberries, and tomatoes. Foods with added salicylates for flavoring may be ice cream, bakery goods (except bread), candy, chewing gum, soft drinks, Jell-O®, jams, cake mixes, and wintergreen flavors. The salts are used as sunburn preventatives and antiseptics.

SALICYLIC ACID • Methyl Salicylate. Aveeno Cleansing Bar for Acne. Buf-Puf Medicated Acne Pads. Calicylic Creme. Clearasil. Clear Away. Compound W. Derma-Soft Cream. Freezone. Noxzema Clear-Ups. Occlusal. Off-Ezy Wart Removal. Oxy Clean Medicated Pads. DuoFilm Liquid. DuoPlant Gel. Freezone. MG 217 Psoriasis. Keralyt. Viranol. Sal-Plant. Paplex. Oxipor. Oxy Medicated Pads. P & S Plus Tar Gel. Sebulex. Sebutone. Stri-Dex Dual Textured Maximum Strength Pads. Wart-Off Wart Remover. Trans-Plantar. Beta-Hydroxides. Occurs naturally in wintergreen leaves, sweet birch, and other plants. Synthetically prepared by heating phenol with carbon dioxide. It has a sweetish taste and is used as a preservative and antimicrobial. Used externally as an antiseptic ingredient, fungicide, and skin-sloughing ingredient. It is used as a preservative and antimicrobial at 0.1 to 0.5 percent in skin softeners, face masks, hair tonics, deodorants, dandruff preparations, protective creams, hair dye removers, and suntan lotions and oils. It is antipruritic (anti-itch). It is also used in making aspirin *(see)*. It is used as a keratolytic *(see)* drug applied topically to treat acne to slough the skin. It can be absorbed through the skin. Absorption of large amounts may cause vomiting, abdominal pain, increased respiration, acidosis, mental disturbances, and skin rashes in sensitive individuals. Avoid contact with face, genitals, and mucous membranes. The Food and Drug Administration issued a notice in 1992 that salicylic acid, while useful for removing warts, is not effective as an external pain or itch reliever in insect bites and stings, poison ivy, poison sumac, and poison oak OTC drug products. Being widely promoted at this writing in "antiaging" beta-hydroxide products. It is being substituted for the "alpha" in alpha-hydroxide products because it is said to be less irritating to the skin.

SALICYLIDES • Any of several crystalline derivatives of salicylic acid *(see)* from which the water has been removed.

SALIX ALBA • See Willow Leaf Extract.

SALMO • See Salmon Egg Extract and Salmon Oil.

SALMON EGG EXTRACT • The fatty compound from salmon eggs used in cosmetic emollients.

SALMON OIL • Oil from the fish. It is used in emollients.

SALVE • An unctuous adhesive composition or substance applied to wounds or sores; a healing ointment.

SALVIA HISPANICA • See Chia Oil.

SALVIA OFFICINALIS • See Sage Extract.

SALVIA SCLAREA • See Clary.

SAMBUCUS EXTRACT • See Elder Flowers.

SAND • Used as an abrasive.

SANDALWOOD • See Sandalwood Oil.

SANDALWOOD EXTRACT • See Sandalwood Oil.

SANDALWOOD OIL • Used in perfume. It is the pale yellow, somewhat viscous volatile oil obtained by steam distillation from the dried ground roots and wood of the plant *Santalum album*. Has a strong, warm, persistent odor, soluble in most fixed oils. Used in floral, fruit, honey, and ginger ale flavorings for beverages, ice cream, ices, candy, baked goods, and chewing gum. Also used for incense and as a fumigant. May produce skin rash in the hypersensitive, especially if present in high concentrations in expensive perfumes.

SANDARAC GUM • Resin from a plant grown in Morocco. Light yellow, brittle, insoluble in water. Used in tooth cements, varnishes, and for gloss and adhesion in nail lacquers. Also used as an incense. No known toxicity.

SANGUINARIA • **Bloodroot.** Derived from the dried roots and rhizome of the North American herb. The resin is used to soothe the skin, and its reddish juice stanches blood when used in styptic pencils. No known toxicity.

SANICLE • *Sanicula europaea*. A plant grown in Europe and the mountains of Africa and in the Americas. According to an old folk saying, "He who has Sanicle, needeth no surgeon." Since ancient times, it has had a reputation for healing powers. It was used for burns and wounds. It was taken in the form of root tea for skin problems and St. Vitus' dance. Herbalists still recommend it for external use to treat skin diseases and for use in mouthwashes and gargles. A strong decoction of the leaves is used for infections.

SANICULA EUROPAEA • See Sanicle.

SANTALUM ALBUM • See Sandalwood.

SANTALOL • Alcohol from sandalwood used in fragrances. See Sandalwood Oil.

SANTOLINA CHAMAECYPARISSUS • See Lavendar.

SAPINDUS MUKUROSSI • See Soapberry Extract.

SAPONARIA EXTRACT • **Soapwort. Fuller's Herb.** The extract is obtained from *Saponaria officinalis,* a European and middle Asian herb that has a coarse pink or white flower and foams like soap bubbles when scratched. It is substituted for soap in shampoos. No known toxicity.

SAPONIFICATION • The making of soap, usually by adding alkalies to fat with glycerol. To saponify is to convert to soap.

SAPONIN • Any of numerous natural glycosides—natural or synthetic compounds derived from sugars—that occur in many plants such as soapbark, soapwort, or sarsaparilla. Characterized by their ability to foam in water. Yellowish to white, acrid, hygroscopic. In powder form they can cause sneezing. Extracted from soapbark or soapwort and used chiefly as a foaming and emulsifying ingredient and detergent; also used to reduce surface tensions and to produce fine bubble lather in shaving creams, shampoos, bath oils, and dry shampoos. No known skin toxicity.

SARCOSINES • Found in starfish and sea urchins, and also formed from caffeine. Sweetish, crystalline acids used in dentifrices as an antienzyme to prevent tooth decay. Because of their excellent foaming qualities, they are also used in shampoos. No known toxicity.

SARGASSUM • See Algae.

SARSAPARILLA EXTRACT • The dried root from tropical American plants. Used in cola, mint, root beer, sarsaparilla, wintergreen, and birch beer flavorings for beverages, ice cream, ices, candy, and baked goods. Still used for psoriasis; formerly used for the treatment of syphilis. No known toxicity.

SASSAFRAS OIL • Used in dentifrices, perfumes, soaps, and powders to correct disagreeable odors. It is the yellow to reddish yellow volatile oil obtained from the roots of the sassafras. It is 80 percent safrole and has the characteristic odor and taste of sassafras. Applied to insect bites and stings to relieve symptoms; also used as a topical antiseptic and to break up intestinal gas. May produce dermatitis in hypersensitive individuals.

SATUREIA HORTENSIS • See Savory Extract.

SAVORY EXTRACT • An extract of *Satureia hortensis,* an aromatic mint known as summer or winter savory. Used as a spice, particularly in baked goods.

SAW PALMETTO EXTRACT • *Serenoa repens* or *serrulata.* **Sabal. Serenoa.** A common stemless palm of Southern Florida and the Indies. The fruit is used to treat debilitating and wasting conditions, prostatic enlargement, urinary tract infections, as an aphrodisiac, and for body building. Herbalists use it to treat "honeymoon cystitis," urinary tract problems due to frequent sexual activity. The FDA does not recognize it as a drug, but in Germany it is used in over-the-counter treatments for benign prostate enlargement. Saw Palmetto contains anti-inflammatory ingredients, carotene, tannin, and estrogenic substances. It is a strong expectorant.

SCABIOSA EXTRACT • The extract of an Old World herb, *Scabiosa,* used to treat scabies in folk medicine.

S-CARBOXY METHYL CYSTEINE • See Cysteine.

SCHIZANDRA CHINENSIS EXTRACT • An herb used by Chinese women as an aphrodisiac and youth tonic. It is a mild sedative. Also believed to increase stamina. Schizandra has been shown in modern scientific laboratories to protect against the narcotic and sedative effects of alcohol and barbiturates. It is used as a tea. Contraindicated in persons with high blood pressure, epilepsy, and increased pressure on the brain.

SCLEROTIUM GUM • A gum produced by the bacterium *Sclerotium rolfssii.* A waxy mass of fungi and sugars.

SCOPOLAMINE • **Transderm-Scop. Isopto Hyoscine. Twilight Sleep.** An anticholinergic antispasmodic drug used to treat irritable bowel syndrome, Parkinsonism, and other spastic states. It is absorbed through a skin patch to prevent nausea and vomiting associated with motion sickness. Used preoperatively to reduce secretions. Also used in eyedrops to dilate the pupil. Potential adverse reactions include disorientation, restlessness, irritability, dizziness, drowsiness, headache, palpitations, rapid heartbeat, slow heartbeat, dilated pupils, blurred vision, eye sensitivity to light, increased eye pressure, difficulty swallowing, urinary retention, flushing, rash, skin dryness, fever, and depressed respiration. The use of scopolamine hydrobromide in OTC sleep aids was deemed ineffective by the FDA in 1990, and products using it had to reformulate or be banned.

SCROPHULARIA NODODA • See Figwort.

SCULLCAP • See Skullcap.

SCULPTURED NAILS • Methyl and polymethyl methacrylates are used to form synthetic nails. Methyl methacrylate can be highly sensitizing and polymethyl methacrylate weakly so.

SCURVY GRASS EXTRACT • The extract of the leaves and flower stalks of *Cochlearia officinalis*. The bright green leaves of this northerly herb were collected and eaten in large quantities by European seamen to prevent scurvy. The plant has the strong odor of horseradish, to which it is related. No known toxicity.

SCUTELLARIA ROOT EXTRACT • See Skullcap.

SD ALCOHOLS 3-A; 23-H; 38-B; 38-F; 39-B; 39-C; 40; 40-A; 40-B; 40-C146 • All ethyl alcohols denatured in accordance with government regulations. Used as thickeners, solidifiers, and liquefiers. See Denaturant.

SEA SALT EXTRACT • The European market calls this Maris Sal. It is used in bath oils and as a skin conditioner.

SEA SILT EXTRACT • The European market calls this Maris Limus. The extract of marine sediments, it is used as a thickener and abrasive.

SEA WHIP EXTRACT • *Pseudopterogorgia.* **Gorgonian Extract.** An animal with tiny, evenly distributed pores, stemps, and braches that are long and whiplike. It maybe purple, red, orange, yellow, or tan. It is found attached to rocks. Its sexual reproduction is a polyp, which then reproduces asexually by budding to become the parent of a new colony. It has been found to yield a potent anti-inflammatory drug which, at this writing, is being tested as therapy for irritant contact dermatitis.

SEABUCKTHORN EXTRACT • The extract of the fruit of *Hippophae rhamnoides*. A Eurasian maritime shrub having orange-red edible berries and yielding a yellow dye. *See Hippophae rhamnoides.*

SEAROCKET • *Cakile maritima.* A succulent herb found along the sandy shore.

SEAWATER • The European market calls this Maris Aqua.

SEAWEED • See Algae, Carrageenan, and Kelp.

SEBACEOUS GLANDS • Oil glands that provide sebum to coat hair and the stratum corneum *(see)*.

SEBACIC ACID • **Decanedioic Acid.** Colorless leaflets, sparingly soluble in water and soluble in alcohol. Manufactured by heating castor oil with alkalies or by distillation of oleic acid *(see)*. The esters of sebacic acid are used as plasticizers in cosmetics. No known toxicity.

SEBORRHEIC DERMATITIS • Skin inflammation caused by overactivity of the oil glands in the skin. Seborrheic dermatitis is a scaling disorder. Its cause is not well understood. In milder manifestations, it affects the scalp and is commonly called dandruff. In more severe cases, lesions can appear on the face and trunk. The most recent advance in the treatment of seborrheic dermatitis of the scalp is a shampoo containing the active ingredient ketoconazole, an antifungal. Recalcitrant cases may require the use of topical corticosteroids in addition to ketoconazole. Older treatments included the use of coal tar shampoos, most of which are now available over the counter, and shampoos containing selenium sulfide, also primarily OTC products. Salicylic acid solutions may help to remove scales.

SECALE CEREALE • See Rye Flour.

SECHIUM EDULE • Cho Cho. **Vegetable Pear.** Herbalists use it to lower high blood pressure and high cholesterol.

SEDGE ROOT • See Cyperus.

SEDUM ACRE • **Stone Crop. Gold Moss.** Flowers in spring in sunny, sandy soil. Related to houseleek *(see)*. Irritating to the skin in a way similar to pepper. Contains nicotine.

SELENIUM ASPARTATE • The selenium salt of aspartic acid. See Aspartic Acid and Selenium Sulfide.

SELENIUM SULFIDE • **Head and Shoulders Intensive Treatment. Selsun Blue Dandruff Shampoo—Extra Medicated.** Discovered in 1807 in the earth's crust, it is used in antidandruff shampoos and applied to the skin for the treatment of tinea versicolor *(see)*. Can severely irritate the eyes if it gets into them while the hair is being washed. May cause dryness or oiliness of hair or scalp, and rarely increases normal hair loss. Occupational exposure causes pallor, nervousness, depression, garlic odor of breath, gastrointestinal disturbances, skin rash, and liver injury in experimental animals.

SELF-HEAL • *Prunella vulgaris.* A perennial herb native to many countries, it was used by New England settlers to cure "female troubles" and as a tonic. Among its ingredients are volatile oils, bitter principle, and tannin *(see all)*. It is used as an herbal treatment and general tonic and by herbalists as an infusion. Externally, it is used in a poultice as an antiseptic for wounds and to stop bleeding. It is also used to treat diarrhea, sore throat, and hemorrhoids.

SEMPERVIVUM • Plant has irritating properties and the leaves have been found to cause skin rash. See Houseleek.

SENECIO • See Groundsel Extract.

SENEGA EXTRACT • *Polygala senega.* **Snakeroot.** The North American Indians, particularly the Senecas, used this for snakebite. It contains saponins, mucilage, salicylic acid, and resin. It is used by herbalists as an expectorant in the treatment of bronchial asthma. It is also used to stimulate saliva and to treat sore throats and laryngitis. If too much is taken, it irritates the lining of the gut and causes vomiting, according to herbalists.

SENNA, ALEXANDRIA • Flavoring from the dried leaves of *Cassia senna* grown in India and Egypt. Has been used as a cathartic.

SENSITIVITY • Hypersensitivity. An increased reaction to a substance that may be quite harmless to nonallergic persons.

SENSITIZE • To administer or expose to an antigen provoking an immune response so that, on later exposure to that antigen, a more vigorous secondary response will occur.

SENSITIZER • An ingredient that causes an increased reaction to a substance.

SEPIA • See Cuttlefish Extract.

SEQUESTERING INGREDIENT • A preservative that prevents physical or chemical changes affecting color, flavor, texture, or appearance of a product. Ethylenediamine tetraacetic acid (EDTA) is an example. It prevents adverse effects of metals in shampoos.

SERENOA SERRULATA • See Saw Palmetto Extract.

SERICA • See Silk.

SERICIN • A protein isolated from the silkworm. Used in hair and skin conditioners.

SERINE • A nonessential amino acid *(see),* taken as a dietary supplement. It is a constituent of many proteins. See Proteins.

SERPENTARIA EXTRACT • **Snakeroot. Snakeweed.** Extracted from the roots of *Rauwolfia serpentina,* its yellow rods turn red upon drying. Used in the manufacture of resins and as a bitter tonic. No known toxicity when applied to the skin, but can affect heart and blood pressure when ingested.

SERUM ALBUMEN • The major protein component of blood plasma derived from bovines. Used as a moisturizing ingredient.

SERUM PROTEINS • See Serum Albumen.

SESAME • Seeds and Oils. *Sesamum Indicum Oil.* The edible seeds of an East Indian herb that has a rosy or white flower. The seeds, which flavor bread, crackers, cakes, confectionery, and other products, yield a pale yellow, bland-tasting, almost odorless oil used in the manufacture of margarine. The oil has been used as a laxative and skin softener, and contains elements active against lice. It is also used in hair conditioners. Bland taste. May cause allergic reactions, primarily contact dermatitis. The CIR Expert Panel says based on available data, it is safe as a cosmetic ingredient.

SESAMIDOPROPYL BETAINE • See Quaternary Ammonium Compounds.

SESAMIDOPROPYL DIMETHYLAMINE • See Quaternary Ammonium Compounds.

SESAMIDOPROPYLAMINE OXIDE • See Quaternary Ammonium Compounds.

SESQUITERPENE LACTONES • These compounds occur naturally in essential oils, particularly citrus oils. They have little flavor and poor water solubility, and react readily with oxygen to produce off-aroma and off-flavor notes. In recent years, more than 600 plants have been identified as containing these substances, and more than 50 are known to cause allergic contact dermatitis. Among them are arnica, chamomile, and yarrow *(see all).*

SETTING LOTIONS • Wave-setting lotions, which women apply before rolling their hair in rollers or pins, depend on the hair-swelling ability of the water contained in them and the gum film that dries and holds the hair in place. The natural gums commonly used in such preparations are tragacanth, karaya, acacia, and quince seed, as well as sodium alginate from seaweed. Synthetic gums such as methylcellulose *(see)* are also used, but tend to flake when dry. A typical setting lotion may consist of karaya gum dissolved in ethyl alcohol and then mixed with water, glycerin, and perfume. A generally harmless product, but there have been some cases of scalp irritation reported to the FDA.

SHADDOCK EXTRACT • An extract of *Citrus grandis* and named for a seventeenth-century sea captain who brought the seeds back from the East Indies to Barbados. Shaddock is a very large, thick-rinded, pear-shaped citrus fruit related to and largely replaced by the grapefruit. No known toxicity.

SHAMPOOS • Shampoos are of relatively recent origin because people used to wash their hair with soap. The original products were made of coconut oil and castile soap. In 1930, the liquid detergent shampoos were introduced, followed by the cream type, and then the liquid cream shampoos. Today, shampoos are packaged in plastic tubes or bottles, aerosol cans, jars, and glass. They have various special purposes, such as mending split ends or curing dandruff. They contain a variety of ingredients ranging from eggs to herbs. A soap shampoo today still may contain about 25 percent coconut oil, some olive oil, about 15 percent alcohol, and 50 percent glycerol and water. The soapless shampoo cream may contain 50 percent sodium lauryl sulfate, some sodium stearate *(see both),* and about 40 percent water. The liquid shampoo is the most popular today and usually contains a detergent such as triethanolamine dodecylbenzene sulfonate, ethanolamide of lauric acid *(see both),* perfume, and water. Cream shampoos may have the same ingredients as the liquid in different proportions to obtain a cream, and they usually contain lanolin. Special shampoos contain such things as dehydrated egg powder or herbs. Opacifying ingredients such as stearyl and cetyl alcohol *(see both)* may be added to the cream lotion types. Various sequestering ingredients *(see)* may be used to make the water soft to remove the film and to make the hair shinier. Various finishing ingredients, such as mineral oil and lanolin, may be added to make the hair lustrous. Water-absorbing materials such as glycerin and sorbitol *(see)* are used as conditioning ingredients; these two increase the water absorption of the hair and make it more pliable and less brittle. Preservatives such as *p*-hydroxybenzoic acid and sodium hexametaphosphate *(see both)* may also be used. Ingestion of detergents can cause gastric irritation. Shampoos are among the most frequently cited in complaints to the FDA. Reports include eye irritation, scalp irritation, tangled hair, swelling of hands, face, and arms, and split and fuzzy hair.

SHARK-LIVER OIL • A rich source of Vitamin A believed to be beneficial to the skin. A brown fatty oil obtained from the livers of the large predatory fish. Used in lubricating creams and lotions. No known toxicity.

SHAVE GRASS • See Horsetail.

SHAVING CREAMS • Dry hair is hard and difficult to cut with a razor. The object of a shaving cream is to make the hair softer and easier to shave. Brushless shave creams are emulsions of oil and water, really vanishing creams rather than soaps. Not as efficient as the lathering type, they usually require that the beard (or legs) be washed with soap and water. Shaving creams, which must be applied, are soaps with small but copious bubbles known as lather. They can be applied with a brush or with an aerosol. Aerosol shaving creams produce foam. This foam is applied directly to the beard and is the most popular form used today. Some men still use the older shaving creams offered in a cake or stick. The American Medical Association recommends that men with dry or soap-sensitive skin use brushless shave creams that, because of their emollient properties, soothe the skin and do not dry it out. Men with oily skin, on the other hand, should use the lather-type cream applied by aerosol or brush. The AMA also points out that thorough washing and rinsing of the face in hot water or applying a hot wet towel for a few minutes before shaving will soften a beard as well as any cream.

SHAVING LOTIONS • Preshave and After-Shave. Most preshave lotions are designed to be used before shaving with an electric razor. Some are made for a regular razor and usually contain coconut oil, fatty acids, triethanolamine, alkyl arylpolyethylene glycol ether (a dispersant), water, and perfume. Preshave preparations temporarily tighten the skin to facilitate cutting the hairs. Electric razor preshave products may contain aluminum phenolsulfonate, menthol, camphor *(see all)*, water, and perfume dissolved in alcohol. An oily type of preshave lotion may contain isopropyl myristate or isopropyl palmitate *(see both)*, 74.5 percent alcohol, and perfume. After-shave lotions are supposed to soothe the skin, which may have been irritated by shaving. The earliest were merely substitutes for water. At the end of the nineteenth century, talcum powder appeared among men's shaving products. Then barbershop preparations such as bay rum and witch hazel came into use. By 1916, manufacturers were actively promoting men's toiletries, and today perfume is as common in men's products as it is in women's.

After-shave lotions fall into two categories: alcoholic and nonalcoholic. The most common ingredients of the alcoholic type are, in addition to alcohol, glycerin, water, certified color, and perfume. Menthol may be added to give that cool feeling to the skin. Some antiseptics such as quaternary ammonium compounds *(see)* may also be added. Alum may be used for its astringent-styptic effect; also allantoin *(see)* to promote rapid healing of razor nicks. The after-shave nonalcoholic product resembles hand lotion. In fact, hand lotion may be substituted by the consumer. Such products may be prepared from stearic acid, triethanolamine, cetyl alcohol, glycerin *(see all)*, distilled water, and very small amounts of lanolin and a preservative such as *p*-hydroxybenzoic acid *(see)*. Many other fats, waxes, and emulsifying ingredients may be added. Antiseptics and the soothing allantoin, as well as coloring and perfume, may be incorporated into this type of preparation. However, the best beard softener is still water. Reports of problems to the FDA include the product igniting on the face from a lighted cigarette, face irritations, burned skin and peeling, and eye irritation.

SHEA BUTTER • The natural fat obtained from the fruit of the karite tree, *Butyrosperum parkii*. Also called karite butter, it is widely used in moisturizers, suntan gels and creams, cleansing products, indoor tanning preparations, hair conditioners, hair tonics and lipsticks. No known toxicity.

SHEA BUTTER UNSAPONIFIABLES • The fraction of shea butter that is not saponified during processing and is not turned into fatty alcohol.

SHEEP SORREL • *Rumex acetosella*. A small herb common in dry places and having a pleasant, tangy-tasting leaf. Used in "organic" cosmetics.

SHELF LIFE • (Expiration Date). The amount of time for which a cosmetic product is good under normal conditions of storage and use, depending on the product's composition, packaging, preservation, and so forth. Expiration dates are, for practical purposes, rule of thumb, and a product may expire long before that date if it has not been stored and properly handled.

SHELLAC • A resinous excretion of certain insects feeding on appropriate host trees, usually in India. As processed for marketing, the lacca, which is formed by the insects, may be mixed with small amounts of arsenic trisulfide for color and with rosin. White shellac is free of arsenic. Shellac is used as a candy glaze and polish; in hair lacquer and on jewelry and accessories. It is also used as a binder in cosmetics. May cause allergic contact dermatitis. The CIR Expert Panel says based on available data, it is safe as a cosmetic ingredient.

SHELLAC WAX • Bleached refined shellac. See Shellac.

SHEPHERD'S PURSE EXTRACT • **Shepard's Skin Cream. Shepherd's Heart.** Extract of the herb *Capsella bursapastoris*. A member of the mustard family. It is a white-flowered, weedy herb. Its tiny blossoms grow in the form of a cross. Pungent and bitter, it was valued for its astringent properties by early American settlers. Cotton moistened with its juice was used to stop nosebleeds. In an oil-in-water emulsion, it is used as a base for skin preparations. Among its constituents are saponins, choline, acetylcholine, and tyramine *(see all)*. These preparations are used in modern medicine to stimulate neuromuscular function. The herb also reduces urinary tract irritation. It has been shown to contract the uterus and lower blood pressure.

SHIELD FERN • **Buckler Fern.** Extract of the leaves of *Dryopteris felix-mass,* a fern that grows in Bermuda.

SHOREA ROBUSTA • See Damar.

SHORTENINGS • See Salad Oils.

SIENNA • Used to color face powder. It is made from any of the various earthy substances that are brownish yellow when raw and orange-red to reddish brown when burnt. They are in general darker in color and more transparent in oils than ochers. No longer authorized for use in cosmetics by the FDA.

SIGESBECKIA ORIENTALIS • **Indian Weed. Hedge Mustard.** An upright, slightly hairy annual with small, yellow daisylike heads. Found in forested areas. Used to soothe inflammation.

SILANES • A foul-smelling gas that solidifies. It is used in the manufacture of silicones *(see)*.

SILANOLS • Compounds containing hydroxyl groups bound to silicon atoms. See Silica.

SILICA • A white powder, slightly soluble in water, that occurs abundantly in nature and is 12 percent of all rocks. Sand is a silica. Upon drying and heating in a vacuum, hard, transparent, porous granules are formed that are used in absorbent and adsorbent material in toilet preparations, particularly skin protectant creams. Also used as a coloring ingredient. See Silicones.

SILICA GEL • Silicic Acid. White gelatinous substance obtained by the action of acids on sodium silicate *(see)*. Odorless, tasteless, inert, white fluffy powder when dried. Insoluble in water and acids. Absorbs water readily. It is a dehumidifying and dehydrating ingredient, and is used in refrigerants, cosmetics, and waxes. No known toxicity. See Silicates.

SILICATES • Salts or esters derived from silicic acid *(see)*. Any of numerous insoluble complex metal salts that contain silicon and oxygen constitute the largest group of minerals, and with quartz make up the greater part of the earth's crust (as rocks, soils, and clays). Contained in building materials such as cement, concrete, bricks, and glass. No known toxicity.

SILICEOUS EARTH • Purified silica *(see)* obtained by boiling with diluted acid and washing through a filter. Used in face masks. No known toxicity.

SILICIC ACID • Silica Gel. White gelatinous substance obtained by the action of acids on sodium silicate *(see)*. Odorless, tasteless, inert, white fluffy powder when dried. Insoluble in water and acids. Absorbs water readily. Used in face powders, dentifrices, creams, and talcum powders as an opacifier. Soothing to skin. No known toxicity.

SILICONES • Any of a large group of fluid oils, rubbers, resins, and compounds derived from silica *(see)*, and which are water-repellent, skin adherent, and stable over a wide range of temperatures. Used in after-shave preparations, hair-waving preparations, nail driers, hair straighteners, hand lotions, and protective creams. Used commercially in waterproofing and lubrication. No known toxicity when used externally.

SILK • A natural fiber secreted as a continuous filament by *Bombyx mori,* the silkworm. In the raw state, it is coated with gum that is usually removed before spinning. See Silk Amino Acids and Silk Powder.

SILK AMINO ACIDS • The mixture of amino acids *(see)* resulting in liquefying silk. Used in hairsprays. No known toxicity.

SILK POWDER • Coloring ingredient in face powders and soaps obtained from the secretion of silkworms. A white solid that is insoluble in water. Causes severe allergic skin reactions and, when inhaled or ingested, systemic reactions.

SILOXANE • See Silicones.

SILVER • White metal not attacked by water or atmospheric oxygen. Used as a catalyst *(see)* and as a germicide and coloring in cosmetics. Prolonged absorption of silver compounds can lead to grayish blue discoloration of the skin. May be irritating to the skin and mucous membranes. Permanently listed for use in nail polish in amounts not to exceed 1 percent.

SILVER BROMIDE • Yellowish, odorless powder; darkens on exposure to light. Used in photography, as a topical anti-infective ingredient and astringent and in the production of mirror finishing. May cause contact dermatitis.

SILVER FIR EXTRACT • The extract of the bark and needles of the silver fir tree, *Abies alba.*

SILVER FIR OIL • The oil of the silver fir tree, *Abies alba.*

SILVER NITRATE • A germicide, antiseptic, and astringent in cosmetics and a coloring ingredient in metallic hair dyes. Odorless, colorless, transparent, and poisonous. A white crystalline salt, it was used as a nineteenth-century hair dye. It darkens with exposure to light in the presence of organic matter. Silver combines readily with protein and turns brown. Disadvantages are that it may cause unpleasant off-shades and make the hair stiff. It is also adversely affected by permanent waving. On the skin, it may be caustic and irritating. If swallowed, it causes severe gastrointestinal symptoms and frequently death.

SILVER SULFATE • See Silver Nitrate.

SIMETHICONE • An antifoam compound, a silicone oil, white viscous liquid. Used as an ointment base ingredient. A topical drug vehicle and skin protectant. Used medicinally to break up intestinal gas. No known toxicity.

SINGLE FLORALS • A basic type of perfume that has a definite fragrance of one flower, such as lily of the valley, carnation, or rose. This does not mean that only one note (*see* Body-Note) is used. Such perfumes require skillful blending to surround the desired single floral with other notes to give it power and beauty without intruding on the single theme.

SISAL • **Agave Lechuguilla.** A wax and intermediate *(see)* obtained from a plant native to the Mexican desert. The dust is irritating to the respiratory tract and may cause allergic asthma. Skin toxicity unknown.

SKATOLE • Used in perfumery as a fixative *(see)*. A constituent of beetroot, feces, and coal tar. Gives a violet color when mixed with iron and sulfuric acid. No known toxicity in humans.

SKIN BLEACH • There are a variety of products for removing freckles, age spots (chloasma), flat moles, postinflammatory changes, and even naturally dark skin. The original bleaching creams contained ammoniated mercury *(see)*, which has been banned by the FDA except for use as a preservative in eye makeup. Mercury produced some temporary lightening of the skin by causing sloughing of the outer skin, thus reducing the number of dark pigment cells near the surface. Mercury frequently caused allergic reactions and could have had adverse effects internally even though applied only to the skin. More efficient bleaching creams today use hydroquinone *(see)*, which may cause some lightening of the skin in light- but not in dark-skinned blacks. After treatment is stopped, repigmentation almost always occurs. Some powerful hydroquinone products can produce blotches, allergic reactions, and other undesirable side effects. According to the American Medical Association, bleach products are useful for treating limited areas where excessive pigmentation is the result of an abnormal process. For instance, they may be of limited use in treating melasma, "the mask of pregnancy," that is, the excessive skin pigmentation fairly common in pregnant women and women taking birth control pills. The use of bleach cream is a long-term process, and often the only benefit is from the lubricating effect of the cream base, which relieves dryness of the skin. The bases of the creams and ointments are usually petrolatum, mineral oil, lanolin, or vanishing creams of the stearate type *(see all)*. Active ingredients, carriers, and scents include acetic acid, alcohol, bismuth compounds, citric acid, glycerin, hydrogen peroxide, hydroquinone, monobenzone, oxalic acid, potassium carbonate, potassium chlorate, rose water, borate, sugar, benzoin, zinc oxide, and zinc peroxide *(see all)*. Among problems reported to the FDA were symptoms of mercury poisoning, swelling of the face and neck, jerking of hands, skin rash, burns, and stomach distress. Mercury was banned from cosmetics in 1973.

SKIN BRACER • There is little difference between shaving lotions *(see)* and skin bracers. A skin bracer may have a high alcohol content and may also be used as a body refresher after a bath or shower. It is made mostly of water, alcohol, and perfume. Toxicity depends upon ingredients.

SKIN CONDITIONERS • Emollients, humectants, moisturizers, protectants, and soothers.

SKIN FRESHENER • Fresheners are weaker than astringents. They are usually clear liquids designed to make the skin feel cool, tight, and refreshed. May contain about 60 percent witch hazel, about 15 percent camphorated alcohol, 24 percent alcohol, and 1 percent citric acid. May also contain arnica, bay rum, boric acid, chamomile, floral scents, glycerin, lactic acid, magnesia, menthol, lavender oil, phosphoric acid, talc, benzoin, and aluminum salts *(see all)*. Depending upon the ingredients, may cause respiratory or allergic contact dermatitis.

SKIN LIPIDS • Mixture of fats derived from animal skin. Used in skin conditioners.

SKIN TIGHTENERS • Usually bovine serum albumin (BSA) used to make skin feel firmer. Since baby boomers may prefer to have plant-derived products, protein fractions in vegetable extracts are claimed to provide a "tightening effect."

SKULLCAP • *Scutellaria laterifolia.* **Madweed. Mad Dog Scullcap. Quaker Bonnet. Huang Chi.** Grown throughout the world. There are about 90 known species. It was used to cure infertility. Herbalists use it today for relief of epilepsy, convulsions, and withdrawal from drug and alcohol addiction. It is also used as a sedative, and it is used in "organic" cosmetics. Widely used during the nineteenth century to treat nervous diseases, convulsions, neuralgia, insomnia, restlessness, and even tetanus. Modern scientists have found that it stabilizes blood pressure. Skullcap tea is used as a mild tranquilizer. The sedative and antispasmodic properties led to its use in treating rabies and hence its popular name, Mad Dog Scullcap. It was also used to treat delirium tremens, and was given to teething babies. Cases of liver toxicity caused by the use of this herb have been reported to the Centers for Disease Control.

SLIPPERY ELM BARK • Bark from the North American elm. Fragrant and sticky, it contains much mucilage and powder. Mixed with hot water, it forms a fawn-colored mass. Used as a demulcent *(see)*. No known toxicity.

SMILAZ ARISTOLOCHIAEFOLIA • See Sarsaparilla Extract.

SNAKEROOT • Any of numerous plants that have a reputation as remedies for snakebites. Among them, for example, senega *(Polygala senega)*. The North American Indians, particularly the Senecas, used this for snakebite. It contains saponins, mucilage, salicylic acid, and resin. It is used by herbalists as an expectorant in the treatment of bronchial asthma. It also is used to stimulate saliva and to treat sore throats and laryngitis. If too much is taken, it irritates the lining of the gut and causes vomiting, according to herbalists. Various snakeroots are used in "organic" cosmetics.

SOAP • The oldest cleanser, usually a mixture of sodium salts of various fatty acids. In liquid soaps, potassium instead of sodium salts is used. Bar soaps vary in contents from brand to brand, depending on the fats or oils used. Sodium hydroxide makes a strong soap, fatty acids a mild soap. So-called neutral soaps are actually alkaline, with pH around 10 (compared to skin, which is 5 to 6.5 pH) when dissolved in water. Liquid soaps use potassium instead of sodium. Soaps are usually found in toothpastes, tooth powder, and shaving creams. Soap is usually made by the saponification of a vegetable oil with caustic soda. Hard soap consists largely of sodium oleate or sodium palmitate and is used medicinally as an antiseptic, detergent, or suppository. Many people are allergic to soaps. They may also be drying to the skin, irritate the eyes, and cause rashes, depending upon ingredients.

SOAPBERRY EXTRACT • The extract of the fruit of *Sapindus saponaria*. The berries of the tree contain as much as 37 percent saponin *(see)*.

SOAPWORT • *Saponaria officinalis*. **Bouncing Bet. Fuller's Herb. Sheep Weed. Bruise Wort. Saponaria.** A European and middle Asian perennial herb that has a coarse pink or white flower. The name is derived from the fact that, when agitated in water, it lathers. The active principle, saponin, is a detergent. Substituted for soap in shampoos. Soapwort was prescribed by medieval Arab physicians for leprosy and other skin complaints. The leaves yield an extract that has been used to promote sweating as a remedy against rheumatism and to purify the blood. No known toxicity.

SODIUM ACETATE • Sodium Salt of Acetic Acid. A preservative and alkalizer in cosmetics. Transparent crystals highly soluble in water. In industrial forms, it is used in photography and dyeing processes and in foot warmers because of its heat retention ability. Medicinally it is used as an alkalizer and as a diuretic to reduce body water. No known toxicity.

SODIUM ACRYLATE/VINYL ALCOHOL • **Acrylic Acid.** Polymer with vinyl alcohol sodium salt. See Polyvinyl Alcohol.

SODIUM ALGINATE • An emollient used in baby lotions, hair lacquers, wave sets, and shaving creams. It is the sodium salt of alginic acid extracted from brown seaweed. Occurs as a white to yellowish fibrous or granular powder, nearly odorless, and tasteless. Dissolves in water to form a viscous, colloidal solution and is used in cosmetics as a stabilizer, thickener, and emulsifier. No known toxicity.

SODIUM ALPHA-OLEFIN SULFONATES • Used in cosmetics as cleansing agents. The highest concentration is reportedly 16 percent in shampoos and bath and shower products. These ingredients are a mixture of sulfonate salts. Concentrations above 10 percent produced moderate eye irritation and a concentration of 5 percent produced mild eye irritation in rabbits. In animal reproductive studies, fetal abnormalities were noted. Various studies in animals and humans showed irritation and sensitization. The CIR Expert Panel says based on available data, these ingredients are safe up to 2 percent in "leave-on" products.

SODIUM ALUM • See Alum.

SODIUM ALUMINUM ASCORBATE • See Ascorbic Acid.

SODIUM ALUMINUM CHLOROHYDROXYL LACTATE • The sodium salt of lactic acid and aluminum chlorohydrate *(see both)*.

SODIUM ALUMINUM LACTATE • The salt of sodium and aluminum lactate. See Lactic Acid.

SODIUM AMMONIUM PHOSPHATE • Transparent, odorless crystals used as an analytical reingredient.

SODIUM ASCORBATE • See Ascorbic Acid.

SODIUM ASPARTATE • The sodium salt of aspartic acid *(see)*.

SODIUM ARSENATE • Very poisonous, white or grayish powder, it is used in the manufacture of arsenical soap for use on skins, for treating vines against certain scale diseases, and as a topical insecticide for animals. May cause contact dermatitis.

SODIUM BENZOATE • An antiseptic and preservative used in eye creams, vanishing creams, and toothpastes. White, odorless powder or crystals with a sweet antiseptic taste. Once used medicinally for rheumatism and tonsillitis. Now used as a preservative in margarine, codfish, and bottled soft drinks. No known toxicity for external use.

SODIUM BICARBONATE • **Bicarbonate of Soda. Baking Soda.** Used in effervescent bath salts, mouthwashes, and skin-soothing powders. It is an alkali. Its white crystals or powder are used in baking powder as a gastric antacid, as an alkaline wash, and to treat burns. Used also as a neutralizer for butter, cream, milk, and ice cream. Essentially harmless to the skin, but when used on very dry skin in preparations that evaporate, it leaves an alkaline residue that may cause irritation.

SODIUM BISCHLOROPHENYL SULFAMINE • **Sodium Bischlorophenyl.** See Quaternary Ammonium Compounds.

SODIUM BISULFATE • Colorless or white crystals fused in water. Disinfectant, used in the manufacture of soaps, perfumes, foods, and pickling compounds. See Sodium Bisulfite.

SODIUM BISULFITE • **Sodium Acid Sulfite.** An inorganic salt. It is a white powder with a disagreeable taste. It is used as an antiseptic; an antifermentative in cosmetic creams, mouthwashes, bleaches, perfumes, and hair dyes; to treat parasitic skin diseases; and to remove warts. In its aqueous solution, it is an acid. Concentrated solutions are highly irritating to the skin and mucous membranes. Sodium bisulfite can cause changes in the genetic material of bacteria and is a suspected mutagen. Not permitted in meats and other sources of Vitamin B_1. A strong irritant to the skin and tissue. The Select Committee on GRAS substances found it did not present a hazard at present use levels but that additional data would be needed if higher use occurred.

SODIUM BORATE • Used in freckle lotions, nail whiteners, liquefying (cleansing) creams, and eye lotions as a preservative and emulsifier. Hard, odorless powder insoluble in water, it is a weak antiseptic and astringent for mucous membranes. Used also in bath salts, foot preparations, scalp lotions, permanent-wave solutions, and hair-setting lotions. Has a drying effect on the skin and may cause irritation. Continued use of a shampoo containing it will cause the hair to become dry and brittle. The FDA issued a notice in 1992 that sodium borate has not been shown to be safe and effective for stated claims in OTC products, including insect-bite and sting, drug products and in astringent *(see)* drugs. In the diet of rabbits and rats it caused growth retardation. In the diet of male rats it exerted toxic effects on the sex glands as well as infertility. The CIR Expert Panel says based on available data, it is safe as a cosmetic ingredient at less than or equal to 5 percent; however, cosmetic formulations containing free sodium borate at this concentration should not be used on infant skin or injured skin.

SODIUM BROMATE • Inorganic salt. Colorless, odorless crystals that liberate oxygen. Used as a solvent. The CIR Expert Panel *(see)* says based on available data, it is safe as a cosmetic ingredient not to exceed 10.17 percent. See Potassium Bromate for toxicity.

SODIUM BUTYLPARABEN • See Parabens.

SODIUM BUTYOXYETHOXY ACETATE • See Surfactants.

SODIUM C12-15 ALKOXYPROPYL IMINODIPROPIONATE • The sodium salt of propionic acid *(see).*

SODIUM C14-17 ALKYL SEC SULFONATE • See Alcohol and Sulfonated Oils.

SODIUM C12-15 ALKYL SULFATE • See Sulfonated Oils.

SODIUM C12-18 ALKYL SULFATE • The sodium salt of the sulfate of a mixture of synthetic fatty alcohols with 12 to 18 carbons in the alkyl chain. See Sulfonated Oils.

SODIUM C16-20 ALKYL SULFATE • See Sodium C12-15 Alkyl Sulfate.

SODIUM CAPROAMPHOACETATE • See Surfactants.

SODIUM CAPROAMPHOHYDROXYPROPYLSULFONATE • See Quaternary Ammonium Compounds and Surfactants.

SODIUM CAPROAMPHOPROPIONATE • See Quaternary Ammonium Compounds and Surfactants.

SODIUM CAPRYLATE • See Palm Oil.

SODIUM CAPRYLETH-2 CARBOXYLATE • The sodium salt of capryl alcohol. See Surfactants.

SODIUM CAPRYLETH-9 CARBOXYLATE • The sodium salt of capryl alcohol with carboxylic acid. See Surfactants.

SODIUM CAPRYLOAMPHOACETATE • See Surfactants.

SODIUM CAPRYLOAMPHOHYDROXYPROPYLSULFONATE • See Quaternary Ammonium Compounds.

SODIUM C14-16 OLEFIN SULFONATE • See Sulfonated Oils.

SODIUM C11-15 PARETH-7 CARBOXYLATE • See Alkanolamines.

SODIUM C12-15 PARETH-6 CARBOXYLATE • The sodium salt of the organic acid. Used as a gelling ingredient. See Alkanolamines.

SODIUM C12-15 PARETH-7 CARBOXYLATE • The sodium salt of C12-15 Pareth-7 Carboxylic Acid. Used as a gelling ingredient.

SODIUM C12-13 PARETH SULFATE • The sodium salt of sulfated polyethylene glycol ether of a mixture of synthetic alcohols. See Polyethylene Glycol.

SODIUM C12-15 PARETH SULFATE • The sodium salt of a sulfated polyethylene glycol ether of a mixture of fatty alcohols. See Sulfated Oil.

SODIUM CARBONATE • **Soda Ash.** Small, odorless crystals or powder that occurs in nature in ores and is found in lake brines or seawater. Absorbs water from the air. Has an alkaline taste and is used as an antacid and reingredient in permanent wave solutions, soaps, mouthwashes, shampoos, foot preparations, bath salts, and vaginal douches. It is the cause of scalp, forehead, and hand rash when the hypersensitive used cosmetics containing it.

SODIUM CARBONATE PEROXIDE • See Sodium Carbonate.

SODIUM CARBOXYMETHYL CELLULOSE • Used in setting lotions. It is an artificial gum that dries and leaves a film on the hair. Prepared by treating alkali cellulose with sodium chloroacetate. See Cellulose Gums.

SODIUM CARBOXYMETHYL CHITIN • See Chitin.

SODIUM CARBOXYMETHYL DEXTRAN • See Surfactants.

SODIUM CARBOXYMETHYL TALLOW PROPYLPROPYLAMINE • See Tallow.

SODIUM CARRAGEENAN • Sodium salt of carrageenan *(see)*.

SODIUM CASEINATE • The soluble form of milk protein in which casein is partially neutralized with sodium hydroxide and used as a texturizer. GRAS.

SODIUM CASTORATE • The sodium salt of the fatty acids derived from castor oil *(see)*.

SODIUM CELLULOSE SULFATE • See Cellulose.

SODIUM CETEARYL SULFATE • The sodium salt of a blend of cetyl and stearyl alcohol *(see both)* and sulfuric-acid ester. A wax used as a surface-active ingredient *(see)*. On the basis of the animal and clinical data, the CIR Expert Panel *(see)* concludes that it is safe as a cosmetic ingredient.

SODIUM CETETH-13 CARBOXYLATE • See Cetyl Alcohol.

SODIUM CETYL SULFATE • Marketed in the form of a paste. Contains alcohol, sodium sulfate *(see)*, and water. A surface-active ingredient *(see)*. No known toxicity.

SODIUM CHLORIDE • Common table salt. Used as an astringent and antiseptic in mouthwashes, dentifrices, bubble baths, soap, bath salts, and eye lotions. It consists of opaque white crystals. Odorless, with a characteristic salty taste, it absorbs water. Used topically to treat inflamed lesions. Diluted solutions are not considered irritating, but upon drying, water is drawn from the skin and may produce irritation. Salt workers have a great deal of skin rashes. Also reported to irritate the roots of the teeth when used for a long time in dentifrices.

SODIUM CHONDROITIN SULFATE • Present in soft connective tissue, it is abundant in skin arterial walls and heart valves. It is used to reduce fats and as a flexible connector between protein molecules. No known toxicity.

SODIUM CITRATE • White, odorless crystals, granules, or powder with a cool salty taste. Stable in air. Used as a sequestering ingredient *(see)* to remove trace metals in solutions and as an alkalizer in cosmetic products. No known skin toxicity.

SODIUM COCETH SULFATE • See Coconut Oil.

SODIUM COCOAMINOPROPIONATE • See Coconut Oil.

SODIUM COCOAMPHOACETATE • See Surfactants.

SODIUM COCOAMPHOHYDROXYPROPYLSULFONATE • See Surfactants.

SODIUM COCOAMPHOPROPIONATE • See Surfactants.

SODIUM COCOATE • See Coconut Oil.

SODIUM COCOGLYCERYL ETHER SULFONATE • See Coconut Oil.

SODIUM COCO-HYDROLYZED COLLAGEN • The sodium salt of the condensation product of coconut acid chloride and hydrolyzed animal protein. The world "animal" was removed from the ingredient name. See Hydrolyzed Collagen.

SODIUM COCOMONOGLYCERIDE SULFATE • See Coconut Oil.

SODIUM COCOMONOGLYCERIDE SULFONATE • The fatty acids derived from coconut oil *(see)*.

SODIUM COCOYL COLLAGEN AMINO ACIDS • See Coconut Oil and Collagen.

SODIUM COCOYL GLUTAMATE • A softener. See Glutamate.

SODIUM COCOYL HYDROLYZED COLLAGEN • This was formerly called hydrolyzed animal protein, which it is. See Hydrolyzed.

SODIUM COCOYL HYDROLYZED SOY PROTEIN • See Soybean and Coconut Oils.

SODIUM COCOYL ISETHIONATE • The sodium salt of the coconut-fatty acid ester of isethionic acid. Used as a cleansing ingredient. On the basis of the animal and clinical data, the CIR Expert Panel *(see)* concludes that it is safe as a cosmetic ingredient up to 50 percent in "rinse-off" products and at 17 percent in "leave-on" products. See Coconut Oil.

SODIUM COCOYL SARCOSINATE • See Sarcosines.

SODIUM C4-12 OLEFIN/MALEIC ACID COPOLYMER • **Kao Soap.** The sodium salt of a polymer synthesized from C4-12 olefins and maleic anhydride *(see)*. Used as a demulcent.

SODIUM C14-16 OLEFIN SULFONATE • See Sulfonated Oils.

SODIUM C11-15 PARETH-7 CARBOXYLATE • The sodium salt of C11-15 pareth. Used as a gelling ingredient.

SODIUM C12-15 PARETH-6 CARBOXYLATE • The sodium salt of the organic acid. See Alkanolamines.

SODIUM C12-15 PARETH SULFATE • The sodium salt of a sulfated polyethylene glycol ether of a mixture of fatty alcohols. See Sulfated Oils and Polyethylene Glycol.

SODIUM CUMENESULFONATE • A solvent. See Benzene and Phenol.

SODIUM CYCLOPENTANE • See Cyclopentane.

SODIUM DECETH-2 CARBOXYLATE • See Polyethylene Glycol.

SODIUM DECETH SULFATE • See Decyl Alcohol.

SODIUM DECYLBENZENESULFONATE • Used in commercial detergents. May cause skin irritations.

SODIUM DEHYDROACETATE • **Dehydroacetic Acid.** A preservative; white, odorless, powdered, with an acrid taste. Used as a plasticizer, fungicide, and bacteria killer in cosmetics; also as an antienzyme ingredient in dentifrices, allegedly to prevent decay, and a kidney-tube blocking ingredient. Can cause impaired kidney function. Large doses can cause vomiting, ataxia, and confusion. There are no apparent allergic skin reactions. On the basis of the animal and clinical data, the CIR Expert Panel *(see)* concludes that it is safe as a cosmetic ingredient.

SODIUM DERMATAN SULFATE • See Mucopolysaccharides.

SODIUM DEXTRAN SULFATE • See Dextran.

SODIUM DICARBOXYETHYLCOCO PHOSPHOETHYL IMIDAZOLINE • See Coconut Acid.

SODIUM DICETEARETH-10 PHOSPHATE • See Cetyl Alcohol.

SODIUM DIETHYLAMINOPROPYL COASPARTAMIDE • See Coconut Oil and Alcohol.

SODIUM DIHYDROXYCETYL PHOSPHATE • See Cetyl Alcohol.

SODIUM DIHYDROXYETHYL GLYCINATE • See Dioctyl Sodium Sulfosuccinate.

SODIUM DIOLETH-8 PHOSPHATE • See Oleic Acid.

SODIUM DNA • The sodium salt of deoxyribonucleic acid. The genetic code of cells used in "youth" creams.

SODIUM DODECYLBENZENE SULFONATE • A very widely used anionic detergent used in cosmetic bath products and in creams. It may irritate the skin. Will cause vomiting if swallowed. In some animal studies it caused kidney, intestinal, and liver damage when given orally. On the basis of the animal and clinical data, the CIR Expert Panel *(see)* concludes that it is safe as a cosmetic ingredient. See Sodium Lauryl Sulfate.

SODIUM DVB/ACRYLATES COPOLYMER • See Acrylates.

SODIUM ERYTHROBATE • A white, odorless powder used as an antioxidant in cosmetics. No known toxicity.

SODIUM-2-ETHYHEXYLSULFOACETATE • Light, cream-colored flakes, water soluble, good foam-maker, and good in hard water. Used as a solubilizing ingredient, particularly for soapless shampoo compositions. See Quaternary Ammonium Compounds.

SODIUM ETHYLPARABEN • See Parabens.

SODIUM ETHYL-2 SULFOLAURATE • See Lauric Acid.

SODIUM FLUORIDE • Used in toothpastes to prevent tooth decay and as an insecticide, disinfectant, and preservative in cosmetics. Can cause nausea and vomiting when ingested and even death, depending upon the dose. Tooth enamel mottling has also been reported. The Nonprescription Drug Manufacturers Association also expressed opposition to an FDA proposal to mandate disclosure of the net fluoride content in OTC dentifrice products as a means of preventing dental fluorosis (caused by an excess intake of fluoride) in young children. The trade association insisted that there is no current scientific evidence to indicate that fluorides in dentifrices can contribute to dental fluorosis. No known skin toxicity. See also Stannous Fluoride.

SODIUM FORMATE • See Formic Acid.

SODIUM GLUCONATE • Made from glucose by fermentation, a white to yellowish powder, it is used in metal cleaners, paint strippers, bottle-washing preparations, metal plating, and rust removers. Nontoxic.

SODIUM GLUTAMATE • The monosodium salt of the L-form of glutamic acid. See Glutamic Acid.

SODIUM GLYCERETH-1 POLYPHOSPHATE • Sodium salt of a complex mixture of esters of tetraphosphoric acid with some glycerin. See Glycerin.

SODIUM GLYCERYL OLEATE PHOSPHATE • See Glyceryl Monostearate.

SODIUM HEPARIN • See Heparin Salts.

SODIUM HEXETH-4 CARBOXYLATE • See Polyethylene Glycol.

SODIUM HEXYLMETAPHOSPHATE • **Graham's Salt.** Used in bath salts, bubble baths, permanent-wave neutralizers, and shampoos. An emulsifier, sequestering ingredient *(see)*, and texturizer. Used in foods and potable water to prevent scale formation and corrosion. Because it keeps calcium, magnesium, and iron salts in solution, it is an excellent water softener and detergent. No known toxicity to the skin.

SODIUM HYALURONATE • The sodium salt of hyaluronic acid. From the fluid in the eye, it is used as a gelling ingredient. No known toxicity.

SODIUM HYDROGENATED TALLOWOYL GLUTAMATE • See Glutamate and Tallow.

SODIUM HYDROSULFATE • **Sodium Dithionate.** A bacterial inhibitor and antifermentative. Slight odor. White or grayish white, crystalline powder that oxidizes in air. No known toxicity to the skin.

SODIUM HYDROSULFITE • See Sulfites.

SODIUM HYDROXIDE • **Caustic Soda. Soda Lye.** An alkali and emulsifier in liquid face powders, soaps, shampoos, cuticle removers, hair straighteners, shaving soaps, and creams. White or nearly white pellets, flakes, or sticks. Readily absorbs water. Also a modifier for food starch, a glazing ingredient for pretzels, and a peeling ingredient for tubers and fruits. The FDA banned use of more than 10 percent in household liquid drain cleaners. If too much alkali is used, dermatitis of the scalp may occur. Its ingestion causes vomiting, prostration, and collapse. Inhalation causes lung damage.

SODIUM HYDROXYMETHANE SULFONATE • Sodium Formaldehyde Bisulfite. See Formaldehyde.

SODIUM HYDROXYMETHYL GLYCINATE • See Glycinate.

SODIUM HYPOCHLORITE • Made by the addition of chlorine to sodium hydroxide, it is used for bleaching paper pulp and textiles, in water purification, in fungicides, as a swimming pool disinfectant, in laundry products, and as a germicide. Liquid household bleaches such as Purex™ and Clorox™ are approximately 5 percent sodium hypochlorite solutions. It is also a preservative used in the washing of cottage cheese curd and an antiseptic for wounds.

SODIUM IODATE • Used in dusting powder and to soothe the skin. White, crystalline powder. Antiseptic, particularly to the mucous membranes. The safety of this ingredient has not been documented and substantiated according to the CIR Expert Panel *(see),* and the Panel cannot conclude whether sodium is safe in cosmetics.

SODIUM IODIDE • White, odorless, water-absorbing crystals. Slowly becomes brown on exposure to air. See Sodium Iodate.

SODIUM ISETHIONATE • See Sodium Hydroxide.

SODIUM ISOOCTYLENE/MA COPOLYMER • See Maleic Acid and Polymers.

SODIUM ISOSTEARETH-6 CARBOXYLATE • See Isostearic Acid.

SODIUM ISOSTEAROAMPHOACETATE • See Surfactants.

SODIUM ISOSTEAROAMPHOPROPIONATE • See Quaternary Ammonium Compounds.

SODIUM ISOSTEROYL LACTYLATE • The sodium salt of isostearic acid and lactyl lactate. See Stearic Acid and Lactic Acid.

SODIUM LACTATE • Plasticizer substitute for glycerin. Colorless, thick, odorless liquid miscible with water, alcohol, and glycerin. Solution is neutral. No known toxicity.

SODIUM LACTATE METHYLSILANOL • See Silanols.

SODIUM LANETH SULFATE • See Lanolin.

SODIUM LAURAMINOPROPIONATE • See Propionic Acid.

SODIUM LAURATE • See Sodium Lauryl Sulfate.

SODIUM LAURETH-4 CARBOXYLATE • See Polyethylene Glycol and Lauric Acid.

SODIUM LAURETH-5 CARBOXYLATE • See Polyoxyethylene Compounds and Lauric Acid.

SODIUM LAURETH-4 PHOSPHATE • See Sodium Lauryl Sulfate.

SODIUM LAURETH SULFATE • The sodium salt of sulfated ethoxylated lauryl alcohol, widely used as a water softener and in baby and other nonirritating shampoos as a wetting and cleansing ingredient. Has caused eye and skin irritation in experimental animals and in some human test subjects. The irritant effects are similar to those produced by other detergens and is affected by concentration. On the basis of available information, the CIR Panel concludes that it is safe as presently used in cosmetic products. See also Surfactants.

SODIUM LAURETH-5, -7, AND -12 SULFATES • See Sodium Laureth Sulfate.

SODIUM LAURIMINODIPROPIONATE • See Quaternary Ammonium Compounds.

SODIUM LAUROAMPHOACETATE • See Surfactants.

SODIUM LAUROAMPHOHYDROXYPROPYLSULFONATE • See Surfactants.

SODIUM LAUROAMPHO PG-ACETATE PHOSPHATE • See Surfactants.

SODIUM LAUROAMPHOPRIOPIONATE • The safety of this ingredient has not been documented and substantiated according to the CIR Expert Panel *(see)*, and the Panel cannot conclude whether sodium is safe in cosmetics. See Quaternary Ammonium Compounds.

SODIUM LAUROYL COLLAGEN AMINO ACIDS • Formerly called sodium lauroyl animal collagen amino acids, but the name was changed to remove the "animal." See Collagen and Amino Acid.

SODIUM LAUROYL GLUTAMATE • A softener. See Glutamate.

SODIUM LAUROYL HYDROLYZED COLLAGEN • The salt of the condensation product of lauric acid and hydrolyzed collagen. See Hydrolyzed Collagen.

SODIUM LAUROYL ISETHIONATE • **Sodium Lauryl Isethionate.** One of the main ingredients in Dove®, it is a mild synthetic soap. See Surfactants.

SODIUM LAUROYL LACTYLATE • See Lauric Acid.

SODIUM LAUROYL METHYLAMINOPROPIONATE • See Lauric Acid.

SODIUM LAUROYL SARCOSINATE • See Sarcosines.

SODIUM LAUROYL TAURATE • See Surfactants.

SODIUM LAUROYLISETHIONATE • See Sodium Lauryl Sulfate.

SODIUM LAURYL BENZENE SULFONATE • See Sodium Lauryl Sulfate.

SODIUM LAURYL SULFATE • A detergent, wetting ingredient, and emulsifier used in bubble baths, emollient creams, cream depilatories, hand lotions, cold permanent waves, soapless shampoos, and toothpastes. Prepared by sulfation of lauryl alcohol followed by neutralization with sodium carbonate. Faint fatty odor; also emulsifies fats. May cause drying of the skin because of its degreasing ability, and is an irritant to the skin. On the basis of available information, the CIR Expert Panel *(see)* concludes that it is safe as presently used in cosmetic formulations designed for brief use followed by thorough rinsing from the surface of the skin. In products for prolonged contact with skin, concentrations should not exceed 1 percent.

SODIUM LAURYL SULFOACETATE • See Sodium Lauryl Sulfate.

SODIUM LIGNOSULFONATE • The sodium salt of polysulfonated lignin derived from wood. It is used as a dispersing ingredient. A tan, free-flowing powder, it is also used as an emulsifier, stabilizer, and cleaning ingredient. No known toxicity.

SODIUM MAGNESIUM SILICATES • See Silicates.

SODIUM MANNURONATE METHYLSILANOL • See Silanols.

SODIUM/MEA LAURETH-2 SULFOSUCCINATE • See Surfactants.

SODIUM METABISULFITE • An inorganic salt. A bacterial inhibitor. Used as an antifermentative in sugar, and a preservative for fruits and vegetables. See Bisulfites.

SODIUM METABORATE • See Boric Acid.

SODIUM METAPHOSPHATE • **Graham's Salt.** Used in dental polishing ingredients, detergents, water softeners, sequestrants, emulsifiers, food additives, and textile laundering. See Sodium Hexylmetaphosphate.

SODIUM METASILICATE • An alkali usually prepared from sand and soda ash. Used in detergents. Caustic substance, corrosive to the skin, harmful if swallowed, and cause of severe eye irritations. Preserves eggs in egg shampoos.

SODIUM METHYL COCOYL TAURATE • See Ox Bile.

SODIUM METHYL LAUROYL TAURATE • See Surfactants.

SODIUM METHYL MYRISTOYL • See Myristic Acid and Taurine.

SODIUM METHYL OLEOYL TAURATE • See Ox Bile.

SODIUM METHYL PALMITOYL TAURATE • See Surfactants.

SODIUM METHYL STEAROYL TAURATE • See Taurine.

SODIUM METHYL-2 SULFOLAURATE • See Lauric Acid.

SODIUM METHYLNAPHTHALENE SULFONATE • Used in solutions for peeling fruits and vegetables with a water rinse and in detergents. See Sulfonated Oils.

SODIUM n-METHYL-n-OLEYL TAURATE • See Ox Bile.

SODIUM METHYLPARABEN • See Parabens.

SODIUM MONOFLUOROPHOSPHATE • See Sodium Fluoride.

SODIUM MONOUNDECYLENAMIDO MEA-SULFOSUCCINATE • See Dioctyl Sodium Sulfosuccinate, Sulfonated Oils.

SODIUM MYRETH SULFATE • A cleansing and emulsifying ingredient. Data indicating that a shampoo containing 7 percent and 20 percent dilution of this ingredient induced mild to moderate eye irritation in some animal studies. On the basis of animal and clinical data, the CIR Expert Panel *(see)* concludes that it is safe as a cosmetic ingredient in the present practices of use and concentration. See Myristyl Alcohol.

SODIUM MYRISTATE • See Myristic Acid.

SODIUM MYRISTOAMPHOACETATE • See Surfactants.

SODIUM MYRISTOL GLUTAMATE • See Glutamic Acid.

SODIUM MYRISTOYL HYDROLYZED COLLAGEN • See Hydrolyzed Collagen and Myristic Acid.

SODIUM MYRISTOYL ISETHIONATE • See Myristic Acid.

SODIUM MYRISTOYL SARCOSINATE • See Sarcosine.

SODIUM MYRISTYL SULFATE • See Myristyl Alcohol.

SODIUM m-NITROBENZENESULFONATE • The CIR Expert Panel concludes that the data available are insufficient to support the safety of this ingredient as used in cosmetics. See Benzene and Phenol.

SODIUM NONOXYNOL-6 PHOSPHATE OR -9 PHOSPHATE • A complex mixture of esters of phosphoric acid and nonoxynol *(see both)*.

SODIUM NONOXYNOL-1 OR -4 SULFATE • See Sulfonated Oils.

SODIUM OCTYL SULFATE • See Sulfonated Oils.

SODIUM OLEATE • Sodium salt of oleic acid. White powder, fatty odor, alkaline. Used in soaps. No known toxicity.

SODIUM OLEOAMPHOACETATE • See Quaternary Ammonium Compounds.

SODIUM OLEOAMPHOHYDROXYPROPYLSULFONATE • See Quaternary Ammonium Compounds.

SODIUM OLEOAMPHOPROPIONATE • See Quaternary Ammonium Compounds.

SODIUM OLEOYL HYDROLYZED COLLAGEN • Formerly called sodium oleoyl hydrolyzed animal protein. See Proteins and Hydrolyzed.

SODIUM OLEOYL ISETHIONATE • See Sulfonated Oils.

SODIUM OLETH-7 OR -8 PHOSPHATE • The sodium salts of the phosphate esters of oleth used in mild detergents such as baby shampoos. No known toxicity.

SODIUM OLETH SULFATE • See Polyethylene Glycol and Oleyl Alcohol.

SODIUM OLEYL SULFATE • See Surfactants.

SODIUM OXALATE • **Sodium Salt of Oxalic Acid.** White, odorless, crystalline powder used as an intermediate *(see),* in hair dyes, and as a texturizer. Toxic when ingested, and may be irritating to the skin.

SODIUM OXYNOL-2 ETHANE SULFONATE • See Sulfonated Oils.

SODIUM PALM KERNELATE • See Palm Kernel Acids.

SODIUM PALMITATE • Sodium salt of palmitic acid *(see).*

SODIUM PARETH-15-7 OR 25-7 CARBOXYLATE • See Fatty Alcohols.

SODIUM PARETH-23 OR -25 SULFATE • See Fatty Alcohols.

SODIUM PCA • A naturally occurring component of human skin that is believed to be in part responsible for its moisture-binding capacity. It is highly water absorbing and at high humidity dissolves in its own water hydration. Application of this compound to the skin as a humectant *(see)* is claimed to increase softness. On the basis of the animal and clinical data, the CIR Expert Panel *(see)* concludes that it is safe as used in cosmetic formulations but should not be used in cosmetics containing nitrosating agents *(see).*

SODIUM PCA METHYSILANOL • See Sodium PCA.

SODIUM PEG-6 COCAMIDE CARBOXYLATE • See Coconut Oil.

SODIUM PEG-8 COCAMIDE CARBOXYLATE • See Coconut Oil.

SODIUM PEG-3 LAURAMIDE CARBOXYLATE • See Lauric Acid.

SODIUM PERBORATE • White crystals soluble in water, used as a reingredient *(see),* antiseptic, deodorant, bleach, and in dentifrices as a tooth whitener; also in foot baths and detergents. Ulcerations of the mouth have been reported in its use in dentifrices. Strong solutions that are very alkaline are irritating if permitted on the skin.

SODIUM PERCARBONATE • Stable, crystalline powder derived from sodium carbonate and hydrogen peroxide *(see both).* Used as a denture cleaner and mild antiseptic. Toxic by ingestion. See Peroxide.

SODIUM PEROXIDE • Yellowish white powder, absorbs hydrogen and carbon dioxide from air. Derived from carbon dioxide heated in aluminum trays. A strong oxidizing ingredient and irritant. Used to purify water and germicidal soaps.

SODIUM PERSULFATE • Oxidizing ingredient that promotes emulsion used in hair-waving solution. An inorganic salt; a crystalline powder that decomposes in moisture and warmth. Can cause allergic reactions in the hypersensitive. The CIR Expert Panel *(see)* concludes there is not enough information about this ingredient to "support safety" in cosmetics.

SODIUM PHENATE • See Phenol.

SODIUM PHENOLSULFONATE • See Phenol.

SODIUM PHENOXIDE • See Phenol.

SODIUM o-PHENYL PHENATE • **Sodium Salt of o-Phenylphenol.** Antiseptic, germicide, fungicide, and preservative used in cosmetic creams and lotions. Yellow flakes or powder with a slight soap odor. Soluble in water, alcohol, and acetone. A skin irritant. Regarded as more effective than phenol *(see)* and cresol *(see)* because it has greater germ-killing power, may be used in smaller concentrations, and is less irritating to the skin, although it is often considered toxic by some cosmetic companies for use in products.

SODIUM PHOSPHATE • Buffer and effervescent used in manufacture of nail enamels and detergents. White, crystalline or granular powder, stable in air. Without water, it can be irritating to the skin but has no known skin toxicity.

SODIUM PHTHALATE STEARYL AMIDE • See Quaternary Ammonium Compounds.

SODIUM PICRAMATE • **Sodium Salt of Picramic Acid.** A hair colorant. It is a mutagen and a mild sensitizer in animal studies. It may be a mild sensitizer in humans. It is used in hair dyes at concentrations of 0.1 percent to 1 percent. On the basis of the available animal data, the CIR Expert Panel *(see)* concludes that it is safe as a cosmetic ingredient at concentrations not to exceed 0.1 percent. See Picramic Acid.

SODIUM POLYACRYLATE STARCH • See Starch and Acrylates.

SODIUM POLYDIMETHYLGLYCINOPHENOLSULFONATE • See Sulfonated Oils.

SODIUM POLYGLUTAMATE • See Glutamic Acid.

SODIUM POLYMETHACRYLATE • See Acrylates.

SODIUM POLYNAPHTHALENE SULFONATE • See Sulfonated Oils.

SODIUM POLYSTYRENE SULFONATE • See Polystyrene.

SODIUM PROPIONATE • Colorless, or transparent, odorless crystals that gather water in moist air. Used as a preservative in cosmetics and foodstuffs to prevent mold and fungus. It has been used to treat fungal infections of the skin, but can cause allergic reactions. The Food and Drug Administration issued a notice in 1992 that sodium propionate has not been shown to be safe and effective for stated claims in OTC products.

SODIUM PROPYLPARABEN • See Parabens.

SODIUM PYRITHIONE • **Sodium Omadine®.** Sodium salt of pyrithione zinc derivative. Used as a fungicide and bacteria killer. Used in dandruff shampoos to control dandruff and as an antibacterial in soaps and detergents. No known toxicity.

SODIUM PYROPHOSPHATE PEROXIDE • White powder, water soluble, used as a denture cleanser, in dentifrices and household laundry detergents, and as an antiseptic. See Hydrogen Peroxide.

SODIUM RIBOFLAVIN PHOSPHATE • B vitamin containing sodium phosphate *(see)*.

SODIUM RIBONUCLEIC ACID • **SRNA.** The basic instructions in the cell that tell it how to behave. Since it is believed that the RNA in the cell may make mistakes as we age, it is added to some antiaging creams.

SODIUM RICINOLEATE • The sodium salt of ricinoleic acid *(see)*.

SODIUM RICINOLEOAMPHOACETATE • See Quaternary Ammonium Compounds.

SODIUM SACCHARIN • An artificial sweetener in dentifrices, mouthwashes, and lipsticks. In use since 1879. Pound for pound, it is 300 times as sweet as natural sugar but leaves a bitter aftertaste.

SODIUM SALICYLATE • A white, odorless, crystalline powder used in shaving creams and in sunscreen lotions. Becomes pinkish upon long exposure to light; also used to lower fever and kill pain in animals. Mild antiseptic analgesic and preservative. May cause nasal allergy. See Salicylates.

SODIUM SARCOSINATE • The sodium salt of sarcosine. See Sarcosines.

SODIUM SESQUICARBONATE • White crystals, flakes, or powder produced from sodium carbonate. Soluble in water. Used as an alkalizer in bath salts, shampoos, tooth powders, and soaps. Irritating to the skin and mucous membranes. May cause allergic reaction in the hypersensitive.

SODIUM SILICATE • **Water Glass.** An anticaking ingredient preserving eggs, detergents in soaps, depilatories, and protective creams. Consists of colorless to white, or grayish white, crystalline pieces or lumps. These silicates are almost insoluble in cold water. Strongly alkaline. As a topical antiseptic can be irritating and caustic to the skin and mucous membranes. If swallowed, it causes vomiting and diarrhea.

SODIUM SILICOALUMINATE • See Silicates.

SODIUM SOAP • See Sodium Stearate.

SODIUM SOY HYDROLYZED COLLAGEN • Formerly called hydrolyzed animal protein, but the "animal" name was removed. The sodium salt of the condensation product of soya acid chloride and hydrolyzed animal protein. See Collagen.

SODIUM STANNATE • An inorganic salt. White or colorless crystals. Absorbs water from air. Used in hair dyes. No known toxicity.

SODIUM STEARATE • 92.82 percent stearic acid *(see)*. A fatty acid used in deodorant sticks, stick perfumes, toothpastes, soapless shampoos, and shaving lather. A white powder with a soapy feel and a slight tallowlike odor. Slowly soluble in cold water or cold alcohol. Also a waterlike odor. Also a waterproofing ingredient and has been used to treat skin diseases and in suppositories. One of the least allergy-causing of the sodium salts of fatty acids. Nonirritating to the skin. On the basis of the available information, the CIR Expert Panel *(see)* concludes that it is safe as a cosmetic ingredient.

SODIUM STEARETH-4 PHOSPHATE • See Surfactants.

SODIUM STEAROAMPHOACETATE • See Sodium Stearate.

SODIUM STEAROMAMPHOPROPIONATE • See Quaternary Ammonium Compounds.

SODIUM STEAROYL HYDROLYZED COLLAGEN • See Hydrolyzed Collagen.

SODIUM STEAROYL LACTYLATE • See Lactic Acid.

SODIUM STEARYL SULFATE • See Surfactants.

SODIUM STYRENE/ACRYLATES/DIVINYLBENZENE COPOLYMER • An opacifier. See Styrene, Benzene, and Acrylates.

SODIUM STYRENE/ACRYLATES/PEG-10 DIMALEATE COPOLYMER • An opacifier. See Styrenes and Acrylates.

SODIUM STYRENE/PEG-10 MALEATE/NONOXYNOL-10 MALEATE/ACRYLATES COPOLYMER • Opacifier. See Styrene and Acrylates.

SODIUM SULFANILATE • The sodium salt of sulfanilic acid *(see)*. Used as a hair coloring.

SODIUM SULFATE • **Salt Cake.** Occurs in nature as the minerals mirabilite and thenardite. Used chiefly in the manufacture of dyes, soaps, and detergents. Also as a chewing gum base and, used medicinally, to reduce body water. It is a reingredient *(see)* and a precipitant; mildly saline in taste. Usually harmless when applied in toilet preparations. May prove irritating in concentrated solutions if applied to the skin, permitted to dry and then remain. May also enhance the irritant action of certain detergents. Based on the available data, the CIR Expert Panel *(see)* concludes it is safe as used in "rinse-off" formulations, and safe up to 1 percent "leave-on" formulations.

SODIUM SULFITE • An antiseptic, preservative, and antioxidant used in hair dyes. White to tan or pink, odorless or nearly odorless powder having a cooling, salty, sulfurlike taste. It has been used medicinally as a topical antifungal ingredient. It is also used as a bacterial inhibitor in wine brewing and distilled-beverage industries. Also an antifermentative in the sugar and syrup industries and an antibrowning ingredient in cut fruits, and is used in frozen apples, dried fruit, prepared fruit pie mix, peeled potatoes, maraschino cherries, dried fruits, and glacéed fruits. Used to bleach straw, silk, and wool; and as a developer in photography. Products containing sulfites may release sulfur dioxide. If this is inhaled by people who suffer from asthma, it can trigger an asthmatic attack. Sulfites are known to cause stomach irritation, nausea, diarrhea, skin rash, and swelling in sulfite-sensitive people. People whose kidneys or livers are impaired may not be able to produce the enzymes that break down sulfites in the body.

Sulfites may destroy thiamine and consequently are not added to foods that are sources of this B vitamin.

SODIUM SULFONATE • A bubble-bath, clarifying ingredient and a dispersing ingredient used to make shampoos clear. See Sulfonated Oils.

SODIUM TALLAMPHOPROPIONATE • See Quaternary Ammonium Compounds.

SODIUM TALLOW SULFATE • A defoamer, emollient, intermediate *(see)*, and surface-active ingredient. A mixture of sodium alkyl sulfates. See Tallow.

SODIUM TALLOWAMPHOACETATE • See Tallow and Sodium.

SODIUM TALLOWAMPHOPROPIONATE • See Tallow and Sodium.

SODIUM TALLOWATE • The sodium salt of tallow *(see)*. Used in soaps and detergents.

SODIUM/TEA-LAUROYL COLLAGEN AMINO ACIDS • See Collagen and Lauric Acid.

SODIUM/TEA-LAUROYL HYDROLYZED COLLAGEN • Formerly had "animal protein" in its name. It is still a mixture of sodium and triethanolamine salts of the condensation product of undecylenic acid chloride and hydrolyzed animal protein. See Hydrolyzed Protein.

SODIUM/TEA-LAUROYL HYDROLYZED KERATIN • See Hydrolyzed Keratin and Lauric Acid.

SODIUM/TEA-LAUROYL KERATIN AMINO ACIDS • See Keratin and Amino Acids.

SODIUM/TEA-UNDECYLENOYL HYDROLYZED COLLAGEN • Formerly had "animal protein" in the name. It is still a mixture of sodium and triethanolamine salts of the condensation product of undecylenic acid chloride and hydrolyzed animal protein. See Hydrolyzed Animal Protein.

SODIUM THIOGLYCOLATE • The sodium salt of mercaptoacetic acid. See Thioglycolic Acid Compounds.

SODIUM TOLUENESULFONATE • **Methylbenzenesulfonic Acid. Sodium Salt.** An aromatic compound that is used as a solvent. See Benzene.

SODIUM TRIDECETH-3, -6, -7, -12 CARBOXYLATE • The sodium salt of tridecyl alcohol and carboxylic acid. See Tridecyl Alcohol.

SODIUM TRIDECETH SULFATE • Widely used sodium salt of sulfated ethoxylated tridecyl alcohol. Used as an emulsifier. See Tridecyl Alcohol and Sulfates.

SODIUM TRIDECYL SULFATE • See Sulfonated Oils.

SODIUM TRIDECYLBENZENE SULFONATE • A mixture of alkyl benzene sulfonates used as a synthetic detergent. See Sodium Dodecylbenzene Sulfonate.

SODIUM TRIMETAPHOSPHATE • See Sodium Metaphosphate.

SODIUM TRIPOLYPHOSHPATE • STPP. Used in bubble baths and as a texturizer in soaps, it is a crystalline salt, moderately irritating to the skin and mucous membranes. Ingestion can cause violent purging. See Sodium Phosphate.

SODIUM UNDECYLENATE • A sodium salt of undecylenic acid. Occurs in sweat. A topical fungicide. Liquid or crystals with a sweaty odor prepared from castor oil. No known toxicity.

SODIUM UNDECYLENOAMPHOACETATE • See Quaternary Ammonium Compounds.

SODIUM UNDECYLENOAMPHOPROPIONATE • See Quaternary Ammonium Compounds.

SODIUM UROCANATE • The sodium salt of urocanic acid. See Histidine.

SODIUM XYLENE SULFONATE • Used as a solubilizer. An isolate from wood and coal tar. No known toxicity. See Xylene.

SOLANUM DULCAMARA • See Dulcamara Extract.

SOLANUM LYCOCARPUM • See Lycopodium.

SOLANUM LYCOPERISCUM • Tomato Extract.

SOLANUM MELONGENA • See Eggplant.

SOLANUM TUBEROSUM • See Potato Extract.

SOLAR ELASTOSIS • Degeneration and loosening of collagen *(see)* under the skin, frequently resulting from exposure to sunlight over a period of years.

SOLIDAGO ODORA • See Goldenrod.

SOLOMON'S SEAL • *Polygonatum officinale.* A perennial herb, the root was formerly used for its emetic properties and externally for bruises near the eyes, as well as for treatment of tumors, wounds, poxes, warts, and pimples. It was thought to help mend broken bones. In sixteenth-century Italy, it was used in a wash believed to maintain healthy skin. The roots contain allantoin *(see),* used today as an anti-inflammatory and healing ingredient.

SOLUBILITY • The degree to which a chemical can dissolve in a solvent, forming a solution.

SOLUBILIZATION • The process of dissolving in water such substances as fats and liquids that are not readily soluble under standard conditions by the action of a detergent or similar ingredient. Technically, a solubilized product is clear because the particle size of an emulsion is so small that light is not bounced off the particle. Solubilization is used in colognes and clear lotions. Sodium sulfonates *(see)* are common solubilizing ingredients.

SOLUBILIZED VAT BLUE 5 • A vat dye in the form of a soluble sodium salt of a sulfuric acid monoester. Vat dyes are more expensive than ordinary dyes and are used in pastels. See Vat Dyes for toxicity.

SOLUBILIZED VAT DYES • These are the sodium salts of vat dyes. They are comparatively expensive but give excellent penetration and fastness. See Vat Dyes.

SOLUBLE COLLAGEN • The protein source derived from the connective tissue of young animals. It is widely used in skin and hair conditioners. Formerly had "animal" in the name. See Solubilization and Collagen.

SOLUBLE PROTEOGLYCAN • Softened protein with a high sugar content.

SOLUM DIATOMEAE • See Diatomaceous Earth.

SOLUM FULLONUM • See Fuller's Earth.

SOLVENT • A liquid capable of dissolving or dispensing one or more substances. Methyl ethyl ketone is an example of a solvent.

SOLVENT BLACK 3 • A diazo color. See Solvent Dye.

SOLVENT BLUE 35 • Classed chemically as an anthraquinone color *(see)*. See Solvent Dye.

SOLVENT DYE • Generally insoluble in water, but dissolves in varying degrees in different organic media in liquid, molten, and solid forms. These include alcohols, oils, fats, and waxes. The use of a solvent dye depends upon fastness to light and adequate solubility, in powders, resins, and plastic. Can be irritating to the skin.

SOLVENT GREEN 3 • An anthraquinone color *(see)*. The name can be used only when applied to uncertified batches of this color. The CTFA adopted name for certified *(see)* batches is D & C Green No. 6 *(see)*.

SOLVENT GREEN 7 • A pyrene color, the name can be used only for batches of uncertified color. The CTFA adopted name for certified *(see)* batches is D & C Green No. 8 *(see)*. Pyrene is a cancer-causing ingredient.

SOLVENT ORANGE 1 • A monoazo *(see)* dye.

SOLVENT RED 1 • A monoazo *(see)* dye. Also see Solvent Dye.

SOLVENT RED 3 • A monoazo color *(see)*. See also Solvent Dye.

SOLVENT RED 23 • A diazo *(see)* color. The name can be used only for uncertified batches of this color. The CTFA adopted name for certified *(see)* batches is D & C Red No. 17 *(see)*.

SOLVENT RED 24 • **Calico Oil Red.** A diazo *(see)* color. See also Solvent Dyes.

SOLVENT RED 43 • A fluoran color. The sodium salt of this is Acid Red 87. The Solvent Red 43 name can be used only when applied to uncertified batches of color. The CTFA adopted name for certified *(see)* batches is D & C Red No. 21.

SOLVENT RED 48 • A fluoran color. The sodium salt is Acid Red 92. The name Solvent Red 48 can be used only for uncertified batches. The CTFA adopted name for certified *(see)* batches is D & C Red No. 27.

SOLVENT RED 49:1 • A xanthene *(see)* color. It is the stearic acid salt of Basic Violet 10. The name Solvent Red 49:1 can be applied only to batches of uncertified color. The CTFA adopted name for certified *(see)* batches is D & C Red No. 37 *(see)*. The use of this color certified as D & C Red No. 37 has been banned in the United States in cosmetic products. Its use in cosmetics in other countries may also be restricted.

SOLVENT RED 72 • A fluoran color. The name can be applied only to uncertified batches. The CTFA adopted name for certified *(see)* batches is D & C Orange No. 5 *(see)*.

SOLVENT RED 73 • A fluoran color. The sodium salt is Acid Red 95. The name Solvent Red 73 can be applied only to uncertified batches of color. The CTFA adopted name for certified *(see)* batches is D & C Orange No. 10 *(see)*.

SOLVENT VIOLET 13 • An anthraquinone color. The name is applied only to uncertified batches of this color. The CTFA adopted name for certified *(see)* batches is D & C Violet No. 2 *(see)*.

SOLVENT YELLOW 13 • A quinoline color. The name can be applied only to uncertified batches of this color. The CTFA adopted name for certified *(see)* batches is D & C Yellow No. 11 *(see)*.

SOLVENT YELLOW 29 • A diazo *(see)* color.

SOLVENT YELLOW 33 • A quinoline *(see)* color. The CTFA certified name for this color is D & C Yellow No. 11.

SOLVENT YELLOW 44 • An aniline *(see)* color.

SONCHUS OLERACEUS • Milk Thistle. An annual herb with yellow semiflorets, it blossoms in spring and summer and can be found growing by the roadside or in fields all over China. It is eaten in salads in China as well as used in medicine. It reportedly has immunity aids.

SOPHORA JAPONICA • Pagoda Tree. Scholar Tree. The United States Agricultural Research Service renamed the tree "Styphnolobium" instead of "Sophora." Has antibacterial propterties.

SORBETH-6 • See Sorbitol.

SORBETH-20, -30, -40 • See Sorbitol.

SORBETH-6 HEXASTEARATE • See Sorbitol and Stearic Acid.

SORBIC ACID • A white, free-flowing powder obtained from the berries of the mountain ash. Also made from chemicals in the factory. Used in cosmetics as a preservative and humectant. A mold and yeast inhibitor, it is also used in foods and beverages. Used as a replacement for glycerin in emulsions, ointments, embalming fluids, mouthwashes, dental creams, and various cosmetic creams. A binder for toilet preparations and plasticizers. Produces a velevetlike feel when rubbed on skin. Sticky in large amounts. Practically nontoxic but may cause skin irritation in susceptible people. When injected under the skin in 2,600-milligram doses per kilogram of body weight, it caused cancer in rodents. On the basis of available information, the CIR Expert Panel *(see)* concludes that it is safe as presently used in cosmetic formulations.

SORBITAN • A compound from sorbitol that has the water removed.

SORBITAN DIISOSTEARATE • The diester of isostearic acid *(see)* and hexitol.

SORBITAN DIOLEATE • The diester of oleic acid and hexitol anhydrides derived from sorbitol. See Sorbitan Fatty Acid Esters.

SORBITAN DISTEARATE • See Stearic Acid and Sorbitol.

SORBITAN FATTY ACID ESTERS • Mixture of fatty acids *(see)*, esters of sorbitol *(see)*, and sorbitol with the water removed. Widely used in the cosmetics industry as an emulsifier and stabilizer. Also used to prevent irritation from other cosmetic ingredients.

SORBITAN ISOSTEARATE • See Sorbitan Fatty Acid Esters.

SORBITAN LAURATE • Span 20®. Oily liquid insoluble in water, soluble in alcohol and oils. An emulsifier in cosmetic creams and lotions; a stabilizer of essential oils in water. No known toxicity.

SORBITAN OLEATE • Sorbitan Monooleate. An emulsifying ingredient, defoaming ingredient, and plasticizer. No known toxicity.

SORBITAN PALMITATE • Span 40®. Derived from sorbitol *(see)*. An emulsifier in cosmetic creams and lotions, a solubilizer of essential oils in water. Light yellow wax, insoluble in water, soluble in solvents. On the basis of available information, the CIR Panel *(see)* concludes that it is safe as presently used in cosmetic formulations.

SORBITAN SESQUIISOSTEARATE • See Sorbitol and Isostearic Acid.

SORBITAN SESQUIOLEATE • A widely used emulsifier. See Sorbitol and Oleic Acid.

SORBITAN SESQUISTEARATE • See Sorbitan Stearate.

SORBITAN STEARATE • **Sorbitan Monostearate.** An emulsifier in cosmetic creams and lotions, a solubilizer of essential oils in water. Used in antiperspirants, deodorants, cake makeup, hand creams, hair tonics, rouge, and suntan creams. Manufactured by reacting edible commercial stearic acid with sorbitol *(see both)*. Light cream to tan-colored, hard, waxy solid, with a bland odor and taste. Soluble in temperatures above its melting point in toluene, ethanol, methanol, and other. On the basis of available information, the CIR Expert Panel *(see)* concludes that it is safe as presently used in cosmetic formulations.

SORBITAN TRIISOSTEARATE • On the basis of available information, the CIR Expert Panel *(see)* concludes that it is safe as presently used in cosmetic formulations. See Stearic Acid.

SORBITAN TRIOLEATE • On the basis of available information, the CIR Expert Panel *(see)* concludes that it is safe as presently used in cosmetic formulations. See Sorbitol.

SORBITAN TRISTEARATE • An emulsifier and alternate for sorbitan stearate *(see)*. On the basis of available information, the CIR Expert Panel *(see)* concludes that it is safe as presently used in cosmetic formulations.

SORBITOL • A humectant. Gives a velvety feel to skin. Used as a replacement for glycerin in emulsions, ointments, embalming fluid, mouthwashes, dental creams, and various cosmetic creams. A binder for toilet preparations and a plasticizer. Also used in hairsprays, beauty masks, cuticle removers, foundation cake makeup, hand lotions, liquid powders, dentifrices, after-shave lotions, deodorants, antiperspirants, shampoos, and rouge. First found in the ripe berries of the mountain ash; it also occurs in other berries (except grapes), and in cherries, plums, pears, apples, seaweed, and algae. Consists of white hygroscopic powder, flakes, or granules with a sweet taste. It is a texturizing ingredient and a sequestrant. Also used in antifreeze, in foods as a sugar substitute, in writing inks to ensure a smooth flow from the point of the pen, and to increase the absorption of vitamins in pharmaceutical preparations. Medicinally used to reduce body water and for intravenous feedings. No known toxicity if taken externally. However, if ingested in excess, it can cause diarrhea and gastrointestinal disturbances; it may also alter the absorption of other drugs, making them less effective or more toxic.

SORBUS EXTRACT • **Service Tree Extract.** The extract of *Sorbus domestica*. An extract that was used by the American Indians to make a wash for eyes that were sore and blurred from the sun, as from climbing and hiking, and from dust.

SORREL EXTRACT • **Rumex Extract.** An extract of the various species of *Rumex*. The Europeans imported this to the Americas, and the Indians adopted it. Originally the root was used as a laxative and as a mild astringent. It was also used for scabs on the skin and as a dentifrice. It was widely used by American medical circles in this century to treat skin diseases.

SOUTHERN WOOD • *Artemisia abrotanum.* Native to southern Europe and widely grown in English gardens, it belongs to the *Compositae* family. Pliny thought it had aphrodisiac qualities when placed under a mattress. It reputedly made hair grow on bald heads. Used in herbal teas as a sedative. It is also used by herbalists to bring on delayed menstruation, from which it got the nickname "Lad's Love." It is also used to remove threadworms in children. It is used in "organic" cosmetics.

SOY ACID • A mixture of the fatty acids derived from soybean oil *(see).*

SOY FLOUR • See Soybean Oil.

SOY GERM EXTRACT • Formerly called soy extract. See Soybean Oil.

SOY STEROL • See Soybean Oil.

SOY STEROL ACETATE • See Soybean Oil and Acetate.

SOYA HYDROXYETHYL IMIDAZOLINE • See Ethylenediamine and Urea.

SOYAETHYL MORPHOLINIUM ETHOSULFATE • See Soybean Oil and Quaternary Ammonium Compounds.

SOYAMIDE DEA • See Soybean Oil.

SOYAMIDOPROPYL BENZYLDIMONIUM CHLORIDE • See Quaternary Ammonium Compounds.

SOYAMIDOPROPYL DIMETHYLAMINE • See Amides.

SOYAMIDOPROPYL ETHYLDIMONIUM ETHOSULFATE • See Quaternary Ammonium Compounds.

SOYAMINE • See Soybean Oil.

SOYAMINOPROPYLAMINE • See Quaternary Ammonium Compounds.

SOYATRIMONIUM CHLORIDE • **Soya Trimethyl Ammonium Chloride.** See Ammonium Chloride and Soybean Oil.

SOYBEAN • An erect, bushy, hairy legume, *Glycine Max,* native to Asia and extensively cultivated in China, Japan, and elsewhere. Its seeds contain glycerides of linoleic, oleic, linolenic, and palmitic acids. See Soybean Oil.

SOYBEAN FLOUR • Used as a thickener.

SOYBEAN OIL • Extracted from the seeds of plants grown in eastern Asia, especially Manchuria, and the midwestern United States. Used in the manufacture of soaps, shampoos, and bath oils. Pale yellow to brownish yellow. Also used in the manufacture of margarine. Debittered soybean flour contains practically no starch and is widely used in dietetic foods. Soybean oil is used in defoamers in the production of beet sugar and yeast, in the manufacture of margarine, shortenings, candy, and soap. Soybean is used in many products, including MSG, dough mixes, Lea and Perrins Sauce, Heinz's Worcestershire Sauce, La Choy Oriental Shoyu Sauce, soy sauce, salad dressings, pork link sausages, luncheon meats, hard candies, nut candies, milk, and coffee substitutes. It is made into soybean milk, soybean curd, and soybean cheese. About 300 million bushels of soybeans are grown yearly in the United States, one-third more than in China. May cause allergic reactions, including hair damage and acnelike pimples.

SOYBEAN OIL UNSAPONIFIABLES • The fraction of soybean oil that is not saponified (turned into fatty alcohol) in the refining of soybean oil fatty acids.

SOYBEAN PALMITATE • Used as a skin conditioner. See Palmitic Acid and Soybean.

SOYTRIMONIUM CHLORIDE • See Quarternary Ammonium Compounds.

SPANISH MOSS • *Tillandsia usneodides*. **Black Moss. Long Moss. Old Man's Beard.** A plant that forms tufts of hairlike grayish green strands upon the trunks and branches of many trees in the southern United States and West Indies. Used in "organic" cosmetics.

SPANISH PELLITORY EXTRACT • Extract of the root of *Anacyclus pyrethrum*. Used as an insecticidal ingredient.

SPEARMINT OIL • Used in perfumes, perfumed cosmetics, and toothpaste. It is the essential volatile oil obtained by steam distillation from the fresh aboveground parts of the flowering plant grown in the United States, Europe, and Asia. It is colorless, yellow or yellow-green, with the characteristic taste and odor of spearmint. Also used as a flavoring ingredient in food. May cause allergic reactions such as skin rash.

SPEEDWELL • Used in shampoos. It is an herb, a common, hairy perennial grown in Europe, with pale blue or lilac flowers. It has a reputation among herbalists of inducing sweating and restoring healthy body functions; also an expectorant tonic, a treatment for hemorrhages, and a medication for skin diseases. No known toxicity.

SPENT GRAIN WAX • The ingredient made from the extraction of the residual dry grains obtained from the malting process in beer production.

SPERGULARIA RUBRA • **Sandspurry. Sabline roughe. Tissa rubra. Birda rubra.** An herb common in Britain in sandy, gravelly healths near the sea. Flowers all summer. Long used in bladder disease. Soothing to mucous membranes.

SPERMACETI • **Cetyl Palmitate.** Used as a base for ointments and creams, and as an emollient in cleansing creams. Also in shampoos, cold creams, and other creams to improve their gloss and increase their viscosity. Derived as a wax from the head of the sperm whale. Generally nontoxic, but may become rancid and cause irritations.

SPF • **Sun Protectant Factor.** A rating scale indicating how much time you can expose your skin to the sun before you will burn when using a particular sunscreen.

SPHINGOLIPIDS • A group of fats that yield amino glycols. See Glycols.

SPICY BOUQUETS • One of the basic perfume types, they derive their characteristics from spice-giving ingredients, such as cinnamon, clove, vanilla, and ginger, but they may also be characterized by spiciness inherent in the flower notes of the perfume composition.

SPIKE LAVENDER OIL • **French Lavender.** Used in perfumes. A pale yellow, stable oil obtained from a flower grown in the Mediterranean region. A lavender-like odor. Used in cologne and toilet water; blended with lavender oil, soaps, and varnishes. Used also for fumigating, to keep moths from clothes, and in food and beverage flavorings. No known toxicity.

SPIKENARD • *Aralia racemosa.* **Nard.** Used for skin ailments such as acne, rash, and general skin problems. It is also used for coughs, colds, and other chest problems.

SPINACEA OLERACEA • See Spinach Extract.

SPINACH EXTRACT • An extract of the leaves of spinach, *Spinacea oleracea.*

SPINAL CORD EXTRACT • The extract obtained from animal spinal cords.

SPINAL LIPID EXTRACT • The extract of fats from animal spinal cords.

SPIRAEA EXTRACT • **Queen Meadow.** An extract from the flowers of *Spiraea ulmaria.* Contains an oil similar to wintergreen *(see).* The roots are rich in tannic acid *(see).*

SPIRODELA • *Herba spirodelae.* **Fuuping. Duckweed.** Oriental herb used to promote sweating and relieve itching and swelling.

SPIRULINA EXTRACT • An extract of *Spirula,* a many-chambered shell coiled in flat spirals. Occurs in most tropical seas.

SPLEEN EXTRACT • The extract of bovine spleen used in "youth" creams.

SPOTTED DOGFISH SKIN EXTRACT • An extract of the skin of *Scyliorhinus canicula.* Used in "antiaging" products.

SPOTTED HEMLOCK ROOT EXTRACT • An extract of the roots of *Conium maculatum.* See Hemlock Oil.

SPRAY DEODORANT • With antiperspirant action. Usually contains aluminum phenolsulfonate, 10 percent; propylene glycol, 5 percent; alcohol, 85 percent; and perfume. May seriously irritate the eyes, especially if you wear contact lenses. Caution is advised, especially since aerosol is a highly efficient way of delivering materials to the lungs. Dispenses by aerosols *(see).* See Deodorants.

SPRUCE OIL • Colorless to light yellow, pleasant-smelling oil obtained from the needles and twigs of various spruces and hemlocks; used chiefly to scent soaps and cosmetics but also used as a flavoring. No known toxicity. See Hemlock Oil.

SQUALANE • Obtained from the hydrogenation of shark-liver oil. Also occurs in sebum. Used as a fine lubricating oil in cosmetics for the skin and hair.

SQUALENE • Obtained from shark-liver oil. Occurs in smaller amounts in olive oil, wheat germ oil, and rice bran oil. It has a faint agreeable odor, is tasteless and miscible with vegetable and mineral oils, organic solvents, and fatty substances. Also found in human sebum. Insoluble in water. A lubricant and perfume fixative. A bactericide, an intermediate *(see)* in hair dyes, and used in surface-active ingredients. On the basis of available information, the CIR Expert Panel *(see)* concludes that it is safe as presently used in cosmetic formulations.

SQUALI LECUR • See Shark-liver Oil.

STABILIZER • A substance added to a product to give it body and to maintain a desired texture—for instance, the stabilizer alginic acid, which is added to cosmetics.

STACHYS OFFICINALIS • Betony. Lousewort. A common herb of eastern North America and the British Isles, it has been used for centuries to treat diarrhea, and as an astringent, and sedative. An ingredient in wood betony has been found to be active against tuberculosis. Wood betony has been used by herbalists to treat heartburn, gout, nervousness, cough, bladder and kidney stones, asthma, and fatigue. Also is reputedly good for chronic headaches. The root is both emetic and purgative. The leaves contain mild laxative and astringent agents. A tea brewed from the plant is used in the treatment of stomach disorders.

STANNIC CHLORIDE • Tin Tetrachloride. A thin, colorless, fuming caustic liquid, soluble in water, used as a mordant *(see)* in metallic hair dye and as a reingredient *(see)* in perfumes and soaps. May be highly irritating to the eyes and mucous membranes.

STANNOUS CHLORIDE • Tin Dichloride. An antioxidant, soluble in water, and a powerful reducing ingredient, particularly in the manufacture of dyes. May be irritating to the skin and mucous membranes.

STANNOUS FLUORIDE • Tin Difluoride. Fluoristan. Prepared by dissolving tin in hydrofluoric acid. Used in dentifrices as a decay preventative. No known toxicity.

STANNOUS PYROPHOSPHATE • Salt of Tin. It is relatively nontoxic and poorly absorbed from the gastrointestinal tract. Used as a mordant *(see)*. No known toxicity when used externally. See Phosphate.

STAR OF BETHLEHEM • See Ornithogallum Umbellatum.

STARCH • Acid Modified. Pregelatinized and Unmodified. Starch is stored by plants and is taken from wheat, potatoes, rice, corn, beans, and many other vegetable foods. Insoluble in cold water or alcohol but soluble in boiling water. Comparatively resistant to naturally occurring enzymes, and for this reason processors modify starch to make it more digestible. Used in dusting powders, dentifrices, hair colorings, rouge, dry shampoos, baby powders, emollients, and bath salts. Soothing to the skin and used to treat rashes. Used internally as a gruel in diarrhea. Allergic reaction to starch in toilet goods includes stuffy nose and other symptoms due to inhalation. Absorbs moisture and swells, causing blocking and distension of the pores leading to mechanical irritation. Particles remain in pores and putrefy, accelerated by sweat.

STARCH DIETHYLAMINOETHYL ETHER • See Starch.

STARCH/ACRYLATES/ACRYLAMIDE COPOLYMER • See Starch and Acrylic Acid.

STATUS COSMETICUS • A term used to describe patients intolerant of all cosmetics.

STEAPYRIUM CHLORIDE • A quarternary ammonium compound *(see)* used an an antistatic ingredient in hair products.

STEARALKONIUM BENTONITE • See Quaternary Ammonium Compounds.

STEARALKONIUM CHLORIDE • Improves the ability to comb the hair and adds shine. It is used in concentrations of less than 0.1 percent to 5 percent. On the basis of evidence at hand, the Expert CIR Panel *(see)* concludes that it is safe when incorporated in cosmetics in concentrations similar to those presently marketed. See Quaternary Ammonium Compounds.

STEARALKONIUM HECTORITE • Used in a wide variety of cosmetics as a suspending agent. Based upon the available data, the CIR Expert Panel *(see)* concludes that it is safe for use in cosmetics. See Quaternary Ammonium Compounds.

STEARAMIDE • An emulsifier. Colorless leaflets, insoluble in water. No known toxicity. See Stearic Acid.

STEARAMIDE DEA • **Stearic Acid Diethanolamine.** See Stearamide.

STEARAMIDE DIBA STEARATE • An emulsifier. See Stearamide.

STEARAMIDE MEA STEARATE • See Stearamide.

STEARAMIDE MIPA • See Stearmide.

STEARAMIDE OXIDE • A hair conditioner. See Stearamide.

STEARAMIDOETHYL DIETHANOLAMIDE • See Diethanolamine.

STEARAMIDOETHYL DIETHYLAMINE • See Quaternary Ammonium Compounds.

STEARAMIDOETHYL ETHANOLAMINE • See Ethanolamine.

STEARAMIDOPROPYL BETAINE • See Quaternary Ammonium Compounds.

STEARAMIDOPROPYL CETEARYL DIMONIUM TOYSYLATE • See Quaternary Ammonium Compounds.

STEARAMIDOPROPYL DIMETHYLAMINE • See Dimethylamine.

STEARMIDOPROPYL DIMETHYLAMINE LACTATE • See Quaternary Ammonium Compounds.

STEARMIDOPROPYL DIMETHYLAMINE STEARATE • See Quaternary Ammonium Compounds.

STEARAMIDOPROPYL MORPHOLINE • See Quaternary Ammonium Compounds.

STEARAMIDOPROPYL MORPHOLINE LACTATE • See Quaternary Ammonium Compounds.

STEARAMIDOPROPYL PYRROLIDONYLMETHYL DIMONIUM CHLORIDE • See Quaternary Ammonium Compounds.

STEARAMIDOPROPYL TRIMONIUM METHOSULFATE • See Quaternary Ammonium Compounds.

STEARAMIDOPROPYLALKONIUM CHLORIDE • See Quaternary Ammonium Compounds.

STEARAMIDOPROPYLAMINE OXIDE • See Quaternary Ammonium Compounds.

STEARAMINE OXIDE • Used in hair products as foam builder, thickener, stabilizer, and conditioner as well as an antistatic agent. On the basis of the available information, the CIR Expert Panel *(see)* concludes that it is safe as a cosmetic ingredient for "rinse-off" products but for "leave-on" products it should be limited to 5 percent. See Stearic Acid.

STEARATES • See Stearic Acid.

STEARETH-2 • A polyoxyethylene *(see)* ether of fatty alcohol. The oily liquid is used as a surfactant *(see)* and emulsifier *(see)*. On the basis of available information, the CIR Expert Panel *(see)* concludes that it is safe as presently used in cosmetic formulations.

STEARETH-3, -4, -6, -10, -11, -13, -15, -16, -20, -21, -25, -27, -30, -40, -50, -100 • The polyethylene glycol ethers of stearyl alcohol. The number indicates the degree of liquidity; the higher, the more solid. Surfactants and emulsifying ingredients. See Steareth-2.

STEARETH-10 ALLYL ETHER/ACRYLATES COPOLYMER • See Acrylates.

STEARETH-5 STEARATE • See Stearic Acid.

STEARIC ACID • Widely used in deodorants and antiperspirants, liquid powders, foundation creams, hand creams, hand lotions, liquefying creams, hair straighteners, protective creams, shaving creams, and soap. Occurs naturally in butter acids, tallow, cascarilla bark, and other animal fats and oils. A white, waxy, natural fatty acid, it is the major ingredient used in making bar soap and lubricants. A large percentage of all cosmetic creams on the market contain it. It gives pearliness to hand creams. It is also used as a softener in chewing gum base, for suppositories, and as a food flavoring. It is a possible sensitizer for allergic people. The CIR Expert Panel *(see)* concludes that this ingredient is safe for use in cosmetic products. See Fatty Acids.

STEARIC HYDRAZIDE • Used in cosmetic products at concentrations of use of less than 1 percent. Hydrazides and their salts are prohibited for use in cosmetic products by the European Economic Community. The safety of stearic hydrazide has not been documented and substantiated. The CIR Expert Panel *(see)* cannot conclude that this ingredient is safe for use in cosmetic products until the appropriate safety data have been obtained and evaluated. See Stearic Acid.

STEARMIDOETHYL DIETHYLAMINE • See Stearic Acid and Diethylamine.

STEAROAMPHOACETATE • See Quaternary Ammonium Compounds.

STEAROAMPHOCARBOXYGLYCINATE • See Surfactants.

STEAROAMPHODIACETATE • See Quaternary Ammonium Compounds.

STEAROAMPHOHYDROXYPROPYLSULFONATE • See Quaternary Ammonium Compounds.

STEAROAMPHOPROPIONATE • See Stearic Acid and Propionic Acid.

STEARONE • Derived from stearic acid. It is insoluble in water and is used as an antiblocking ingredient. See Stearic Acid.

STEAROXY DIMETHICONE • See Stearic Acid and Dimethicone.

STEAROXYTRIMETHYLSILANE • See Stearic Acid and Silicones.

STEAROYL GLUTAMIC ACID • A hair and skin conditioning ingredient. See Glutamic Acid.

STEAROYL LACTYLIC ACID • See Stearic Acid and Lactic Acid.

STEAROYL SARCOSINE • See Sarcosines.

STEARTRIMONIUM CHLORIDE • The CIR Expert Panel *(see)* concludes, on the basis of animal studies, this ingredient is safe for use in "rinse-off" products, and for use at concentrations of up to 0.25 percent in "leave-on" products. See Quaternary Ammonium Compounds.

STEARTRIMONIUM HYDROLYZED ANIMAL PROTEIN • See Quaternary Ammonium Compounds.

STEARYL ACETATE • The ester of stearyl alcohol and acetic acid *(see both)*.

STEARYL ALCOHOL • **Stenol.** A mixture of solid alcohols prepared from sperm whale oil. Unctuous, white flakes, insoluble in water, soluble in alcohol and ether. Can be prepared from sperm whale oil. A substitute for cetyl alcohol *(see)* to obtain a firmer product at ordinary temperatures. Used in pharmaceuticals, cosmetic creams, for emulsions, as an antifoam ingredient, and a lubricant; also in depilatories, hair rinses, and shampoos. No known toxicity.

STEARYL BEHENATE • The ester of stearyl alcohol and behenic acid *(see both)*.

STEARYL BETAINE • See Surfactants and Stearic Acid.

STEARYL CAPRYLATE • The ester of stearyl alcohol and citric acid *(see both)*.

STEARYL CITRATE • The ester of stearyl alcohol and citric acid *(see both)*.

STEARYL DIMETHICONE • A synthetic wax. See Silicones.

STEARYL ERUCAMIDE • See Quaternary Ammonium Compounds.

STEARYL ERUCATE • See Stearyl Alcohol and Erucic Acid.

STEARYL GLYCYRRHETINATE • The ester of stearyl alcohol and glycyrrhetinic acid *(see both)*.

STEARYL HEPTANOATE • The ester of stearyl alcohol and heptanoic acid. Used as a wax and in skin emollients. On the basis of available information, the CIR Expert Panel *(see)* concludes that it is safe as presently used in cosmetic formulations. See Stearyl Alcohol and Heptanoic Acid.

STEARYL HYDROXYETHYL IMIDAZOLINE • See Quaternary Ammonium Compounds.

STEARYL LACTATE • An emulsifier that occurs in tallow and other animal fats as well as vegetable oils. No known toxicity.

STEARYL OCTANOATE • The ester of stearyl alcohol and 2-ethylhexanoic acid. See Stearyl Alcohol.

STEARYL STEARATE • The ester of stearyl alcohol and stearic acid *(see both)*.

STEARYL STEAROYL STEARATE • See Stearyl Alcohol.

STEARYLDIMETHYL AMINE • See Stearyl Alcohol.

STEARYLDIMONIUM HYDROXYPROPYL HYDROLYZED CASEIN • See Quaternary Ammonium Compounds.

STEARYLDIMONIUM HYDROXYPROPYL HYDROLYZED COLLAGEN • The Quaternary Ammonium Chloride. See Hydrolyzed Collagen.

STEARYLDIMONIUM HYDROXYPROPYL HYDROLYZED KERATIN • See Quaternary Ammonium Compounds and Hydrolyzed Keratin.

STEARYLDIMONIUM HYDROXYPROPYL HYDROLYZED SILK • See Quaternary Ammonium Compounds and Silk.

STEARYLDIMONIUM HYDROXYPROPYL HYDROLYZED VEGETABLE PROTEIN • See Quaternary Ammonium Compounds and Hydrolyzed Vegetable Protein.

STEARYLDIMONIUM HYDROXYPROPYL HYDROLYZED WHEAT PROTEIN • See Quaternary Ammonium Compounds and Wheat Germ.

STEARYLTRIMONIUM HYDROXYETHYL HYDROLYZED COLLAGEN • See Hydrolyzed Collagen.

STEARYLTRIMONIUM METHOSULFATE • See Quaternary Ammonium Compounds.

STEARYLVINYL ETHER/MA COPOLYMER • A polymer of stearylvinyl ether and maleic anhydride *(see).*

STEROIDS • Class of compounds that includes certain drugs of hormonal origin, such as cortisone, used to treat the inflammations caused by allergies. Glucocorticoids reduce white blood-cell production, prostaglandins, and leukotrienes *(see both).* Natural and synthetic steroids have four rings of carbon atoms but have different actions according to what is attached to the rings. Cortisone and oral contraceptives are steroids. The following toxic effects, all of which relate to the length and level of dosage, may occur: susceptibility to infection, osteoporosis, muscle weakness and wasting, diabetes, high blood pressure due to sodium and water retention, weight gain, edema, bruising, moon face, psychotic reactions, hairiness, menstrual disturbance, pancreatitis, cataracts, and growth retardation.

STEROL • Any class of solid complex alcohols from animals and plants. Cholesterol is a sterol and is used in hand creams. Sterols are lubricants in baby preparations, emollient creams and lotions, emulsified fragrances, hair conditioners, hand creams, and hand lotions. No known toxicity.

STIFFENING INGREDIENT • An ingredient to add body to shaving soaps and creams. Many of the gums, such as karaya and carrageenan *(see),* are used for this purpose.

STILLINGIA • Chinese Tallow Tree. Queen's Root. Yaw Root. Dried roots of a southeastern United States plant. An acrid resin; fixed and volatile oils. Used as a drying oil in cosmetics. Formerly used medicinally to induce vomiting. No known toxicity in cosmetics.

ST. JOHN'S WORT • See Saint John's Wort.

STONEROOT • Horse Balm. Used for its constituents of resin, saponin, and tannic acid *(see all).* An erect, smooth perennial; a strong scented herb of eastern North America with pointed leaves. It produces a chocolate-colored powder with a peculiar odor and bitter astringent taste. Soluble in alcohol. No known toxicity.

STORAX • Styrax. Sweet Oriental Gum. Used in perfumes. It is the resin obtained from the bark of an Asiatic tree. Grayish brown, fragrant semiliquid, containing styrene and cinnamic acid *(see both).* Once used in medicine as a weak antiseptic and as an expectorant. Also used in food and beverage flavorings. Moderately toxic when ingested. Can cause urinary problems when absorbed through the skin. Can cause skin irritation, welts, and discomfort when applied topically. A common allergen.

STPP • See Sodium Tripolyphosphate.

STRAMONIUM • Thorn Apple. Jimsonweed. Stinkweed. Used in antiperspirants for its antiperspirant properties. Obtained from the dried leaves and flowering tops of a plant grown in Europe, Asia, and the United States. Leaves contain 0.25 to 0.45 percent alkaloids consisting of atropine, hyoscyamine, and scopolamine. It is used medicinally to treat intestinal spasms, asthma, and Parkinson's disease. No known toxicity.

STRATUM CORNEUM • The outermost, horny cell layer of your skin, which serves to retain body water and prevent the entry of chemical irritants.

STRAWBERRY EXTRACT • See Strawberry Juice.

STRAWBERRY JUICE • Fresh, ripe strawberries are reputed to contain ingredients that soften and nourish the skin. Widely used in natural cosmetics today. No scientific evidence of benefit or harm.

STRAWFLOWER EXTRACT • The extract of *Helichrysum italicum,* grown for its bright yellow, strawlike flowers. Used in coloring.

STREPTOMYCIN • Sulfate. An antibiotic active against streptococcal infections. May cause skin reactions.

STRONTIUM DIOXIDE • **Strontium Peroxide.** A white, odorless, and tasteless powder derived by passing oxygen over hot strontium. Used as a bleaching ingredient and antiseptic. It is highly flammable and explosive.

STRONTIUM HYDROXIDE • Used chiefly in making soaps and greases in cosmetics. Colorless, water-absorbing crystals or white powder. Absorbs carbon dioxide from the air. Very alkaline in solution. Also used in refining beet sugar and separating sugar from molasses. Irritating when applied to the skin.

STRONTIUM SULFIDE • Used in depilatories, it is less irritating than sodium sulfide and more efficient than calcium sulfide. It is a sulfur compound that occurs free or in combination, such as gypsum; found most often in volcanic areas. It is a gray powder with the odor of hydrogen sulfide and is slightly soluble in water. May cause skin rash, irritation, and hair breakage.

STRYCHNINE • A powerful poison from the seeds of *Nux-vomica.* It is toxic by ingestion and inhalation.

STYPTIC PENCIL • A cylindrical stick composed of potassium aluminum sulfate, glycerin, and talc. It has an astringent effect, tending to contract or bind. Designed to check blood flow, primarily from razor nicks. May sting but is nontoxic.

STYRAX • See Storax.

STYRENE • Obtained from ethylbenzene by taking out the hydrogen. Colorless to yellowish, oily liquid with a penetrating odor. Used in the manufacture of cosmetic resins and in plastics. May be irritating to the eyes and mucous membranes, and in high concentrations, it is narcotic.

STYRENE/ACRYLAMIDE COPOLYMER • An opacifier. See Acrylates.

STYRENE/ACRYLATE COPOLYMER • An opacifier. See Acrylates.

STYRENE/ACRYLATE/AMMONIUM METHACRYLATE COPOLYMER • A polymer *(see)* of styrene and a monomer of acrylic acid, methacrylic acid, or one of their esters. Used in liquid eyeliners. See Styrenes and Acrylates.

STYRENE/ACRYLIC ACID COPOLYMER • See Styrene and Acrylates.

STYRENE/MA COPOLYMER • See Styrene and Maleic Acid.

STYRENE/PVP COPOLYMER • Prepared from vinyl pyrrolidone and styrene monomers, it is used in liquid eyeliners as a carrier for color. See Styrene and Polyvinylpyrrolidone.

SUBCUTANEOUS • Under the skin.

SUCCINIC ACID • **Butanedioc acid.** Occurs in fossils, fungi, lichens, etc. Prepared from acetic acid *(see)*. Odorless; very acid taste. The acid is used as a plant-growth retardant. Used as a germicide and mouthwash, and in perfumes and lacquers; also used as a buffer and neutralizing ingredient. Has been employed medicinally as a laxative. No known toxicity in cosmetic use. Large amounts injected under the skin of frogs kills them.

SUCCINIC ANHYDRIDE • A starch modifier. See Succinic Acid.

SUCROSE • **Sugar. Cane Sugar. Saccharose.** A sweetening ingredient and food, a starting ingredient in fermentation production, a preservative and antioxidant in the pharmacy, a demulcent, and a substitute for glycerin *(see)*. Workers who handle raw sugar often develop rashes and other skin problems. When it oxidizes with sweat, sugar draws water from the skin and causes chapping and cracking. Infections, erosions, and fissures around the nails can occur. No known toxicity in cosmetics.

SUCROSE ACETATE ISOBUTYRATE • A denaturant for rubbing alcohols *(see both)*.

SUCROSE BENZOATE • See Benzoic Acid.

SUCROSE BENZOATE/SUCROSE ACETATE ISOBUTYRATE/BUTYL BENZYL PHTHALATE COPOLYMER • The condensation polymer of sucrose benzoate, sucrose acetate isobutyrate, and butyl benzyl phthalate monomers. Used as a film.

SUCROSE BENZOATE/SUCROSE ACETATE ISOBUTYRATE/BUTYL BENZYL PHTHALATE/METHACRYLATE COPOLYMER • The condensation product of sucrose benzoate, sucrose acetate isobutyrate, butyl benzyl phthalate, and methyl methacrylate monomers. Used as a film. See Acrylates.

SUCROSE COCOATE • See Coconut Acid and Sucrose.

SUCROSE DILAURATE • See Lauric Acid.

SUCROSE DISTEARATE • A mixture of sucrose and lauric acid *(see both)*.

SUCROSE LAURATE • A mixture of sucrose and lauric acid *(see both)*.

SUCROSE MYRISTATE • See Myristic Acid and Sucrose.

SUCROSE OCTAACETATE • A preparation from sucrose *(see)*. A synthetic flavoring. Used in adhesives and nail lacquers; a denaturant for alcohol. No known toxicity.

SUCROSE OLEATE • See Oleic Acid and Sucrose.

SUCROSE PALMITATE • See Palmitic Acid and Sucrose

SUCROSE POLYLAURATE • See Lauric Acid and Sucrose.

SUCROSE POLYOLEATE • See Oleic Acid and Sucrose.

SUCROSE POLYSTEARATE • See Stearic Acid and Sucrose.

SUCROSE RICINOLEATE • See Ricinoleic Acid and Sucrose.

SUCROSE STEARATE • A mixture of sucrose and stearic acid *(see both)*.

SUCROSE TETRASTEARATE TRIACETATE • See Stearic Acid and Sucrose.

SUCROSE TRIBEHENATE • See Behenic Acid and Sucrose.

SUCROSE TRISTEARATE • See Stearic Acid and Sucrose.

SUDAN III • Oil Red. Oil Scarlet. Solvent Red 23. A reddish brown powder used in coloring for waxes, oils, stains, dyes, and resins. May cause contact dermatitis.

SUGAR • See Sucrose.

SUGAR MAPLE • *Acer Saccharinum Extract.* Used as a flavoring and skin conditioner.

SULFAMIC ACID • A cleaning ingredient in cosmetics and used in the manufacture of hair dyes and lakes *(see).* A strong, white, crystalline acid used chiefly as a weed killer, in cleaning metals, and as a flameproofing and softening ingredient. Moderately irritating to the skin and mucous membranes.

SULFANILIC ACID • Grayish-white crystals made from aniline and sulfuric acid *(see both).* Used in dyes and medicines as an antibacterial.

SULFATED CASTOR OIL • See Sulfated Oil and Castor Oil.

SULFATED GLYCERYL OLEATE • Produced by adding sulfuric acid to glyceryl oleate. See Sulfated Oil and Glyceryl Oleate.

SULFATED OIL • Sulphated Oil. A compound to which a salt of sulfuric acid has been added to help control the acid-alkali balance.

SULFATED OLIVE OIL • See Sulfated Oil and Olive Oil.

SULFATED PEANUT OIL • See Sulfated Oil and Peanut Oil.

SULFIDES • Inorganic sulfur compounds that occur free or in combination with minerals. They are salts of a weak acid and are used as hair-dissolving ingredients in depilatories. They are skin irritants and may cause hair breakage.

SULFITES • Sodium, Potassium, and Ammonium. Preservatives, antioxidants, and antibrowning ingredients used in foods. Many packaged foods including fresh and frozen cellophane-wrapped fruits and vegetables, processed grain foods (crackers and cookies), and citrus-flavored beverages contain sulfites; however, the highest levels occur in potatoes (any peeled variety), dried fruits (apricots and white raisins), and shrimp and other seafoods, which are sprayed after unloading on the dock.

Sulfites can cause serious and even fatal reactions in persons sensitive to them. Such adverse responses include acute asthma attacks, loss of consciousness, anaphylactic shock, diarrhea, and nausea occurring soon after ingesting sulfiting ingredients. There have been 17 deaths that the FDA has determined were "probably or possibly" associated with sulfites. A citizens' petition was submitted by the Center for Science in the Public Interest, Washington, D.C., on October 28, 1982, that asked the agency to restrict the use of sulfiting ingredients to a safe residue level in food or require labels on those food products in which sulfiting ingredients must be used at higher levels to perform essential public health functions.

The California Grape and Tree Fruit League lobbied for the continued GRAS status of sulfiting ingredients used in sulfur dioxide fumigation within specific limitations. The group also wanted the continuation of sulfites as an ingredient to treat fresh grapes. Stating that the compound is essential to the marketing, transport, storage, and export of table grapes, the group claimed lack of any known substitute for the gaseous compound effective in preventing mold-rot and other storage fungi and in prolonging storage life. A spokesperson for the Wine Institute, which represents 460 domestic wine makers, said that many of the sulfur compounds in wine are natural parts of fermentation, but they also are added to many wines.

The FDA reviewed sulfiting ingredients in 1983. As part of the review, the agency proposed a reaffirmation of the GRAS status of sulfur dioxide, sodium bisulfite, sodium sulfite, and sodium and potassium metabisulfite *(see all),* but with specific use limitations. The FDA banned the use of the preservative on fresh fruits and vegetables in 1986. The FDA decided in 1988 against extending its ban on the use of sulfites to a variety of foods sold in supermarkets and served in restaurants, including wine, dried fruit, some seafood, and condiments. Sulfites must be declared on the labels of wine and packaged foods sold in supermarkets when they are added in excess of 10 parts per million.

Despite reports of severe or even fatal reactions to sulfites, there are six sulfiting ingredients currently listed as GRAS chemical preservatives. They are sulfur dioxide, sodium sulfite, sodium and potassium bisulfite, and sodium and potassium metabisulfite *(see all).* Under the current listing, sulfiting ingredients may be used as preservatives in any food, except meat or food that is a recognized source of Vitamine B_1 (thiamine). The FDA prohibits the use of sulfites in foods that are important sources of Vitamine B_1, such as enriched flour, because sulfites destroy the nutrient. You have to be cautious about "prepared" products in general if you are sulfite-sensitive. For example, lemon juice from a lemon may be fine, but bottled lemon juice may contain sodium bisulfite. When dining in a restuarant, you have to have a lot of faith in your waiter if you are allergic to sulfites. Foods, especially potato products and some canned foods served in restaurants, could contain sulfites. You can ask but you may not receive a proper answer.

SULFONAMIDE FORMALDEHYDE • A solvent in nail polish and the most frequent cause of nail polish dermatitis, which generally affects the neck and eyelids. Sulfonamide is the amide of sulfonic acid. See Formaldehyde and Sulfonamide Resins.

SULFONAMIDE RESINS • **Sulfanilamide.** The use of sulfonamides dates back to 1934, when the dye prontosil was shown to cure certain infections caused by bacteria. Sulfonamides are bacteria-killers and are used to inhibit germ growth in cosmetics. They are also used to contribute depth, gloss, flow adhesion, and water resistance to films in nail lacquers. They may cause allergic reactions.

SULFONATED OILS • **Sulfated.** Prepared by reacting oils with sulfuric acid. Used in soapless shampoos and hairsprays as an emulsifier and wetting ingredient. Shampoos containing sulfonated oils were first manufactured in 1880 and were effective in hard or soft water. Sulfonated oils strip color from both natural and colored hair and can bring out streaks. Sulfated castor oil has been used to remove all types of dye. Applied to hair and heated, it is used as a hair treatment. Sulfonated oils are used in hair tonics that remain on the hair as hairdressings. May cause drying of the skin.

SULFOSUCCINIC ACID • From sulfur and succinic acid. Used as a surfactant *(see)* and a solubilizing agent.

SULFUR • **Brimstone.** A mild antiseptic in antidandruff shampoos, dusting powders, ointments, and permanent-wave solutions. Occurs in the earth's crust in the free state and in combination. Used in hair tonic to stimulate the scalp and in acne creams and lotions. Also a stimulant to healing when used on skin rashes; derivatives are used in depilatories. May cause irritation of the skin. A case of death was reported following absorption through the scalp of a cold-wave solution containing free sulfur. Death was attributed to acute, hydrogen-sulfide poisoning. The Food and Drug Administration issued a notice in 1992 that sulfur has not been shown to be safe and effective for stated claims in OTC products, including those for treatment of poison ivy, poison sumac, and poison oak and sulfur (sublimed) in products to kill lice. Sulfur has also been banned for use in diaper rash, fever blister, and cold sore products because it has not been shown to be safe and effective for its stated claims.

SULFUR TAR COMPLEX • **Tricosulfan®.** The product obtained from the distillation of wood of various species of fir and treated with sulfur.

SULFURIC ACID • **Oil of Vitriol.** A clear, colorless, odorless, oily acid used to modify starch and to regulate acidity/alkalinity. It is very corrosive and produces severe burns on contact with the skin and other body tissues. Diluted sulfuric acid has been used to stimulate appetite. It is used as a topical caustic in cosmetic products. If ingested undiluted, it can be fatal.

SULFURIZED JOJOBA OIL • A mixture of sulfur and jojoba oil *(see both)*.

SUMAC • *Rhus glabra.* **Sumach.** A number of this genus possess poisonous properties. *Rhus* is found growing wild in all parts of the United States. The bark and fruit are astringent. Sumac berries are used as a gargle in decoction form for the chest pain of angina. The decoction was also gargled for throat irritations and to help asthmatics breathe easier. The high tannin *(see)* content in the berries explains why it was used for diarrhea. The root was chewed by some North American Indians for mouth sores. It is used in "organic" cosmetics.

SUNBURN LOTION • Includes Creams and Sprays. Serious sunburn requires medical attention and the use of oils, including butter, is not recommended. However, there are a number of soothing lotions, creams, and sprays for mild sunburn on the market. A common formula includes mineral oil, 10 percent; lanolin, 2.5 percent; propylene glycol, 2.5 percent; triethanolamine, 5.0 percent *(see all);* and water, distilled, 80 percent.

SUNFLOWER SEED EXTRACT • An extract of the seed of *Hellanthus annuus.* Used in skin creams.

SUNFLOWER SEED OIL • Widely used oil obtained by milling the seeds of the large flower produced in Russia, India, Egypt, and Argentina. A bland, pale yellow oil, it contains amounts of Vitamin E *(see* Tocopherols) and forms a "skin" after drying. Used in food and salad oils, and in resin and soap manufacturing. In many "antiaging" products. No known toxicity.

SUNFLOWER SEED OIL GLYCERIDE • See Sunflower Seed Oil and Glycerides.

SUNSCREEN PREPARATIONS • Preparations to prevent painful sunburn that encourage a change in pigmentation (a tan) have a large market. Suntan creams (emulsions) may contain para-aminobenzoic acid, mineral oil, sorbitan stearate, poloxamers *(see all),* and 62 percent water. A suntan ointment may contain petrolatum, stearyl alcohol, mineral oil, sesame oil, and calcium stearate *(see all).* A suntan lotion may contain methyl anthranilate, propylene glycol, ricinoleate, glycerin *(see all),* and about 65 percent alcohol and 10 percent water. A suntan oil may contain salicylates, about 40 percent sesame oil *(see both),* and 55 percent mineral oil. Sunscreen preparations may also contain alcohol, *p*-aminobenzoic acid and derivatives, benzyl salicylate, cinnamic acid derivatives, and coumarin *(see all).* A common suntan oil formula includes 2-ethyl hexyl salicylate, 5 percent; sesame oil, 40 percent; mineral oil, about 55 percent; perfume; color; and an antioxidant. Complaints to the FDA concerning sunscreen preparations include rash, blisters, burns, yellowed skin, and even death. The newer brands of sunscreens available protect against UVA rays of the sun, which tan, and UVB rays, which burn. They are called broad-spectrum sunscreens, and they list the UVA blocker, oxybenzone, among their ingredients. A few new sunscreens also block the infrared heat rays, which, according to Dr. Albert Kligman of the University of Pennsylvania Medical School, may also damage the skin. The maximum protection means choosing an SPF 15 broad-spectrum product that's also formulated to block infrared heat rays. Some sunscreens also claim water resistance that lasts for up to 50 minutes. It has become common practice to add sunscreening ingredients to cosmetics to protect against the adverse effects of ultraviolet rays. In a study done at Case Western Reserve University, Cleveland, Ohio, it was shown that cosmetic preparations containing sunscreening ingredients are protective against the sun's rays and should therefore be encouraged. In 1993, the FDA fixed the upper limit for the Sun Protection Factor (SPF) at 30, a decision that undercut efforts by leading marketers to increase ranges into the 40s and beyond with products for children and consumers especially sensitive to solar radiation. The new regulations also curb to some degree the label warnings, discarding the liberal old "prevents cancer of the skin" to versions of "Sun Alert: the sun causes skin damage. Regular use of sunscreens over the years may reduce the chance of skin damage, some types of skin cancer, and other harmful effects due to the sun."

The FDA was believed to be influenced by epidemiologists who maintain it is not very healthy for light-complexioned people to expose themselves to long-term UV radiation, even when protected by sunscreens deemed to be effective. The epidemiologists believe the rising toll of melanoma may well be attributed to the desire to acquire tans at a time when UVA radiation is growing more destructive because of thinning of the ozone layer.

SUNSET YELLOW • A monoazo color. The name can be used only when applied to batches of uncertified color. The CTFA adopted name for certified *(see)* batches is FD & C Yellow No. 6 *(see).*

SUNTAN PREPARATIONS • See Sunscreen Preparations.

SUPEROXIDE DISMUTASE • A copper-containing protein enzyme that decomposes oxygen.

SURFACE-ACTIVE INGREDIENT • Any compound that reduces surface tension when dissolved in solution. There are three types: detergents, wetting ingredients, and emulsifiers. See all three.

SURFACTANTS • These are wetting ingredients. They lower water's surface tension, permitting it to spread out and penetrate more easily. These surface-active ingredients are classified by whether or not they ionize in solution and by the nature of their electrical charges. There are four major categories—anionic, nonionic, cationic, and amphoteric. Anionic surfactants, which carry a negative charge, have excellent cleaning properties. They are stain and dirt removers in household detergent powders and liquids and in toilet soaps. Nonionic surfactants have no electrical charge. Since they are resistant to hard water and dissolve in oil and grease, they are especially effective in spray-on oven cleaners. Cationic surfactants have a positive charge. These are primarily ammonia derivatives and are antistatic and sanitizing ingredients used as friction reducers in hair rinses and fabric softeners. Amphoteric surfactants may be either negatively charged or positively charged, depending on the activity or alkalinity of the water. They are used for cosmetics where mildness is important, such as in shampoos and lotions.

SURMA • A lead-based eye cosmetic used by Chinese women. Medical personnel are campaigning to inform the women about the danger of the cosmetic.

SUTILAINS • Enzymes obtained from the bacteria *Bacillus subtillis.*

SWEET ALMOND OIL • *Prunus Amygdalus dulcis.* Used in perfumes and in the manufacture of fine soaps and emollients. Expressed from the seeds of a plant. Colorless or pale yellow, oily liquid, almost odorless, with a bland taste. Insoluble in water. No known skin toxicity. On the basis of available information, the CIR Expert Panel *(see)* concludes that it is safe as presently used in cosmetic formulations. See Bitter Almond Oil.

SWEET BAY OIL • Used in perfumes. It is the yellow-green volatile oil from the leaves of the laurel. No known toxicity.

SWEET BIRCH • See Methyl Salicylate.

SWEET CHERRY EXTRACT and OIL • *Prunis avium.* A tall pyramidlike Eurasian tree with reddish-brown bark, white flowers, and fruits that are often small and bitter in the wild but have been cultivated into sweet-flavored cherries. The extract is used in flavorings and in organic cosmetics. The oil is used as a skin conditioning ingredient.

SWEET CLOVER EXTRACT • The extract of various species of *Melilotus,* grown for hay and soil improvement. It contains coumarin *(see)* and is used as a scent to disguise bad odors.

SWEET FLAG • See Calamus Root Extract.

SWEET GRASS EXTRACT • The extract of *Hierochloe borealis.* Any of various grasses of sweet flavor or odor such as manna grass or holy grass.

SWEET MARJORAM OIL • Marjoram Pot. Used in perfumery and hair preparations. The natural extract of the flowers and leaves of two varieties of the fragrant marjoram. Also a food flavoring. No known toxicity.

SWEET VIOLET EXTRACT • The extract of the flowers of *Viola odorata* of Eurasia and North Africa, which is the source of many of the commercially developed violets. Used in perfumery.

SWERTIA EXTRACT • The extract of flowers, leaves, and stems of various species of *Swertia*. A small genus of herbs found in the western United States. Has a thick, bitter-tasting root and dull-colored flowers. Used as a wax.

SYLVIC ACID • See Abietic Acid.

SYMPHTUM OFFICIALE • See Comfrey.

SYNTHETIC BEESWAX • A mixture of alcohol esters.

SYNTHETIC CANDELILLA WAX • See Swertia Extract and Candelilla Wax.

SYNTHETIC CARNAUBA • See Carnauba Wax.

SYNTHETIC HECTORITE • See Hectorite.

SYNTHETIC JAPAN WAX • See Japan Wax.

SYNTHETIC JASMINE • See Cinnamic Aldehyde.

SYNTHETIC JOJOBA OIL • See Jojoba Oil.

SYNTHETIC SPERMACETI • Widely used substitutes for spermaceti *(see)*.

SYNTHETIC WAX • A hydrocarbon wax derived from various oils.

SYRINGA VULGARIS • See Lilac.

T

TABEBUIA • Lapacho. Pau D'arco • Tabecuia heptaphylla or impetiginosa. The inner bark of a tree in the forests of Brazil, it was used by Brazilian Indians for the treatment of cancer. Contains quinones and lapachol. It also is used to treat fungal and parasitic infections, and to aid digestion. Also reportedly lowers blood sugar. It is now being studied in Brazil to treat cancers, including leukemia.

TAGETES • Meal, Extract, and Oil. The *meal* is the dried, ground flower petals of the Aztec marigold, a strong-scented, tropical American herb, mixed with no more than 0.3 percent ethoxyquin, a herbicide and antioxidant. The *extract* is taken from tagetes petals. Both the meal and the extract are used to enhance the yellow color of chicken skin and eggs. They are incorporated in chicken feed, supplemented sufficiently with the yellow coloring xanthophyll. The coloring has been permanently listed since 1963 but is exempt from certification. The *oil* is extracted from the Aztec flower and used in fruit flavorings for beverages, ice cream, ices, candy, baked goods, gelatin, desserts, and condiments. No known toxicity.

TALC • French Chalk. The main ingredient of baby and bath powders, face powders, eye shadows, liquid powders, protective creams, dry rouges, face masks, foundation cake makeups, skin fresheners, foot powders, and face creams. Gives a slippery sensation to powders and creams. Talc is finely powdered native magnesium silicate, a mineral. It usually has small amounts of other powders such as boric acid or zinc oxide added as a coloring ingredient. Prolonged inhalation can cause lung problems because it is similar in chemical composition to asbestos, a known lung irritant and cancer-causing ingredient.

TALCUM POWDER • Talc-based powders have been linked to ovarian cancer. In Boston's Brigham and Women's Hospital, of 215 women with ovarian cancer, 32 had used talcum powder on their genitals and sanitary napkins. Talc easily works its way up the reproductive tract. Eventually, a few particles reach the ovary and may set the stage for cancer. All factors considered in the study, the risk of ovarian cancer was raised to 3.28 times greater for women who use talc than for women who don't. Daniel Cramer, M.D., the obstetrician-gynecologist who wrote of the findings in the journal *Cancer,* said further studies are needed before doctors could recommend that women should not use talc but said that he, himself, advises patients to use other products such as cornstarch-based powders or creams. Talcum powder has been reported to cause coughing, vomiting, or even pneumonia when it is used carelessly and inhaled by babies. See Talc.

TALL OIL • **Liquid Rosin.** A by-product of the pine wood pulp industry and used to scent shampoos, soaps, varnishes, and fruit sprays. "Tall" is Swedish for "pine." Dark brown liquid; acrid odor. A fungicide and cutting oil. It may be a mild irritant and sensitizer. On the basis of available information, the CIR Expert Panel *(see)* concludes that it is safe as presently used in cosmetic formulations.

TALL OIL ACID • A mixture of rosin *(see)* and fatty acids recovered from tall oil *(see).* Used as a surfactant and cleansing ingredient.

TALL OIL BENZYL HYDROXYETHYL IMIDAZOLINIUM CHLORIDE • See Quaternary Ammonium Compounds and Tall Oil.

TALL OIL GLYCERIDES • A mixture of glycerides derived from tall oil. See Glycerides and Tall Oil.

TALL OIL HYDROXYETHYL IMIDAZOLINE • See Tall Oil and Imidazoline.

TALL OIL STEROL • See Phytosterols.

TALLAMIDE DEA • See Tall Oil.

TALLAMPHOPROPIONATE • See Tall Oil.

TALLOW • The fat from the fatty tissue of bovine cattle and sheep in North America. Used in shaving creams, lipsticks, shampoos, and soaps. White, almost tasteless when pure, and generally harder than grease. May cause eczema and blackheads. On the basis of available information, the CIR Expert Panel *(see)* concludes that it is safe as presently used in cosmetic formulations

TALLOW ACID • See Tallow.

TALLOW AMIDE • See Tallow.

TALLOW AMIDE DEA and MEA • See Tallow.

TALLOW AMIDOPROPYLAMINE OXIDE • See Tallow.

TALLOW AMINE • See Tallow.

TALLOW AMINE OXIDE • See Tallow.

TALLOW GLYCERIDES • A mixture of triglycerides (fats) derived from tallow.

TALLOW HYDROXYETHYL IMIDAZOLINE • See Tallow and Imidazoline.

TALLOW IMIDAZOLINE • See Tallow.

TALLOW TRIMONIUM CHLORIDE • Tallow. Trimethyl Ammonium Chloride. See Quaternary Ammonium Compounds.

TALLOWAMIDOPROPYL BETAINE • See Quaternary Ammonium Compounds.

TALLOWAMIDOPROPYL HYDROXYSULTAINE • See Quaternary Ammonium Compounds.

TALLOWAMINOPROPYLAMINE • See Quaternary Ammonium Compounds.

TALLOWAMPHOACETATE • See Quaternary Ammonium Compounds.

TALLOWETH-6 • See Tallow.

TAMARIND EXTRACT • The extract of *Tamarindus indica,* a large tropical tree grown in the East Indies and Africa. Preserved in sugar or syrup, it is used as a natural fruit flavoring. The pulp contains about 10 percent tartaric acid. No known toxicity.

TAMARINDUS INDICA • See Tamarind Extract.

TANACETUM CINERARIIFOLIUM • See Pyrethrins.

TANGERINE OIL • The oil obtained by expression from the peels of the ripe fruit from several related tangerine species. Reddish orange, with a pleasant orange aroma. Used in blueberry, mandarin, orange, tangerine, and other fruit flavorings for beverages, ice cream, ices, candy, baked goods, gelatin desserts, and chewing gum. Used in "organic" cosmetics. A skin irritant. GRAS.

TANG KUEI EXTRACT • The extract of the roots of *Angelica sinensis.* See Dong Quai.

TANNIC ACID • Used in sunscreen preparations, eye lotions, and antiperspirants. It occurs in the bark and fruit of many plants, notably in the bark of the oak and sumac, and in cherry, coffee, and tea. Used medicinally as a mild astringent, and when applied it may turn the skin brown. Also used in food flavorings. Tea contains tannic acid, and this explains its folk use as an eye lotion. Excessive use in creams or lotions by hypersensitive persons may lead to irritation, blistering, and increased pigmentation. Low toxicity orally, but large doses may cause gastric distress. The FDA issued a notice in 1992 that tannic acid has not been shown to be safe and effective as claimed in OTC digestive aid products, fever blister treatment products, and products to treat poison ivy, poison oak, and poison sumac. Tannic acid glycerite in astringent *(see)* drugs and tannic acid in diaper rash, fever blister, and cold sore drugs were also on the list.

TANNIN • Any of a broad group of plant-derived phenolic compounds characterized by their ability to precipitate proteins. Some are beneficial and some are toxic, depending upon their source. Tannins in herbs are astringents *(see).* They are soothing to the skin and mucous membranes. They can bind to the tissues of the intestines and reduce diarrhea and internal bleeding. Herbalists use them to treat burns and for wound healing. See Tannic Acid.

TANSY • *Tanacetum vulgare.* **Bitter Buttons. Parsley Fern.** A native of Greece, tansy is widespread in the United States in gardens and along highways. During the fifteenth century, it was used in a tea for gas, children's colic, and abdominal cramps, gout, and even for the plague. It was used for centuries by young girls in tea to alleviate slow and painful menstruation. It was considered a laxative, a gentle stimulant to digestion, and even a sedative. The plant is still listed in the United States Pharmacopeia chiefly for its use as a tea to avert colds, a cold decoction to be used during convalescence from fevers and jaundice, to get rid of worms, and externally for use on bruises, tumors, and inflammations. If too much of tansy is taken, it can result in vomiting, convulsions, and death.

TAPIOCA STARCH • Used as a thickener.

TARAKTOGENOS KURZII • See Chaulmoogra Oil.

TARAXUM OFFICINALE • See Dandelion Leaf and Root.

TAR OIL • The volatile oil distilled from wood tar, generally from the family *Pinaceae*. Used externally to treat skin diseases, the principle toxic ingredients are phenols and naphthalenes. Toxicity estimates are hard to make because even the U.S. Pharmacopeia does not specify the phenol content of official preparations. However, if ingested, it is estimated that one ounce would kill. See Pine Tar Oil, which is a rectified tar oil used as a licorice flavoring.

TARO • *Colocasia esculenta*. **Elephant's Ear. Dasheen.** A starchy root grown throughout the tropics for its edible starch. It has to be peeled to remove its poisonous outer covering. Used to make the Hawaiian dish poi. Used in "organic" cosmetics.

TARRAGON • Used in perfumery to improve the note *(see)* of chypre-type perfumes *(see)*. Derived from the dried leaves of a small, European perennial, wormwood herb. Pale yellow oil grown for its aromatic, pungent foliage. Also used in making pickles and vinegar. No known toxicity.

TARS • An antiseptic, deodorant, and bug killer. Any of the various dark brown or black bituminous, usually odorous, viscous liquids or semiliquids obtained by the destructive distillation of wood, coal, peat, shale, and other organic materials. Used in hair tonics and shampoos and as a licorice food flavoring. May cause allergic reactions.

TARTARIC ACID • Effervescent acid used in bath salts, denture powders, nail bleaches, hair-grooming aids, hair rinses, depilatories, and hair coloring. Widely distributed in nature in many fruits but usually obtained as a by-product of winemaking. Consists of colorless or translucent crystals or a white, fine-to-granular, crystalline powder that is odorless and has an acid taste. In strong solutions it may be mildly irritating to the skin.

TARTRAZINE • **FD and C Yellow No. 5.** Bright orange-yellow powder used in foods, drugs, and cosmetics and as a dye for wool and silk. Those allergic to aspirin are often allergic to tartrazine. Allergies have been reported in persons eating sweet corn, soft drinks, and cheese crackers—all colored with Yellow No. 5. It is derived from coal tar.

TAURINE • An amino acid found in almost every tissue of the body, and is especially high in human milk. Most infant soy-protein formulas are now supplemented with taurine. Taurine is almost absent from vegetarian diets. It is believed necessary for healthy eyes, and it is an antioxidant. It is also used as a nutritional supplement in feed for growing chicks. Some researchers theorize irregular heartbeat is characteristic of lack of blood to the heart and may be partly due to loss of intracellular taurine. Much like magnesium, taurine affects membrane excitability by normalizing potassium flux in and out of the heart muscle cells. Supplementation may prevent digitalis-induced arrhythmias.

TBS • See Tribromsalan.

TCC • See Triclocarban.

TDI OXIDIZED MICROCRYSTALLINE WAX • Microcrystalline wax *(see)* that has been treated with toluene *(see)*. Used as a thickener.

TEA- • The abbreviation for triethanolamine.

TEA • The leaves, leaf buds, and intermodes of plants having leaves and fragrant white flowers, prepared and cured to make an aromatic beverage. Cultivated principally in China, Japan, Ceylon, and other Asian countries. Tea is a mold stimulant, and its tonic properties are due to the alkaloid caffeine; tannic acid *(see)* makes it astringent. Used by natural cosmeticians to reduce puffiness around the eyes. A cotton or gauze pad is dampened with a weak solution of tea and placed on the eyelids. One then lies down for five to ten minutes. No known toxicity.

TEA EXTRACT • See Chinese Tea Extract.

TEA SORBATE • See Triethanolamine and Sorbic Acid.

TEA TREE OIL • The essential oil obtained from the leaves of an Australian tree. Light yellow. Used as a germicide in cosmetics. Eleven to 13 times as powerful as carbolic acid. Penetrates the skin quickly, and accelerates the healing of skin disorders. No known toxicity.

TEA-ABIETOYL HYDROLYZED COLLAGEN • The salt of the condensation product of abietic acid chloride and hydrolyzed animal protein. The "animal" was taken out of this ingredient's name. Used as a skin conditioner. See Hydrolyzed Protein.

TEA-ACRYLATES/ACRYLONITROGENS COPOLYMER • See Acrylates.

TEA-C12-15 ALKYL SULFATE • See Triethanolamine, Alcohols, and Sulfate.

TEA-COCOATE • The triethanolamine *(see)* soap derived from coconut fatty acids *(see)*. No known toxicity.

TEA-COCOYL GLUTAMATE • A softener. See Coconut Acid and Glutamic Acid.

TEA-COCOYL HYDROLYZED COLLAGEN • See Hydrolyzed Animal Protein Derivative and Anionic Surfactants.

TEA-COCYL SARCOSINATE • See Cocoyl Sarcosine.

TEA-DODECYLBENZENESULFONATE • See Sulfonated Oils.

TEA-EDTA • See Ethylenediamine Tetraacetic Acid.

TEA-HYDROCHLORIDE • The salt of hydrochloric acid *(see)*.

TEA-HYDROGENATED TALLOWOYL GLUTAMATE • A softener. See Glutamate.

TEA-HYDRIODIDE • See Iodide.

TEA-ISOSTEARATE • See Triethanolamine and Isostearic Acid.

TEA-LACTATE • See Triethanolamine and Lactic Acid.

TEA-LANETH-5 SULFATE • See Surfactants.

TEA-LAURAMINOPROPIONATE • See Quaternary Ammonium Compounds.

TEA-LAURETH SULFATE • See Anionic Surfactants.

TEA-LAUROYL COLLAGEN AMINO ACIDS • Protein enhancer for cosmetic creams. See Hydrolyzed Protein.

TEA-LAUROYL GLUTAMATE • A softener. See Glutamate.

TEA-LAUROYL KERATIN AMINO ACIDS • See Keratin Amino Acids.

TEA-LAUROYL LACTYLATE • See Lauric Acid and Triethanolamine.

TEA-LAUROYL SARCOSINATE • See Sarcosines.

TEA-LAURYL BENZENE SULFONATE • See Surfactants.

TEA-LAURYL SULFATE • A cleansing ingredient and emulsifier. On the basis of available information, the CIR Expert Panel *(see)* concludes that it is safe without significant irritation at a final concentration not exceeding 10.5 percent. Greater concentrations may cause irritation, especially if allowed to remain in contact with the skin for significant periods of time. See Sodium Lauryl Sulfate.

TEA-MYRISTAMINOPROPIONATE • See Surfactants.

TEA-MYRISTATE • See Myristic Acid and Surfactants.

TEA-MYRISTOL HYDROLYZED COLLAGEN • See Hydrolyzed Animal Protein and Surfactants.

TEA-OLEAMIDO PEG-2 SULFOSUCCINATE • Triethanolamine and succinic acid *(see both)*.

TEA-OLEATE • **Triethanolamine Oleate.** See Oleic Acid and Ethanolamines.

TEA-OLEOYL HYDROGENATED COLLAGEN • The hydrolyzed collagen is the triethanolamine salt of the condensation product of oleic acid and hydrolyzed collagen.

TEA-OLEOYL SARCOSINATE • See Oleic Acid and Sarcosines.

TEA-PALM KERNEL SARCOSINATE • See Palm-Kernel Oil and Sarcosines.

TEA-PALMITATE • See Palmitic Acid.

TEA-PCA • See Ethanolamines.

TEA-PEG-3 COCOAMIDE SULFATE • See Surfactants.

TEA-SALICYLATE • See Salicylic Acid and Triethanolamine.

TEA-STEARATE • See Triethanolamine and Stearic Acid.

TEA-SULFATE • See Triethanolamine and Sulfuric Acid.

TEA-TALLATE • See Fatty Acids and Tall Oil.

TEA-TRIDECYLBENZENESULFONATE • See Surfactants.

TEA-UNDECYLENOYL HYDROLYZED COLLAGEN • See Hydrolyzed Protein.

TECOMA CURIALIS EXTRACT • See Lapacho Extract.

TELPHAIRIA PEDATA OIL • **Oyster Nut Oil.** Used as an emollient and cover-up.

TERATOGEN • From the Greek *terat* (monster) and Latin *genesis* (origin): the origin or cause of a monster—or defective fetus.

TEREPHTHALYLIDENE DICAMPHOR SULFONIC ACID • An ultraviolet slight absorber. See Sulfonic acid.

TERMINALIA CATAPPA • Belongs to a large family of tropical trees and shrubs. See Almond Oil.

TERPENELESS OILS • An essential oil from which the terpene components have been removed by extraction and fractionation, either alone or in combination. The terpeneless grades are more highly concentrated than the original oil. Removal of the terpenes is necessary to inhibit spoilage, particularly of oils derived from citrus. See Terpenes.

TERPENES • A class of unsaturated hydrocarbons *(see)*. Its removal from products improves their flavor and gives them a more stable, stronger odor. However, some perfumers feel that the removal of terpenes destroys some of the original odor. Has been used as an antiseptic. No known toxicity.

TERPINEOL • A colorless, viscous liquid with a lilaclike odor, insoluble in mineral oil and slightly soluble in water. It is primarily used as a flavoring ingredient but is also employed as a denaturant to make alcohol undrinkable. It has been used as an antiseptic. It can be a sensitizer.

TERPINYL ACETATE • Colorless liquid, odor suggestive of bergamot and lavender. Slightly soluble in water and glycerol. Derived by heating terpineol with acetic acid *(see both)*. Used as a perfume and flavoring ingredient. No known toxicity.

TERPINYL FORMATE • **Formic Acid.** A synthetic fruit-flavoring ingredient. Derived by heating terpineol with formic acid *(see both)*. Used as a synthetic fruit-flavoring ingredient for beverages, ice cream, ices, candy, liqueurs, and baked goods. See Turpentine for toxicity.

TERPINYL PROPIONATE • A synthetic fruit-flavoring ingredient, colorless with a lavender odor. Derived by heating terpineol with propionic acid *(see both)*. Used as a synthetic fruit-flavoring ingredient for beverages, ice cream, ices, candy, and baked goods. See Turpentine for toxicity.

TERTIARY BUTYLHYDROQUINONE • **TBHQ.** This antioxidant was put on the market after years of pressure by food manufacturers to get it approved. It contains the petroleum-derived butane and is used either alone or in combination with the preservative-antioxidant butylatedhydroxyanisole (BHA) and/or butylated hydroxytoluene (BHT). Application to the skin may cause allergic reactions.

TESTICULAR EXTRACT • Extract of bovine testicular tissue.

TESTICULAR HYDROLYSATE • The testicular hydrolysate of animal testicular tissue. Used in skin creams.

TESTOSTERONE • It stimulates target tissues to develop normally in androgen-deficient men. It is used to treat eunuchs and male hormonal change symptoms. It is used for breast engorgement in nonnursing mothers and to treat breast cancer in women one to five years postmenopausal. Potential adverse reactions in women include acne, edema, oily skin, weight gain, hairiness, hoarseness, clitoral enlargement, changes in libido, flushing, sweating, and vaginitis with itching. In males before puberty, premature epiphyseal closure, priapism, growth of body and facial hair, phallic enlargement; after puberty, testicular atrophy, scanty sperm, decreased ejaculatory volume, impotence, enlargement of breast, and epididymitis. In both sexes, edema, gastroenteritis, nausea, vomiting, diarrhea, constipation, change in appetite, bladder irritability, jaundice, liver toxicity, and high levels of calcium.

TETRABROMOFLUORESCEIN • Eosine Yellow. A red color with a yellowish or brownish tinge prepared by adding bromine fluorescein *(see)*. Used to make lipstick indelible and to color nail polish. It may cause photosensitivity *(see)*, and has caused inflamed lips and respiratory and gastrointestinal symptoms. Tetrabromofluorescein is also used to dye wool, silk, and paper.

TETRABUTYOXYPROPYL TRISILOXANE • An emollient. See Silicones.

TETRACAINE • Pontocaine. Pontocaine Eye. A local anesthetic introduced in 1932 for sprain or saddle block in delivery of a baby. It is ten times as strong as procaine. Onset is in 15 minutes, and the duration of effect is up to three hours. Potential adverse reactions include skin reactions and swelling.

TETRACHLOROETHYLENE • Perchloroethylene. A colorless, nonflammable liquid with a pleasant odor, made from acetylene and chlorine. Used as a solvent in cosmetics. Used medicinally for hookworm. Narcotic in high doses. Has a drying action on the skin and can lead to adverse skin reactions.

TETRADECENE • An emollient. See Decanoic Acid.

TETRADECYLEICOSANOL • See Myristic Acid and Arachadonic Acid.

TETRADECYLEICOSYL STEARATE • See Stearic Acid and Myristic Acid.

TETRADECYLOCTADECANOL • See Octanoic Acid and Alcohol.

TETRAETHYLTHIURAM DISULFIDE • Thiram. An agricultural chemical found to be a degerming ingredient when incorporated in soap. A disinfectant, insecticide, fungicide, and bacteria killer. May cause irritation of nose, throat, and skin. Also may be harmful if swallowed or inhaled. One should not breathe the spray or mist and should avoid contact with eyes, skin, or clothing. Causes allergic skin reactions.

TETRAHYDROFURAN • Solvent derived from furan for natural and synthetic resins, particularly vinyls, protective coatings, adhesives, and printing inks. Toxic by ingestion.

TETRAHYDROFURFURYL ACETATE • See Furfural.

TETRAHYDROFURFURYL ALCOHOL • A liquid that absorbs water and is flammable in air. A solvent for cosmetic fats, waxes, and resins. Mixes with water, ether, and acetone. Mildly irritating to the skin and mucous membranes. See Furfural.

TETRAHYDROGERANYL HYDROXYL STEARATE • See Stearic Acid and Hydroxylation.

TETRAHYDROXYPROPYL ETHYLENEDIAMINE • Clear, colorless, thick liquid, a component of the bacteria-killing substance in sugarcane. It is strongly alkaline and is used as a solvent and preservative. It may be irritating to the skin and mucous membranes and may cause skin sensitization.

TETRAMETHYL DECYNEDIOL • See Fatty Alcohols.

TETRAMETHYLAMMONIUM CHLORIDE • See Quaternary Ammonium Compounds.

TETRAPOTASSIUM PYROPHOSPHATE • TKPP. A sequestering, clarifying, and buffering ingredient for shampoos. Produced by molecular dehydration of dibasic sodium phosphate. Insoluble in alcohol. A water softener in bath preparations. No known toxicity.

TETRASELMIS SUECICA • Extract of a sea plankton.

TETRASODIUM DICARBOXYETHYLSTEARYL SULFOSUCCINANATE • See Surfactants.

TETRASODIUM EDTA • **Sodium Edetate.** Powdered sodium salt that reacts with metals. A sequestering ingredient and chelating ingredient *(see both)* used in cosmetic solutions. Can deplete the body of calcium if taken internally. No known toxicity on the skin. See Ethylenediamine Tetraacetic Acid.

TETRASODIUM ETIDRONATE • See Tetrasodium EDTA.

TETRASODIUM PYROPHOSPHATE • **TSPP.** A buffering and chelating ingredient *(see both)*. Also used in dentifrices. See Sodium Pyrophosphate Peroxide.

TEUCRIUM SCORODONIA • See Germander Extract.

TEXTURIZER • A chemical used to improve the texture of various cosmetics. For instance, in creams that tend to become lumpy, calcium chloride *(see)* is added to keep them smooth.

TFC • **Tricloflucarban.** A disinfectant used in cosmetics. No known toxicity.

THAUMATOCOCCUS DANIELLII • **Thaumatin.** A mixture of intensely sweet-tasting proteins extracted from the fruit of a West African plant, *Thaumatococcus daniellii*. It has about 2000 to 3000 times the sweetness of sugar. It does contain calories. The fruits of the plant have been used for centuries by the West Africans as a source of sweetness. It is also sold in Japan. Because of problems with stability, taste profile, and compatibility, thaumatin is used primarily as a flavor enhancer, at levels below the sweet-taste threshold. It is awaiting approval in the United States.

THENOYL METHIONATE • An amino acid compound used to treat hair.

THEOBROMA OIL • **Cacao Butter. Cocoa Butter.** Yellowish white solid with chocolatelike taste and odor. Derived from the cacao bean. Widely used in confections, suppositories, pharmaceuticals, soaps, and cosmetics. No known toxicity, but may cause allergic reactions in the sensitive.

THEOBROMINE • The alkaloid found in cocoa, kola nuts, tea, and chocolate products, closely related to caffeine. It is used as a diuretic, smooth muscle relaxant, heart stimulant, and blood-vessel dilator in medications. See Theobroma Oil.

THEOPHYLLINE • A white powder, soluble in water. Occurs in tea. Its current use in cosmetics has not been revealed. However, it is a smooth muscle relaxant, heart stimulant, and diuretic (reduces body water). It can cause nausea and vomiting if ingested. The toxic dose in man is only 2.9 milligrams per kilogram of body weight.

THIABENDAZOLE • A mold retardant used on animal feed, apples, bananas, beef, citrus fruit, lamb, milk, pears, pheasants, pork, potato-processing waste, rice hulls. FDA limits are 0.1 ppm in cattle, goats, sheep, pheasant, and swine; 0.05 ppm in milk; 33 ppm in dried apple pomace; 150.0 ppm in dry or wet grape pomace; 30 ppm in potato-processing waste; and 8 ppm in rice hulls when used for animal feed. Moderately toxic by ingestion.

THIAMINE HCL • Vitamin B₁. A white, crystalline powder used in emollients and as a dietary supplement in prepared breakfast foods, peanut butter, milk, and noodle products. Acts as a helper in important energy-yielding reactions in the body. Practically all commercial Vitamin B₁ is synthetic. The vitamin is destroyed by alkalies and alkaline drugs. No known toxicity.

THIAMINE NITRATE • B vitamin. A white, crystalline powder used as a diet supplement and to enrich flour. No known toxicity. GRAS.

THICKENERS • Substances to add body to lotions and creams. Those usually employed include such natural gums as sodium alginate and pectins.

THIMEROSAL • Mercurochrome. The metallo-organic compound also called Merthiolate. Used as a bacteriostat and fungistat in eye preparations. May cause allergic reaction from either the mercury or the salicylates in the compound.

2,2′-THIOBIS (4-CHLOROPHENOL) • See Phenol.

THIOCYANATE • Colorless or white crystals derived from cyanide. Used in animal feed to stimulate growth.

THIODIGLYCOL • See Thioglycolic Acid Compounds.

THIODIGLYCOLAMIDE • See Quaternary Ammonium Compounds.

THIODIPROPIONIC ACID • An acid freely soluble in hot water, alcohol, and acetone. Used as an antioxidant in general food use. Used also for soap products and polymers (see) of ethylene. GRAS.

THIOGLYCEROL • Used in soothing skin lotions. Prepared by heating glycerin (see) and alcohol. Yellowish, very viscous liquid, with a slight sulfur odor. Used to promote wound healing. No known toxicity.

THIOGLYCOLIC ACID COMPOUNDS • Prepared by the action of sodium sulfohydrate on sodium chloroacetate. A liquid with a strong unpleasant odor; mixes with water and alcohol. The ammonium and sodium salts are used in permanent wave solutions and as a hair straightener. The calcium salts are used in depilatories, hair-waving solutions, and lotions. Thioglycolates can cause hair breakage, skin irritations, severe allergic reactions, and pustular reactions.

THIOINDIGOID DYE • See Vat Dyes and Indigo.

THIOKOL® • One of the first synthetic elastomers (see), it is used in face masks and nail enamels and in the manufacture of rubbers and resins. No known toxicity.

THIOLACTIC ACID • Used in depilatories and hair-waving preparations. See Thioglycolic Acid Compounds.

THIOLANEDIOL • An antibacterial. See Phenol.

THIOMALIC ACID • See Malic Acid.

THIOMORPHOLINONE • See Morpholine.

THIONYL CHLORIDE • Pale yellow or red liquid with suffocating odor. Used in pesticides and plastics. Strong irritant to the skin.

THIOSALICYLIC ACID • Sulfur yellow flakes, slightly soluble in hot water. Used in the manufacture of cosmetic dyes. No known toxicity.

THIOTAURINE • An antioxidant. See Taurine.

THIOUREA • White, lustrous crystals with a bitter taste made by heating ammonium thiocyanate. Used in photography, dyes, hair preparations, and as a mold inhibitor. A carcinogen. May not be used in food products. Skin irritant. Allergenic.

THIOXANTHINE • See Xanthene.

THIRAM • see Tetraethylthiuram Disulfide.

THISTLE • *Carduus marianus. Cnicus benedictus. Sonchus oleraceus.* **Sow Thistle. Holy Thistle.** Several thistles were used as medicinal herbs, including holy thistle. Holy thistle is a native of Greece and Italy and is an annual. Sow thistle, a vile-smelling weed, appeared in English medicine in 1387 and was mentioned frequently since then as a tonic. It is used in "organic" cosmetics.

THREONINE • An essential amino acid *(see);* the last to be discovered (1935). Prevents the buildup of fat in the liver. Occurs in whole eggs, skim milk, casein, and gelatin.

THUJA OIL • See White Cedar Leaf Oil.

THUNDER GOD VINE • *Tripteryqium wilfordii Hook F.* **Lei Gong Tang.** The Chinese have been using the root medicinally for centuries to treat arthritis, systemic lupus erythematosus, chronic hepatitis, and a variety of skin disorders. Researchers at the University of Texas have applied to the FDA for permission to administer an extract of the vine root to treat rheumatoid arthritis.

THYME • Used to flavor toothpastes and mouthwashes, and to scent perfumes, after-shave lotions, and soap. It is a seasoning from the dried leaves and flowering tops of the wild, creeping thyme grown in Eurasia and throughout the United States. Used as a flavoring in cough medicines. May cause contact dermatitis and hay fever.

THYMOL • Used in mouthwashes and to scent perfumes, after-shave lotions, and soap. Obtained from the essential oil of lavender, origanum oil, and other volatile oils. It destroys mold, preserves anatomical specimens, and is a topical antifungal ingredient with a pleasant aromatic odor. It is omitted from hypoallergenic cosmetics because it can cause allergic reactions.

THYMUS EXTRACT • The extract of animal thymus gland, an organ in the chest that helps to activate the body's defenses against infections. Used in skin creams.

THYMUS HYDROXYLATE • The hydrolysate of animal thymus derived by acid, enzyme, or other method of hydrolysis. See Thymus Extract.

TIARE FLOWER • The flower obtained from *Gardenia tahitensis.* See Gardenia.

TILIA TOMENTOSA • See Linden Extract.

TILIA VULGARIS • See Linden Extract.

TILLIA AMERICANA • See Basswood Extract.

TILLIA CORDATA • See Linden Extract.

TILLIA PLATYPHYLLOS • See Linden Extract.

TILLANDSIA USNEODIDES • See Spanish Moss.

TIN CHLORIDE • See Stannous Chloride.

TIN OXIDE • A coloring ingredient in cosmetics. A brownish black powder insoluble in water. No known toxicity.

TINCTURE • A solution in alcohol of the flavors derived from plants obtained by mashing or boiling.

TINCTURE OF BENZOIN • See Benzoin.

TINEA VERSICOLOR • An eruption of tan or brown patches on the skin of the trunk, often appearing white in contrast with tan skin after exposure to the summer sun.

TIOXOLONE • Prepared from resorcinol *(see)*. Used in dandruff shampoo.

TIPA • The abbreviation for Triisopropanolamine.

TIPA-LAURETH SULFATE • See Surfactants.

TIPA-LAURYL SULFATE • See Surfactants.

TIPA-STEARATE • See Stearic Acid.

TISANE • An infusion of dried leaves or flowers that is used as a beverage or a mild medicine.

TITANIUM DIOXIDE • The greatest covering and tinting power of any white pigment used in bath powders, nail whites, depilatories, eye liners, white eye shadows, antiperspirants, face powders, protective creams, liquid powders, lipsticks, hand lotions, and nail polish. Occurs naturally in three different crystal forms. Used chiefly as a white pigment and as an opacifier; also a white pigment for candy, gum, and marking ink. No known toxicity when used externally. In high concentrations the dust may cause lung damage. Permanently listed for general cosmetic coloring in 1973.

TITANIUM HYDROXIDE • See Titanium Dioxide.

TOAD FLAX • *Linaria vulgaris.* **Yellow Toad Flax. Snap Dragon. Butter and Eggs. Ramsted.** A woody herb native to Europe and introduced in North America and Great Britain, it is valued for both external and internal use. It is employed to treat hemorrhoids and skin diseases. The flowers are sometimes mixed with vegetable oils to make a liniment. Taken internally, an infusion of the leaves has been used by herbalists to eliminate kidney stones. Toad flax is reportedly both diuretic and cathartic.

TOBACCO EXTRACT • Extract of Nicotiana Tabacum *(see)*.

TOCOPHERETH 5-18 • Antioxidants. See Tocopherol.

TOCOPHEROL • **Vitamin E.** An antioxidant in baby preparations, deodorants, and hair-grooming aids. Obtained by the vacuum distillation of edible vegetable oils. Used as a dietary supplement and as an antioxidant for essential oils, rendered animal fats, or a combination of such fats with vegetable oils. Helps form normal red blood cells, muscle, and other tissues. Protects fat in the body's tissues from abnormal breakdown. Experimental evidence shows Vitamin E may protect the heart and blood vessels and retard aging.

TOCOPHERYL SUCCINATE • **Vitamin E Succinate.** Obtained by the distillation of edible vegetable oils and used as a dietary supplement and as an antioxidant for fats and oils. No known toxicity.

TOILET SOAP • A mild, mostly pure soap made from fatty materials of high quality, usually by milling and molding to form cakes. Usually contains an emollient *(see),* perfume, color, and stabilizer with preservatives. More pleasant to use and less drying to the skin.

TOILET WATER • The scent is similar to that of perfume, but it does not last as long and is not as strong or as expensive. Usually made by adding a large amount of alcohol to the perfume formula. In Europe it is called "lotion"—8 ounces of perfume oil per gallon as compared to 20 to 24 ounces per gallon for perfumes. Considered moderately toxic if swallowed. Skin reactions depend upon ingredients.

TOLERANCE • The ability to live with an allergen.

TOLU BALSAM • Extract and Gum. Extract from the Peruvian or Indian plant. Contains cinnamic acid and benzoic acid *(see both)*. Used in butter, butterscotch, cherry, and spice flavorings for beverages, ice cream, ices, candy, baked goods, and chewing gum. The gum is used in fruit, maple, and vanilla flavorings for beverages, ice cream, ices, candy, baked goods, and syrups. Mildly antiseptic, and may be mildly irritating to the skin.

TOLUENE • Used in nail polish up to 50 percent. Obtained from petroleum or by distilling Tolu balsam. Used chiefly as a solvent. Resembles benzene but is less volatile, flammable, or toxic. May cause mild anemia if ingested, and is narcotic in high concentrations. Being tested at the U.S. Frederick Cancer Research Center for possible cancer-causing effects. It can cause liver damage and is irritating to the skin and respiratory tract. While halogenated hydrocarbons like toluene are assumed responsible for health risks, long-term effects of low-level exposure to them have been found in at least 20 cities where toluene is present in the drinking water. See Toluene Sulfonamide/Formaldehyde Resin (TSAFr). On the basis of available information, the CIR Panel *(see)* concludes that it is safe as presently used in cosmetic formulations

TOLUENE-2, 4-DIAMINE • See Toluene.

TOLUENE-3, 4-DIAMINOTOLUENE • An intermediate chemical in the manufacture of polyurethanes; dyes for textiles, fur, and leather, varnishes, pigments, and hair dyes. In a National Cancer Institute study, it caused liver cancer when fed to rats and mice, as well as breast cancer in female rats. In tests, a closely related compound, 2,4-toluenediamine, had the greatest absorption through the scalp of the hair dyes tested. See Phenylenediamine.

TOLUENE SULFONAMIDE/FORMALDEHYDE RESIN • **TSAFr.** It is used as a "nail strengthener" or hardener, and to improve adhesion and gloss. There is supposed to be no free formaldehyde in this widely used formula. Large cosmetic manufacturers stopped producing nail hardeners with free formaldehyde in the 1960s because of the frequent adverse reactions reported. This compound is a strong sensitizer while in the liquid state but not when solidified; therefore, if it doesn't touch the skin while being applied, even a person sensitive to the ingredients may not have a reaction. Those allergic to this common ingredient of nail polishes almost always have allergic reactions on the eyelids, the sides of the neck, and around the mouth and almost never on the hands. On the basis of available information, the CIR Expert Panel *(see)* concludes that it is safe as presently used in cosmetic formulations.

TOLUENE SULFONIC ACID • See Toluene.

o-TOLYL BIGUANIDE • See Toluene.

p-TOLYL ACETATE • **p-Cresyl Acetate.** A synthetic butter, caramel, fruit, honey, nut, and spice flavoring for cosmetics and beverages, ice cream, ices, candy, baked goods, chewing gum, and gelatin. No known toxicity.

TOLYLALDEHYDE • Colorless liquid from benzene. Used in perfumes and flavorings. See Tolu Balsam.

TOMATO EXTRACT • **Tomatine.** Extract from the fruit of the tomato, *Solanum esculentum.* Used as a fungicide and as a precipitating ingredient. Nontoxic.

TOMATO OIL • *Solanum Lycopersicum.* Oil from tomatoes used as a skin conditioning ingredient.

TONER • In cosmetics, an organic pigment that is used at full strength. For example, D & C Red No. 7 *(see).*

TONKA • **Tonka Bean. Coumarouna Bean.** Black, brownish seeds with a wrinkled surface and brittle, shiny or fatty skins. A vanillalike odor and a bitter taste. Used in the production of natural coumarin *(see),* flavoring extracts, and toilet powders.

TOOTHPASTE • See Dentifrices.

TOP COAT • Same ingredients as in base coat *(see)* so as to give the nail enamel a greater gloss and to help prevent chipping.

TOP-NOTE • The first impression of a fragrance upon the sense of smell. The most volatile part of the perfume. It is one of the most important factors in the success of the perfume, but does not persist after the first sniff.

TORMENTIL • *Potentilla procumbens. P. tormentilla.* **Septfoil.** Hippocrates used it for skin problems. The earliest citation of this plant in England appeared in 1387 recommending it for toothaches. Tormentil is a powerful astringent. Through the years it came to be used for piles, fevers, canker sores, and to relieve pain. It is used by herbalists as a gargle for sore throats and sore mouths. Supposedly a piece of cloth soaked in a decoction of it covering a wart will cause the growth to turn black and fall off. The same decoction is recommended for sores and ulcers. A fluid extract of the root is used by herbalists to stop bleeding of the gums and of cuts. The root contains more tannin *(see)* than oak bark.

TORREYA CALIFORNICA • See Nutmeg.

TOSYLAMIDE/EPOXY RESIN • A widely used resin in nail polish and other manicuring preparations. See Acrylates.

TOUCH-ME-NOT • See Impatiens.

TRAGACANTH • See Gum Tragacanth.

TRAILING ARBUTUS EXTRACT • The extract of the leaves of *Epigaea repens.* See Arbutus Extract.

TRANSLUCENT POWDER • Because it contains more titanium dioxide *(see)* than other face powders, translucent makeups are actually more opaque. But other than that, they contain the same ingredients.

TREE MOSS • *Climacium.* Lichen that grows on trees. Used in fragrances and flavors.

TREHALOSE • A sugar that yields glucose *(see)* on hydrolysis, and this is obtained from trehala, ergot of rye, and many fungi in which it is stored.

TRETINOIN • **Vitamin A Retinoic Acid. Retin-A.** A prescription cream, gel, or solution introduced in 1973 to treat severe acne and fine wrinkles from sun-damaged skin. Clinically, according to researchers at Emory University Medical School, Atlanta, Georgia, patients experience decreased wrinkling, improved texture, and pinkening of sallow skin. However, the changes induced by topical tretinoin extend beyond a cosmetic. Microscopic, ultrastructural, and biochemical alterations, the researchers say, indicate that topical tretinoin is a significant medical therapy and requires medical supervision. Potential adverse reactions include a feeling of warmth, slight stinging, local redness, peeling, chapping, swelling, blistering, crusting, and temporary increase or decrease in pigmentation and acne. Contact with eyes and mouth should be avoided. Topical preparations containing sulfur, resorcinol, or salicylic acid increase risk of skin irritation and should not be used with tretinoin. Contraindicated in hypersensitivity to any tretinoin components. Should be used with caution in eczema. Increased sensitivity to wind and cold may occur. No medicated cosmetics should be used. Over-the-counter versions could be on the market someday.

TRIACETIN • Glyceryl Triacetate. Primarily a solvent for hair dyes. Also a fixative in perfume and used in toothpaste. A colorless, somewhat oily liquid with a slight fatty odor and a bitter taste. Obtained from adding acetate to glycerin *(see both)*. Soluble in water and miscible with alcohol. No known toxicity in above use. Large subcutaneous injections are lethal to rats.

2,5,6-TRIAMINO-4-PYRIMIDINOL SULFATE • A hair coloring.

TRIARACHIDIN • Made from glycerin and arachidic acid *(see both)*, it is used as a skin conditioning ingredient and thickener.

TRIBEHENIN • Glyceryl Tribenenate. See Behenic Acid and Glyceryl.

TRIBROMSALAN • TBS. 3,4',5-Tribromosalicylanilide. Used in medicated cosmetics; an antiseptic and fungicide. Irritating to the skin, and may cause allergic reaction when skin is exposed to the sun. Salicylanilide is an antifungal compound used to treat ringworm. TBS is contained in the most popular soaps to kill skin bacteria. Used as a germicide, frequently replacing hexachlorophene *(see)*.

TRIBUTYL CITRATE • The triester of butyl alcohol and citric acid *(see both)*, it is a pale yellow, odorless liquid used as a plasticizer, antifoam ingredient, and solvent for nitrocellulose. Low toxicity.

TRI (BUTYLCRESYL) BUTANE • Used as a stabilizer. See Phenol.

TRICALCIUM PHOSPHATE • The calcium salt of phosphate *(see)*. A polishing ingredient in dentifrices; also an anticaking ingredient in table salt and vanilla powder, and a dietary supplement. No known toxicity. See Calcium Phosphate.

TRICAPRIN • See Decanoic Acid.

TRICETEARETH-4, or -5 PHOSPHATE • See Phosphoric Acid and Surfactants.

TRICETETHS • Emulsifiers. See Cerearic Acid.

TRICETYL PHOSPHATE • A wax. See Phosphoric Acid and Cetyl Alcohol.

TRICETYLMONIUM CHLORIDE • See Quaternary Ammonium Compounds.

TRICHLOROACETIC ACID • A topical preparation containing salicylic acid; used to treat warts.

TRICHLOROETHANE • Used in cosmetics as a solvent and degreasing ingredient. Nonflammable liquid. Insoluble in water and absorbs some water. Less toxic than carbon tetrachloride, which is used in fire extinguishers. Trichloroethane solutions are irritating to the eyes and mucous membranes, and in high concentrations can be narcotic. Can be absorbed through the skin. Inhalation and ingestion produce serious symptoms, ranging from vomiting to death.

TRICHLOROETHYLENE • TCE. Residue in decaffeinated coffee powder. Used in metal degreasing, as a solvent for fats, waxes, dyeing, dry cleaning, refrigerant, and heat exchange liquid, fumigant, paint thinner, and as a solvent in adhesives and for spice oleoresins. Moderate exposure can cause symptoms similar to alcohol inebriation, and its analgesic and anesthetic properties make it useful for short operations. High concentrations have a narcotic effect. Deaths have been attributed to irregular heart rhythm. Tests conducted by the National Cancer Institute showed that this chlorinated hydrocarbon caused cancer of the liver in mice. Now being studied by NTP as a carcinogen.

TRICHODESMA ZEYLANICUM OIL • Sea Bloom. See Algae.

TRICLOCARBAN • Trichlorocarbanilide. TCC. A bacteria killer and antiseptic in soaps, medicated cosmetics, deodorants, and cleansing creams. Prepared from aniline *(see)*. In May 1983, it was revealed that tests for this soap ingredient were falsified and that rat deaths were not reported. The reasons for the deaths were not confirmed.

TRICLOSAN • A broad-spectrum antibacterial ingredient that is active primarily against some types of bacteria. It is used in deodorant soaps, vaginal deodorant sprays, and other cosmetic products as well as in drugs and household products. Its deodorant properties are due to the inhibition of bacterial growth. Can cause allergic contact dermatitis, particularly when used in products for the feet.

TRICONTANYL PVP • See Polyvinylpyrrolidone.

TRICRESYL PHOSPHATE • TCP. A plasticizer in nail polishes and a strengthener in lubricants. Colorless or pale yellow liquid. Can cause paralysis many days after exposure. For instance, in 1960, approximately 10,000 Moroccans became ill after ingesting cooking oil adulterated with turbojet engine oil containing 3 percent TCP. Can be absorbed through the skin and mucous membranes, causing poisoning. Persons sensitive to the plasticizer in eyeglass frames may develop a skin rash from tricresyl. Toxic dose in man is only 6 milligrams per kilogram of body weight.

TRIDECETH-2, -3, -5, -7, -9, -10, -12, -15, -20, -50 • See Polyethylene Glycols. The number signifies the viscosity.

TRIDECETH-4, -7, OR -19 CARBOXYLIC ACID • A surfactant *(see)*. See also Polyoxyethylene and Carboxylic Acid.

TRIDECETH-3 OR -6 PHOSPHATE • See Phosphoric Acid and Polyethylene Glycol. The number signifies viscosity.

TRIDECYL ALCOHOL • Derived from tridecane, a paraffin hydrocarbon obtained from petroleum. Used as an emulsifier in cosmetic creams, lotions, and lipsticks. No known toxicity.

TRIDECYL BEHENATE • Skin conditioning ingredient. See Behenic Acid.

TRIDECYL COCOATE • A skin conditioning ingredient. See Coconut Oil.

TRIDECYL SALICYLATE • See Salicylates.

TRIDECYL STEARATE • See Stearic Acid.

TRIDECYL STEAROYL STEARATE • See Stearic Acid.

TRIDECYL TRIMELLITATE • See Trimellitic Acid.

TRIDECYLBENZENE SULFONIC ACID • See Sulfonamide Formaldehyde.

TRIDETH-3 • See Tridecyl Alcohol.

TRIDETH-6, -10, -12 • See Tridecyl Alcohol.

TRIERUCIN • Made from glycerin and erucic acid *(see both)* used as a skin conditioning ingredient and also used as a thickener.

TRIETHANOLAMINE • A coating ingredient for fresh fruit and vegetables and widely used in surfactants *(see)* and as a dispersing ingredient and detergent in hand and body lotions, shaving creams, soaps, shampoos, and bath powders. Its principal toxic effect in animals has been attributed to overalkalinity. Gross pathology has been found in the gastrointestinal tract in fatally poisoned guinea pigs. It is an irritant. It has been found, in tests in Italy at the University of Bologna, to be the most frequent sensitizer among the common emulsifiers used in cosmetics. On the basis of available information, the CIR Expert Panel *(see)* concludes that it is safe as presently used in cosmetic formulation but in products intended for prolonged contact with the skin, the concentration should not exceed 5 percent and be used only in "rinse-off" products. Should not be used with nitrosating agents *(see)*.

TRIETHANOLAMINE DODECYLBENZENE SULFONATE • **Linear.** Made from ethylene oxide and used in bubble baths and soapless shampoos. May be mildly irritating to the skin. See Ethanolamines.

TRIETHANOLAMINE-d-1-2-PYRROLIDONE-5-CARBOXYMETHYLATE • **Triethanolamine.** A colorless liquid, soluble in water, and used as a soap base and oil emulsifier. See Ethanolamines.

TRIETHANOLAMINE STEARATE • Made from ethylene oxide. Used in brilliantines, cleansing creams, foundation creams, hair lacquers, liquid makeups, fragrances, liquid powders, mascara, protective creams, baby preparations, shaving creams and lathers, and preshave lotions. A moisture absorber, viscous, used in making emulsions. Cream-colored, turns brown on exposure to air. May be irritating to the skin and mucous membranes, but less so than many other amines *(see)*.

TRIETHANOLAMINE TRISODIUM PHOSPHATE • Made from ethylene oxide and used in cuticle softeners. May be mildly irritating to the skin. See Ethanolamines.

TRIETHONIUM HYDROLYZED COLLAGEN ETHOSULFATE • See Hydrolyzed Animal Protein and Quaternary Ammonium Compounds.

TRIETHYL CITRATE • **Citric Acid. Ethyl Citrate.** A plasticizer in nail polish. Odorless, practically colorless, bitter; also used in dried egg as a sequestering ingredient *(see)* and to prevent rancidity. Citrates may interfere with laboratory tests for blood, liver, and pancreatic function, but there is no known skin toxicity.

TRIETHYLENE GLYCOL • Used in stick perfume. Prepared from ethylene oxide and ethylene glycol *(see both)*. Used as a solvent. See Polyethylene Glycol for toxicity.

TRIFOLIUM PRATENSE • See Clover.

TRIFLUOROMETHYL C1-4 ALKYL DIMETHICONE • See Silicones.

TRIGONELLA FOENUM-GRAECUM • See Fenugreek Seed.

TRIHEPTANOIN • See Heptanoic Acid.

TRIHYDROXY STEARIN • Isolated from cork and used as a thickener. No known toxicity.

TRIHYDROXYBENZENE • See Benzene.

TRIHYDROXYMETHOXYSTEARIN • Used as a skin conditioner, a solvent, and a thickener in cosmetic formulations at concentrations up to 5 percent. On the basis of available information, the CIR Expert Panel *(see)* concludes that it is safe as presently used in cosmetic formulations. See Stearic Acid.

TRIIODOTHYRONINE • Possesses 5 times the activity of the thyroid drug L-thyroxine, used in thyroid replacement therapy. It increases the metabolic rate and oxygen consumption of animal tissues.

TRIISOCETYL CITRATE • See Citric Acid.

TRIISOCETYL STEARATE • Made from citric acid and isocetyl alcohol *(see both)*. Used as a skin conditioning ingredient. On the basis of the available animal and human data, the CIR Expert Panel *(see)* concludes that this ingredient is safe as used in cosmetics.

TRIISOPALMITIN • A skin conditioning ingredient made from palmitic acid and glycerin.

TRIISONONANOIN • See Glycerin and Nonanoic Acid.

TRIISOPROPANOLAMINE • A crystalline white, solid. A mild base used as an emulsifying ingredient. No known toxicity.

TRIISOPROPYL TRILINOLEATE • See Isopropyl Alcohol and Trilinoleic Acid.

TRIISOSTEARIN • See Glycerin and Isostearic Acid.

TRIISOSTEARYL TRILINOLEATE • See Isostearyl Alcohol and Trilinoleic Acid.

TRILANETH-4 PHOSPHATE • See Lanolin Alcohols.

TRILAURIN • See Lauric Acid.

TRILAURYL CITRATE • See Lauryl Alcohol and Citric Acid.

TRILAURYLAMINE • See Lauryl Alcohol.

TRILINOLEIC ACID • **Trimer Acid.** See Linoleic Acid.

TRILINOLEIN • The triester of glycerin and linoleic acid *(see both)*.

TRIMAGNESIUM PHOSPHATE • **Magnesium Phosphate. Tribasic.** Occurs in nature as the mineral bobierite. A white, crystalline powder, it absorbs water and is used in cosmetics as an alkali. No known toxicity.

TRIMELLITIC ACID • Colorless crystals from coal. Used in the manufacture of plastics, dyes, adhesives, and polymers.

TRIMETHYLHEXANOL • See Hexanol.

TRIMETHYLOLPROPANE TRICAPRYLATE/TRICAPRATE • See Caprylic Acid.

TRIMETHYLOLPROPANE TRIISOSTEARATE • See Propane and Isostearic Acid.

TRIMETHYLOLPROPANE TRIOCTANOATE • See Propane and Octanoic Acid.

TRIMETHYLPENTANEDIOL/ISOPHTHALIC ACID/TRIMELLITIC ANHYDRIDE COPOLYMER • See Copolymers.

TRIMETHYLSILOXYSILICATE • See Silicates.

TRIMETHYLSILYLAMODIMETHICONE • See Silicones.

TRIMYRISTIN • **Glyceryl Trimyristate.** Solid triglyceride of myristic acid that occurs in many vegetable fats and oils, particularly in coconut oil and nutmeg butter. White to yellowish gray, it is used as an emollient in cold creams and for shampoos. No known toxicity.

TRIOCTANOIN • See Octanoic Acid and Glyceryl.

TRIOCTYL CITRATE • See 1-Octanol and Citric Acid.

TRIOCTYLDODECYL CITRATE • See Citric Acid and Dodecanoic Acid.

TRIOLEIN • **Glyceryl Trioleate.** From the Palestine olive and one of the chief constituents of nondrying oils and fats used in cosmetics. Colorless to yellowish, tasteless, odorless. Used in cosmetic creams and oils. No known toxicity.

TRIOLEIN PEG-6 ESTERS • See Esters and Triolein.

TRIOLETH-8 PHOSPHATE • Derived from phosphoric acid and oleyl alcohol *(see both)*.

TRIOLEYL PHOSPHATE • Used as an emulsifier. No known toxicity. See Oleyl Alcohol.

TRIPABA PANTHENOL • See Panthenol and PABA.

TRIPALMITIN • Occurs in fats and is prepared from glycerol and palmitic acid *(see both)*. Insoluble in water. See palmitic acid for toxicity.

TRIPHENYL PHOSPHATE • A noncombustible substitute for camphor in celluloid. Colorless; insoluble in water. Stable, fireproof, and used as a plasticizer in nail polish. Causes paralysis if ingested and skin rash in hypersensitive people. Inhalation of only 3.5 milligrams per kilogram of body weight is toxic to humans.

TRIPHENYL TRIMETHICONE • See Silicones.

TRIPHENYLMETHANE GROUP • **Tritan.** Certified dyes made from the reduction *(see)* of carbon tetrachloride and benzene with aluminum chloride. Very soluble in water, affected by light and alkalies. Among the triphenylmethane group are FD & C Blue No. 1 and FD & C Green Nos. 1, 2, and 3. See Colors for toxicity.

TRIPOLYPHOSPHATE • A buffering ingredient in shampoos. A phosphorus salt. Used to soften water, as an emulsifier, and as a dispersing ingredient. Can be irritating because of its alkalinity. May cause esophageal stricture if swallowed. Moderately irritating to the skin and mucous membranes. Ingestion can cause violent vomiting.

TRIPOTASSIUM EDTA • See Edetate Disodium and Potassium.

TRIPROPYLENE GLYCOL CITRATE • See Propylene Glycol.

TRIRICINOLEIN • Made from glycerin and ricinoleic acid *(see both)*, it is used as a skin conditioning ingredient and a thickener.

TRISEBACIN • The ester of glycerin and sebacic acid.

TRIS (HYDROXYMETHYL) NITROMETHANE • Crystals from ethyl acetate and benzene *(see both)*. Soluble in alcohol. Inhibits bacterial growth in water systems, cutting oils, nonprotein glues, and sizings. Irritating to the skin and mucous membranes. May release formaldehyde *(see)*.

TRIS (NONYLPHENYL) PHOSPHITE • See Phenol.

TRISODIUM EDTA • See Tetrasodium EDTA.

TRISODIUM HEDTA • Mineral suspending ingredients. See Sequestering Ingredients.

TRISODIUM HYDROXY EDTA • See Tetrasodium EDTA.

TRISODIUM HYDROXYETHYL ETHLENEDIAMINETRIACETATE • See Tetrasodium EDTA.

TRISODIUM LAUROAMPHO PG-ACETATE PHOSPHATE CHLORIDE • See Quaternary Ammonium Compounds.

TRISODIUM NTA • See Sequestering Ingredients.

TRISODIUM PHOSPHATE • Obtained from phosphate rock. Highly alkaline. Used in shampoos, cuticle softeners, bubble baths, and bath salts for its water-softening and cleaning actions. Phosphorous was formerly used to treat rickets and degenerative disorders, and is now used as a mineral supplement for foods; also in incendiary bombs and tracer bullets. Can cause skin irritation from alkalinity.

TRISTEARIN • Present in many animal and vegetable fats, especially hard ones like tallow and cocoa butter, it is used in surfactants, quaternary ammonium compounds, and emollients. No known toxicity.

TRISTEARYL CITRATE • The triester of stearyl alcohol and citric acid *(see both)*.

TRISTEARYL PG-PHOSPHATE DIMONIUM CHLORIDE • See Quaternary Ammonium Chloride.

TRIS (TRIBUTOXYSILOXY) METHYLSILANE • See Silanes.

TRITICUM VULAGRE • See Wheat Bran.

TRIUNDECANOIN • See Glyceryl and Undecanoic Acid.

TROMETHAMINE • Made by the reduction *(see)* of nitro compounds, it is a crystalline mass used in the manufacture of surface-active ingredients *(see)*. Used as an emulsifying ingredient for cosmetic creams and lotions, mineral oil, and paraffin wax emulsions. Used medicinally to correct an overabundance of acid in the body. No known toxicity.

TROMETHAMINE ACRYLATES/ACRYLONITROGENS COPOLYMER • See Acrylates.

TROMETHAMINE MAGNESIUM ALUMINUM SILICATE • See Silicates.

TROPAEOLUM MAJUS • See Indian Cress Extract.

TRUE FIXATIVE • This holds back the evaporation of the other materials. Benzoin is an example. See Fixative.

TRYPSIN • An enzyme formed in the intestine. It is administered as a drug in the treatment of indigestion.

TRYPTOPHAN • A tremendous amount of research is now in progress with this amino acid *(see)*. First isolated in milk in 1901, it is now being studied as a means to calm hyperactive children, induce sleep, and fight depression and pain. Although it is sold over the counter, it is not believed to be completely harmless and has been suspected of being a co-carcinogen and affecting the liver when taken in high doses. In cosmetics, it is used to increase the protein content of creams and lotions. No known toxicity in cosmetics.

TSAFr • Abbreviation for toluene sulfonamide/formaldehyde resin *(see)*.

TUBEROSE OIL • Derived from a Mexican bulbous herb commonly cultivated for its spike of fragrant, white, single or double flowers that resemble small lilies. Tuberose oil is used in perfumes. Can cause allergic reactions.

TUMERIC • See Turmeric.

TUNA EXTRACT • The extract of the fish species *Thunnus*. See Fish Oil.

TURKEY-RED OIL • One of the first surface-active ingredients *(see)*. Used in shampoos. Contains sulfated castor oil. It has been used to obtain bright, clear colors in dyeing fabrics. See Sulfonated Oils.

TURMERIC • **Tumeric.** Derived from an East Indian herb. An aromatic, pepperlike, but somewhat bitter, taste. The cleaned, boiled, sun-dried, pulverized root is used in coconut, ginger ale, and curry flavorings for puddings, condiments, meats, soups, and pickles; also for yellow coloring for sausage casings, oleomargarine, shortening, and marking ink. The extract is used in fruit, meat, and cheese flavorings for beverages, condiments, meats, soup bases, and pickles. The oleoresin *(see)* is obtained by extraction of one or more of the solvents acetone, ethyl alcohol, ethylene dichloride *(see all)*, and others. It is used in spice flavorings for condiments, meats, pickles, and brine. Both turmeric and its oleoresin have been permanently listed for coloring food since 1966. No known toxicity. GRAS.

TURNERA DIFFUSA • See Damiana Leaves.

TURNIP EXTRACT • The extract of *Brassica rapa*. Biennial herbs with thick root. Has a hairy skin.

TURPENTINE • Any of the various resins obtained from coniferous trees. A yellowish, viscous exudate with a characteristic smell, it is a natural solvent composed of pine oils, camphenes, and terpenes. It is used as a solvent, thinner for paints, varnishes, and lacquers, as a rubber solvent, in insecticides, and in wax-based polishes. The volatile components of turpentine, pinene, and carene, may be hazardous to the lungs. Turpentine is readily absorbed through the skin. Irritating to the skin and mucous membranes and can cause allergic reactions. In addition, it is a central nervous system depressant. Death is usually due to respiratory failure. As little as 15 milliliters has killed children.

TURPENTINE GUM • A solvent in hair lotions, waxes, perfume soaps, and to soothe skin. It is the oleoresin from a species of pines. Also a food flavoring. Readily absorbed through the skin. Irritating to the skin and mucous membranes. In addition to being a local skin irritant, it can cause allergic reactions.

TURTLE OIL • The oil of *tartarouchos,* used in emollients. At one time there was a great deal of hype about the antiwrinkle benefits of this ingredient but, as pointed out, it never did much for a turtle's skin.

TUSSILAGO FARFARA • See Coltsfoot.

TYRAMINE • A derivative of tyrosine *(see)*, it is a chemical present in mistletoe and many common foods and beverages. It raises blood pressure but usually causes no problem because enzymes in the body hold it in check.

TYROSINE • Widely distributed amino acid *(see)*, termed nonessential because it does not seem to be necessary for growth. It is used as a dietary supplement. It is a building block of protein and is used in cosmetics to help creams penetrate the skin. No known toxicity.

U

UBIQUINONES • **Coenzyme Q.** A group of quinones *(see)* used as antioxidants and skin conditioning ingredients in cosmetics. Some are naturally occurring and many are synthetic. Coenzyme Q is a naturally occurring antioxidant nutrient and a cofactor in the energy production of the cell. It is chemically similar to Vitamins E and K, and its use in medicine to aid muscle function in diseases such as multiple sclerosis and heart failure is still being studied. It is also being tested as an adjunctive treatment for breast cancer in Denmark. Biotin *(see)* is another example.

UDDER EXTRACT • The extract of animal udder used in moisturizers.

ULEX EUROPAEUS • **Gorse.** Extract of a spiny, evergreen shrub with yellow flowers. This common plant is often used for fuel and fodder. See Furze Extract.

ULMUS FLUVA • See Slippery Elm.

ULTRAMARINE, BLUE, GREEN, PINK, RED, AND VIOLET • Colorings permanently listed for external use only, including in the area of the eye, in 1976. See Colors.

ULVA LACTUCA • See Algae.

UMBILICAL EXTRACT • The extract of the umbilical cords of animals. Used in moisturizers.

UNCARIA GAMBIR • See Catechu Black.

UNDARIA PINNATIFIDA • **Sea Blackberry.** A pesty seaweed that is native to the Japan Sea and that has spread to the Australian coastline. In Japan it is known as wakame and is cultivated as a food plant. See Kelp.

2, 3-UNDECADIONE • A synthetic butter-flavoring ingredient for beverages, ice cream, ices, candy, and baked goods. No known toxicity.

γ-UNDECALACTONE • **Peach Aldehyde.** Colorless to light yellow liquid with a peachy odor. Derived from undecylenic acid with sulfuric acid. A synthetic fruit flavoring, colorless or yellow, with a strong peach odor. Used for beverages, ice cream, ices, candy, baked goods, gelatin desserts, and chewing gum. Used also in perfumery. No known toxicity.

UNDECANAL • A synthetic flavoring ingredient. Colorless to slightly yellow, with a sweet, fatty odor. Used in lemon, orange, rose, fruit, and honey flavorings for beverages, ice cream, ices, candy, baked goods, and chewing gum. No known toxicity.

9-UNDECANAL • A synthetic citrus and fruit flavoring for beverages, ice cream, ices, candy, baked goods, and chewing gum. No known toxicity.

10-UNDECANAL • A synthetic citrus, floral, and fruit flavoring ingredient for beverages, ice cream, ices, and candy. No known toxicity.

UNDECANOIC ACID • A topical antifungal. See Undecylenic Acid.

1-UNDECANOL • Colorless liquid with a citrus odor used in perfumery and as a flavoring. See Undecylenic Acid.

2-UNDECANOL • Antifoaming ingredient, perfume fixative, and plasticizer. See Undecylenic Acid.

2-UNDECANONE • A synthetic flavoring ingredient that occurs naturally in rue and hops oil. Used in citrus, coconut, peach, and cheese flavorings for beverages, ice cream, ices, candy, baked goods, and puddings. No known toxicity.

10-UNDECEN-1-YL ACETATE • A synthetic citrus and fruit flavoring ingredient for beverages, ice cream, ices, candy, and baked goods. No known toxicity.

UNDECETH-5 • The polyethylene glycol derivative of undecyl alcohol *(see)*. See also Polyethylene Glycol.

UNDECYL ALCOHOL • A synthetic lemon, lime, orange, and rose flavoring ingredient for beverages, ice cream, ices, candy, and baked goods. No known toxicity.

UNDECYLENAMIDE DEA • A fungicide, it is a mixture of ethanolamides *(see)* of undecylenic acid *(see)*.

UNDECYLENAMIDE MEA • A fungicide, it is a mixture of ethanolamides of undecylenic acid.

UNDECYLENAMIDOPROPYL BETAINE • See Quaternary Ammonium Compounds.

UNDECYLENAMIDOPROPYLAMINE • See Quaternary Ammonium Compounds.

UNDECYLENIC ACID • **Caldesene. Cruex. Desenex. Pedi-Dri. Decylenes. Quinsana Plus. Kool Foot. Ting Spray. Undoguent.** Occurs in sweat. Obtained from ricinoleic acid *(see)*. A liquid or crystalline powder, with an odor suggestive of perspiration or citrus. Used as a fungicide, in perfumes, as a flavoring, and as a lubricant additive in cosmetics. An antifungal and antibacterial ingredient used to treat athlete's foot, jock itch, and ringworm of the body except nails and hairy areas. Potential adverse reactions include skin irritation in hypersensitive persons. Ointments, creams, and liquids are used as primary therapy in very mild conditions or as prophylactic ingredients especially in moist areas. Powders with a cornstarch base may be preferred over those with a talc base. Avoid inhaling and contact with the eyes or other mucous membranes. Should not be applied on blistered, raw, or oozing skin or over deep or puncture wounds. Patients with impaired circulation, including diabetics, should consult a physician before using. If the skin problem does not clear up in a month or it gets worse, consult your physician.

UNDECYLENOYL COLLAGEN AMINO ACIDS • The treatment of animal collagen with acid to obtain amino acids. Used as a protein additive.

UNDECYLENOYL PEG-5 PARABEN • See Parabens and Polyethylene Glycol.

UNDECYLENYL ALCOHOL • Colorless liquid with a citrus odor. Used in perfumes. It is combustible but has a low toxicity.

UNDECYLIC ACID • See Undecylenic Acid.

UNDECYLPENTADECANOL • See Fatty Alcohols.

UNSAPONIFIABLE OLIVE OIL • The oil fraction that is not broken down in the refining of olive fatty acids.

UNSAPONIFIABLE RAPESEED OIL • The oil that is not broken down in the refining of rapeseed oil fatty acids.

UNSAPONIFIABLE SHEA BUTTER • The fraction of shea butter that is not broken down during processing.

UNSAPONIFIABLE SOYBEAN OIL • The fraction of soybean oil that is not broken down in the refining recovery of soybean oil fatty acids.

UREA • **Carbamide.** A product of protein metabolism excreted from human urine. Used in yeast food and wine production up to 2 pounds per gallon. It is used to "brown" baked goods such as pretzels, and consists of colorless or white, odorless crystals that have a cool salty taste. An antiseptic and deodorizer used in liquid antiperspirants, ammoniated dentifrices, roll-on deodorants, mouthwashes, hair colorings, hand creams, lotions, and shampoos. Medicinally, urea is used as a topical antiseptic and as a diuretic to reduce body water. Its largest use, however, is as a fertilizer, and only a small part of its production goes into the manufacture of other urea products. The final report to the FDA of the Select Committee on GRAS Substances stated in 1980 that it should continue its GRAS status with no limitations other than good manufacturing practices.

UREA-D-GLUCURONIC ACID • See Glucuronic Acid.

UREA-FORMALDEHYDE RESIN • **UFFI.** A large class of resins, the mixture of urea and formaldehyde *(see both)* were the first colored plastics made. They are used in dinnerware, interior plywood, flexible foams, and insulation. Urea-formaldehyde foam insulations may release formaldehyde during decomposition and have been cited for releasing free formaldehyde to the indoor air. The level of formaldehyde released by the foam reportedly decreases over one to three years. The adverse health effects of UFFI are hotly debated. People exposed to UFFI in buildings report shortness of breath, headache, stuffy nose, irritated eyes, cough, frequent "colds," rash, fatigue, sore throat, and vomiting. See Formaldehyde.

UREA PEROXIDE • When used in over-the-counter drugs, the established name for this ingredient is carbamide peroxide. A strong oxidizing ingredient, it is used for softening wax.

UREASE • An enzyme that hydrolyzes urea *(see)* to ammonium carbonate *(see)*.

URIC ACID • White, odorless, tasteless crystals. It forms the end product of nitrogen metabolism of birds and scaly reptiles. It is present in small amounts in human urine. Used in the manufacture of chemicals.

UROCANIC ACID • Skin conditioner and sunscreen. Prepared from histidine *(see)*. The CIR Expert Panel *(see)* says there is insufficient data to conclude that this ingredient is "safe for use in cosmetics." Because of this, sunscreens containing urocanic acid should not be used by consumers when trying to minimize the potential of increased sun sensitivity due to AHA use. The safety of this ingredient has not been documented and substantiated. The CIR Expert Panel *(see)* cannot conclude whether it is safe for use in cosmetic products until the appropriate safety data have been obtained and evaluated.

URTICA DIOICA • See Nettles.

USNEA BARBATA • See Lichen Extract.

USNIC ACID • Antibacterial compound found in lichens. Pale yellow, slightly soluble in water. No known toxicity.

V

VA • Abbreviation for vinyl acetate *(see)*.

VA/BUTYL MALEATE/ISOBORNYL ACRYLATE COPOLYMER • The copolymer of vinyl acetate, butyl maleate, and isobornyl acrylate monomers. See Vinyl Polymers.

VA/CA COPOLYMER • Binder, hair fixative, and emulsifier. An epidemiological study of hairdressers, who would inhale more VA/CA than the average person, did not show lung problems. On the basis of available information, the CIR Expert Panel *(see)* concludes that it is safe as presently used in cosmetic formulations. See Vinyl Acetate.

VACCINIUM ANGUSTIFOLIUM • See Bilberry Extract.

VACCINIUM MACROCARPON • See Cranberry.

VACCINUM MYRTILLUS • See Bilberry Extract.

VA/CROTONATES COPOLYMER • A polymer of vinyl acetate and one or more monomers consisting of crotonic acid or any of its simple esters. See Vinyl Polymers and Crotonic Acid.

VAGINAL DEODORANTS • **Feminine Hygiene Sprays.** Introduced in 1966, vaginal deodorant sprays have grown very popular. Marketed as mists or powders in aerosol sprays and widely advertised as products to keep women feeling "feminine," they are designed to prevent "feminine odor" and to give that "clean feeling." Classified as cosmetics, these deodorants did not need clearance for the ingredients. Reports to the FDA of irritations and other problems from the sprays within the last two years include bladder infections, burning, itching, swelling, rash, boils in the vaginal area, and blood in the urine. Physicians recommend soap and water as more beneficial than the sprays, and that concentrating chemicals, including perfumes, in one area is not wise because of the possibility of allergic reactions and irritations. Ingredients in vaginal deodorants include emollients such as glycerides, myristate, polyoxyethylene derivatives, perfumes, and propellants. Some sprays, in addition, contain an antibacterial. The allergic and skin reactions may not only occur in the women who use these products but also in their male partners who are exposed to the ingredients during sexual relations. Among some of the problem spray ingredients identified were benzalkonium chloride, chlorhexidine, isopropyl myristate, and perfume.

VALERIAN • The extract of *Valeriana officinalis.* A perennial native to Europe and the United States, it was reputed to be a love potion. Its vapor was found to kill the bacillus of typhoid fever after 45 minutes. The herb has been widely studied in Europe and Russia, and the major constituents, the valepotriate, have been reported to have marked sedative, anticonvulsive, blood pressure–lowering, and tranquilizing effects. It has been used for centuries to treat panic attacks. In Germany, valerian preparations have been used for more than a decade to treat childhood behavioral disorders, supposedly without the side effects experienced with pharmaceuticals for that purpose. It has been reported that it also helps concentration and energy. Prolonged use of valerian may result in side effects such as irregular heartbeat, headaches, uneasiness, nervousness, and insomnia. Very large doses may cause paralysis. See Valeric Acid.

VALERIANA OFFICINALIS • See Valerian.

VALERIC ACID • Used in the manufacture of perfumes. Occurs naturally in apples, cocoa, coffee, oil of lavender, peaches, and strawberries. Colorless, with an unpleasant odor. Usually distilled from the roots of valerian *(see)*. It is used also as a synthetic flavoring, and some of its salts are used in medicine. No known toxicity.

VALINE • An essential amino acid *(see)*. Occurs in the largest quantities in fibrous protein. It is indispensable for growth and nitrogen balance. Used in suntan lotions. No known toxicity in cosmetics, but the FDA has asked for further study of this ingredient as a food additive.

VANCIDE FP • See Captan.

VANILLA EXTRACT • Used in perfumes and flavorings. Extracted from the fullgrown unripe fruit of the vanilla plant of Mexico and the West Indies. Also a food flavoring and scent made synthetically from eugenol *(see);* also from the waste of the wood pulp industry. One part vanillin equals 400 parts vanilla pods. The lethal dose in mice is 3 grams (30 grams to the ounce) per kilogram of body weight. A skin irritant that produces a burning sensation and eczema. May also cause pigmentation of the skin.

VANILLA PLANIFOLIA EXTRACT • See Vanilla Extract.

VANILLIN • Used in perfumes. Occurs naturally in vanilla and potato parings but is an artificial flavoring and scent made synthetically from eugenol *(see);* also from the waste of the wood pulp industry. One part vanillin equals 400 parts vanilla pods. The lethal dose in mice is 3 grams (30 grams to the ounce) per kilogram of body weight. A skin irritant that produces a burning sensation and eczema. May also cause pigmentation of the skin.

VANISHING CREAM • An emollient cream that creates the feeling of vanishing when rubbed on the skin. See Emollients.

VASELINE® • **Petroleum Jelly. Petrolatum. Paraffin Jelly.** Used in cold creams, emollient creams, conditioning creams, wax depilatories, eyebrow pencils, eye shadows, liquefying creams, liquid powders, nail whites, lipsticks, protective creams, baby creams, and rouge. While usually soothing to the skin, it may cause allergic reactions, particularly in creams and hairdressings, because it is a derivative of petroleum.

VAT DYES • Water-soluble aromatic organic compounds. They dissolve in water when vatted with an alkaline solution of the reducing *(see)* ingredient sodium hydrosulfite. Good fastness. Considered low in toxicity.

VAT RED 1 • An indigoid color. The certified name of this color is D & C Red No. 30. See Vat Dyes.

VA/VINYL BUTYL BENZOATE CROTONATES COPOLYMER • A polymer of vinyl acetate, vinyl *t*-butylbenzoate, and one or more monomers of crotonic acid or one of its simple esters. See Vinyl Polymers.

VEGETABLE GLYCERIDES PHOSPHATE • A skin conditioner. See Vegetable Oils.

VEGETABLE GUMS • Includes derivatives from quince seed, karaya, acacia, tragacanth, Irish moss, guar, sodium alginate, potassium alginate, ammonium alginate, and propylene glycol alginate. All are subject to deterioration and always need a preservative. The gums function as liquid emulsions; that is, they thicken cosmetic products and make them cream. No known toxicity other than allergic reactions in hypersensitive persons.

VEGETABLE OILS • Peanut, sesame, olive, and cottonseed oil obtained from plants and used in baby preparations, cleansing creams, emollient creams, face powders, hair-grooming aids, hypoallergenic cosmetics, lipsticks, nail creams, shampoos, shaving creams, and wave sets. No known toxicity.

VERATALDEHYDE • Derived from petroleum. Has the odor of vanilla beans. Used in perfumery.

VERBASCUM THAPSUS • See Mullein Extract.

VERBENA EXTRACT • Has a characteristic odor; insoluble in water. Used as a perfume ingredient. See Terpenes.

VERONICA EXTRACT • Extract of the flowering herb Veronica, a small herb of wide distribution that has pink or white flowers. Used in perfumery.

VETIVER OIL • **Vetiverol. Khus-Khus.** Stable, brown to reddish brown oil from the roots of a fragrant grass. Used in soaps and perfumes, it has an aromatic to harsh, woodsy odor. No known toxicity.

VETIVER RECTIFIED • Perfume ingredient. See Vetiver Oil.

VETIVEROL • See Vetiver Oil.

VETIVERYL ACETATE • See Vetiver Oil.

VIBURNUM EXTRACT • **Haw Bark. Black Extract.** Extract of the fruit of a hawthorn shrub or tree. Used in fragrances and in butter, caramel, cola, maple, and walnut flavorings for beverages. Has been used as a uterine antispasmodic. No known toxicity.

VICIA FABA • See Faba Bean Extract.

VINCA MAJOR • See Periwinkle Extract.

VINEGAR • Used for hundreds of years to remove lime soap after shampooing. It is a solvent for cosmetic oils and resins. Vinegar is about 4 to 6 percent acetic acid. Acetic acid occurs naturally in apples, cheese, grapes, milk, and other foods. No known toxicity, but may cause an allergic reaction in those allergic to corn.

VINYL ACETATE • A starch modifier not to exceed 2.5 percent in modified starch *(see)*. Vapors in high concentration may be narcotic; animal experiments show low toxicity.

VINYL BROMIDE • A flame retardant. A cancer-causing ingredient.

VINYL CAPROLACTAM/PVP/DIMETHYLAMINOETHYL METHACRYLATE COPOLYMER • See Vinyl Polymers.

VINYL CHLORIDE • Banned in aerosol cans for hairsprays and deodorants in 1974. It is a proven cause of liver cancer in workers who work with the compound.

VINYL POLYMERS • Includes resins used in false nails and nail lacquer preparations. A major class of polymer *(see)* material widely used in the plastics, synthetic fibers, and surface coatings. Such materials are derived from the polymerization of vinyl groups, which include vinyl acetate and vinyl chloride. Vinyls are made from the reaction between acetylene and certain compounds such as alcohol, phenol, and amines. Inhalation of 300 parts per million is toxic in man.

VINYL PYRROLIDONE • See Polyvinylpyrrolidone.

VINYLDIMETHICONE • See Silicones and Vinyl Polymers.

VIOLA TRICOLOR • See Pansy.

VIOLET EXTRACT • **Flowers and Leaves.** Green liquid with typical odor of violet. It is taken from the plant widely grown in the United States. Used in perfumes, face powders, and for coloring inorganic pigments. May produce skin rash in the allergic.

VISCUM ALBUM • See Mistletoe.

VISNAGA VERA EXTRACT • A plant related to celery *(see)*.

VITAMIN A • A yellow, viscous liquid insoluble in water. Used in lubricating creams and oils for its alleged skin-healing properties. Can be absorbed through the skin. Its absence from the diet leads to a loss in weight, retarded growth, and eye diseases. Too high a level can cause the skin to turn yellow and can cause birth defects and pressure on the brain. See also Retinoids and Retin-A.

VITAMIN B$_2$ • See Riboflavin.

VITAMIN B$_6$ • **Pyridoxine hydrochloride.** A colorless or white crystalline powder added to evaporated milk base in infant foods. Present in many foodstuffs. Especially good sources are yeast, liver, and cereals. A coenzyme that helps in the metabolism of amino acids *(see)* and fat. Permits normal red blood cell formation. The final report to the FDA of the Select Committee on GRAS Substances stated in 1980 that it should continue its GRAS status with no limitations other than good manufacturing practices. The FDA is doing a toxicology search on this additive.

VITAMIN C • See Ascorbic Acid.

VITAMIN D$_2$ • **Calciferol.** A pale yellow, oily liquid, odorless, tasteless, insoluble in water. Used for its alleged skin-healing properties in lubricating creams and lotions. The absence of Vitamin D in the food of young animals can lead to rickets, a bone-affecting condition. It is soluble in fats and fat solvents, and is present in animal fats. Absorbed through the skin, its value in cosmetics has not been proven. No known toxicity to the skin.

VITAMIN E • See Tocopherol.

VITAMIN E ACETATE • See Tocopherol.

VITAMIN E SUCCINATE • See Tocopherol.

VITAMIN K • Recommended Daily Allowance for Adults has not been established, but the safety and adequate daily dietary intake level is listed at 0.07 to 0.14 mg. It is necessary for blood clotting. Current research seems to indicate it helps maintain bone mass in the elderly and prevents osteoporosis. Vitamin K antagonizes the action of anticoagulants and has been used as an antidote in managing overdosages or excessive responses to the latter.

VITILIGO • **Leukoderma.** Irregular white patches of skin, sometimes streaks of white or gray hair due to lack of pigment. Usually, there is a family tendency to develop this condition. The white patches are most noticeable when surrounded by deeply tanned skin. It is not a systemic but merely a cosmetic condition.

VITAVERIA ZIZANOIDES • See Vetiver Oil.

VITIS VINEFERA • See Grape Leaf Extract.

VITREOSCILLA FERMENT • An extract of the bacterial culture derived from Vitreoscilla.

VITULUS • **Calf Blood** or **Calf Skin Extract.**

VOLATILE OILS • Volatility in oils is the tendency to give off vapors, usually at room temperature. The volatile oils in plants such as peppermint or rose produce the aroma. The volatile oils in plants stimulate the tissue with which they come into contact, whether they are inhaled, ingested, or placed on the skin. They can relax or stimulate, irritate or soothe, depending upon their source and concentration.

W

WALNUT EXTRACT • *Juglans nigra.* An extract of the husk of the nut of *Juglans* species, used in walnut flavorings and for brown coloring. The fruit is used by herbalists to promote strength and weight gain and to treat skin diseases, including eczema, herpes, and psoriasis. The bark is used to treat constipation. No known toxicity.

WALNUT LEAVES • Used in hair products for "split ends." See Walnut Extract.

WALNUT OIL • See Walnut Extract.

WALNUT SHELL POWDER • The ground shell of English walnuts, *Juglans regia.* See Walnut Extract.

WATER • The major constituent of all living matter and the ingredient used most in the cosmetic industry. Because of this fact, the industry fought labeling that required listing ingredients in descending order since water would be first most of the time. However, listing in descending order is now required. It is important that water used in cosmetics be sterile to avoid contamination of the product. Manufacturers may also have to soften water in some areas because of the high mineral content that may affect the texture and appearance of the finished product.

WATER CHESTNUT EXTRACT • The extract of the seeds of *Eleocharis dulcis,* which has an edible nutlike fruit. See Cyperus.

WATER LILY • *Nymphea alba.* **Water Rose.** Cultivated in pools, this beautiful and romantic flower was used in folk medicine to depress sexual function.

Externally, white and yellow water lilies were used to treat various skin disorders such as boils, inflammations, tumors, and ulcers.

WATERCRESS EXTRACT • Extract obtained from *Nasturtium officinalis,* a water-loving plant. Used in emollients for oily skin.

WATERMELON • *Citrullus vulgaris.* Succulent fruit of the gourd family, native to tropical Africa, and under cultivation on every continent. The sweet, juicy fruit may be red, white, or yellow. Used in "organic" cosmetics.

WAVE SET • See Setting Lotions.

WAXES • Obtained from insects, animals, and plants. Waxes have a wide application in the manufacture of cosmetics. Beeswax, for instance, is a substance secreted by the bee's special glands on the underside of its abdomen. The wax is glossy and hard but plastic when warm. Insoluble in water but partially soluble in boiling alcohol. Used in hair-grooming preparations, hair straighteners, as an epilatory (hair pull) to remove unwanted hair, and as the traditional stiffening ingredient *(see)* in lipsticks. Wax esters such as lanolin or spermaceti *(see both)* differ from fats in being less greasy, harder, and more brittle. Waxes are generally nontoxic to the skin but may cause allergic reactions in the hypersensitive, depending upon the source of the wax.

WETTING INGREDIENT • Any of numerous water-soluble ingredients that promote spreading of a liquid on a surface or penetration into a material such as skin. It lowers surface tension for better contact and absorption.

WHEAT AMINO ACIDS • Used in hair and skin conditioners. See Wheat Germ and Amino Acids.

WHEAT BRAN • The broken coat of *Triticum aestivum.* See Wheat Germ.

WHEAT BRAN LIPIDS • An extract of the coat of wheat. See Wheat Germ.

WHEAT FLOUR • Milled from the kernels of wheat, *Triticum aestivum.* Used as an abrasive and thickener. See Wheat Starch.

WHEAT GERM • *Triticum vulgare.* The golden germ of the wheat is high in Vitamin E. It is used by organic cosmeticians to make a face mask to counteract dry skin. Here is the formula: Crush ¼ cup wheat germ plus 1 tablespoon sesame seeds with a mortar and pestle or with the back of a spoon. Add 2 tablespoons of fresh olive oil and mix well. Spread on face and neck. Leave on for 10 minutes. Remove with lukewarm water. Then rinse with cold water. Apply a rinse of chilled witch hazel *(see).* In low concentrations, it has not been found to cause sensitization. On the basis of available information, the CIR Expert Panel *(see)* concludes that it is safe as presently used in cosmetic formulations. See Tocopherol.

WHEAT GERM EXTRACT • Widely used extract of wheat germ used in "antiaging" and other emollients. See Tocopherol.

WHEAT GERM GLYCERIDES • See Tocopherol and Glycerides.

WHEAT GERM OIL • *Triticum vulgare.* Used in hair conditioners, emollients, and solvents. On the basis of available information, the CIR Expert Panel *(see)* concludes that it is safe as presently used in cosmetic formulations. See Tocopherol.

WHEAT GERM OIL UNSAPONIFIABLES • See Saponification.

WHEAT GERM PROTEIN • The protein derived from wheat germ used in shampoos and emollients.

WHEAT GERMAMIDOPROPYL BETAINE • See Quaternary Ammonium Compounds.

WHEAT GERMAMIDOPROPYL DIMETHYLAMINE • See Quaternary Ammonium Compounds.

WHEAT GERMAMIDOPROPYL DIMETHYLAMINE HYDROLYZED COLLAGEN • The wheat germ salt of hydrolyzed collagen. See Quaternary Ammonium Compounds.

WHEAT GERMAMIDOPROPYL DIMETHYLAMINE HYDROLYZED WHEAT PROTEIN • See Quaternary Ammonium Compounds.

WHEAT GERMAMIDOPROPYL DIMETHYLAMINE LACTATE • See Quaternary Ammonium Compounds.

WHEAT GERMAMIDOPROPYL ETHYDIMONIUM ETHOSULFATE • See Quaternary Ammonium Compounds.

WHEAT GLUTEN • Used in powders and creams as a base. A mixture of proteins present in wheat flour and obtained as an extremely sticky, yellowish gray mass by making a dough and then washing out the starch. It consists almost entirely of two proteins, gliadin and glutenin. It contributes to the porous and spongy structure of bread. No known toxicity.

WHEAT STARCH • A product of cereal grain. It swells when water is added. Used as a demulcent, emollient, and in dusting and face powders. May cause allergic reactions such as red eyes and stuffy nose.

WHEY PROTEIN • Obtained from the thin, watery part of milk separated from the curds, it is used in emollients. No known toxicity.

WHITE • Inorganic pigments are widely used to "color" cosmetics white. The most widely used are zinc oxide and titanium dioxide to whiten face powders. Also used are gloss white (aluminum hydrate), barium sulfate (blanc fixe), and alumina *(see all)*.

WHITE CEDAR LEAF OIL • **Oil of Arborvitae.** Stable, pale yellow volatile oil obtained by steam distillation from the fresh leaves and branch ends of the eastern arborvitae. Has a strong camphoraceous and sagelike scent. Used as a perfume and scent for soaps and room sprays. Also used as a flavoring ingredient. Soluble in most fixed oils. See Cedar for toxicity.

WHITE GINGER EXTRACT • The extract of the roots of Hawaiian white ginger, *Hedycium coronarium koenig.* See Ginger.

WHITE LILY EXTRACT • Extract of the bulbs of *Lilium candidum.* Edible bulbs that were made into soup by the Indians, the lily is used in perfumery.

WHITE MUSTARD EXTRACT • The pulverized seeds of *Brassica alba,* native to southern Europe and western Asia and naturalized in the United States. It is used medically to cause vomiting, and in cosmetics as a counterirritant *(see).* It is irritating to the skin, however, and can cause burns that are slow to heal.

WHITE NETTLE EXTRACT • Obtained from the flowers of *Lamium album.* See Nettles.

WHITE OAK BARK • *Quercus alba.* The extract of *Quercus alba.* Contains tannic acid, quercitol, resin, pectin, and levulin. Used as an astringent.

WHITE SAPONARIA • *Gypsophila paniculata.* A cleansing ingredient. See Saponaria.

WHOLE DRY MILK • The solid residue produced by the dehydration of cow's milk.

WILD AGRIMONY EXTRACT • **Extract of Wild Pansy.** The extract of the herb *Potentilla anserina.* The Indians used to crush the leaves to treat boils and swellings. By the late 1800s, the wild pansy was being ground up and used to treat many skin diseases, including impetigo, skin ulcers, and scabies.

WILD CHERRY • See Wild Cherry Bark.

WILD CHERRY BARK • **Wild Black Cherry Bark.** The dried stem bark of *Prunus serotina,* collected in autumn in North America. Used in lipsticks and cherry flavorings for food and medicines. Also used as a sedative and expectorant medicinally. No known toxicity.

WILD GINGER • *Asarum heterotropoides.* **Xi Xin.** The root is used by Chinese herbalists to treat menstrual problems and congestion in the lungs and nose. Its warm, pungent action relieves spasms. The American wild ginger is not as strong as the Chinese. The Chinese can be mildly toxic.

WILD INDIGO ROOT • **Baptisia. Bastard Indigo.** A wild uncultivated plant of North America with showy yellow or blue flowers. Used as a coloring. No known toxicity.

WILD MARJORAM EXTRACT • Extract of the flowering ends of *Origanum vulgare.* Yellow or greenish yellow liquid containing about 40 percent terpenes *(see).* Used in perfumery. See Marjoram Oil.

WILD MINT EXTRACT • Extract of the leaves and tender twigs of *Mentha arvensis.* The Cheyenne Indians prepared a decoction of the ground leaves and stems of wild mint and drank the liquid to check nausea. Pulegone and thymol *(see)* are derived from an oil of wild mint. Its odor resembles peppermint.

WILD MINT OIL • See Wild Mint Extract.

WILD PANSY • See Agrimony Extract.

WILD SARSAPARILLA EXTRACT • The extract of the roots of *Aralia nudicaulis.*

WILD THYME EXTRACT • *Thymus serpillium.* The flowering tops of the plant grown in Eurasia and throughout the United States. The dried leaves are used in emollients and fragrances, and as a seasoning in foods. Has also been used as a muscle relaxant. No known toxicity.

WILD YAM ROOT • *Dioscorea paniculata* or *Dioscorea villosa.* **Colicroot. Rheumatism Root. Chinese Yam.** Japanese researchers in 1936 discovered glycoside saponins of several Mexican yam species from which the steroid saponin *(see),* primarily diosgenin, could be derived. These derivatives were then converted to progesterone, an intermediate in cortisone production. Steroid drugs derived from diosgenin include corticosteroids, oral contraceptives, androgens, and estrogens. American herbalists for more than two centuries used wild yam root to treat painful menstruation, ovarian pain, cramps, and problems of child-birth. Wild yam root has also been used to treat gallbladder pain and ease the passage of gallstones. Wild yam root reputedly can also lower blood cholesterol and blood pressure. The most widely prescribed and popular birth control pill in the world, desogen, is made from the wild yam, confirming what the ancient Mexican women knew all along: They used wild yam as a contraceptive.

WILLOW BARK EXTRACT • See Salicylates and Willow Leaf Extract.

WILLOW LEAF EXTRACT • The extract of the leaves of the willow tree species *Salix*. The willow has been used for its pain-relieving and fever-lowering properties since ancient Greece. The American Indians used willow baths to cool fevers and indeed, the extract of willows contains salicylic acid, a close cousin of aspirin.

WINTERGREEN EXTRACT • An extract of the leaves of *Gaultheria procumbens*. See Wintergreen Oil.

WINTERGREEN OIL • **Menthyl Salicylate.** Used in toothpaste, tooth powder, and perfumes. Obtained naturally from betula, sweet birch, or teaberry oil. Present in certain leaves and bark, but usually prepared by treating salicylic acid with methanol *(see both)*. Also used as a food and beverage flavoring. Wintergreen is a strong irritant. Ingestion of relatively small amounts may cause severe poisoning and death. Average lethal dose in children is 10 milliliters and in adults 30 milliliters. It is very irritating to the mucous membranes and skin, and can be absorbed rapidly through the skin.

WISTERIA • Used in perfumes. The extract from the Asiatic, mostly woody vines of the family that produces showy blue, white, purple, and rose flowers. No known toxicity.

WITCH HAZEL • One of the most widely used cosmetic ingredients, it is a skin freshener, local anesthetic, and astringent made from the leaves and/or twigs of *Hamamelis virginiana*. Collected in the autumn. Witch hazel has an ethanol content of 70 to 80 percent and a tannin content of 2 to 9 percent. Witch hazel water, which is what you buy at the store, contains 15 percent ethanol. See Ethanol for toxicity.

WOOD POWDER • Ground wood consisting of mainly cellulose *(see)* and lignin. Used as an abrasive, absorbent, and thickener.

WOODRUFF • **Master of the Woods.** Used in perfumes and sachets. Made of the leaves of an herb grown in Europe, Siberia, North Africa, and Australia. It is a symbol of spring, and has a clean fresh smell. No known toxicity.

WOOL FAT • Crude lanolin *(see)*.

WOOL WAX ALCOHOLS • **Wool Fat.** Chemically more like a fat than a wax, it is the deposit sheep make on their wool. Used as emollients. See Lanolin Alcohols.

WORMSEED OIL • **Chenopodium Oil.** Colorless or yellowish oil with a penetrating odor and bitter taste. Distilled from the seeds and leaves of *Chenopodium ambrosiodies anthelminticum*. It is used to combat worms.

WORMWOOD • *Artemisia absinthium*. **Absinthe.** A perennial herb native to the Ural Mountains, it was taken to Egypt very early in recorded history and was listed in Ebers Papyrus as useful for headaches and for eliminating pinworms, two uses still prescribed by herbalists. Because it was used to expel tapeworms and other intestinal worms, it was called "wormwood." In Europe and North America, it was believed to counteract poison. It was recommended for insomnia, jaundice, indigestion, sprains, bruises, and inflammations. Herbalists today recommend an infusion of the leaves and stems to stimulate appetite and soothe stomach pains. In large and/or repeated doses, it is a narcotic poison, causing headache, trembling, and convulsions. Ingestion of the volatile oil or of the liquor, absinthe, distilled from wormwood, may cause gastrointestinal symptoms, nervousness, stupor, coma, and death. The use of absinthe is banned in many nations.

WRINKLE REMOVERS • Periodically, the cosmetic industry comes up with a magic ingredient that will prevent or cure wrinkles. Among such ingredients in recent years was serum albumen (from bulls) and estrogen. Another wrinkle remover contained some unidentified ingredients that irritated the skin so that it "puffed up" and the wrinkles "filled out." Turtle oil, natural proteins, and polyunsaturates, among many others, were supposed to feed aging skin, but there is no apparent biochemical or physiological activity in any of them. The companies really went wild in the mid-eighties when Christiaan Barnard, M.D., the pioneer South African heart surgeon, lent his name to a Swiss product with "glycel" and mysterious ingredients that reversed the aging process in the skin. Other competitors came out with similar claims. Ironically, around the same time, physicians reported that Retin-A, a Vitamin A derivative, actually did have some wrinkle-reducing effects. See Retin-A and Tretinoin. It is difficult for the Federal Trade Commission and the FDA to get after promoters of wrinkle creams. By the time the agencies get the manufacturers to court, it has taken several years and a great deal of money and manpower. Then all the manufacturers have to do is open up under different names or change the names of their products and start selling wrinkle creams all over again. The constant advertising that wrinkles are bad also has its deleterious effects on the psyche of women who may have them.

X

XANTHAN GUM • A gum produced by a pure culture fermentation of a carbohydrate with *Xanthomonas campestris*. Also called corn sugar gum. Widely used as a thickener, an emulsifier, and a stabilizer. No known toxicity

XANTHENE • Colorants are divided into acid and basic groups. Xanthenes are the second largest category of certified colors. The acids are derived from fluorescein. The quinoid acid type is represented by FD & C Red No. 3, erythrosine, used frequently in lipsticks. The phenolic formulations, often called "bromo acids," are represented by D & C Red No. 2, used to "stain" lips. The only basic type certified is D & C Red No. 19, also called Rhodamine B.

XANTHINES • Occurs in animal organs, blood, urine, yeast, potatoes, coffee beans, and tea. First isolated from gallstones. Xanthines are found in chocolate, coffee, tea, and many drugs such as aminophyllin and caffeine *(see)*. They stimulate the brain, heart, and muscles. They act as diuretics to reduce body fluid and also dilate the heart's blood vessels.

XANTHOPHYLL • **Vegetable Lutein.** A yellow coloring originally isolated from egg yolk, now isolated from petals of flowers. Occurs also in colored feathers of birds. One of the most widespread carotenoid alcohols (a group of red and yellow pigments) in nature. Provisionally listed for use in food. Although carotenoids can usually be turned into Vitamin A, xanthophyll has no Vitamin A activity.

XANTHOXYLUM AMERICANUM • See Zanthoxylum.

XERODERMA • Dry skin.

XIMENIA AMERICANA • A widely distributed family of tropical shrubs and trees. An essential oil, it has a scent like sandalwood *(see)* and is used in fragrances.

XYLENE • Since xylene is an aromatic hydrocarbon, as is chlorine, it warrants further investigation as a cancer-causing ingredient. There has been no definite association, but it is toxic by inhalation or ingestion. Used as a solvent.

XYLENE SULFONIC ACID • A mixture of aromatic acids. See Surfactants.

XYLITOL • Formerly made from birchwood, but now made from waste products from the pulp industry. Xylitol has been reported to have diuretic effects but this has not been substantiated. It is used in chewing gum and as an artificial sweetener. It has been reported to sharply reduce cavities in teeth but costs more than sugar. FDA preliminary reports cited it as a possible cancer-causing ingredient.

XYLOCAINE® • **Lidocaine.** Used in after-shave lotions. A local anesthetic that interferes with the transmission of nerve impulses, thereby effecting local anesthetic action. Recommended by manufacturers for topical use on mucous membranes only. Can cause allergic reactions. Not permitted in cosmetics in Switzerland.

XYLOSE • A flavoring agent.

Y

YAM • *Dioscorea paniculata.* **Colicroot. Rheumatism Root. Chinese Yam.** Japanese researchers in 1936 discovered glycoside saponins of several Mexican yam species from which the steroid saponin *(see)*, primarily diosgenin, could be derived. These derivatives were then converted to progesterone, an intermediate in cortisone production. Steroid drugs derived from diosgenin include corticosteroids, oral contraceptives, androgens, and estrogens. American herbalists for more than two centuries used wild yam roots to treat painful menstruation, ovarian pain, and cramps, and problems of childbirth. Wild yam root has also been used to treat gallbladder pain and ease the passage of gallstones. Wild yam root reputedly can also lower blood cholesterol and blood pressure. The most widely prescribed and popular birth control pill in the world, desogen, is made from the wild yam, confirming what the ancient Mexican women knew all along: They used wild yam as a contraceptive. Yam is used in "organic" cosmetics.

YARA YARA • **Methoxy naphthalene.** Leaflets from ether. Used in the manufacture of cosmetics as a solvent. See Naphthalene.

YARROW • A strong scented, spicy, wild herb used in astringents and shampoos. Its astringent qualities have caused it to be recommended by herbalists for greasy skins. According to old herbal recipes, it prevents baldness when the hair is washed regularly with it. Used medicinally as an astringent, tonic, and stimulant. May cause a sensitivity to sunlight and artificial light, in which the skin breaks out and swells.

YEAST • A fungi that is a dietary source of folic acid. It produces enzymes that will convert sugar to alcohol and carbon dioxide. Used in skin conditioners. No known toxicity.

YEAST EXTRACT • See Yeast.

YEAST PALMITATE • A derivative of yeast and palmitic acid (see both) used as a hair fixative and skin conditioner.

YELLOW CURLED DOCK • *Rumex crispus.* **Curly Dock. Out-Sting.** One of the most common wayside plants, the yellow dock flourished on wasteland. The herb has antibacterial properties. English children use it as an antidote for a nettle sting. It was once used as a primary treatment for scurvy and anemia, probably because of its high iron content. A tincture is used by herbalists to relieve coughs and sore throats. It is also recommended by herbalists for skin diseases, arthritis, piles, and lung and gallbladder problems. It is used in "organic" cosmetics. It contains ingredients similar to those in cascara (see). The leaves also contain oxalic acid, which can be toxic.

YELLOW DOCK • See Yellow Curled Dock.

YELLOW NO. 5 • All foods containing this coloring, which is the most widely used color additive in food, drugs, and cosmetics, are supposed to identify it on the label. The FDA ordered this so that those allergic to it could avoid it. See also Tartrazine and Salicylates.

YERBA SANTA FLUID EXTRACT • **Holy Herb. Mountain Balm. Consumptive's Weed. Bear's Weed. Gum Bush.** An extract of the leaves of *Eriodictyon californicum.* A fruit flavoring in commercial products derived from evergreen shrubs grown in California, the American Indians smoked or chewed the leaves of this plant as a treatment for asthma. It is still used by herbalists as an expectorant to treat bronchial congestion, asthma, and hay fever. Yerba is also used by herbalists to treat chronic genitourinary tract inflammations and to mask the bitter taste of drugs.

YLANG-YLANG OIL • A light yellow, very fragrant liquid obtained in the Philippines from flowers. Used for perfumes and as a food and beverage flavoring. May cause allergic reactions.

YOGURT • A dairy product produced by the action of bacteria or yeast on milk. No known toxicity. Supposedly has emollient properties.

YOGURT FILTRATE • Obtained by removing insoluble matter from fermented skim milk.

YUCCA EXTRACT • **Mohave Extract. Joshua Tree. Adam's Needle.** Derived from a southwestern United States plant and used as a base for organic cosmetics as a hair fixative and as a root beer flavoring for beverages and ice cream. *Yucca glauca,* often called Mojave Yucca or Soap Weed, was used by the Indians of the Southwest to treat burns and abrasions. Modern scientists at the Brooks Industries, South Plainfield, N.J., report that it increases cell growth and is an anti-irritant.

Z

ZANTHOXYLUM • *Xanthoxylum.* **Ash Bark. Toothache Tree. Angelica Tree.** The dried bark or berries of this tree, which grows in Canada and south of Virginia and Missouri, is used to ease the pain of toothaches and stomachaches, and as an antidiarrheal medicine. No known toxicity. A member of the rue family.

ZEA MAYS • See Corn Oil.

ZEDOARY • Obtained from the rhizome of *Curcuma zedoaria,* an East Indian plant. It is used as a bitters and ginger ale flavoring for beverages. Long used as a stimulant in folk medicine. No known toxicity. GRAS.

ZEIN • Used in face masks, nail polishes, and as a plasticizer. It is the principal protein in corn. Obtained as a yellowish powder by extracting corn gluten with an alcohol; also used to make textile fibers, plastics, printing inks, varnishes, and other coatings and adhesives. No known toxicity.

ZEOLITE PROCESS • Water softeners of this type utilize salt to cause an exchange to take place between the calcium and magnesium ions in the water and sodium ions from the salt. With this method, hardness can be reduced substantially, and the water takes on a slippery feeling.

ZINC • A white brittle metal insoluble in water and soluble in acids or hot solutions of alkalies. Widely used as an astringent for mouthwashes and as a reducing ingredient *(see).* Ingestion of the salts can cause nausea and vomiting. It can cause contact dermatitis.

ZINC ACETATE • The zinc salt of acetic acid *(see).* Used in medicine as a dietary supplement and as a cross-linking ingredient for polymers *(see).* For toxicity, see Zinc Salts.

ZINC ACETYLMETHIONATE • See Zinc and Methionine.

ZINC ASPARTATE • See Zinc and Aspartic Acid.

ZINC BORATE • The inorganic salt of zinc oxide and boric oxide, it is used as a fungistat and mildew inhibitor. See Zinc Salts.

ZINC BROMIDE • Absorbs water. It is used in photography and in emulsions. See Bromides.

ZINC CARBONATE • A cosmetic coloring ingredient, it is a crystalline salt of zinc occurring in nature as smithsonite. See Zinc for toxicity.

ZINC CHLORIDE • **Butter of Zinc.** A zinc salt used as an antiseptic and astringent in shaving creams, dentifrices, and mouthwashes. Odorless and water absorbing; also a deodorant and disinfectant. Can cause contact dermatitis and is mildly irritating to the skin. Can be absorbed through the skin.

ZINC CITRATE • See Zinc and Citric Acid.

ZINC CYSTEINATE • An organic salt that is used as a preservative. See Cystein.

ZINC DNA • The zinc salt of DNA *(see)*.

ZINC FORMALDEHYDE SULFOXYLATE • See Formaldehyde and Zinc.

ZINC GLUCONATE • See Zinc and Gluconic Acid.

ZINC GLUTAMATE • The zinc salt of glutamic acid *(see)*.

ZINC HYDROLYZED COLLAGEN • "Animal" was removed from this ingredient's name but not from the ingredient. See Hydrolyzed Collagen.

ZINC LAURATE • See Zinc and Lauric Acid.

ZINC MYRISTATE • The zinc salt of myristic acid *(see)*.

ZINC NEODECANOATE • The zinc salt of neodecanoic acid *(see)*.

ZINC OLEATE-STEARATE • A white, dry, greasy powder, insoluble in water, soluble in alcohol. An antiseptic and astringent in cosmetic creams. Used medicinally to treat eczema and other skin rashes. No known toxicity.

ZINC OXIDE • **Flowers of Zinc.** Used to impart opacity to face powders, foundation creams, and dusting powders. A creamy white ointment used medicinally as an astringent, antiseptic, and protective in skin diseases. Zinc is believed to encourage healing of skin disorders. It is insoluble in water. In cosmetics it is also used in baby powder, bleach and freckle creams, depilatories, face packs, antiperspirants, foundation cake-makeup, nail whiteners, protective creams, rouge, shaving creams, and white eye shadow. Workers suffer skin eruptions called "zinc pox" under the arm and in the groin when working with zinc. Zinc pox is believed to be caused by the blocking of the hair follicles. Because of its astringent qualities, zinc oxide may be unsuitable for dry skins. Generally harmless, however, when used in cosmetics. Permanently listed as a coloring in 1977. The FDA proposed a ban in 1992 for the use of zinc oxide to treat insect bites and stings because it has not been shown to be safe and effective for stated claims in OTC products, including in astringent *(see)* drug products.

ZINC PCA • The zinc salt of PCA.

ZINC PENTADECENE TRICARBOXYLATE • See Zinc and Carboxylic Acid.

ZINC PEROXIDE • **Zinc Superoxide.** Disinfectant, antiseptic, deodorant, and astringent applied as a dusting powder alone or with talc or starch. White to yellowish white powder. Liberates hydrogen peroxide, a bleach. It is used in bleach and freckle creams and medicinally as a deodorant for festering wounds and skin diseases. No known toxicity.

ZINC PHENOLSULFONATE • A phenol that is used as a topical astringent when mucous membranes are inflamed. Also used in deodorants. Mild redness was observed in a 28-day skin tests. Rats exposed to a spray containing this ingredient for 13 weeks had depressed brain, liver, testes, and organ/body weight ratios. On the basis of available information, the CIR Expert Panel *(see)* concludes that it is safe as presently used in cosmetic formulations See Phenols.

ZINC PYRIDINETHIONE • Zinc Pyrithione. An antidandruff ingredient that is reportedly damaging to nerves. A bactericide and fungicide used in antidandruff products. A rare sensitizer but may cross-react with ethylene diamine, piperazine, or hydrochloride derivatives *(see all)*.

ZINC RESINATE • The zinc salt of rosin *(see)*.

ZINC RICINOLEATE • The zinc salt of ricinoleate *(see)*. Used as a fungicide, emulsifier, and stabilizer.

ZINC ROSINATE • The zinc salt of rosin *(see)*.

ZINC SALICYLATE • A zinc salt used as an antiseptic and astringent in dusting powders and antiperspirants. White, odorless needles or crystalline powder. It is omitted from hypoallergenic cosmetics. Causes both skin irritations and allergic reactions.

ZINC SALTS • These salts, if ingested, can produce irritation or corrosion of the gastrointestinal system with pain and vomiting. Used widely in the cosmetic industry in soaps and deodorants, creams, dentifrices, shaving preparations, and astringents. Zinc chloride *(see)* appears to be more corrosive and more toxic than the sulfate. A few grams of the chloride have killed an adult, although recovery has been reported after ingestion of 90 gm. See Zinc Sulfate and Zinc Ricinoleate.

ZINC STEARATE • Zinc Soap. A mixture of the zinc salts of stearic and palmitic acids *(see both)*. Widely used in cosmetic preparations because it contributes to adhesive properties. Also used as a coloring ingredient. Baby powders of 3 to 5 percent zinc are water repellent and prevent urine irritation. Zinc soap is also used in bath preparations, deodorants, face powders, hair-grooming preparations, hand creams, lotions, and ointments. It is used in tablet manufacture and in pharmaceutical powders and ointments. Inhalation of powder may cause lung problems and produce death in infants from pneumonitis, with lesions resembling those caused by talc but more severe. No known toxicity on the skin. On the basis of the available information, the CIR Expert Panel *(see)* concludes that it is safe as a cosmetic ingredient.

ZINC SULFATE • White Vitriol. The reaction of sulfuric acid with zinc. Mild crystalline zinc salt used in shaving creams, eye lotions, astringents, styptics, and in gargle spray, skin tonic, and after-shave lotion. Used medicinally as an emetic. Irritating to the skin and mucous membranes. May cause an allergic reaction. Injection under the skin of 2.5 milligrams per kilogram of body weight caused tumors in rabbits.

ZINC SULFIDE • An inorganic zinc salt used as a white pigment and as a fungicide. See Zinc Salts.

ZINC SULFOCARBOLATE • See Zinc Sulfate.

ZINC UNDECYLENATE • A zinc salt. Occurs in sweat. Used to combat fungus in cosmetics and on the skin. Made by dissolving zinc oxide *(see)* in diluted undecylenic acid *(see)*. Has an odor suggestive of perspiration. No known toxicity. See Antiperspirants.

ZINC YEAST DERIVATIVE • The derivative of yeast with zinc.

ZINGIBER OFFICINALE • See Ginger.

ZIRCONIUM • Discovered in 1789. Bluish black powder or grayish white flakes used as a bonding ingredient and abrasive; also used in the preparation of dyes. High-quality zirconium is used as a pigment toner and solvent. Mildly acidic, it has been used in body deodorants and antiperspirants. Zirconium hydroxide is used in nail whiteners. Low systemic toxicity, but a disease of the skin has been reported in users of a deodorant containing sodium zirconium lactate. Manufacturers voluntarily removed zirconium from spray antiperspirants in 1976 because the element was found harmful to monkey lungs. The FDA has said that zirconium is safe in formulations other than sprays. Zirconium oxide and zirconium silicate are no longer authorized for use as colorings.

ZIRCONIUM CHLOROHYDRATE • See Zirconium.

ZIRCONIUM DIOXIDE • See Zirconium.

ZIRCONIUM SILICATE • See Zirconium.

ZIRCONYL CHLORIDE • **Zirconium Oxychloride.** Used to make other zirconium compounds and to precipitate acid dyes. Acts as a solvent. Mildly acidic. It has been used in deodorants and antiperspirants, but because of skin bumps, particularly under the arm, it has been discontinued.

ZIRCONYL HYDROXYCHLORIDE • Colorless powder that absorbs moisture. See Zirconium.

ZIZIPHUS • A large genus of American and Asian shrubs. See Lotus.

APPENDIX A: COMMON LABEL WARNINGS — PAY ATTENTION!

For halocarbon or hydrocarbon propellants, such as aerosol hairsprays or deodorants, the following is required:

- Warning—Use only as directed. Intentional misuse by deliberately concentrating and inhaling the contents can be harmful or fatal.

- All cosmetics in self-pressurized containers, such as shaving creams, must have specifically worded warnings against spraying near the eyes, puncturing, incinerating, storing, and intentionally misusing.

- Keep out of reach of children is also required for all products in pressurized containers. In case of products intended for use by children, such as foaming soap, the phrase "except under adult supervision" may be added.

- Detergent bubble-bath products should have: may irritate skin and the urinary tract through excessive use or prolonged exposure. The labeling instructs you to discontinue the product if rash, redness, or itching occurs, to consult your physician if irritation persists, and to keep out of reach of children.

- Feminine deodorant sprays intended for use in the genital area—are for external use only and should not be applied to broken, irritated, or itching skin. A physician should be consulted if persistent unusual odor or discharge occurs. The statement instructs users to discontinue immediately if rash, irritation, or discomfort develops. Labeling on self-pressurized containers must state that the product should be sprayed at least 8 inches from the skin.

- Coal-tar, color-containing, hair-dye products. The label, except in professional beauty salons, must read that it contains ingredients that may cause skin irritation on certain individuals, and a preliminary test, according to the products accompanying directions, should first be made. Users are cautioned not to dye eyelashes or eyebrows because doing so may cause blindness. In addition, the ammonia, soaps, detergents, conditioning agents, and dyes in hair-dye products are all strong eye irritants and could also cause allergic reactions in other areas.

- Depilatories and hair straightener are highly alkaline; if they are used incorrectly, they may cause serious skin irritations.

- Shampoos, rinses, and conditioners can cause eye problems that range from irritation to permanent damage. If the eye cornea is scratched or otherwise damaged, a contaminated product could cause infection.

- Nail builders (elongators, extenders, hardeners, and enamels) can cause irritation, inflammation, and infection of the nail bed and nail fold (where the nail meets the finger) due to residual traces of the methylacrylate monomers. Also, nail hardeners and enamels often contain formaldehyde and formaldehyde-releasing preservatives, which may cause allergic reactions in people who are sensitive to them. In addition, the solvents or plasticizers may be irritating. Nail enamels that are also nail hardeners cause the most problem. Their high resin *(see)* content or low concentration of plasticizer seals the nail surface to air and makes the nail too brittle. Another frequent problem is flammability during and shortly after application.

- Flammable products such as aerosol hairsprays containing alcohol and isobutane *(see both)* propellants include caution statements on the label. The label also usually cautions about avoiding heat, fire, and smoking during use until the product is fully dried.

- Baby powder, if accidentally inhaled by the baby in large amounts, can block the infant's lungs and cause suffocation.

- Fluoride toothpastes are supposed to carry a controversial warning that they should be kept out of the reach of children under 6 years of age, and if you accidentally swallow more than used for brushing, seek professional assistance or contact a Poison Control Center immediately. The FDA's own package-size limitations are designed to prevent fluoride poisoning, and the toothpaste manufacturers have a way of giving the message such as putting it inside the package so that it is easy to ignore.

- The law allows a manufacturer to ask the FDA to grant "trade secret" status for a particular ingredient. If the FDA grants the request, the substance does not have to be listed on the label.

APPENDIX B:
NAIL SAFETY

- If you are going to have your nails done professionally, choose a salon that has a state license and a state inspection certificate.

- The technician should be licensed and the license should be posted.

- Make sure the salon is clean and sterilizes manicure implements. Autoclaving (heat sterilization) is best or chemical sterilization.

- You should have a fresh bowl of soap waters in which to soak your nails and a new nail file.

- Make sure the manicurist washes hands before beginning work on your hands.

- Nail hardeners often contain formaldehyde which can be irritating to the skin or cause allergic reactions. The product should contain no more than 5 percent formaldehyde.

- You should be provided with nail shields which restrict application just to the nail tip.

- If you suspect you may be sensitive to materials in artificial nails, have only one nail done as a test and wait a few days to see if a reaction develops.

- Never apply an artifical nail if your natural nail or skin around it is infected or irritated. Let the infection heal first.

- Read the directions for do-it-yourself nails before applying them, and follow the directions carefully. Save the ingredient list for your doctor in case you have an allergic reaction or other injury.

- Treat your artifical nails with care. They may be stronger than your own but they still can break and separate. Try not to bump or knock them. Find new ways to do ordinary tasks, like using a pencil to dial or depress the numbers on the phone.

- If an artifical nail separates, dip the fingertip into rubbing alcohol to clean the space between the natural and artificial nails before reattaching the artificial nail. This will help prevent infection.

- Never use household glues for nail repairs. Use only products intended for nail use, and follow directions.

- Don't wear artificial nails for longer than three months at a time. Remove them for one month to give nails a rest.

- Keep nail glue and other poisonous substances out of the reach of children.

BIBLIOGRAPHY

Allen, Linda. *The Look You Like.* Chicago: American Medical Association, Committee on Cutaneous Health and Cosmetics, 1971.

Castro, Miranda. *The Complete Homeopathy Handbook.* New York: St. Martin's Press, 1990.

CIR (Cosmetic Ingredient Review) Compendium, Washington, D.C., 1998.

Color Additive Status List. Food and Drug Administration, 1992.

Done, Alan. *Toxic Reactions to Common Household Products.* Paper read at the Symposium on Adverse Reactions sponsored by the Drug Service Center for Disease Control, December 1976, San Francisco.

Ellenhorn, Matthew J., and Barceloux, Donald G. *Medical Toxicology: Diagnosis and Treatment of Human Poisoning.* New York: Elsevier Science Publishing Company, 1988.

Fisher, Alexander A. *Contact Dermatitis,* 3rd. ed. Philadelphia: Lea & Febiger, 1986.

Gordon, Lesley. *A Country Herbal.* New York: Mayflower Books, 1980.

Gosselin, Robert, M.D., Ph.D.; Smith, Robert, Ph.D.; and Hodge, Harold, Ph.D., D.Sc., with Braddock, Jeannette. *Clinical Toxicology of Commercial Products.* Baltimore: The Williams & Wilkins Co., 1984.

Greenberg, Leon A., and Lester, David. *The Handbook of Cosmetic Materials.* New York: Interscience Publishers, 1954.

Hawley's Condensed Chemical Dictionary, 11th ed. Revised by N. Irving Sax and Richard J. Lewis, Sr. New York: Van Nostrand Reinhold, 1987.

Hoffman, David. *The New Holistic Herbal,* Rockport, Mass.: Element, Inc., 1991.

Investigation Operations Manual. Washington, D.C.: Food and Drug Administration, 1992.

International Business Communications Second Annual International Industry Conference: Drug Discovery and Development Approaches to Cosmeceuticals, Short Hills, N.J., February 12–13, 1998.

Juo Pei-Shaw, Ph.D. *Concise Dictionary of Biomedicine and Molecular Biology.* Boca Raton, Fl.: CRC Press, 1995.

Kahn, Julius. "Hypo-Allergenic Cosmetics." NARD *Journal* (February 20, 1967).

Kamm, Minnie Watson. *Old-Time Herbs for Northern Gardens.* Boston: Little Brown & Co., 1938.

Kibbe, Constance V. *Standard Textbook of Cosmetology,* rev. ed. Bronx, N.Y.: Milady Publishing Corp., 1981.

Loprieno, N., Chairman, Scientific Committee on Cosmetology of the European Communities. *Guidelines for Safety Evaluation of Cosmetics Ingredients Food and Chemical Toxicology.* The Scientific Committee on Cosmetology of the Commission of The European Communities Department of Environmental Sciences. Great Britain: Pergamon Press Ltd., 1995.

March, Cyril, M.D., and Fisher, Alexander, M.D. *Cutaneous Reactions to Cosmetics.* Chicago: American Medical Association, 1965.

Martin, Eric W., et al. *Hazards of Medications.* Philadelphia: J. B. Lippincott Co., 1971.

The Merck Index, 8th, 9th, and 10th editions. Rahway, N.J.: Merck, Sharp and Dohme Research Laboratories, 1983.

The Merck Manual, 15th edition. Edited by Robert Berkow, M.D. Rahway, N.J.: Merck, Sharp and Dohme Research Laboratories, 1987.

Miall, L. Mackenzie, and Sharp, D. W. A. *A New Dictionary of Chemistry,* 4th ed. New York: John Wiley & Sons, Inc., 1968.

Mindell, Earl R., Ph.D. *Earl Mindell's Herb Bible.* New York: Fireside Books, 1992.

Mowrey, Daniel B. *The Scientific Validation of Herbal Medicine.* New Canaan, Conn.: Keats Publishing, Inc., 1986.

Physicians' Desk Reference. Oradell, N.J.: Medical Economics, 1988.

Principles of Cosmetics for Dermatologists. St. Louis: C. V. Mosby Co., 1982.

Prospective Study of Cosmetic Reactions, 1977–1980. North American Contact Dermatitis Group, Journal of the American Academy of Dermatology, Vol. 6, No. 5: May 1982.

Steadman's Medical Dictionary, 25th ed. Baltimore: The Williams & Wilkins Col, 1990.

Stehlin, Dori, "Cosmetic Safety More Complex Than at First Blush," *FDA Consumer,* December 1992.

Suspected Carcinogens: A Subfile of the NIOSH Toxic Substance List. Rockville, Md.: Tracor Jitco, Inc., U.S. Department of Health, Education and Welfare, 1975.

Suspected Carcinogens: A Subfile of The Registry of Toxic Effects of Chemical Substances. Cincinnati: U.S. Department of Health, Education and Welfare, Public Health Services, Center for Disease Control, 1976.

Tierra, Michael, C.A., N.D. *The Way of Herbs.* New York: Pocket Books, 1990.

Toxicity Testing: Strategies to Determine Needs and Priorities. Washington, D.C.: National Research Council: National Academy Press, 1984.

Webster's Third New International Dictionary, Chicago: G. & C. Merriman Co., 1966.

Weiner, Michael, Ph.D. *Weiner's Herbal 1990 Edition,* Mill Valley, CA.: Quantum Books, 1990.

Wenniger, John A. and G. N. McEwen, Jr., Ph.D., J. D. *CTFA Cosmetic Ingredient Dictionary and Handbook.* 7th ed. Washington, D.C.: The Cosmetic, Toiletry, and Fragrance Association, 1997.

White, John Henry. *A Reference Book of Chemistry,* 3rd ed. New York: Philosophical Library, 1965.

Winter, Ruth. *Cancer-Causing Ingredients: A Preventive Guide,* New York: Crown Publishers, Inc., 1979.

_____. *A Consumer's Dictionary of Household, Yard and Office Chemicals,* Crown Publishers, 1992.

_____. Winter, Ruth. *A Consumer's Dictionary of Medicines: Prescription, Nonprescription and Herbal,* Crown Publishers, 1994.

_____. Winter, Ruth. *A Consumer's Guide to Medicines in Food,* Crown Publishers, 1995.